European Manual of Medicine

T0384423

Hans-Jörg Oestern · Otmar Trentz
Selman Uranues
(Editors)

Wolfgang Arnold
Uwe Ganzer
(Series Editors)

Head, Thoracic, Abdominal, and Vascular Injuries

Trauma Surgery I

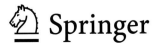 Springer

Editors

Prof. Hans-Jörg Oestern, MD
Allgemeines Krankenhaus Celle
Klinik für Unfall- und
Wiederherstellungschirurgie
Siemensplatz 4
29223 Celle
Germany
sekretariat.unfallchirurgie@akh-celle.de

Univ. - Prof. Selman Uranues, MD
Medizinische Universität Graz
Auenbruggerplatz 15
8036 Graz
Austria
selman.uranues@medunigraz.at

Prof. Otmar Trentz, MD
UniversitätsSpital Zürich
Forschungsabteilung Chirurgie
Klusweg 18
8032 Zürich
Switzerland
otmartrentz@yahoo.com

Series Editors

Prof. Wolfgang Arnold, MD
Director emeritus
Department of Otorhinolaryngology
Head & Neck Surgery
Klinikum rechts der Isar
Technical University of Munich
Munich
Germany
w.arnold@lrz.tum.de

Prof. Uwe Ganzer, MD
Director emeritus
Department of Otorhinolaryngology
Head & Neck Surgery
University of Düsseldorf
Düsseldorf
Germany
uwe.ganzer@arcor.de

ISBN 978-3-540-88121-6   e-ISBN 978-3-540-88122-3
DOI 10.1007/978-3-540-88122-3
Springer Heidelberg Dordrecht London New York

Library of Congress Control Number: 2010937981

© Springer-Verlag Berlin Heidelberg 2011

Cover design: eStudioCalamar, Figueres/Berlin

Printed on acid-free paper

Springer is part of Springer Science+Business Media (www.springer.com)

Foreword of the Series Editors

The *European Manual of Medicine* was founded on the idea of offering resident as well as specialized clinicians the latest and most up-to-date information on diagnosis and treatment in Europe. In contrast to existing textbooks, the *European Manual of Medicine* aims to find a consensus on the demands of modern European medicine based on the "logbooks" recommended by the Union of European Medical Societies (UEMS). Therefore, for each discipline those diagnostic and therapeutic principles that are generally considered best practice are presented as "recommended European standards."

To fulfill these demands we – together with Springer – recruited editors who are well established and recognized in their specialties. For each volume at least three editors from different European countries were invited to contribute the high clinical and scientific standards of their discipline to their book.

Wherever possible the volume editors were asked to follow a standardized structure for each chapter so as to provide readers quick and easy access to the material. High-quality illustrations and figures serve to provide additional useful information. Detailed references allow interested readers to further investigate areas of individual interest.

The series editors wish to express their sincere gratitude to Springer-Verlag, especially to Gabriele Schroeder and Stephanie Benko for their support and assistance in the realization of this project from the early stages.

The fifth volume of our *European Manual of Medicine* series is dedicated to trauma surgery and will be published in three parts. The first part presented here focuses on cranial, thoracic, abdominal and vascular trauma. The following two parts will deal with trauma of the skeletal system and joints, of peripheral nerves and soft tissues, as well as with the special care needed by trauma patients, handling complications, pain management, and principles of rehabilitation.

One of the main aims of this volume is to provide, especially, trainees with a comprehensive yet condensed guide to the core knowledge required in this broad surgical field and also give them the ability to work in their specialty throughout the European Union.

The volume editors Prof. Hans-Jörg Oestern (Celle, Germany), Prof. Otmar Trentz (Zürich Switzerland) and Prof. Selman Uranues (Graz, Austria), – who are leading European experts in trauma surgery, – recruited contributors from different European countries to compile a textbook that fulfills our original concept of the *European Manual of Medicine* series.

Munich
Düsseldorf
Fall 2010

Wolfgang Arnold
Uwe Ganzer

Preface

Internationally, trauma is at the top, if not the very top of the list of causes of death under the age of 50 years. At the same time, enormous developments continue to be made in diagnostics and treatment, while the field of trauma/acute/emergency surgery undergoes exciting and dramatic expansion and restructuring, with the establishment of new surgical specialties. At this crucial juncture, it is desirable to work in the direction of bringing evidence-based order and uniformity into the trauma care system.

This first volume in the "Trauma Surgery" series deals with cranial, thoracic, abdominal, and vascular trauma. These injuries frequently fulfill the criteria for "lethal trauma" and are often camouflaged by more obvious associated lesions. Even though the emergency and trauma surgeon may need the support of organ-focused specialists for the definitive surgical care of many of the addressed injuries, he or she must be able to detect the full trauma pattern, set priorities, and perform at least the most urgent damage-control procedures. The organ-focused specialist, moreover, may have had only sporadic exposure to critical organ lesions and the respective handbooks may provide only marginal coverage of trauma issues.

Target groups of this volume are general and trauma surgeons looking for an up-to-date outline of surgical trauma care or preparing for the EBSQ-Trauma exam. The contributing authors are all highly experienced trauma surgeons or specialists in their fields with strong trauma commitment. They are drawn in part from the professional environment of the editors, and in part from the distinguished faculty of AAST and ESTES congresses.

Progress is made when established techniques are challenged and know-how is transmitted to critical colleagues. In this sense, the editors hope that surgeons, whether young or established, will scrutinize the given recommendations, apply them, and pass on their suggestions for improving them.

We express our sincere gratitude to all the authors who contributed to this volume for sharing their extraordinary experience in the field of trauma.

Special appreciation also is due to Springer Publishing and in particular to Gabriele Schroeder for initiating and publishing this volume of "Trauma Surgery." Finally, we are very much indebted to Stephanie Benko for her support of both the editors and the authors.

Celle, Graz, and Zurich   Hans-Jörg Oestern
Fall 2010   Otmar Trentz
                                                                              Selman Uranues

Contents

Traumatic Brain Injury

H.-G. Imhof and P. Lenzlinger

1.1 Introduction

Trauma of the head is a common cause of morbidity and mortality and continues to be an enormous public health problem. Tagliaferri and colleagues [391] compiling data from 23 European reports including findings from national studies from Denmark, Sweden, Finland, Portugal, Germany, and from regions within Norway, Sweden, Italy, Switzerland, Spain, Denmark, Ireland, the U.K., and France derived an aggregate hospitalized plus fatal traumatic brain injury (TBI) incidence rate of about 235 per 100,000, an average mortality rate of about 15 per 100,000, and a case fatality rate of about 11 per 100. Prevalence is estimated to reach a 317 per 100,000 persons living in Denmark with a work-precluding TBI sequelae in 1989 [97].

The highest incidence of TBI occurs in men aged 15–24 years, and is the leading cause of death among people younger than 45 years [3, 177, 200].

While various mechanisms may cause TBI, the most common causes include motor vehicle accidents (e.g., collisions between vehicles, pedestrians struck by motor vehicles, bicycle accidents), falls, assaults, sports-related injuries, and penetrating trauma. The percentages of TBI from external causes varied considerably from one European country to any other. In Southern Europe, road traffic crashes constitute the

vast majority of cases. Falls are the leading cause of trauma in Northern Europe [167, 383, 387]. Thirty five to 50% of TBI patients are under the influence of alcohol [372]. Trauma of the head is common in children too: Annually, 280 children/100,000 population require hospitalization for 24 h or more. Mild TBI accounts for 82.7% of admissions. Each year, approximately 15% of children admitted with TBI will have a moderate or severe brain injury. Falls account for 60% of TBI admissions among under 5 years of age, and nonaccidental injuries account for 8.7% of TBI admissions for children under 2 years of age [154].

Ninety to 95% of all TBIs are considered mild [256, 391, 419]. European study of the TBI severity ratio of hospitalized patients was about 22:1.5:1 for mild vs. moderate vs. severe cases, respectively.

About 60% of the brain-injured patients have an additional other injury that may add to the severity of cases and may worsen outcome [258, 360, 377].

The incidence of cervical spine trauma in moderately or severely head-injured patients ranges from 4% to 8%. Head-injured patients sustaining MVA (motor vehicle accident)-related trauma and those with an initial GCS (Glasgow coma scale) score less than or equal to 8 are at the highest risk for concomitant cervical spine injury. A disproportionate number of these patients sustain high cervical injuries, the majority of which are mechanically unstable and involve a spinal cord injury [161].

Gennarelli [126] and colleagues analyzed the causes, incidence, and mortality in 16,524 patients (one third of the trauma center patients) with injury to the brain or skull and compared them to patients without head injury. Relative to its incidence, patients with head injury composed a disproportionately high percentage (60%) of all the deaths. Overall mortality of patients with head injury (18.2%) was three times higher than if no head injury was present (6.1%). This

H.G. Imhof (✉)
Department of Neurosurgery, University Hospital Zürich
Rämistrasse 100, 8091 Zürich, Switzerland
e-mail: hans-georg.imhof@access.uzh.ch

P. Lenzlinger
Department of Traumasurgery, University Hospital Zürich
Rämistrasse 100, 8091 Zürich, Switzerland
e-mail: philipp.lenzlinger@bluewin.ch

H.-J. Oestern et al. (eds.), *Head, Thoracic, Abdominal, and Vascular Injuries*,
DOI: 10.1007/978-3-540-88122-3_1, © Springer-Verlag Berlin Heidelberg 2011

mortality was only mildly influenced by extracranial injuries except when minor and moderate head injuries were accompanied by very severe – Abbreviated Injury Scale (AIS) levels 4 to 6 [25] – injuries elsewhere. The cause of death in head-injured patients was approximated and it was found that 67.8% were due to head injury, 6.6% due to extracranial injury, and 25.6% due to both. Head injury is thus associated with more deaths (3,010 vs. 1,972) than all other injuries and causes almost as many deaths (2,040 vs. 2,170) as extracranial injuries. Because of its high mortality, head injury is the single largest contributor to trauma center deaths.

Outcome in head injuries is influenced by accompanying extracranial injuries only if producing hypotension or hypoxia affecting cerebral metabolism – mortality rise from 12.8% to 62% – and if the head injury is minor in relation to the extracranial injuries [68, 72, 127, 337, 359].

1.2 Traumatic Insults

Head injury is a nonspecific term, which includes clinically evident external injuries to the face, scalp (as lacerations, contusions, abrasions), and calvarium (fractures) and may or may not be associated with traumatic brain injury. Traumatic brain injury (TBI) is more properly defined as an alteration in brain function manifest as confusion, altered level of consciousness, seizure, coma, or focal sensory or motor neurologic deficit resulting from blunt or penetrating force to the head. Neurologic damage from TBI does not occur entirely at the moment of impact, but evolves over the ensuing hours and days [291, 298].

1.2.1 Mechanisms of Traumatic Brain Injury: Primary Insult

Traumatic brain injury is the consequence of a sudden impulsive or impact loading to the head – "*the primary insult*" – during which energy (impulse) is transmitted to the head, which undergoes sudden acceleration, deceleration, or rotation, or a combination of all. The result will be deformation of tissue by tissue compression, tissue stretching, or tissue shear: produced when tissue slides over other tissue. Brain damage after head injury can be classified by its time course.

1.2.1.1 Primary Brain Damage

Primary damage is a *mechanical damage*, occurring at the moment of the primary insult and is thought to be irreversible. In treatment terms, this type of injury can best be treated through avoidance, or blunting of the impact through safety devices.

The principal mechanisms of head injury are due to the two phenomena of acceleration [125, 291, 298] and contact.

Impulsive Loading

Acceleration results from a sudden motion without significant physical contact, resulting in intracranial and intracerebral pressure gradients and shear, tensile, and compressive strains [86].

The nonimpact phenomena cause both subdural hematoma resulting from tearing of bridging veins and diffuse damage to axons (diffuse axonal injury, DAI) attributed mainly to shear and tensile strain, with regard to death, the two worst types of head injury [121, 124].

Indirect transmission of energy to the head results in either translation, rotation, or a combined movement of the brain relatively to the skull and the dura mater (with falx cerebri and tentorium cerebelli).
Translation: Translation causes focal lesions

- Cortical contusions (gliding contusions; contrecoup contusions), cortical laceration
- Subdural hematoma

Rotation: Sudden angular acceleration/deceleration generates shear forces in the brain that may cause *diffuse damage* to axons (diffuse axonal injury, DIA) and blood vessels. [4, 123]. These injuries decrease gradually from the surface to the center of the brain [214].

Impact Loading Contact phenomena result from an object striking the head resulting in *focal lesions*

- Bruise, abrasio, lacerations, and hematoma of the scalp
- Skull fracture
- Extradural hematoma
- Some types of cerebral contusion
- Intracerebral hemorrhage

These injuries can be closed if continuity of the scalp and mucous membranes is maintained or open (Synonym: compound) if the scalp or mucous membranes are lacerated to the bone. In a penetrating head injury, the dura underlying a compound skull fracture is lacerated (direct communication between environment and cerebrospinal fluid (CSF) compartment).

Mostly, indirect transmission of energy to the head is combined with the much more frequent direct transmission, for example in a fall with subsequent dashing against the ground. [123, 140].

Static Loading

A static force – acting mostly bitemporal – slowly deforms the cranium resulting in the very rare crushing injury.

Contrary to the dynamic loading injuries, either rapid deformation of the brain and migration or coup and contrecoup injuries from shearing strain occur [136, 252].

1.2.1.2 Secondary Brain Damage

A secondary brain damage (injury) is *nonmechanical damage*. This secondary injury is a direct result of the primary injury and is a response to the primary injury and other contributing factors. The secondary injury is best defined as the pathophysiological response of the brain that follows the primary injury and that is often described as a cascade of events that is triggered by the primary impact, which lead to further injury and damage. Secondary injury may include conditions such as excitotoxicity, inflammation, and dysautoregulation and result in the brain swelling and intracranial hypertension frequently observed after TBI [204, 265].

If the primary injury is coupled with second insults, the extent and magnitude of the secondary injury (damage) response is most likely worsened by the second insults that follow (Table 1.1).

1.2.2 Mechanisms of Traumatic Brain Injury: Secondary Insult

A secondary insult, by definition, is an "additional insult" that follows the primary injury, but is not a direct

Table 1.1 Morphologic classification of traumatic head/brain injury

Impulsive loading
Translation
• Cortical contusions, cortical laceration or "burst lobe"
• Subdural hematoma
Rotation
• Diffuse damage to axons (diffuse axonal injury, DIA) and blood vessels
Impact loading
• Bruise, abrasio, lacerations, and hematoma of the scalp
• Skull fracture
• Extradural hematoma
• Some types of cerebral contusion
• Intracerebral hemorrhage

result of that primary injury. This would include such situations as hypovolemia, hypotension, hypoxia [67, 68, 127, 220], and/or hyperthermia that, although they may be a result of the trauma – especially in multiple organ injury – are not caused by the primary injury to the brain itself but can contribute to the worsening of the secondary response of the primary injury. A common second insult is the raised intracranial pressure [265].

These secondary insults may themselves be insufficient to cause any neurological injury, but, in combination with the primary trauma, may markedly worsen the final extent of damage. Secondary insults very often cause a reduction of the cerebral blood flow. Reversibility of this damage depends on the extent and the duration of this impairment [185, 295].

Outcome from head injury depends on the nature and severity of the primary lesion, and the manifestations of secondary brain damage of extra- and intracranial origin (see Sects. 1.3.3 and 1.3.4) [239]. Systemic hypotension and intracranial hypertension are the only independent risk factors for mortality that can be readily treated during the initial management of patients with severe head injuries [261] (Table 1.2).

1.3 Clinical Assessment of TBI

Central nervous system (CNS) injury may be an isolated injury, or it may occur in patients with multiple trauma.

Table 1.2 Systemic secondary insults and intracranial secondary insults to the brain [229]

Systemic secondary insults	
Hypoxemia	Hypoxia, apnea, hypoventilation, chest wall injury, hemothorax, bronchospasm, airway obstruction, lung contusion, pneumothorax, aspiration pneumonitis, anemia, carbon monoxide poisoning
Hypotension	Hypovolemia, hemorrhage, pharmacologic causes, myocardial contusion, pericardial tamponade, arrhythmia, cardiac arrest, cardiac failure, sepsis, pneumothorax, spinal cord injury
Hypercapnia	Respiratory depression/obstruction
Hypocapnia	Hyperventilation (spontaneous or induced)
Hyperthermia	Hypermetabolism, stress response, infection
Hyperglycemia	Intravenous dextrose, stress response
Hypoglycemia	Inadequate nutrition, insulin infusion
Hyponatremia	Insufficient intake, excess losses, hypotonic fluids
Hypoproteinemia	Malnutrition, starvation
Intracranial secondary insults	
Intracranial hypertension and/or brain shift	Hematoma, edema, vascular engorgement, hydrocephalus
Seizures	Cortical brain injury
Vasospasm	Traumatic subarachnoid hemorrhage
Infection	Skull base fracture, compound depressed skull fracture

In all multitrauma cases, patients must be treated according to the advanced trauma life support (ATLS) protocols (i.e., airway, breathing, circulation, disability [ABCD]) because any patient will die much more quickly from systemic injuries than from CNS injuries [345].

1.3.1 Assessment According to ATLS

Adherence to (national) algorithms (guidelines) relevant to the assessment [311] and management of accident victims [188] optimizes operational sequence and thereby has a significant impact on head injury care outcomes [106, 302, 345, 414]. Advanced Trauma Life Support (ATLS) is a widely applied algorithm [14, 36].

The premise of the ATLS program is to treat the greatest threat to life first. The ABCDE establishes an order for evaluations and treatments with the most time-critical interventions performed early. Evaluation and treatment are performed simultaneously, beginning with systems that pose the most immediate threat to life if damaged.

In neurotrauma-surgery, stabilizing life threats imply stopping intracranial bleeding, evacuation of intracranial hematomas, and limiting of contamination of compound wounds. The surgeon may need to insert an intracranial pressure (ICP) monitor in the emergency room so that ICP can be monitored at the earliest opportunity and continued during the subsequent management in the operating room and ICU. The mortality and morbidity of acute extradural and subdural hematomas are time-dependent [75, 325]. Emergency craniotomy should be commenced preferably within 30 min of arrival of the patient in the trauma center and has to be performed at the same time as a laparotomy or a thoracotomy.

1.3.1.1 Primary Survey

The first and key part of the assessment of patients presenting with trauma is called the primary survey – a focused physical examination directed at identifying and treating life-threatening conditions present in a trauma patient. Primary survey and resuscitation occur simultaneously.

The ABCDE approach sets an order for evaluations and treatments with the most time-critical interventions performed early

a. Airway maintenance with cervical spine protection
b. Breathing and ventilation
c. Circulation with hemorrhage control
d. Disability: Neurologic function is evaluated for major deficits involving the brain and spinal cord
e. Exposure and environment

Radiological examination: chest, pelvis, lat spine X-ray (other areas as indicated), skull X-ray, and CT head scan

Disability

Neurologic function is evaluated for major deficits involving the brain and spinal cord. During the primary survey, a minineurologic examination is carried out, directed toward a rapid determination of the presence and severity of gross neurologic deficits [349], especially those that may require urgent surgery. The examination includes the exploration and judgment of

a. Level of consciousness
b. Assessment of pupillary function and
c. Lateralized extremity weakness.

Minineurologic examination has a high interobserver agreement [40], allows to classify the degree of severity of the TBI (see Sect. 1.3.2), and is designed to detect evolving of secondary brain damage. Guidelines based on these criteria are widely used for clinical decision-making.

Assessment of Level of Consciousness

The level of consciousness has to be assessed after the patient has been resuscitated and stabilized. It is classified according the Glasgow Coma Scale [395] – a physiologic measure of level of consciousness – and its derivative, the Glasgow Coma Score (GCS).

The scale comprises three tests: eye, verbal, and motor responses. The three values separately as well as their sum are considered. The lowest possible GCS (the sum) is 3 (deep coma or death), while the highest is 15 (fully awake person) (Tables 1.3 and 1.4).

The *Glasgow Coma Score* is the sum of eye opening (E 1–4), verbal response (V 1–5), and the best motor response (M 1–6). Total scores of 8 or below indicate a true coma and severe brain injury.

Intubation and severe facial/eye swelling or damage make it impossible to test the verbal and eye responses. In these circumstances, the score is given as 1 with a modifier attached, e.g., "E1c" where c=closed, or "V1t" where t=tube. A composite might be "GCS 5tc." This would mean, for example, eyes closed because of swelling=1, intubated=1, leaving a motor score of 3 for "abnormal."

The GCS can provide a useful single figure summary and a basis for systems of classification, but contains less information than a description of the three

Table 1.3 Glasgow coma scale: adult patients

Best eye response (E)	
1	No eye opening
2	Eye opening in response to pain
3	Eye opening to speech
4	Eyes opening spontaneously
Best verbal response (V)	
1	No verbal response
2	Incomprehensible sounds (moaning, no words)
3	Inappropriate words (no conversational exchange)
4	Confused (responding to questions coherently, some disorientation and confusion)
5	Oriented (responding coherently and appropriately to questions)
Best motor response (M)	
1	No motor response
2	Extension to pain (decerebrate response[a])
3	Abnormal flexion to pain (decorticate response[b])
4	Flexion/Withdrawal to pain
5	Localizes to pain (moves towards painful stimuli[c])
6	Obeys commands

[a] Adduction of arm, internal rotation of shoulder, pronation of forearm, extension of wrist, decerebrate response
[b] Adduction of arm, internal rotation of shoulder, pronation of forearm, flexion of wrist, decorticate response
[c] Flexion of elbow, supination of forearm, flexion of wrist when supra-orbital pressure applied; pulls part of body away when nail bed pinched

responses separately. The three responses of the scale, not the total score, should therefore be used in describing, monitoring, and exchanging information about individual patients [173]. Accurate determination of the admission GCS is important because the number of intracranial abnormalities and the need for neurosurgical interventions are inversely related to the admission GCS [80, 135].

Alcohol intoxication does not result in clinically significant changes in GCS score for patients with blunt TBI. Hence, alterations in GCS score after TBI should not be attributed to alcohol intoxication, as doing so might result in inappropriate delays in monitoring and therapeutic interventions [372, 384].

Table 1.4 Glasgow coma scale: pediatric patients [322]

Eye opening score	>1 Year	0–1 Year	
4	Opens eyes spontaneously	Opens eyes spontaneously	
3	Opens eyes to a verbal command	Opens eyes to a shout	
2	Opens eyes in response to pain	Opens eyes in response to pain	
1	No response	No response	
Best motor response score	>1 Year	0–1 Year	
6	Obeys command	N/A	
5	Localizes pain	Localizes pain	
4	Flexion withdrawal	Flexion withdrawal	
3	Flexion abnormal (decorticate)	Flexion abnormal (decorticate)	
2	Extension (decerebrate)	Extension (decerebrate)	
1	No response	No response	
Best verbal response score	>5 Years	2–5 Years	0–2 Years
5	Oriented and able to converse	Uses appropriate words	Cries appropriately
4	Disoriented and able to converse	Uses inappropriate words	Cries
3	Uses inappropriate words	Cries and/or screams	Cries and/or screams inappropriately
2	Makes incomprehensible sounds	Grunts	Grunts
1	No response	No response	No response

The GCS has limited applicability to children, especially below the age of 36 months (where the verbal performance of even a healthy child would be expected to be poor). Consequently, the Pediatric Glasgow Coma Scale, a separate yet closely related scale, was developed for assessing younger children

Assessment of Pupillary Function, Oculocephalic Testing, and Oculovestibular Testing [32]

- The pupils should be examined after the patient has been resuscitated and stabilized. Bilaterally dilated and fixed pupils may be the result of inadequate cerebral vascular perfusion. If the time of inadequate has not be too long, return of pupillary response may occur promptly.
- Attention has to be paid on the differences between left and right eye: Notation of pupil size, equality, and response to bright light: unilateral or bilateral fixed pupils/unilateral or bilateral dilated pupils/fixed and dilated pupils. A difference in diameter of more than 1 mm is abnormal. Light reactivity has to be evaluated for the briskness of response. A fixed pupil is defined as no response.
- A mild dilatation of the pupil and a sluggish pupillary reaction is an early sign of temporal lobe herniation. Bilateral mitotic pupils occur in the early stages of central herniation. Continued herniation causes wider dilatation of the pupils and paralysis of its light responses.
- In a patient with a dilated pupil from the onset of injury, an improving level of consciousness and appropriate ocular muscle weakness is to surmise a damage of the oculomotor nerve, a mydriatic pupil (6 mm or more) may occur with direct trauma of the globe of the eye [69].
- Oculocephalic testing: Before performing oculocephalic testing, the status of the cervical spine must be established. If a cervical spine injury has not been excluded reliably, oculocephalic testing should not be performed.
- In oculocephalic testing (doll's eyes), the head, elevated to 30° from horizontal, is turned by grasping and rotating briskly the jaw in a patient with open eyelids. Similar as doll's eyes move when the head is turned, the eyes of the patient deviate to the contralateral side assuming the brain stem is intact. With brain stem injury in the region of the lateral gaze centers, the eyes do not move (negative doll's eyes).

- Oculovestibular testing [32]: Before performing oculovestibular testing, the presence of an intact tympanic membrane has to be assessed. Oculovestibular testing is performed on the patient supine with the head elevated to 30° from horizontal to bring the horizontal semicircular canal into the vertical position. Ten to 20 cc iced saline (20 cc syringe) is injected slowly into the external auditory channel, which alters the endolymphatic flow. In alert patients, there results a fast nystagmus away from the irrigated ear and a slow compensatory nystagmus toward the irrigated side. As the level of consciousness declines, the fast component of nystagmus fades gradually. Thus, in unconscious patients, only the slow phase of nystagmus may be evaluated. This means that the injury causing coma must be rostral to the reticular activating system in the upper brainstem.
- With a unilateral frontal lobe injury, the eyes of the patient are deviated toward the side of injury prior to caloric testing. Cold-water irrigation of the opposite ear results in a normal response to caloric testing (i.e., eye deviation toward the irrigated side) because the injury is in the frontal region and spares the pontine gaze centers.
- This is in contrast to a pontine injury causing the eyes to deviate away from the side of injury: In this situation, cold-water irrigation of the contralateral ear does not cause the gaze to deviate toward the irrigated ear because the pontine gaze centers are compromised.
- A disconjugate response to caloric testing suggests an injury to either the third or sixth cranial nerves or an injury to the MLF, resulting in an internuclear ophthalmoplegia. If caloric testing causes the eyes to move disconjugately in the vertical direction, this is a skew deviation, a lesion in the brainstem is present.

Lateralized Extremity Weakness

Tone and muscle strength is assessed by comparing the left extremities with the right ones. In patients not obeying orders, the motor examination is limited to an assessment of asymmetry in the motor examination findings. A consistent asymmetry between right- and left-sided responses strongly point to a structural lesion.

1.3.1.2 Secondary Survey

The secondary survey of patients according to the ATLS principles is a detailed examination and assessment of the system with the goal of identifying all traumatic injuries and directing further treatment, performed after immediate life threats are assessed and stabilized.

Findings of the secondary survey provide baseline for comparison for subsequent reassessments. At any given moment, the depth of the examination is dependent on the patient's level of arousal and attention span.

Special neurosurgical assessment includes:

- History
- Local findings
- Extended neurological exam
- Completion of radiological examination

History

A focused history has to be obtained. If only limited conversation is possible, history covers essential information: allergies, medications, past medical history, last meal, and events of the injury ("AMPLE").

The following information has to be asked of the patient and/or accompanying persons and prehospital personnel, respectively:

- Injury description: overall cause of injury, mechanism of injury (fall, vehicular crash (driver or car passenger, pedestrian), assault), neurologic and cardiorespiratory status at the scene.
- Amnesia (retrograde and/or anterograde), loss of consciousness (LOC), seizures, and early signs observed by others.
- History of drugs or alcohol, both prior to and at the time of injury. Other medical disease, previous head injury, and ocular conditions.

Prehospital personnel has to be asked:

- Has the patient talked before becoming unconscious. If so, there is some secondary cause of a poor neurological state, e.g., hypoxia, hypotension, intracranial hematoma.
- Were the pupils equal or unequal at the scene of the injury? (Initial equality with change to inequality suggests a lateralized mass lesion.)
- About the cardiorespiratory status at the accident site and response to resuscitation.

Simply knowing the history allows one to estimate the risks of complications to be expected: Unclear or ambiguous accident history, high-energy accident, seizure, coagulation disorders, age < 2 years and age > 60 are rated as risk factors for intracranial complications. To be injured in a fall instead of a vehicle crash quadruples the risk of harboring an intracranial hematoma [148].

Local Status

External signs of injury to the head have to be specifically looked for: Scalp injuries (contusion, laceration, bruise), eye injury, ear, and nose (bleeding, escape of cerebrospinal fluid (CSF)), indication of skull fracture (skull impression, raccoon eyes (periorbital ecchymosis), battle sign (retroauricular ecchymosis), and facial fractures). Trauma above the clavicles are rated as risk factors for intracranial complications [156].

Neurologic Status

The result of the initial neurologic examination is only the starting point for judging further development of the consequences of the sustained trauma.
Mental status:

- State of consciousness (awareness and responsiveness to the environment and the senses);
- Appearance and general behavior; mood;
- Orientation with reference to time, place, and person; comprehension; ability to pay attention
- Memory
- Speech and language function

Cranial nerves:

- In sufficiently alert patients, eye movements and pupillary reaction can be assessed easily. In conscious patients, serial quantitation in each eye is important. In patients with depressed consciousness, oculocephalic and oculovestibular responses are to be evaluated.
- Eyelid strength and function; visual function; peripheral vision;
- Strength of facial musculature;
- The gag reflex;
- Tongue and lip movements;
- Ability to smell and taste;
- Hearing; and sensation in the face, head, and neck.

Motor exam:

Power, tone, and fine coordination of the limbs.
The results are to be classified:
0/5: no contraction
1/5: muscle flicker, but no movement
2/5: movement possible, but not against gravity (test the joint in its horizontal plane)
3/5: movement possible against gravity, but not against resistance by the examiner
4/5: movement possible against some resistance by the examiner
5/5: normal strength

Reflexes:
Deep tendon reflexes; Babinski response
Coordination and gait:

Sensory exam:
Sensation of pain, temperature, pressure, and position

Risk Factors

In patients suffering from mild TBI, these signs and symptoms are rated as risk factors for intracranial complications after mild traumatic brain injury [420] indicating computed tomographic scanning of the head imperatively (see Sect. 1.4.2) (Table 1.5).

Table 1.5 Risk factors [419]

• Unclear or ambiguous accident history
• Continued posttraumatic amnesia
• Retrograde amnesia longer than 30 min
• Trauma above the clavicles including clinical signs of skull fracture (skull base or depressed skull fracture)
• Severe headache
• Focal neurological deficit
• Seizure
• Age < 2 years
• Age > 60
• Coagulation disorders
• High-energy accident
• Intoxication with alcohol/drugs

Facial/cervical-spinal fractures, unexplained neurologic deficit, anisocoria, lateral neck soft tissue injury, are risk factors for blunt cerebrovascular injury (BCVI)

Radiological Examination

Need for radiological examination (plain X-ray skull, computed tomography, magnetic tomography, angiography) is judged following clinical guidelines (see Sect. 1.4).

1.3.2 Classification of TBIs

Traumatic brain injury is widely classified on the basis of the Glasgow Coma Score (GCS-Score) quantified on arrival at hospital, based on the Glasgow Coma Scale [395] (see Sect. 1.3.1) (Table 1.6).

Classification of severity of TBI based on GCS scores is important both when outcome is to be forecast and proposals and guidelines concerning management

Table 1.6 Classification of traumatic brain injury (EFNS) [419]

Classification	
Mild	GCS = 13–15
Category 0	GCS = 15
	No LOC, no PTA, = head injury, no TBI
	No risk factors[a]
Category 1	GCS = 15
	LOC < 30 min, PTA < 1 h
	No risk factors
Category 2	GCS = 15 and risk factors present[a]
Category 3	GCS = 13–14
	LOC < 30 min, PTA < 1 h
	With or without risk factors present[a]
Moderate	GCS = 9–12
Severe	GCS ≥ 8
Critical	GCS = 3–4, with loss of pupillary reactions and absent or decerebrate motor reactions

Admission Glasgow Coma Scale Score (GCS) and clinical characteristics modified from the Dutch, Scandinavian, and American classification systems (Teasdale and Jennett, 1974; Stein and Spettell, 1995; Maas et al., 1997; Ingebrigtsen et al., 2000; Twijnstra et al., 2001)
TBI, traumatic brain injury; *GCS*, Glasgow Coma Scale; *LOC*, loss of consciousness; *PTA*, posttraumatic amnesia
[a] Risk factors for intracranial complications after mild traumatic brain injury (Table 1.5)

of patients are to be published. The perspective is neurosurgical and concerned with acute management, especially the early detection of intracranial hematomas. This classification does not concern itself with the controversy about the extent and basis of any neuropsychological sequelae of mild head injury. Every patient surviving a traumatic brain injury may suffer from subtle neurologic, cognitive, and psychological deficits causing significant and long-lasting disability.

Minor traumatic brain injury (Synonym: concussion, mild head injury, minor brain injury, minor head trauma, minor TBI) is defined as a nonpenetrating trauma in a patient presenting with a GCS Score 13–15 on admission to hospital [324]. To differentiate a brain injury from a scalp bruise or a skull injury, the occurrence of a transient loss of consciousness (LOC) or a period of amnesia has been taken as a "conditio sine qua non."

Irrespective of the GCS score, a patient is considered having sustained a serious head injury if he exhibits one of the following

- Unequal pupils
- Unequal motor examination
- An open head injury with leaking CSF or exposed brain tissue
- Neurologic deterioration
- Depressed skull fracture

while neurologic deterioration includes any of the following:

- Increase in severity of headache or an extraordinarily severe headache
- An increase in the size of one pupil
- Development of weakness on one side
- Increasing confusion or worsening of the level of consciousness

Classification of severity of TBI based on GCS scores is important both when outcome is to be prognosed (see Sect. 1.3.4) and when proposals and guidelines concerning managing patients (see Sects. 1.4.2 and 1.5) are to be defined. Each single class has to be as homogeneous as possible. Clinical experience disclosed has shown a wide heterogeneity (Table 1.7) in injury severity within the group "minor TBI" (GCS 13–15): The frequencies of skull fractures (diagnosed in plain skull X-ray) and pathological CT-findings rise proportionally with declining GCS, explaining the different prognosis within the group of "Minor Head Injury."

Table 1.7 Cranial fractures/intracranial abnormalities and the GCS [80]

Cranial fractures and the GCS						
GCS	No. of Patients	% of Fractures				
15	90/2,398	3.8				
14	78/796	9.8				
13	31/176	18.0				
Intracranial abnormalities on computed tomographic scan and the GCS						
GCS	Pathol.		Lesions			
Score	CT	%	contusion	aEDH	aSDH	Edema	SAH
15	95/2,179	4	39	6	23	2	36
14	118/775	16	63	14	29	0	54
13	48/173	28	30	7	15	6	12

In a prospective, consecutive, unselected cohort of MHI patients, the incidence of positive CT scans was 38%. Seven percent of this cohort required neurosurgical intervention. Six percent showed neurological deterioration and there was one death in this series [403].

While Stein [376] proposed to classify patients presenting with a GCS Score 13 as having sustained a moderate head injury, the Neurotraumatology Committee of the World Federation of Neurosurgical Societies (NCWFNS) proposed [356] that acute head-injured patients previously described as minor, mild, or trivial are defined as "mild head injury," and that further groups are recognized and classified (Table 1.8). A similar concept is proposed by the European Federation of Neurological Societies [420].

With low-risk mild injury, the risk of intracranial hematoma requiring surgical evacuation is definitively less than 0.1:100, medium risk mild injury in the range of 1–3:100, and with high-risk mild head injury in the range 6–10:100 [356]. But even mild traumatic head injury – defined as short-term loss of consciousness and/or amnesia as a result of skull trauma in a patient presenting in the emergency department with a GCS15 and normal neurological findings [8] – may become problematic. Out of 1,000 patients arriving at hospital with mild head injury, about 80 will show pathological findings on CT, 1 will die, and 9 will require surgery or other intervention [6]. When studying clinical publications concerning head injury, it is most important to identify the meaning of expressions like "mild," "minor," or "moderate."

Table 1.8 Criteria proposed by the NCWFS for classification and diagnosis of patients with mild head injury [356]

	Low risk	Medium risk	High risk
GCS	15	15 with clinical findings	14 or 15 with neurodeficits or skull fracture or risk factors with/without clinical findings
Clinical findings	No	1. Amnesia	1. Amnesia
		2. Diffuse headache	2. Diffuse headache
		3. Vomiting	3. Vomiting
		4. Loss of consciousness	4. Loss of consciousness
Neurodeficits	No	No	Yes
Skull fracture	No	No	Yes
Risk factors	No	No	1. Coagulopathy
			2. Age > 60 years
			3. Previous neurosurgery
			4. Pretrauma epilepsy
			5. Alcohol and/or drug misuse
Imaging	No	CT scan or SR	CT scan

CT, computer tomography; *GCS*, Glasgow coma scale; *NCWFS*, Neurotraumatology Committee of the World Federation of Neurosurgical Societies; *SR*, skull radiography

1.3.3 Outcome After TBI

1.3.3.1 Outcome Scales

The Glasgow Outcome Scale [179] is the most often used method for categorizing the functional status of a patient after having sustained TBI. The clearly defined categories are as follows (Table 1.9):

Because of limitations recognized in the use of the GOS, an *extended eight-point scale* (GOS E) in which the last three categories on the GOS are divided into upper and lower bands was proposed [397]. More sensitive to change in mild to moderate TBI is the "Modified Rankin Scale" (Table 1.10).

Table 1.9 Glasgow outcome scale [179]

Score
5 – Full recovery (i.e. the resumption of normal life even though there may be minor neurologic or psychological deficits);
4 – Moderate disability (i.e., disabled, but independent in daily life);
3 – Severe disability (i.e., conscious but disabled with the patient being dependent for daily support [for _8 h per day] due to mental or physical disability);
2 – Vegetative state (i.e., the patient being unresponsive and speechless for weeks or months after the injury);
1 – Dead, which included 30-day all-cause mortality and 1-year disease-specific mortality.

Table 1.10 Modified Ranking scale [317]

Score
0 – No symptoms at all
1 – No significant disability despite symptoms; able to carry out all usual duties and activities
2 – Slight disability; unable to carry out all previous activities, but able to look after own affairs without assistance
3 – Moderate disability; requiring some help, but able to walk without assistance
4 – Moderately severe disability; unable to walk without assistance and unable to attend to own bodily needs without assistance
5 – Severe disability; bedridden, incontinent and requiring constant nursing care and attention
6 – Dead

1.3.3.2 Mild (GCS 15–13) TBI: Outcome

Mild TBI is defined as GCS 13–15 at admission [324] or as a modification "transient loss of consciousness without major complications and not requiring intracranial surgery" [213].

In a historical cohort study including all residents with any diagnosis suggestive of TBI (35% were pediatric; 55% were adult; only 9% were elderly), traumatic brain injuries have been classified as mild TBI in up to 90% of patients admitted to hospital. The proportions of those patients who died within 6 months of injury increased with increasing age, ranging from 0% in young to 9% in elderly patients [109].

In adults having sustained a minor TBI (GCS score of 13–14 or a GCS score of 15 and a risk factor), CT shows traumatic lesions in about 10%. One year disease-specific mortality was 3.2% [367]. In pediatric trauma patients, an admission GCS of 14 or 15 and a normal neurologic exam and maintenance of consciousness does not preclude significant rates of intracranial injury [362].

A common sequel of mild TBI is the postconcussion syndrome. This syndrome refers to a large number of symptoms and signs that may occur alone or in combination following usually mild head injury. The most common complaints are headaches, dizziness, fatigue, irritability, anxiety, insomnia, loss of consciousness and memory, and noise sensitivity [100].

Although nearly all patients initially report cognitive problems, somatic complaints, and emotional malaise, these postconcussion symptoms resolve by the 3-month follow-up examination. A single uncomplicated minor head injury (only transient loss of consciousness without major complications and not requiring intracranial surgery) produces no permanent disabling neurobehavioral impairment in the great majority of patients who are free of preexisting neuropsychiatric disorder and substance abuse [213].

Nevertheless, it has to be realized that the terms "minor" or "mild" can be misleading because the sequelae that often follow such injuries can cause significant detriment to psychosocial and interpersonal functioning [194, 419].

1.3.3.3 Moderate (GCS 12–9) TBI: Outcome

Moderate head injury results in mortality and substantial morbidity intermediate between those of severe and minor head injury. Unlike minor head injury, the principal predictors of outcome after moderate head injury are measures of the severity of injury. Patients with moderate head injury and subdural hematoma have a very poor outcome: In a study by Rimel et al., 65% died or were severely disabled and none made a good recovery as measured by the Glasgow Outcome Scale [324]. At 3 months, about 40% (38%) of the moderate head injury patients had made a good recovery. Within the good recovery category, however, there was much disability as headache (93%), memory difficulties (90%), difficulties with activities of daily living (87%), and only 7% of the patients were asymptomatic. Sixty-six per cent of the patients previously employed had not returned to work [324]. In a study by Vitaz et al., in terms of looking at the long-term outcome (about 2 years) following moderate TBI, the majority of patients made a good functional recovery with almost 90% having GOS of 4 or 5 and being able to perform greater than 75% of their activities of daily living (ADLs) without assistance. However, such scoring systems are crude and tend to underestimate the impact that such injuries may have on a patient's life, since in this patient population is a high incidence of subjective, cognitive, and mental complaints. Only 74% of patients working full-time before their injury returned to such levels of employment (at the time of last follow-up). Although the GCS in most of these patients returned to nearly normal, this does not equate to normal function. In fact, even the GOS is limited in its ability to portray the extent of deficits that affect these patients [417].

1.3.3.4 Severe (GCS 8–3) TBI: Outcome

Not surprisingly, mortality following severe TBI increases significantly when compared with moderate injury. The outcome of severe head injury was prospectively studied in 746 patients with severe head injury (defined as a Glasgow Coma Scale (GCS) score of 8 or less following nonsurgical resuscitation). The overall mortality rate for the 746 patients was 36%, determined at 6 months postinjury. As expected, the mortality rate progressively decreased from 76% in patients with a postresuscitation GCS score of 3 to approximately 18% for patients with a GCS score of 6, 7, or 8. Among the patients with nonsurgical lesions (overall mortality rate, 31%), the mortality rate was higher in those having an increased likelihood of elevated intracranial pressure as assessed by the computerized tomography findings. In the 276 patients undergoing craniotomy, the mortality rate was 39% [242]. In their series of patients surviving severe TBI more than 3 years (76% of the cohort) Skandsen and colleagues (362) qualified, 3% of patients to be in a vegetative state. Twenty-eight were severely (GOSE 3: 22% lower level, 6% upper level) and 39% moderately disabled (GOSE 4: 22% lower level, 17% upper level), respectively. Twenty-seven made a good recovery (GOSE 5: 10% lower level, 17% upper level).

In children having sustained severe TBI, mortality was found lowest in the 5- to 10-year-old group (at discharge about 15%/at 1 year about 20%) and highest in infants and preschoolers (at discharge about 40%/at 1 year about 60%) [215].

1.3.4 Predictors of Outcome

Accurate assessment of prognosis [283] is important when making decisions about the use of specific methods of treatment, in deciding whether or not to withdraw treatment and counseling patients and relatives. Improvement in accuracy occurs when there is agreement between age, clinical indices indicating the severity of brain injury (GCS (motor score), and pupillary reactivity) and the results of investigation and imaging studies, particularly intracranial pressure (ICP) and computed tomography (CT) scanning. Nevertheless, an estimate of a patient's prognosis should never be the only factor in influencing clinical decisions. All the more because an outcome prognosis of patients with severe head injury has limited accuracy when made within the first 24 h after injury.

Even with sophisticated clinical and radiological technologies or application of mathematical models, it is impossible to predict outcome on the first day after the accident with sufficient accuracy to guide early management [191] and to say with certainty what will be the future course of events in an individual patient.

The working group convened by the Brain Trauma Foundation, the American Association of Neurological Surgeons, the Neuro-trauma Committee of the World Health Organization, and the Brain Injury Association to evaluate the literature on prognostic indicators in head injury, has developed a model for making recommendations, adhering to the concepts of evidence-based practice. Having searched and qualitatively evaluated the appropriate literature according to criteria intended to establish study strength, specific prognostic indicators were then examined separately.

1.3.4.1 Age

Age is an extremely important primary determinant of both mortality and morbidity following isolated traumatic brain injury (TBI) [275, 396, 418]. Older patients following isolated TBI have poorer functional status at discharge and make less improvement at 1 year when compared with all other patients [37]. These worse outcomes occur despite what appears to be less severe TBI as measured by a higher GCS on admission. Differences in outcome begin to appear even in patients between 45 and 59 years [224].

There is an increasing probability of poor outcome with increasing age, in a stepwise manner. Despite some contradictions, most literature supports indicate that children fare better than adults who have severe brain injury. The significant influence of age on outcome cannot be explained by the increased frequency of systemic complications or intracerebral hematomas with age. Thus, increasing age is a strong independent factor in prognosis with a significant increase in poor outcome above 60 years of age [63]. The CRASH-study found age to be the strongest predictor of outcome in high income countries [78].

1.3.4.2 Admission GCS Score

The initial GCS score may give an erroneous view of the likelihood of salvage [240]. In the TCDB group, 42% of patients had a GCS score of 3 at the first evaluation, which fell to 21.5% following nonsurgical resuscitation. The GCS score following resuscitation (postresuscitation GCS) is closely associated with the outcome [242]. In multiple injured patients, the combination of GCS and Injury Severity Score (ISS, an anatomical scoring system that provides an overall score for patients with multiple injuries [26, 300, 311]) correlate with outcome better than do any of the three measures alone [112].

The two most important problems are the reliability of the initial assessment, and its lack of precision for prediction of a good outcome if the initial GCS score is low. There is an increasing probability of poor outcome with a decreasing Glasgow Coma Score (GCS) in a continuous, stepwise manner: If the initial GCS score is reliably obtained and not tainted by pre-hospital medications or intubation, approximately 20% of the patients with the worst initial GCS score will survive and 8–10% will have a functional survival (GOS 4–5) [62].

Glasgow coma score was the strongest predictor of outcome in low-middle income countries [78] and age was the strongest predictor, while the absence of pupil reactivity was the third strongest predictor in both regions.

1.3.4.3 Pupils

It is important to be certain that pupils are not fixed by drugs or direct injury to the globe. Bilaterally absent pupillary light reflex is a very strong predictor of fatal outcome [240, 338]. Patients with abnormal pupil prior to and following resuscitation fared better (34.3% dead or vegetative) than if one pupil became abnormal for at least one observation following resuscitation (50% dead or vegetative) [242].

The pupillary diameter and the pupiloconstrictor light reflex are the two parameters that have been studied extensively in relation to prognosis. Accurate measurement of pupil diameter or the constrictor response or the duration of the response has not been performed in studies on traumatic brain-injured individuals – for lack of a standardized measuring procedure. The following is recommended [65]:

1. Pupillary light reflex for each eye should be used as a prognostic parameter.
2. The duration of pupillary dilation and fixation should be documented.
3. A pupillary size greater than 4 mm is recommended as the measure for a dilated pupil [17].
4. A fixed pupil should be defined as no constrictor response to bright light.
5. Right or left distinction should be made when the pupils are asymmetric.
6. Hypotension and hypoxia should be corrected before assessing pupils for prognosis.
7. Direct orbital trauma should be excluded.
8. Pupils should be reassessed after surgical evacuation of intracranial hematomas.

Following GCS and age, the absence of pupil reactivity was the third strongest predictor.

1.3.4.4 Hypotension and Hypoxia

Hypotension and to a lesser extent hypoxia – frequent consequence of multiple injuries – play a major role in determining the outcome of patients with severe head injury [53, 253].

A systolic blood pressure of less than 90 mmHg was found to have a 67% positive predictive value (PPV) for poor outcome and, when combined with hypoxia, a PPV of 79% PPV resulted. Hypotension, occurring at any time from injury through the acute intensive care course, has been found to be a primary predictor of outcome for severe head injury. Hypotension is repeatedly found to be one of the five most powerful predictors of outcome and is generally the only one of these five that is amenable to therapeutic modification. A single recording of a hypotensive episode is generally associated with a doubling of mortality and a marked increase in morbidity from a given head injury. The estimated reduction in unfavorable outcome that would result from the elimination of hypotensive secondary brain insults is profound [64].

1.3.4.5 Intracranial Pressure

The importance of intracranial hypertension in determining the outcome of head-injured patients is well known and has been confirmed in a large clinical trial [187, 379]. Vik and colleagues [415] comment on a significant relationship between the dose of ICP, the worst Marshall CT score, and patient outcome (see Chap. 2).

1.3.4.6 Mechanism of Injury

Pedestrians fare particularly poorly. In this group, the frequency of shock and hypoxia as a consequence of multiple injuries is frequent [53, 242].

1.3.4.7 Computed Tomography

The Marshall CT classification (see Sect. 1.4.2.1 and Table 1.13) has strong predictive power, but greater discrimination can be obtained if the individual CT parameters underlying the CT classification are included in a prognostic model [231, 232]. Consequently, for prognostic purposes, Maas and colleagues recommend the use of individual characteristics rather than the CT

classification. Performance of CT models for predicting outcome in TBI can be significantly improved by including more details of variables and by adding other variables to the model. Such models should include the following characteristics: status of basal cisterns, shift, tSAH, and/or IVH and presence of mass lesions with differentiation between EDH versus intradural lesions [231]. CT scan features as early indicators of prognosis in severe traumatic brain injury are presented in Tables 1.11 and 1.12, respectively.

Table 1.11 Early indicators of prognosis in severe traumatic brain injury, CT scan features: Conclusions [62]

A. The following features of the parameter were supported by Class I and strong Class II evidence have at least a 70% positive predictive value (PPV) in severe head injury?
a. Presence of abnormalities on initial computed tomography (CT) examination
b. CT classification
c. Compressed or absent basal cisterns
d. Traumatic subarachnoid hemorrhage (tSAH):
• Blood in the basal cisterns
• Extensive tSAH
B. Parameter measurement:
1. How should measurements be performed?
• Compressed or absent basal cisterns measured at the midbrain level.
• tSAH should be noted in the basal cisterns or over the convexity.
• Midline shift should be measured at the level of the septum pellucidum.
2. When should it be measured?
• Within 12 h of injury
• The full extent of intracranial pathology, however, may not be disclosed on early CT examination.
3. Who should measure it?
• A neuroradiologist or other qualified physician, experienced in reading CT-scans of the brain
Particularly relevant in terms of prognosis were found to be:
a. Status of basal cisterns
b. tSAH
c. Presence and degree of midline shift
d. Presence and type of intracranial lesions

Table 1.12 CRASH head-injury prognostic models [78]

The following characteristics on computed tomography were strongly associated with the outcomes in addition to the predictors included in the basic models:

- Presence of petechial hemorrhages,

- Obliteration of the third ventricle or basal cisterns,

- Subarachnoid bleeding,

- Midline shift, and

- Nonevacuated hematoma.

Obliteration of the third ventricle and midline shift were the strongest predictors of mortality at 14 days, and nonevacuated hematoma was the strongest predictor of unfavorable outcome at 6 months.

1.3.4.8 Laboratory Parameters

Increasing values of glucose are associated with poorer outcome as are low values of Hb, platelets, and pH while sodium demonstrated a U-shaped relation to outcome, with low levels being more strongly related to poorer outcome. Effects were strongest for increasing levels of glucose [412].

1.3.4.9 Combinations of Several Predictive Characteristics

Combinations of several predictive characteristics were proposed as an indicator of prognosis [72, 274]. The model correctly predicted outcome into one of the four outcome categories in 78% of cases (specifically accurate predictions). If predictions into an outcome category adjacent to the actual outcome were accepted, this model was accurate in 90% of cases (grossly accurate predictions) [72].

Prognostic models that include simple variables may be used as an aid to estimate mortality and severe disability in patients with traumatic brain injury [78, 79, 167].

These prognostic models may be used as an aid to estimate mortality at 14 days and death and severe disability at 6 months in patients with traumatic brain injury (TBI). The predictions are based on the average outcome in adult patients with Glasgow coma score (GCS) of 14 or less, within 8 h of injury, and can only support – not replace – clinical judgment. Although individual names of countries can be selected in the models, the estimates are based on two alternative sets of models (high income countries or low and middle income countries).

1.4 Technical Assessment of TBI

When traumatic brain injuries are categorized according to Rimel (GCS score 15–13: minor head injury), most of the victims of TBI (about 85%) are low-risk patients (see Sect. 1.3.2) [324]. However, a normal neurologic exam and maintenance of consciousness does not preclude significant rates of intracranial injury in trauma patients. Even if the Glasgow Coma Scale score is 15, intracranial lesions cannot be completely excluded clinically on head-trauma patients who have loss of consciousness or amnesia, regardless of age, mechanism of injury, or clinical findings [6].

Patients presenting a mild head injury are at the greatest risk of inadequate diagnosis and treatment [196]. The most serious complication of TBI is the occurrence of an intracranial mass lesion, i.e., a hematoma within the skull vault [351]. Without effective surgical management, an intracranial hematoma may transform an otherwise benign clinical course with the expectation of recovery, into to a situation where death or permanent vegetative survival is imminent. The primary goal of initial management in MTBI is therefore to identify the patients at risk for intracranial abnormalities and especially those who may need neurosurgical intervention.

Accordingly, several guidelines were designed, some of which were based on a previously published decision algorithm the Dutch guidelines on the New Orleans criteria, the criteria proposed by the National Institute for Clinical Excellence ([401]; see Sect. 1.4.2) on the Canadian CT head rule, and the guidelines proposed by the European Federation of Neurological Societies (EFNS) on both the New Orleans criteria and the Canadian CT head rule [366].

These Guidelines frame proposals concerning clarification of TBI and resulting consequences in managing (dismission of ER; need in-hospital care) the patient [7, 8, 104, 156, 170, 229, 230, 356, 377, 410, 420] (see Sect. 1.5).

1.4.1 Skull Radiography (SR)/Cervical Spine

Skull radiography is useful for imaging of calvarial fractures, penetrating injuries, and radiopaque foreign bodies. Four standard views have to be obtained: An AP view, a Towne's view, and two lateral views (to permit the film to focus on one side at a time). In assessing traumatic brain injury, the diagnostic yield of SR is small, a fracture is to be diagnosed in only 1.5–4% of the plain skull X-rays [176, 248], depressed fractures or fractures in penetrating head injuries in only about 1% [102].

Isolated skull fractures are not rather threatening injuries and by itself have few clinical consequences, except in cases of basal skull fractures involving cerebral vessels [254] and in depressed skull fractures. However, the presence of a skull fracture indicates that significant enough impact occurred to cause brain trauma: The demonstration of a skull fracture increases the risk of significant intracranial hemorrhage fivefold [159, 264].

The primary goal of initial management of the huge number of victims of mild and moderate TBI – about 85% of victims of TBI in this huge group (about 80%) of patients is to identify those patients at risk for intracranial abnormalities and especially those who may need neurosurgical intervention. To screen these patients, the Society of British Neurological Surgeons had proposed an algorithm based on skull X-rays [335].

However, 90% of skull fractures are not associated with an intracranial injury, and 44% of patients harboring an intracranial hemorrhage have no skull fracture. By excluding skull radiography for low-risk patients, no intracranial injury would have been missed [159, 249]. Additionally, fractures of the skull are not diagnosed as accurately as supposed: Thillainayagam and colleagues noted that casualty officers diagnosed 66 fractures of the skull on radiographs but 27 of these were subsequently reported by a radiologist as not being fractures. Of the 45 fractures reported by the radiologist, 6 had been missed by the casualty officer [402]. Thiruppathy and Muthukumar [403] noted that CT-scan had a greater chance of detecting a skull fracture than routine skull radiography.

Since computed tomography scanning is widely available in the emergency departments of most hospitals, importance is no longer attached to skull X-rays [401]. Most likely, skull radiography are conducted in the assessment of depressed fractures and if in children abuse is suspected [407].

Assessing cervical spine injury on plain X-rays have become less important. Plain radiography alone is not sufficiently sensitive as the definitive investigation, and radiographs obtained in the acute trauma setting are often technically unsatisfactory. Additionally, among children, variations in osseous development may create additional confusion [306]. Recommendation for assessment includes the use of flexion/extension lateral cervical spine fluoroscopy with static images obtained at extremes of flexion and extension if normal findings are observed on the initial plain X-ray films and CT scans [152].

1.4.2 Computed Tomography

Accurate radiographic diagnosis is a cornerstone of the clinical management and outcome prediction of the head-injured patient. Computed tomography with its ability to rapidly image the trauma patient is the initial imaging modality of choice in severe acute craniocerebral trauma [314]. In head-injured patients, CT is used for the detection of intracranial hemorrhage, mass effect (including brain herniation), ventricular size and configuration, skull fractures, displaced bone fragments, foreign bodies, intracranial air, etc [293, 294]. Accompanying injuries of the cervical spine can be assessed without changing position of the patient [306].

A multidetector-row CT-scanner allows true three-dimensional imaging and may be used as a screening test for blunt cerebrovascular injury (see Sect. 1.4.4). Besides morphologic imaging, cerebral imaging techniques can provide detailed hemodynamic and metabolic information over multiple regions of interest (xenon CT and CT perfusion). However, they are limited by two serious disadvantages: they are only able to provide snapshot images of the brain and they require the transfer of critically ill patients to specialized imaging facilities [76].

Using a multislice CT scanner (16 up to 128 array), a spiral head CT scan with an effective slice thickness of 0.75 to 1 mm is acquired. The raw data is reconstructed at a slice thickness of 4 mm and a distance between slices of 4 mm (4/4) in 3 planes (axial/coronal/sagittal) and with adequate windowing for soft tissue and bone, respectively (possibly an additional intermediate setting for the detection of a thin layer of subdural or epidural blood against the dense calvarium). In cases where basal skull or midface fractures are suspected but not seen on the above reconstructions, high-resolution reconstructions (2/2 or 1/1) may be performed selectively.

CT should be performed as soon as possible, to assess the possible need for surgical intervention and intracranial pressure management. Critically injured patients can be monitored within the scanner with relative ease [303] in patients with craniocerebral trauma.

Scout views must be carefully studied for fractures, which may be missed on axial imaging if they run parallel with the scan plane. For severe brain injury where the patient is intubated, the entire cervical spine should be included in the scan.

It is mandatory that the first series are without the use of intravenous iodinated contrast agents. The majority of acute traumatic intracranial lesions can be adequately assessed without the use of intravenous iodinated contrast agents. Contrast helps to enhance lesions not clearly discernible on conventional computed tomography such as arteriovenous fistulae, occlusion of major cerebral arteries (see Sect. 1.4.4), and highly vascular membranes around chronic subdural hematomas.

1.4.2.1 CT-Classification of TBI

According to the proposals of Marshall and colleagues, CT are classified on a system relaying on radiographic markers of cerebral swelling (focal or global) or mass lesions to gauge severity of injury [243] (Table 1.13).

Computed tomography allows not only diagnosis of the primary lesion but also identification of additional

Table 1.13 CT-Classification of TBI [243]

Diffuse Injury I:	Includes all diffuse head injuries where there is no visible pathology;
Diffuse Injury II:	Includes all diffuse injuries in which the cisterns are present, the midline shift is less than 5 mm, and/or there is no high- or mixed-density lesion of more than 25 cc; may include bone fragments and foreign bodies
Diffuse Injury III:	Includes diffuse injuries with swelling where the cisterns are compressed or absent and the midline shift is 0–5 mm with no high- or mixed-density lesion of more than 25 cc
Diffuse Injury IV:	Includes diffuse injuries with a midline shift of more than 5 mm and with no high- or mixed-density lesion of more than 25 cc
Evacuated mass lesions:	Any lesion surgically evacuated
Nonevacuated mass lesions:	High or mixed density lesions >25 cc, not surgically evacuated

features that affect outcome, such as midline shift (MLS), traumatic subarachnoid hemorrhage, obliteration of the basal cisterns, thickness of the blood clot, and hematoma volume [66].

1.4.2.2 Initial Assessment: Indication for CT Scanning

The necessity to perform CT in severely head-injured patients (GCS 8–3) is beyond discussion. In minor (GCS 15–13) and moderate (GCS 12–9) traumatic brain injury – about 85–90% of victims of TBI - the indication to perform CT-scans is less clear. Algorithms with a high sensitivity for detecting injuries that require neurosurgical intervention are needed to identify the few patients at risk within the large number of patients suffering from mild and moderate TBI.

Smits and colleagues [366] compared six European guidelines. The results showed

a. That only those guidelines proposed by the European Federation of Neurological Societies (EFNS) have 100% sensitivity for the identification of neurocranial complications after a minor head injury.
b. A sensitivity of 100% in the identification of neurocranial complications after minor head injury can be reached only by scanning virtually all patients with a minor head injury.
c. The criteria for the use of CT in patients with a minor head injury as set forth by the United Kingdom National Institute for Clinical Excellence (NICE) have the highest potential to reduce the number of CT scans performed while still having reasonable sensitivity for the identification of patients with neurocranial complications or who require neurosurgical intervention after minor head injury (Tables 1.14 and 1.15).

Having tested the clinical performance of NICE [401] variables in adult patients, Fabbri and colleagues stated that the variables selected by NICE recommendations, when applied to a typical broad sample of emergency medicine, are a reliable, clinically sensible tool in predicting significant outcomes in patients with mild head injury and are resource saving [104]. As therapeutically consequential – defined as either a directed intervention or a poor Glasgow Outcome Scale score – these CT abnormalities are to be judged [22] (Table 1.16):

Table 1.14 Head injury: criteria for immediate request for CT scan of the head (NICE) [400]

For adults:

Criteria for immediate request for CT scan of the head (adults)

- GCS less than 13 on initial assessment in the emergency department.
- GCS less than 15 at 2 h after the injury on assessment in the emergency department.
- Suspected open or depressed skull fracture.
- Any sign of basal skull fracture (hemotympanum, "panda" eyes, cerebrospinal fluid leakage from the ear or nose, Battle's sign).
- Posttraumatic seizure.
- Focal neurological deficit.
- More than one episode of vomiting.
- Amnesia for events more than 30 min before impact.

Criteria for immediate request for CT scan of the head provided patient has experienced some loss of consciousness or amnesia since the injury (adults)

- Age 65 years or older.
- Coagulopathy (history of bleeding, clotting disorder, current treatment with warfarin).
- Dangerous mechanism of injury (a pedestrian or cyclist struck by a motor vehicle, an occupant ejected from a motor vehicle, or a fall from a height of greater than 1 m or five stairs).

For children:

Criteria for immediate request for CT scan of the head (children)

- Loss of consciousness lasting more than 5 min (witnessed).
- Amnesia (antegrade or retrograde) lasting more than 5 min.
- Abnormal drowsiness.
- Three or more discrete episodes of vomiting.
- Clinical suspicion of nonaccidental injury.
- Posttraumatic seizure but no history of epilepsy.
- GCS less than 14, or for a baby under 1 year GCS (pediatric) less than 15, on assessment in the emergency department.
- Suspicion of open or depressed skull injury or tense fontanelle.

- Any sign of basal skull fracture (hemotympanum, "panda" eyes, cerebrospinal fluid leakage from the ear or nose, Battle's sign).
- Focal neurological deficit.
- If under 1 year, presence of bruise, swelling, or laceration of more than 5 cm on the head.
- Dangerous mechanism of injury (high-speed road traffic accident either as pedestrian, cyclist, or vehicle occupant, fall from a height of greater than 3 m, high-speed injury from a projectile or an object).

Table 1.15 Urgency in performing CT imaging of the head (NICE) [400]

Criteria for CT scan to be performed within 1 h of receipt of request by radiology department

- GCS less than 13 on initial assessment in the emergency department.
- GCS less than 15 at 2 h after the injury.
- Suspected open or depressed skull fracture.
- Any sign of basal skull fracture (hemotympanum, "panda" eyes, cerebrospinal fluid leakage from the ear or nose, Battle's sign).
- More than one episode of vomiting in adults; three or more episodes of vomiting in children.
- Posttraumatic seizure.
- Coagulopathy (history of bleeding, clotting disorder, current treatment with warfarin) providing that some loss of consciousness or amnesia has been experienced; patients receiving antiplatelet therapy may be at increased risk of intracranial bleeding, though this is currently unquantified – clinical judgment should be used to assess the need for an urgent scan in these patients.
- Focal neurological deficit

Criteria for CT scan to be performed within 8 h of injury

- Amnesia for events more than 30 min before impact (the assessment of amnesia will not be possible in preverbal children and is unlikely to be possible in any child aged under 5 years).
- Age 65 years or older providing that some loss of consciousness or amnesia has been experienced.
- Dangerous mechanism of injury (a pedestrian struck by a motor vehicle, an occupant ejected from a motor vehicle or a fall from a height of greater than 1 m or five stairs) providing that some loss of consciousness or amnesia has been experienced.

Table 1.16 CT abnormalities considered to be important from a neurosurgical therapeutic standpoint [22]

- Mass effect (sulcal effacement)
- Basal cistern compression or midline shift
- Substantial epidural hematoma or subdural hematoma (>1 cm in width, or causing mass effect)
- Pneumocephalus
- Bilateral hemorrhage of any type
- Extensive subarachnoid hemorrhage
- Substantial cerebral contusion (>1 cm in diameter, or >1 site of contusion)
- Signs of herniation
- Hemorrhage in the posterior fossa
- Depressed or diastatic skull fracture
- Diffuse cerebral edema
- Diffuse axonal injury

1.4.2.3 Repeated CT Scanning

Knowing that controversy exists as to the role of a routine repeat head computed tomography (CT) for patients with traumatic brain injury and an initially abnormal head CT, the following recommendation can be given. Patients with any head injury (mild, moderate, or severe) should undergo a repeat head CT after neurologic deterioration, because it leads to intervention in over one third of patients. Routine repeat head CT is indicated for patients with a GCS score ≥ 8, as results might lead to intervention without neurologic change [44].

In patients with an MHI (defined as the loss of consciousness or posttraumatic amnesia with a Glasgow Coma Scale (GCS) score of greater than or equal to 13) and a normal neurologic examination, repeat cranial CT appears unlikely to result in a change in management or neurosurgical intervention and should not be indicated therefore [361].

1.4.3 Magnetic Resonance Tomography

1.4.3.1 Structural Imaging

Magnetic Resonance Tomography (MRI) is the method of choice for evaluating the full extent of brain injury. MR imaging is more sensitive than CT in the detection of small SDHs and tentorial and interhemispheric SDHs and detects a number of intracranial injuries that are difficult to detect on CT: Diffuse axonal injury, brainstem injury, and deep gray matter injury. Detection of these injuries can be helpful in determining causes of previously unexplained neurological deficits [129]. Because of the technical difficulties of transporting critically ill patients and problems with equipment compatibility (ferromagnetic implants), MRI is not routinely used in the acute phase of TBI [85]. MR imaging generally serves as a problem-solving tool for questions that cannot be answered by CT, for example to evaluate an unexplained neurologic deficit – and later on to assess the degree of brain injury.

In patients with mild traumatic brain injury (MTBI), routine MRI techniques unveil nonspecific abnormalities, which show a trend towards correlation with poor performance in attention and executive function. However, with conventional sequences, abnormal MRI does not predict a poor long-term outcome and is therefore not routinely indicated in the clinical management of patients with mild TBI [165].

In contrast, Diffusion-weighted imaging (DWI) is able to demonstrate lesions that are not visualized with conventional MR sequences [166] and the signal intensity on DWI correlates with modified Rankin (outcome) score (see Sect. 1.3.3), but a poor correlation with initial Glasgow Coma Score (GCS) [341]. Diffusion tensor MR imaging (DTI) can provide in vivo information on integrity of white matter structures and connectivity (fiber tracking) and correlates with prognosis too [117, 373].

Magnetic resonance angiography (MRA) may be used in some patients with TBI to assess for arterial injury or venous sinus occlusion [314].

1.4.3.2 Functional Imaging

Besides structural imaging, MR can provide data concerning physiological derangements: MRI and MR spectroscopy (MRS) are able to provide detailed hemodynamic and metabolic information over multiple regions of interest. These imaging modalities are helpful in defining the extent of injury, evidence of cerebral ischemia, and predicting outcome [76]. However, they cannot be used to track the course of brain injury over time or guide neuroprotective treatment strategies in real time (snapshot images, prolonged scanning time, transportation).

1.4.3.3 Clearance of the Cervical Spine in Blunt Trauma

MRI may be necessary for completing evaluation of the cervical spine, as plain radiographs and cervical CT scan failed to detect significant ligamentous injuries [309]. A magnetic resonance image that did not disclose anything abnormal can conclusively exclude cervical spine injury and is established as a gold standard for clearing the cervical spine in a clinically suspicious or not evaluatable blunt trauma patient. An accurate number of false-positive MRI scans cannot be determined [271]. However, clearing of the cervical spine using MRI should only be performed if a high index of suspicion exists for a ligamentous injury, which was not conclusively diagnosed using a spine CT scan.

1.4.4 Cerebral Angiography

Cerebral angiography has a role in diagnosis and management of traumatic vascular injuries such as pseudoaneurysms and dissection [85, 93], typically occurring with penetrating trauma [182], basal skull fracture (especially fractures of the clivus of the sella turcica–sphenoid sinus region [107, 254]), or trauma to the neck. Furthermore, angiography is indicated if there is a suspicion that the cause of accident may be a rupture of a preexisting vascular malformation (cerebral aneurysm or arteriovenous malformation) or that the accident has caused rupture of a preexisting vascular malformation. To assess vessel pathology, intraarterial and intravenous digital subtraction angiography (iaDSA, ivDSA), computed tomography angiography (CTA), and magnetic resonance angiography (MRA) are available. Intraarterial digital subtraction angiography is the gold standard for assessing cerebral vessels selectively.

1.4.4.1 Intra-Arterial Digital Subtraction-Angiography (iaDSA)

The best imaging modality for screening is DSA, although noninvasive modalities such as CT angiography and MR angiography are reasonable options. Contrary to CTA, MRA, and the ivDSA, intraarterial DSA allows imaging of a single vessel by selective catheterization of the desired vessel. With iaDSA, only

brief seconds of patient cooperation are necessary to image arterial anatomy [375]. Intraarterial DSA should be performed only in a center where interventional neuroradiology is routinely performed.

1.4.4.2 Computed Tomography Angiography

Multislice spiral computed tomography angiography (MSCTA) is an excellent test with which to screen for injury of cerebral vessels [29], especially in patients considered to be too unstable for more time-consuming investigations and frequently allows complete avoidance or deferral of catheter angiography [119]. MSCTA allows one to compute three-dimensional reconstructions of the vessel system. In subtle exploration, superposition of the vessels may be a disadvantage. However, it is a debatable point if CTA technology cannot reliably diagnose or exclude blunt carotid/vertebral artery injury (BCVI). Twenty percent of CTAs are either not evaluable or suboptimal. Until more data are available and the technique is standardized, the current trend towards using CTA to screen for and/or diagnose these rare but potentially devastating injuries is dangerous [234]. Massive maxillofacial hemorrhage may be secondary to facial or skull fracture.

1.4.4.3 Magnetic Resonance Angiography (MRA)

As MRA is well suitable for imaging cerebral vessels, on direct comparison to four vessel iaDSA specificity and sensitivity of MRA has found to be low. Additionally, due to the technical difficulties of transporting critically ill patients and problems with equipment compatibility, MRI is not routinely used in the acute phase of TBI [85, 266, 314].

1.4.4.4 Recommendation

Angiography is recommended in perforating brain injuries (an orbitofacial or pterional injury) where a vascular injury – a traumatic intracranial aneurysm (TICA) or arteriovenous fistula – is suspected. Patients with an increased risk of vascular injury include cases in which the wound's trajectory passes through or near the Sylvian fissure, supraclinoid carotid, cavernous sinus, or a major venous sinus, particularly in patients harboring an intracerebral hematoma. The development of substantial and otherwise unexplained subarachnoid hemorrhage or delayed hematoma should also prompt consideration of a vascular injury and of angiography [284].

1.4.5 Electroencephalography

Electroencephalography (EEG) measure the electrical activity of the brain. The test is noninvasive and simply involves the placement of recording electrodes on a person's scalp (see Chap. 2).

EEGs are not always obtained after TBI. They are most useful when there is a concern that a patient might have had or is at risk of having seizures. EEGs have very little ability to predict outcome after a TBI.

Seizures occur in about 20% of patients with TBI during ICU treatment as shown by continuous electroencephalography (cEEG) studies on the NICU. Many of these seizures are of the nonconvulsive variety and cannot be detected clinically, and some occur despite the use of prophylactic phenytoin at adequate serum concentrations. Continuous EEG generates large quantities of data and systems must be developed, which are able to reduce the data volume and flag up potential abnormalities. One methodology, which has shown potential, is the use of alpha variability in cEEG recordings to predict outcome after TBI [404].

1.4.5.1 Evoked Potentials (EP)

While EEGs measure the brain's natural or spontaneous electrical activity, evoked potentials measure the brain's electrical activity in response to stimulation. This stimulation can be visual (visual evoked potentials), sounds (auditory evoked potentials), or electrical stimuli to the skin (somatosensory evoked potentials).

This test is most useful in patients who are still unconscious; there is evidence that in these situations, the test can provide some information about future outcome [144].

1.4.5.2 Electrophysiologic Examination

In the initial assessment of patients suffering from moderate or severe TBI, electrophysiologic examination have no weight.

However, both electroencephalography and evoked potentials (somatosensory evoked potentials (SEP) and brain auditory evoked potential (BAEP) are of importance in the phase of the intensive care environment [269, 390, 404] (see Chap. 2).

1.4.6 Lumbar Puncture

Although generally considered innocuous, there may be considerable danger when lumbar puncture [88] is performed in the presence of increased intracranial pressure, especially when a mass lesion is present (characteristic findings on the brain CT scan): Midline shift, loss of suprachiasmatic and basilar cisterns, posterior fossa mass, loss of the superior cerebellar cistern, loss of the quadrigeminal plate cistern [183].

Therefore, in acute traumatic brain injury, lumbar puncture is contraindicated for lack o diagnostic significance and because of the danger of transtentorial herniation in the presence of a mass lesion. Herniation is a complication of lumbar puncture that occurs in the presence of an intracranial mass lesion or increased intracranial pressure. Signs of uncal or tonsillar herniation typically develop within 2 h of a lumbar puncture when this complication occurs.

Lumbar puncture should not be performed

- If the IVth ventricle and the quadrigeminal cistern are not visualized by neuroimaging [331].
- In a patient with posterior fossa signs without obtaining a cranial MR scan first to be certain there is no mass lesion [331].
- In acute trauma to the spinal column

- In cutaneous infections in the region of the puncture site

Lumbar puncture is contraindicated in patients with/on

- Increased intracranial pressure due to space occupying lesions
- Drug-induced coagulopathy therapy and those with platelet counts of less than 50,000 until anticoagulation is reversed and platelet counts corrected to avoid the complication of an epidural or subdural hematoma [331].
- Signs of lumbar epidural abscess or subdural empyema because of the risk of introducing infection into the subarachnoid space [331].

- In the presence of spinal subarachnoid block because the withdrawal of fluid can worsen the neurological deficit [331].

Later on LP is mandatory – CT scan has to confirm that no compression of basal cistern exists

- When conceiving suspicion of CSF infection
- When a lumbar drainage has to substitute a ventricular catheter to a lumbar drainage.

1.4.7 Intracranial Pressure Monitoring

Monitoring of intracranial pressure (ICP) is accepted as an important means to recognize impending complications (worsening of intracranial pathology and surgical mass lesions), especially in patients not assessable neurologically but also as the only mean by which therapy can be selectively monitored (see Chap. 2). Furthermore, ICP data are found to be useful in predicting outcome [238].

Based on the Monro--Kellie hypothesis stating that the cranial compartment is incompressible (a near rigid container) and the intracranial volume is fixed, the ICP is basically the consequence of the actual volume of the cerebrospinal fluid (CSF) and the actual volume of the intracranial blood [V i/c = V (brain) + V (cerebrospinal fluid) + V (blood)] [400].

In patients suffering from TBI, cerebral edema and/or mass lesions (additional volume) cause an exponential rise in ICP, resulting in brain tissue compression, shift of brain structures, and reduction of the cerebral perfusion pressure (CPP: $MABD_{CCA}$ – ICP) [204].

1.4.7.1 Indication for Intracranial Pressure Monitoring

Recommendation [41]: Intracranial pressure should be monitored in all salvageable patients with a severe traumatic brain injury (GCS 3–8 after resuscitation)) and an abnormal computed tomography scan (CT revealing hematomas, contusions, herniation, or compressed basal cisterns (level II, "recommendation")).

Option [41]: ICP monitoring is indicated in patients with severe TBI with a normal CT scan if two or more of the following features are noted at admission: age over 40 years, unilateral or bilateral motor posturing, or systolic blood pressure <90 mmHg.

Even if the benefit of ICP monitoring seems obvious, doubt is harbored about this recommendation [9]. It is hypothesized that BTF criteria for ICP monitoring in blunt TBI do not identify patients who are likely to benefit from it [358].

1.4.7.2 Method

A pressure transduction device for ICP monitoring can be placed in the epidural, subdural, subarachnoid, parenchymal, or ventricular location (see Sect. 1.7.1.3), available are different types of pressure transduction systems (fluid coupled, strain gauge and fiber-optic, and pneumatic catheter tip pressure transducer devices).

Ventricular pressure measurement is considered as the reference standard for ICP monitoring. ICP measurement by parenchymal mirco strain gauge pressure transduction is estimated as equivalent to the ventricular ICP. Fluid coupled epidural devices or subarachnoid bolts and pneumatic epidural devices are less accurate than ventricular ICP monitors. Ventriculostomies not only allow for monitoring of ICP but also for drainage of CSF, which is effective in decreasing the ICP [132].

1.4.7.3 Complications

The potential risk of catheter misplacement, infection, hemorrhage [31, 120], and obstruction can be lowered/avoided by choosing alternative sites for ICP monitoring. Nevertheless, each type of pressure transduction system and intracranial location of the monitor has a profile of potential complications – hemorrhage, infection, and malfunction (see Chap. 2).

1.5 Minor Traumatic Brain Injury

Minor (Synonym: mild) traumatic brain injury (MTBI) is defined as the consequence of blunt (nonpenetrating) impact with sudden acceleration, deceleration, or rotation of the head with a GCS score of 13–15 [321] on admission to hospital. The primary goal of initial management of the considerable number (up to 90%), of patients suffering from MTBI (390) is to identify the few patients at risk for intracranial abnormalities and especially those who may need neurosurgical intervention (Table 1.17).

Table 1.17 Management of patients suffering from MTBI (13–15) (EFNS) [419]

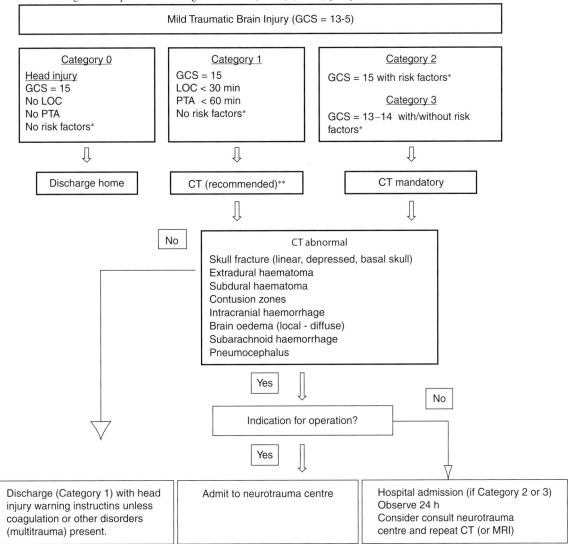

This guideline on mild traumatic brain injury [420] – analogical recommendations are (were) given by the "World Federation of Neurosurgical Societies" [356] (Table 1.18) and by the "Scandinavian Guidelines for Initial Management of Minimal, Mild, and Moderate Head Injuries" [170] – postulate: "Skull radiography is of insufficient value in the detection of intracranial abnormalities in patients with MTBI" (Grade A, recommendation), and stated "CT is the gold standard for the detection of intracranial abnormalities and is a safe method for home triage."

Fabbri and colleagues [103], validating the WFNS proposal for diagnosis and management of patients attending the emergency department for mild head injury concluded: CT scan is the gold standard for early detection serious complications in MTBI. Only low-risk mild injury patients – those with a Glasgow Coma Score (GCS) of 15 and without a history of loss of consciousness, amnesia, vomiting, or diffuse headache – do not need a CT. In these patients, the risk of intracranial hematoma requiring surgical evacuation is definitely less than 0.1:100. Geijerstam and Britton [7] searched the literature for case reports on adverse outcomes in patients with mild head injury where acute computed tomography (CT) findings had been normal. They found very few cases where an early adverse event occurred after normal acute CT in patients with mild head injury and stated: "The strongest scientific evidence available at this time shows that a CT strategy is a safe way to triage patients for admission." Patients

Table 1.18 Criteria proposed by the NCWFS for classification, diagnosis, and treatment of patients suffering from MTBI (13–15) [356]

	Low risk	Medium risk	High risk
GCS	15	15 with clinical findings	14 or 15 with neurodeficits or skull fracture or risk factors with/without clinical findings
Clinical findings	No	1. Amnesia	1. Amnesia
		2. Diffuse Headache	2. Diffuse headache
		3. Vomiting	3. Vomiting
		4. Loss of consciousness	4. Loss of consciousness
Neurodeficits	No	No	Yes
Skull fracture	No	No	Yes
Risk factors	No	No	1. Coagulopathy
			2. Age > 60 years
			3. Previous neurosurgery
			4. Pretrauma epilepsy
			5. Alcohol and/or drug misuse
Imaging	No	Ct scan or SR	CT scan
Disposition	Home	In hospital (3–6 h after CT or 24 h after SR), followed by home observation	In hospital (24–48 h), followed by home observation

CT, computer tomography; *GCS*, Glasgow coma scale; *NCWFS*, Neurotraumatology Committee of the World Federation of Neurosurgical Societies; *SR*, skull radiography

with a cranial CT scan, obtained on a helical CT scanner, that shows no intracerebral injury and who do not have other body system injuries or a persistence of any neurologic finding can be safely discharged from the emergency department without a period of either inpatient or outpatient observation [223].

1.6 Moderate and Severe Traumatic Brain Injury

Management of traumatic brain injury aims to prevent secondary injuries and to damp their impact to the brain, respectively. Also, the tolerance of the brain against second injuries should be ameliorated with MTBI-patients, which implies to realize the rather low probability of an intracranial mass lesion in time (see Sect. 1.5).

With patient suffering from moderate or severe TBI damage control implies [23, 188]

- Ensuring of an adequate perfusion of the brain
- Arresting of intracranial bleeding, evacuation of intracranial hematomas, limiting of contamination

of compound wounds, and controlling ICP, respectively [334]

- Controlling neurologic injury, acute respiratory failure, organ failure, anemia, coagulopathy, thermal dysregulation, sepsis, unnecessary fluid administration, damage control sequelae, and acid--base imbalance and more medical complications [308]. Elaboration on medical and neurosurgical management are set forth in Chap. 2 and in Sect. 1.7, respectively.

1.7 Traumatic Brain Injury: Neurosurgical Management

The essence of damage control in neurotraumatology implies arresting of intracranial bleeding, evacuation of intracranial hematomas, limiting of contamination of compound wounds, and controlling ICP, respectively.

Prompt evacuation of intracranial hematomas is a cornerstone of damage control. Emergency craniotomy should be commenced preferably within 30 min of arrival of the patient in the trauma center and definitely before 60 min after arrival [334].

In closed head injuries, there is a high incidence of temporal and frontal contusions and tearing of midline bridging veins in severe brain injury associated with mass lesions requiring operation. The basic craniotomy trauma flap therefore should be generous enough and placed so as to permit one to deal quickly with the most frequently found disorder without further operative extension for additional exposure. In order to accomplish this, the exposure should provide adequate access

- To decompress the epidural and subdural space;
- To debride contused cerebral tissue (anterior temporal and frontal lobes and orbital gyri) and
- To remove associated intracerebral hematomas as necessary;
- To control hemorrhage from avulsed bridging veins to the sagittal sinus and from temporal lobe to transverse sinus and petrosal sinus;
- To control hemorrhage from the skull base,
- To pack sinuses as necessary,
- To repair potential cerebral spinal fluid fistulae;
- To explore and manage lesions of vascular and neural elements at the base as necessary

In performing corresponding surgical procedures, the use of surgical loupes combined with a head lamp or an operating microscope is mandatory.

Prophylactic antibiotics

The goal of prophylactic antibiotics is to reduce the incidence of postoperative wound infection (surgical site infection, SSI). There is a great deal of evidence showing that antibiotic prophylaxis is statistically significantly better than either placebo or no treatment for clean nonimplant surgery. The chosen antibiotic needs to be effective against *Staphylococcus aureus* as well as other Gram-positive cocci and Gram-negative bacilli. Prophylaxis starts 60 min prior to incision and is repeated for 24 h [292]. In preventing postoperative meningitis, antibiotic prophylaxis is a matter of debate [219].

1.7.1 Standard Procedures

1.7.1.1 Standard or Generic (Standard) Head Trauma Craniotomy

The standard craniotomy flap is recommended for evacuation of acute epidural, subdural, and intracerebral

hematomas and contusions [143]. It significantly improves outcome in severe TBI with refractory intracranial hypertension resulting from unilateral frontotemporoparietal contusion with or without intracerebral or subdural hematoma [181].

Anesthesia

The procedure is performed in general anesthesia. Routine determination of the coagulation status should be performed in all patients with traumatic brain injury [151] – platelets, fibrinogen, and fibrin split products together with prothrombin time (PT) and activated partial thromboplastin time/correction of abnormal clotting factors.

Positioning

The patient is positioned supine. The thorax and head are elevated 10° to improve venous return. The head is rotated in such a way that the (ipsilateral) zygoma is the highest point, then the vertex is tilted towards the floor (in order to bring the skull base into maximal line of view), and the head is positioned either on the donut or in a rigid skull fixation device. The latter is mandatory in patients with an unstable C-spine fracture. Attention has to be directed to maintenance of adequate venous return in patients when the head is rotated.

Preparing

The scalp is shaved completely and prepared antiseptically before the skin incision is outlined in ink (Fig. 1.1). To avoid injuring the frontal branches of the facial nerve and/or the superficial temporal artery, the incision is placed close to the tragus, starting at the superior border of the zygomatic arch. In planning the skin flap, the existing skin lacerations are to be considered.

Draping

An adherent sterile plastic drape is placed over the operation field, and a windowed waterproof sheet laid on the top of this, secured by a second plastic drape.

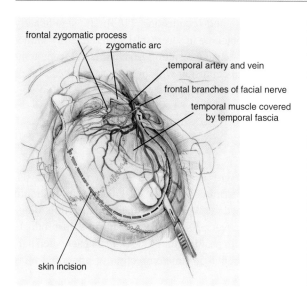

Fig. 1.1 Standard head trauma craniotomy: Dissection of the skin-galea flap

Scalp Incision

The skin incision starts anterior to the tragus at the temporal portion of the zygomatic arch preauricularly and is carried superiorly and posteriorly over the ear.

If the patient has been deteriorating rapidly prior to operation, an *immediate subtemporal decompression* is warranted: The portion of the incision just anterior to and above the ear is opened first, down through the temporalis muscle to bone (Fig. 1.23). A burr-hole is made and a small craniectomy is quickly performed and the dura is opened in a linear cruciate fashion. An extra-axial or temporal lobe clot will express itself partially from the site and thus lead to a reduction of brain shift and intracranial pressure. Afterwards, the formal craniotomy may then be completed with less haste.

Otherwise, the skin incision is carried posteriorly around the parietal bone to the midline, where it is brought anteriorly on the midline down to the forehead (Fig. 1.1). Thereby, the galea has to be cut but not the periosteum and temporal fascia. For scalp hemostasis, mosquito hemostats or hemostatic scalp clips are applied. The galea is separated in a plane through the loose areolar tissue of the scalp from the pericranium and temporalis fascia within 4 cm of the orbital rim, then the skin-galea flap is turned and fixed with fish hooks.

The fat pad over the deep temporal fascia (containing the frontal branch of the facial nerve) is gently pushed down to the zygoma. Thereafter, the

periosteum and the temporal fascia are incised as shown in Figs. 1.2 and 1.3. The periosteum and the temporal muscle are scraped off the bone, the latter moved backwards out of the temporal fossa and fixed.

Standard head trauma craniotomy: Dissection of the pericranium

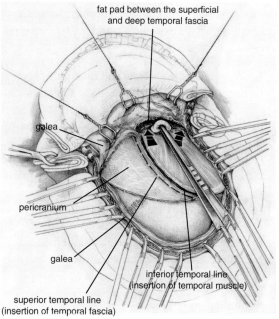

Fig. 1.2 Standard head trauma craniotomy: Dissection of the pericranium

Standard head trauma craniotomy: Dissection of the temporal muscle

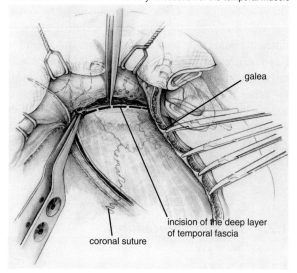

Fig. 1.3 Standard head trauma craniotomy: Dissection of the temporal muscle

Craniotomy

The burr-holes are placed with regard to the existing fracture lines. Thereby, one has to mind to place paramedian burr-holes 2–3 cm lateral to the midline. In each burr-hole, the dura is freed from the overlying inner table with a slim and blunt dissector (a specially designed dural separator), then the bone is turned using a Gigli saw or a craniotome and breaking of the temporal base after the pterion has been grooved with a drill (Fig. 1.4). To gain access to the floor of the anterior and middle cranial fossa, the remainder of the pterion and the squamous temporal bone is removed with a highspeed drill and a rongeur as is the lateral portion of the lesser wing of the sphenoid bone. Thereby, the meningo-orbital artery (an anastomotic branch of the ophthalmic artery to the frontal branch of middle meningeal artery) is coagulated and cut through (Figs. 1.5 and 1.6). It is important to reach the floor of both the middle and anterior fossa to lessen strangulation of the swollen temporal and posterior frontal lobe when herniating out of the operative site postoperatively. Additionally, a temporal decompression remains even in cases where the bone flap is replaced. If the skull base is fractured, attention has to be given not to remove basal bone fragments and thereby tearing vessels and nerves.

Standard head trauma craniotomy: Removal of the pterional bone flap

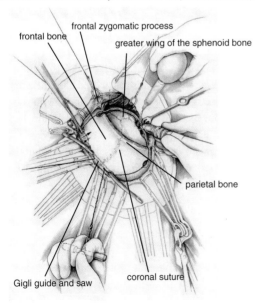

Fig. 1.4 Standard head trauma craniotomy: Removal of the pterional bone flap

Standard head trauma craniotomy:Enlargement of the bony entrance

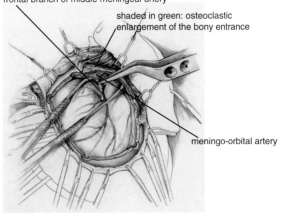

Fig. 1.5 Standard head trauma craniotomy: Enlargement of the bony entrance

Standard head trauma craniotomy: Removal of the lesser wing of the spenoid bone.

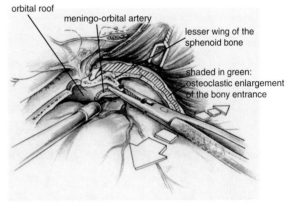

Fig. 1.6 Standard head trauma craniotomy: Removal of the lesser wing of the sphenoid bone

Dural Opening

The dura is opened in a semicircular fashion around the Sylvian fissure. The veins bridging from the Sylvian veins to dural veins have to be preserved. The opening of the dura may be completed by adding one or two additional incisions directed postero-medially (Fig. 1.7). Dural bleeding is controlled by bipolar coagulation. Surgery should be used sparingly in a patient who has just undergone surgical mass decompression to relieve or prevent increased intracranial pressure.

Fig. 1.7 Standard head
trauma craniotomy: Dural
opening

Standard head trauma craniotomy: Dural opening

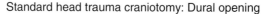
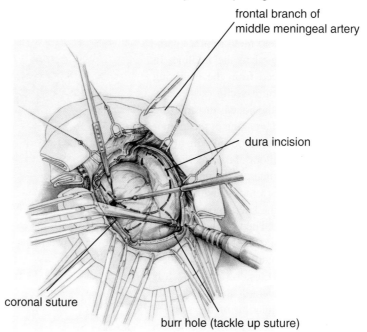

frontal branch of
middle meningeal artery

dura incision

coronal suture

burr hole (tackle up suture)

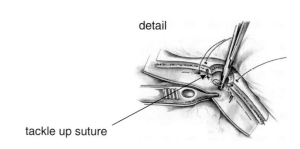

detail

tackle up suture

Dural Closure

ICP-monitor: Before closing the dura, a ventricular catheter (connected to an extradural strain gauge or with a fiber-optic or micro strain gauge device) is installed contralaterally to the bone flap (see Sect. 1.4.7). If this is difficult (because of the shift or a very narrow compressed anterior horn), a fiber-optic device is placed intraparenchymally.

The dura is reapproximated then with a continuous (4–0 monofilament slowly resorbable) suture. A dural closure keeps postoperative extradural bleeding out of the subarachnoid space, reduces the chance of CSF leaks, isolates possible wound infections, reduces herniation of brain tissue from the craniotomy site, and prevents cortical adhesions to soft tissues – the latter is especially important, if the bone flap is not put back to allow better decompression of the swollen brain. To achieve a complete closure of the dura and to allow

expansion of the swelling brain, a pericranium patch graft or a synthetic dura patch graft may be required.

Small diameter holes are drilled along the margin of the bone edge using a power drill and the dura is tacked to the bone edges. Tacking sutures should be placed only through the outer layer of the dura (Fig. 1.7). One or two central tack-up sutures are placed, and the knots will be tied after the bone flap has eventually been put back (Fig. 1.8).

Bone Flap/Skin Closure

Whenever possible, the bone flap is replaced and is fixed in place with suture material using the same holes that are used for the tenting suture. However, if the surface of the brain passes the level of the inner table, the bone flap should not be replaced. The removed bone flap can be frozen [168] or placed in the abdominal or

Standard head trauma craniotomy: Closure of the dura and putting back of the bone flap

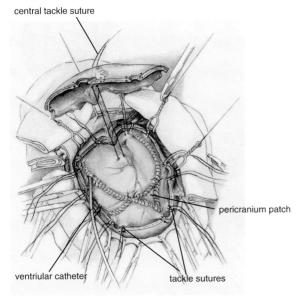

central tackle suture

pericranium patch

ventriular catheter   tackle sutures

Fig. 1.8 Standard head trauma craniotomy: Closure of the dura and putting back of the bone flap

thigh subcutaneous tissues [364]. The need for subsequent surgical bone replacement and the syndrome of the trephined [111] can be prevented by applying the hinge technique during the initial procedure [134].

The temporal muscle is fixed with several sutures to the periosteum. A subgaleal drain is used and the scalp is closed in a two-layer fashion.

CT within 24 h following the craniotomy is mandatory. The preoperatively started antibiotic prophylaxis may be continued postoperatively until removal of intraventricular drains. The subgaleal drain is removed after 24–48 h, the skin sutures after 5–6 days. If the bone flap because of swelling of the brain was not put back, as a rule replantation takes place after 3–6 months.

1.7.1.2 Burr-Hole Exploration

Availability of modern CT technique has limited the need for diagnostic trephination largely. However, exploratory burr-holes are to be considered in patients who have had a precipitous downhill course with mydriasis, in patients in whom the course of the head injury is such that a hematoma is common (falls or assaults), and to exclude a contralateral mass lesion in

patients developing sudden massive brain swelling intraoperatively. In deteriorating patients, trephination should be done on the side of the enlarged pupil, if there is no mydriasis the first burr-hole is placed on the side of the skull fracture [15].

With the patient in supine position, the head – shaved totally – is placed on a donut headrest or on a horseshoe headrest and properly draped, thereby allowing changing of the position of the head during the procedure to get access to the contralateral side.

The burr-holes are placed according to the neurologic symptoms (i.e., pupil reactivity/diameter, lateralized extremity weakness, see Sect. 1.3). The skin is incised on an imaginative incision required for a standard craniotomy: the frontal burr-holes 3 cm from the midline and 5 cm above the eyebrow, temporal 1 cm in front of the ear and 1 cm over the zygomatic arch, posteroparietal 3 cm from the midline and behind the level of the ear (Fig. 1.9). If no epidural clot was located, the dura is opened to explore for subdural clots.

If either an epi- or a subdural hematoma is diagnosed, the corresponding burr-hole is enlarged and as much of the hematoma as possible is aspirated providing temporary decompression before the procedure goes on as described in Sect. 1.7.1.1.

If the exploration was negative, burr-holes are placed on the contralateral side. Finally, if the exploration over both hemispheres is negative (and CT scan is not available), the patient is placed in prone position and two additional burr-holes are placed in the occipital bone over the cerebellar hemispheres. Whether or not a mass lesion has been evacuated, CT scanning has to follow the procedure as soon as possible [90].

Anesthesia: Local anesthesia may be used, general endotracheal anesthesia is preferred.

1.7.1.3 Ventriculostomy

Good clinical practice recommends that ventriculostomies [143, 299] and other intracranial pressure (ICP) monitors should be placed under sterile conditions to closed drainage systems, minimizing manipulation and flushing. There is no support for routine catheter exchanges as a means of preventing cerebrospinal fluid (CSF) infections (42). No consensus exists regarding the use of Antibiotic prophylaxis with ICP monitors and external ventricular drainage [313]. For patients with ventriculostomy, duration of catheter insertion strongly predicts infection [110].

Fig. 1.9 Position of the exploratory burr-holes

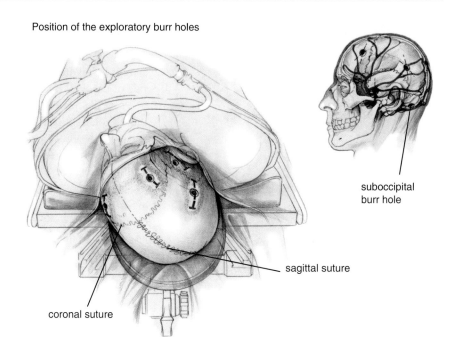

Position of the exploratory burr holes

suboccipital
burr hole

sagittal suture

coronal suture

Frontal Ventriculostomy

With the patient in supine position, the head – placed on a doughnut headrest and shaved locally – a burr-hole is placed 1 cm anterior to the coronal suture on the right side and in the ipsilateral mid-pupillary plane, left-sided only when either a scalp laceration, depressed fracture, or suspected mass lesion is present on the right. The dura is coagulated and incised crosswise, then the underlying cortex is coagulated avoiding cortical vessels and then punctured. Alternatively, a twist drill hole can be made, the dura and the underlying cortex then punctured blindly.

The flexible ventriculostomy catheter stabilized by the intrinsic mandrin is directed in a plane to the medial canthus of the ipsilateral eye and approximately 2 cm anterior to the external auditory meatus (Fig. 1.10). In the depth of 5–6.5 cm, the resistance of the ventricular wall is felt, CSF escapes when the frontal horn of the lateral ventricle is entered. A manometric reading of CSF pressure is made, then the ventricular catheter is connected with a strain gauge. In situations in which a small, tight CSF compartment exists, only a minimal amount of CSF drainage may be noted.

If the catheter reveals no CSF, additional passes toward the nasion, then toward the contralateral medial canthus, are made. The catheter is tunneled through

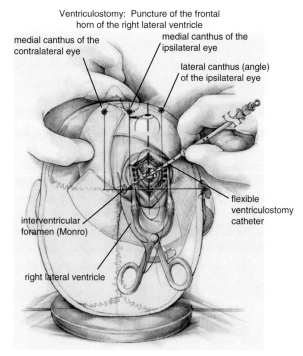

Ventriculostomy: Puncture of the frontal
horn of the right lateral ventricle

medial canthus of the
contralateral eye

medial canthus of the
ipsilateral eye

lateral canthus (angle)
of the ipsilateral eye

flexible
ventriculostomy
catheter

interventricular
foramen (Monro)

right lateral ventricle

Fig. 1.10 Ventriculostomy: Puncture of the frontal horn of the right lateral ventricle

the scalp to a second incision and secured to the skin with a suture. The skin incisions are closed in layers.

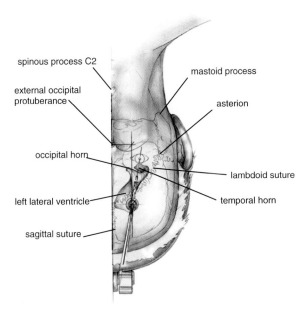

spinous process C2

mastoid process

external occipital
protuberance

asterion

occipital horn

lambdoid suture

left lateral ventricle

temporal horn

sagittal suture

Fig. 1.11 Ventriculostomy: Puncture of the occipital horn of the left lateral ventricle

Parieto-Occipital Ventriculostomy

A twist drill hole or a burr-hole is placed 9 cm rostral to the inion and 3 cm lateral to the midline (Fig. 1.11). The subsequent procedure is the same as with frontal ventriculostomy whereby the catheter is passed anteriorly toward the mid pupillary line. The ventricle should be encountered within 4–5 cm of the outer table of the skull.

Anesthesia: Local anesthesia may be used.

1.7.1.4 Intra/Postoperative Problems/Complications

Intraoperative Brain Swelling (IOS)

Hemispheric brain swelling after traumatic brain injury occurs in almost all patients with severe head injury. Patients with bilateral brain swelling (diffuse Injury III [243]) were found to have a high risk of increased ICP (63.2%). Acute SDH hematoma is the lesion most frequently associated with massive cerebral swelling. Intraoperative brain swelling is far more common in patients with the lowest GCS scores and those with one or more fixed, dilated pupils, suggesting a relationship to prior hypoperfusion.

The causes of massive IOS may be cytotoxic edema or vascular engorgement (as for instance in venous sinus obstruction) [13, 227] and a consequence of anesthesiologic problems (disconnection of the endotracheal tube, obstruction of venous outflow), respectively. An evolving mass lesion may simulate IOS.

Consequence: Herniation (through the craniotomy opening, tentorial (lateral or central), underneath the falx or into the foramen magnum (tonsillar), respectively).

Therapy: The patient is hyperventilated to achieve a $PaCO_2$ of 25–30 mmHg (3.3–4 kPa). Mannitol 1–2 g/kg or Lasix 20–40 mg may be given intravenously. If these efforts do not reduce the swelling, 500–1,000 mg of pentobarbital is given by slow IV infusion.

Search for an etiology: anesthesiologic problem? mass lesion (such as a contralateral epidural hematoma)? When no mass lesion is diagnosed: wide craniectomy without replacement of the bone flap (see Sect. 1.7.1.1).

Intraoperative Bleeding

a. With penetrating head injuries causing vessel damage and with depressed skull fractures over a lacerated sinus, severe intraoperative bleeding is to be expected. Uncontrollable intraoperative hemorrhage may be encountered during evacuation of an acute subdural hematoma, when the tamponade effect on the venous bleeding source is relieved. Coagulopathy occurs frequently in TBI and is more pronounced in patients with severe injuries. Routine determination of the coagulation status should therefore be performed in all patients with traumatic brain injury [151].

Consequence: Arterial hypotension

Therapy: Arterial hypotension is corrected by volume replacement using crystalloids and colloids as well as vasopressors (e.g., norepinephrine and dobutamine). It is of utmost importance to search for the source of hemorrhage and to adequately correct any underlying coagulation disorder by substituting red blood cells, fresh frozen plasma, and isolated coagulation factors as e.g., fibrinogen or factor XIII and possibly recombinant factor VII, where indicated.

b. Bleedings in previously unsuspected sites (as contralaterally), starting from fracture lines, torn meningeal vessels, and small cortical or parenchymal contusions may arrive when the tamponading effect of the initial mass lesion is relieved.

Consequence: Growing intracranial (ipsi- or contralateral) additional mass lesion causing herniation.
Therapy: Localizing (with the help of ultrasound imaging and/or exploratory burr-holes) [17] and eventually evacuation of the suspected mass lesion.

Air Embolism [27, 227]

Intraoperative venous air embolism (fall in end-tail pCO_2) machinery sound in the precordial Doppler can occur in any position where there is an open vein and a gradient in venous pressure between the operative site and the heart [172]. Venous sinuses exposed to air during craniotomy are noncollapsible making this type of surgery higher risk. However, VAE during neurosurgery is not exclusive to the sitting position and has frequently been reported in the prone and supine positions. VAE has been reported in 10–17% of craniotomies performed in the prone position [116].

Pulmonary dysfunction after severe head injury may be caused by air embolism [192].

Therapy Anesthetist: Change to a Trendelenburg position (patients head lowered), bilateral jugular vein compression, aspiration of air from the right atrium using a 20-mL syringe, oxygenation with FiO_2 0.1, administration of vasopressors and volume expanders.

Surgeon: flooding the surgical field with normal saline and putting a saline soaked gauze held over the craniotomy site, finally identify the site of injured vessel (incised dural veins and veins in calvarial bone), and stop venous bleeding/oozing.

1.7.1.5 Postoperative Problems/Complications

Early, if not immediate, postop CT after emergency craniotomy for head trauma appears to be warranted. Paci [301] and colleagues report a significant incidence of unexpected findings on postop CT and encountered avoidable delays in treatment of new or recurrent findings: 7.0% patients required a second craniotomy in the 2 days after their initial operation; in 3.0% of patients, postop CTs were obtained between 4.2 h and 21.1 h after initial craniotomy, and an earlier postop

CT would most likely have prevented a significant delay in operation. Findings in these patients included recurrent SDH or EDH, new SDH or EDH in, and intraparenchymal hemorrhage. Neither neurologic examination nor postop intracranial pressure monitoring reliably predicted the presence of new or recurrent hemorrhage or other significant findings [301].

Postoperative Reaccumulation of Intracranial Hematomas

Second hematomas at the operation site requiring a second procedure are predominantly extradural. Postcraniotomy hematoma is frequent with coagulopathy and has a higher incidence in patients with evidence of alcohol intake and preoperative mannitol administration. In patients not amenable to neurologic assessment, monitoring of ICP may allow early detection of recurrent clot [47] as can repeated postoperative CT scanning.

Therapy: Depends on actual size of the hematoma and its space-occupying effect: Conservative therapy or recraniotomy and evacuation (see Sect. 1.7).

Delayed Traumatic Intracranial Hematomas (DITCH) and Evolving Contusions

Delayed intracranial hematomas: Delayed intracranial hematomas can develop at sites other than the initial evacuated hematoma, even contralaterally, when the tamponading effect of the mass has diminished.

Traumatic intracerebral hemorrhage refers to the appearance of hemorrhage (usually within 48 h of head trauma but even after 8 days) [128] that were normal in appearance or nearly so on the CT scan taken shortly after injury. Neurologic deterioration is common but is not universally the rule. The frequency of delayed traumatic intracerebral hemorrhage is variable but is reported to occur in 1–8% of patients with severe head injury. The pathogenesis is multifactorial and may result from one or more of the following: coagulation abnormalities, necrosis of blood vessels in areas of brain injury, dysautoregulation, and release of tamponade effect with evacuation of extra-axial hematomas. Outcome is poor, and most series report a mortality of 50% or higher [77]. Clotting disorders can provoke occurrence of delayed intracranial hemorrhage. Delayed posttraumatic hematoma or hemorrhagic contusion may form at a different site from the first craniotomy [128].

With penetrating head injuries, delayed traumatic intracerebral hemorrhage may be a consequence of a rupture of a traumatic cerebral aneurysm.

Evolving ("blowing") contusion [355]: Patients with SAH on early CT are those at highest risk for associated evolving contusions. In patient suffering from ASDH, CT scans performed within 3 h from the insult demonstrated associated parenchymal damage in about 25% while CT scans repeated in the following day showed additional parenchymal lesions in 50%. Patients with traumatic subarachnoid hemorrhage (tSAH) on early CT are those at highest risk for associated evolving contusions [355].

ICP monitoring and repeated postoperative CT scanning offers earlier diagnosis.

Therapy: Depends from the actual size of the hematoma and its space-occupying effect: Conservative therapy or recraniotomy and evacuation (see Sect. 1.7).

Postoperative Intracranial Hypertension

Raised intracranial pressure may be a very early event after traumatic brain injury, but in most cases, especially when contusions and edema develop over time, ICP will worsen over succeeding days [380].

Intracranial hypertension is a frequent finding following evacuation of an acute SDH. These hematomas are often associated with multiple small contusions causing swelling and edema. In the category of evacuated mass lesions, two thirds of the patients were found to present with intracranial hypertension, in one third – all patients with midline shift >5 mm but no high – or mixed density lesions >25 cc (diffuse injury IV [243]) – ICP was refractory to treatment [310].

Intracranial hypertension may be a consequence of compromised venous outflow (e.g., because of adverse position of the head/patient, a depressed fractures with a bony fragment compressing a venous sinus) or of systemic problems causing elevated intrathoracic pressure.

Therapy: ICU-treatment (see Chap. 2)and decompressive craniectomy eventually (see Sect. 1.7.1.1) [1, 145, 181].

Posttraumatic Hydrocephalus

Surgical

Early hydrocephalus is caused by an obstruction of the CSF pathway (foramen Monroe, third ventricle, aqueduct or fourth ventricle) by coagula [280].

Ventricular dilatation following severe head trauma (GCS <8) may be either a manifestation of brain atrophy or of active, symptomatic ventricular dilatation. The latter is to be considered in young patients presenting surgical flap tension or CSF accumulation, added neurological deficits or ceased further clinical improvement after initial improvement. The distinction between atrophy and potentially treatable hydrocephalus cannot be made on the basis of conventional computerized tomographic (CT) or magnetic resonance (MR) scanning [40, 307].

To its development contribute meningitis, traumatic subarachnoid hemorrhage, posterior fossa mass, supratentorial clot with contralateral ventricular dilatation, and craniotomy. In two series, the frequency of shunting procedure was 0.2% and 0.7%, respectively. Licata and colleagues found that even patients in coma may benefit from a shunt procedure [55, 218].

Therapy: CSF drainage (in the acute phase; later on a shunt treatment).

Hygroma

Adult traumatic subdural hygroma is considered a delayed traumatic lesion, a consequence of arachnoid tear and CSF influx into the subdural space followed by compromised CSF dynamics [1, 207, 435].

Therapy: When causing a significant mass effect, hygromas are to be drained.

Chronic Subdural Hematoma

Over time, a small acute SDH may come to be a slowly growing chronic SDH.
Therapy: see Sect. 1.7.2.6.

Infection

Scalp infection; bone flap osteitis; brain abscess and subdural empyema; meningitis

Penetrating brain injuries are associated with a high rate of infection, both early infections and delayed abscesses. Some of the risk factors for infection following penetrating brain injury include extensive bony destruction, persistent CSF leak, and an injury pathway that violates an air sinus.

Risk factors for postoperative infections after craniotomy: Cerebrospinal fluid leakage, surgical diagnosis; no antibiotic prophylaxis; early reoperation [197]. Most important risk factors:

- Monitoring of ICP and further parameters by use of intradural devices is the most important risk factor. The risk of infection may be as high as 10–17% and is proportional to the duration of monitoring [160]. CSF leakage and manipulation of the system affect negatively.
- Postoperative CSF leakage [197].

Therapy: Debridement and water-tight closure; removal of bone flap; evacuation; antibiotics.

Sinking Skin Flap Syndrome (Syndrome of the Trephined)

With an extensive skull defect, the overlying skin flap is usually sunken, progressive, and sometimes neurologic deterioration may appear. The deterioration is thought to be caused by the force of the atmospheric pressure and also by the in-and-out displacement of the brain through the skull defect. The symptomatology can possibly be arrested or even reversed by cranioplasty [111, 343].

Medical Complications (see Chap. 2)

- Disturbances of serum electrolytes,
- Coagulopathy (DIC),
- Pulmonary compromise (pneumonia, ARDS),
- Septicemia (10%), hypotension),
- Posttraumatic vasospasms,
- Seizures (60),
- Intracranial infection,
- Gastro-intestinal mucosal erosion,
- Cardiac rhythm abnormalities,
- Protein-calorie malnutrition, and
- Complications related to immobility [308].

1.7.2 Specific Lesions

1.7.2.1 Scalp Injury

Synonym: Bruise (contusion), abrasion, laceration, scalp defect, cephalohematoma

Definition

- Scalp contusion: A bruise (bleeding into the skin without an overlying cut or abrasion) of the scalp with no internal damage (galea aponeurotica intact).
- Scalp lacerations, gashes, tears, cuts: gap in the dermis or underlying tissues and galea aponeurotica of the scalp.
- Traumatic avulsion of the Scalp: small partial losses with an intact or destroyed pericranium.
- Total scalp avulsions.

Etiology/epidemiology: Scalp injuries are very common and are often present in patients requiring emergency care for blunt trauma and in almost every patient with severe head injury. Most lacerations are the result of the skin hitting an object, or an object hitting the skin with force.

Clinical presentation/symptoms: Bleeding, swelling, tenderness. The actual condition of the casualty depends on the location and the seriousness of the accompanying brain lesions.

Complications: Scalp lesions have to rise suspicion of additional head injuries. Intracranial suppuration may result from secondary infection through emissary veins, calvarial foramina, fracture lines, or surgical openings in the bone resulting in intracranial infections (epidural abscess, subdural empyema, septic sinus thrombosis, brain abscess) [138].

A skull fracture may be present in the area of laceration but not necessarily right below it. Missing an open skull fracture may entail severe infectious complications when the dura is torn.

Some scalp lacerations are severe enough to cause hypovolemic shock and acute anemia. If the patient arrives in shock, the perfusion pressure may be low, and there may be minimal active scalp bleeding. Under such circumstances, the scalp wound may be initially dismissed as trivial. However, as the blood pressure returns toward normal, bleeding from the scalp wound becomes more profuse [409]. Scalp wounds have to be secured when definitive management has to be postponed [389].

Diagnostic Procedures

In injured patients, the scalp has to be examined carefully. Small penetrating wounds as stab wounds or gunshot wounds for example can be missed readily in the absence of a leading history. The position of the scalp lesion may point towards the location of a possible brain injury.

Recommended European Standard: *Clinical assessment* according to ATLS.

Exploring of the scalp laceration; when a skull fracture or an intracranial injury is supposed, a CT scan is performed.

Additional/useful diagnostic procedures :None

Therapy

Conservative treatment
Recommended European Standard: None
Surgical treatment
Recommended European Standard
Surgical treatment aims at hemostasis, infection prophylaxis, and primary closure. Massive bleeding from a torn superficial temporal or an occipital artery is treated as an emergency. Moreover, the timing of scalp repair is not crucial. If the patient is harboring a mass lesion, the scalp can be repaired after evacuation of the mass. Large localized hematomas of the subgaleal space may be aspirated, thereby minimizing the chance of formation of an encapsulated seroma. To prevent unexpected strong bleeding, foreign matter and bony fragments should not be mobilized outside of the operating theater.

Useful additional therapeutic strategies: Tetanus prophylaxis according to immune status of the patient

Differential Diagnosis

Simple scalp laceration has to be differentiated from a penetrating head injury. Subperiosteal hematomas may pretend depressed skull fractures.

Prognosis/Outcome

Simple scalp wounds usually heal without problems; large skin defects are treated according to the principles of plastic surgery.

Surgical Principles

Wound closure should be done under sterile conditions with particular attention paid to galeal approximation. Before infiltration with local anesthetic, the wound is controlled exactly concerning CSF leak and extrusion of brain substance.

Technique: Whether hair should be shaved or not is at the discretion of the surgeon. Scalp lacerations have to be thoroughly cleaned. Foreign material and devitalized or contaminated tissue from or adjacent to the lesion is removed until surrounding healthy tissue is exposed. The laceration is explored assiduously (self-retaining retractors, high intensity light, hemostasis) to make sure there is no underlying fracture or penetrating injury.

In view of the potentially contaminated nature of the wounds, closure in a single layer (including the galea) with a synthetic monofilament suture is recommended. If this is not possible, reconstructive techniques are used, the proper choice is affected by several factors – the size and location of the defect, the presence or absence of periosteum, the quality of surrounding scalp tissue, the presence or absence of hair, location of the hairline, and patient comorbidities, etc. [158, 210].

Surgical complication (see Sect. 1.7.1.4)

Noticeable scarring
Wound dehiscence
Infection

Special Remarks

Type of anesthesia
With the exception of large scale wounds, scalp wounds are treated under local anesthesia.

1.7.2.2 Skull Fracture (Fig. 1.CT-1a)

Definition
A skull fracture is a break or split in one or more of the bones in the skull caused by a head injury.
Types of skull fractures:
Skull fractures are defined referring to their

- Localization: vault or base (see Sect. 1.7.2.2.2)
- Shape: linear, depressed (in children possibly "ping-pong fracture"), or comminuted

Fig. 1.CT-1 (**a**) Skull x-ray lateral: Linear fractures in the temporal-temporoparietal region. (**b**) Computed tomography (**b1**: coronar, native, bone window, **b2**: brain window): Open depressed skull fracture frontal parasagittal (blow of a hammer), depressed bony fragments; air under the medial bony rim; falx; anterior horns of cerebral ventricles (with a cavum verge as a variation)

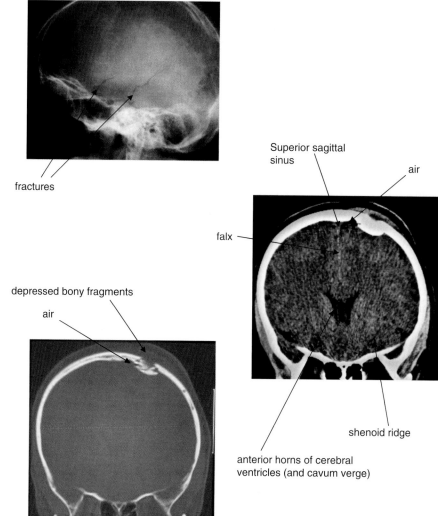

- Accompanying injuries:

  - Scalp (or mucosa of the paranasal sinuses) intact: closed fracture (synonym: simple fracture)
  - Scalp (or mucosa of the paranasal sinuses) overlaying the fracture lacerated: open fracture (synonym: compound fracture)
  - Dura: laceration/tearing of the dura resulting in open fractures in a direct communication between environment and CSF/brain. Both in closed and in compound depressed skull fracture, the dura may be intact, contused, or lacerated. Penetrating and perforating head injury are per definition combined with an open (compound) skull fracture and a lacerated dura (see Sect. 1.7.2.9)

Special forms of skull fractures

- Depressed skull fracture: A comminuted skull fracture impressed more than the thickness of the skull table. The underlying dura may be intact, contusioned, or torn (see Sect. 1.7.2.2.1).
- Cranial burst fracture: A widely diastatic skull fracture associated with dural laceration and extrusion of cerebral tissue outside the calvaria beneath an unbroken scalp (in children possibly resulting in a growing fracture).
- Crushing fracture: A fracture caused by static loading (the head pinched between two objects) (see Sect. 1.7.2.2.2).

Etiology/epidemiology: Skull fractures most commonly result from a traumatic force impacting on the head directly. Affected are patients of all ages and with a variety of types of trauma including motor vehicle accidents, falls, and assaults.

Linear fracture results from low-energy blunt trauma over a wide surface area of the skull. Depressed skull fractures are the result from a high-energy direct blow to a small surface area of the skull with a blunt object.

The most common type of fracture are simple linear fractures of the vault. Preferential sites are the thin squamous temporal and parietal bones over the temples. Fractures of the skull base are considerably less common, scoring high are the petrous temporal ridge, the cribriform plate, and the roof of orbits, the inner parts of the sphenoid wings, the sphenoid sinus, and the foramen magnum.

A fracture by itself is of little significance. However, it indicates that significant enough impact occurred to cause brain trauma increasing the risk of intracranial hemorrhage fivefold. Cranial fracture is the only independent significant risk factor in predicting intracranial hematomas [57].

Clinical presentation/symptoms: In patients suffering from a skull fracture who are fully alert at presentation, the frequency of posttraumatic vomiting is doubled [282]. Scalp is mostly with bruise, contusion, abrasio, or laceration, with possibly visible deformity or depression in the head or face. Leaking cerebrospinal fluid from the scalp laceration is strongly indicative of penetrating injury (dura torn).

Complications: Fracture crossing a vascular channel, venous sinus groove, or a suture may cause epidural hematoma, arterial or venous sinus thrombosis/occlusion [434], and sutural diastasis, respectively.

The presence of a cranial fracture is associated with a higher incidence of intracranial lesions, neurological deficit, and poorer outcome [57, 353]. In patients with minor head injury (MHI) and a skull fracture, the probability of intracerebral hemorrhage (ICH) is about five times higher than in patients without a skull fracture [159]. Cranial fracture was found to be the only independent significant risk factor in predicting intracranial hematomas in a cohort of adolescents [57]. In children, an interposition of leptomeningeal tissue within the bony gap may lead to a growing fracture.

Diagnostic Procedures

Imaging: Skull radiography (SR) is useful for imaging of calvarial fractures, penetrating injuries, and radiopaque foreign bodies. Any linear area of increased bone density should be considered probable depressed fracture (see Sect. 1.4.1). However, with plain skull X-ray, fractures of the skull are not diagnosed as accurately as supposed [402]. Computed tomography has a greater chance of detecting a skull fracture than routine skull radiography [403].

Recommended European Standard

Clinical Assessment → second survey (ATLS).

Imaging: ([401], NICE): Both patients presenting with a GCS score of 14 points or less and patients presenting with a GCS score of 15 in the presence of risk factors are to be scanned. Helical computed tomography (three window-level settings without the use of intravenous iodinated contrast agents, reconstructions in three planes) should be obtained immediately after the patient is stabilized using standard advanced trauma life support (ATLS) guidelines (see Sect. 1.4.2).

Additional/useful diagnostic procedures: Cranial burst fracture: MR imaging allows early diagnosis of a skull fracture associated with acute cerebral extrusion [96].

Therapy

Conservative therapy

Recommended European Standard: Adults with simple linear fractures who are neurologically intact do not require any intervention. For treatment of tangential head wounds, depressed fractures of the vault, and basal fractures: see Sects. 1.7.2.9.1, 1.7.2.2.1, and 1.7.2.2.2, respectively.

Surgical treatment

Recommended European Standard

Compound calvarial fractures require debridement and wound care (see Sect. 1.7.2.1); For depressed skull fractures and fractures of the skullbase, respectively, see Sects. 1.7.2.2.1 and 1.7.2.2.2.

Useful additional therapeutic strategies: Open fractures, if contaminated, may require antibiotics in addition to tetanus toxoid [315].

Differential Diagnosis

Vascular channel or indentation.

By computed tomography, the presumed diagnosis of a skull fracture is to be validated without any doubt.

Prognosis/Outcome

Prognosis depends on concomitant brain injury.

Surgical Principles

See Sects. 1.7.2.2.1 and 1.7.2.2.2, respectively.

Special Remarks

Type of anesthesia

When a fracture of the skull base is suspected, insertion of a nasogastric tube should be avoided. The orogastric route is preferred, as there have been cases of intracranial nasogastric tube placement in the presence of cribriform plate fractures [189].

1.7.2.2.1 Depressed Skull Fracture (Fig. 1.CT-1b1, b2)

Definition

A skull fracture is defined depressed if the outer table of one or more of the fractured segments lies below the level of the inner table of the surrounding intact skull. Comminution of fragments starts from the point of maximum impact and spreads centrifugally. Minimally depressed fractures are less than the thickness of the bone.

Closed/open (compound) fracture: A depressed fracture may be open (compound) or closed (simple). By definition, there is either a skin laceration over the fracture or the fracture runs through a paranasal or petrosal sinus or through the middle ear structures, resulting in communication between the external environment and the cranial cavity. Open fractures may be clean or contaminated.

Dura: Both in closed and in compound depressed skull fracture the dura may be intact, contused, or lacerated.

Special types of depressed fractures:

- "Pond" or "ping-pong ball" type fracture. Usually seen in young children, this type of depressed skull fracture is resembling the indentation that can be produced with the finger in a ping-pong ball; when elevated, it resumes and retains its normal position.

- Depressed skull fracture overlaying a venous sinus
- Depressed bitable frontal sinus fracture (see Sect. 1.7.2.2.2)
- Tangential missile wound (see Sect. 1.7.2.9)

Etiology/epidemiology

A depressed skull fracture is the consequence of a dash of a fairly small blunt object – such as a hammer, a baseball bat, or a golf ball – with a large amount of kinetic energy against the head. Assault and road traffic accidents are the most common cause [12, 413]. About 80% of depressed fractures are open fractures.

The incidence of depressed skull fractures is estimated to be 20 per 1,000,000 population per year, 75–90% of which are comminuted and compound (scalp or air sinus involvement) [39]. If bone fragments are intruded more than 5 mm, the dura is usually torn. Most of the depressed fractures are over the frontoparietal region because the bone is thin and the specific location is prone to an assailant's attack. Because the scalp is mobile, the area of depression may not underlie the laceration.

Compared with linear fractures, depressed fractures are more commonly associated with parenchymal injury – contusions, dural sinus injuries, and intracranial hematomas – than linear fractures. Persistent neurologic deficits and death is not a rare outcome [12, 39], but even with marked depression of fragments, intracranial injury may be insufficient to produce unconsciousness.

In newborns, "ping-pong" depressed fractures are secondary to the baby's head impinging against the mother's sacral promontory during uterine contractions [95]. Depressed skull fractures in infants originate from neglect, fall, or abuse. Most of the fractures seen in children are a result of falls and bicycle accidents. In adults, fractures typically occur from motor vehicle accidents or violence [205].

Bitable frontal sinus fracture is the consequence of an enormous amount of force. Motor vehicle crashes are the most common cause, followed by falls and assaults. Accordingly, these fractures are mostly combined with orbital roof fractures, zygomatic complex fractures, and intracranial lesions: Pneumocephalon and frontal contusions are often. Suffering from local brain damage, these patients present in relatively good neurologic grades; in the series of Lee and colleagues [209], 66% of patients were graded mild TBI (see Sect. 1.7.2.2.2).

Clinical presentation/symptoms

Mostly, a scalp laceration is present. With the dura torn, cerebrospinal fluid or brain tissue may ooze out of the wound. The actual condition of the casualty depends on the location and the seriousness of the accompanying brain lesions. To be of clinical significance, a free fragment of bone should be depressed greater than the adjacent inner table of the skull. The extent of the impression is not to be judged clinically.

Complications

Misdiagnosis: When judged clinically, depressed skull fractures may be missed (relocatability of the scalp with respect to the skull).

Bleeding: "Exploration" of the injury with mobilizing of bone fragments may initiate a severe bleeding.

Intracranial hypertension: Depressed skull fracture overlying the major venous sinuses may lead to chronic intracranial hypertension as a late manifestation of sinus venous compression and infection [178, 433].

CSF leak: Comminuted fractures of the frontal skull base are nearly always combined with dural tears.

Infection: Postoperative infection rate is about 8–10% and is significantly associated with brain contusion and dural tear [12, 178].

Posttraumatic seizure/posttraumatic epilepsy: The risk of late posttraumatic seizures depends both on the GCS score and on the amount and the location of the parenchymal injuries. It is highest in moderate TBI (GCS score 9–12) and with biparietal contusions [98] and subdural hematoma [19, 180, 398].

Diagnostic Procedures

Imaging: Computed tomography is the first choice. Exploration of the skull in the region of the scalp laceration may fail to reveal a fracture. In plain skull radiographs, a depressed fracture is suspected from the appearance of double density or circular fracture. Air in the subdural space or in the ventricles is evidence of a tear or a laceration of the dura.

Recommended European standard

Clinical assessment according to ATLS.

Imaging: Both patients presenting with a GCS score of 14 points or less and patients presenting with a GCS score of 15 in the presence of risk factors are to be scanned [52, 401]. Helical computed tomography should be obtained immediately after the patient is stabilized using standard advanced trauma life support (ATLS) guidelines (see Sect. 1.4.2).

Additional/useful diagnostic procedures

A preoperative angiogram (preferable iaDSA, eventually CT- or MR-angiography) with venous flow phase is recommended whenever CT has shown a depressed fracture overlaying a venous sinus. Data regarding both position and extent of obstruction affect decisions regarding the surgical procedure (see below "Controlling dural venous sinus injury").

Therapy

In closed depressed skull fractures where no piece of bone is depressed greater than the adjacent inner table of the skull, no surgery (elevation) is required [413]. Based on an extensive study of the relevant literature (1975–2001), the Surgical Management of Traumatic Brain Injury Author Group [52] recommend the following treatment options:

Conservative treatment

Recommended European Standard

Except obligatory debridement (removal of foreign material and devitalized tissue) of the skin, patients with open (compound) depressed cranial fractures may be treated nonoperatively – supposed there is no clinical or radiographic evidence of dural penetration,

- No significant intracranial hematoma
- No depression greater than 10 mm
- No frontal sinus involvement
- No gross cosmetic deformity
- No wound infection
- No pneumocephalon
- No gross wound contamination. Under these conditions, conservative management of closed (simple) depressed cranial fractures is a treatment option [52]. A neurologically stable patient with a closed depressed fracture over an intact venous sinus should be observed. A patient with an open depressed fracture over a patent and not compromised venous sinus who is neurologically stable should undergo skin debridement without elevation of the fracture [91, 143].

Surgical treatment

Recommended European Standard

If these conditions are not present, operative treatment is recommended. Also, patients with open (compound) cranial fractures depressed greater than the thickness of the cranium should undergo operative intervention. Operative debridement reduces the incidence of infection. Thereby, early operation is recommended to reduce the incidence of infection.

In the absence of gross wound infection at the time of presentation, immediate replacement of bone fragments seems not to increase the incidence of infection if surgery is performed expeditiously, and this replacement eliminates the need for subsequent cranioplasty and its inherent risks and complications. No controlled data exist to support the timing of surgery or the use of one technique over another.

Elevation and debridement is recommended as the surgical method of choice. Primary bone fragment replacement is a surgical option in the absence of wound infection at the time of surgery. If the sinus is compromised, urgent elevation of the depressed fragment is required if the patient is neurologically unstable (mass lesion, severe bleeding) [91, 143].
Useful additional therapeutic strategies

Antibiotic prophylaxis/seizure prophylaxis: Both prophylactic medication of antibiotics and prophylactic medication of antiepileptic medication are discusses controversially. The author group [52] recommends that all management strategies for open (compound) depressed fractures should include antibiotics.

Differential Diagnosis

A tear in the temporal fascia may be erroneously interpreted clinically as a depressed fracture of the temporal squama. By computed tomography, the presumed diagnosis of a depressed skull fracture is to be validated without any doubt.

Prognosis/Outcome

Morbidity and mortality is related to the most part to the severity of the central nervous injury rather than to the depression itself. With infection, a significantly higher incidence of persistent neurological deficit, late epilepsy (defined as seizures longer than 1 week from injury), and death has been observed [12, 178].

Surgical Principles

The dura should be opened and the brain inspected even though there is no evidence of a dura laceration. When the brain has been contused and pulped, necrotic brain should be resected leaving clean edges. Depressed fractures over a venous sinus require special attention. The decision to operate such fractures is based on the neurological status of the patient, the exact location of the sinus involved, and the degree of venous flow compromise.

Immediate replacement of bone fragments in compound depressed skull fractures does not increase the risk of infectious complications [430]. If skull defects are reconstructed subsequently, alloplastic material, autogenous bone grafts, and resorbable bone plates cross-linked with bone matrix protein may be used [71, 346].
Technique

The positioning of the patient and the localization of the craniotomy depends on the site of the fracture. Parieto-occipital and suboccipital fractures are elevated in prone or park bench position. The extent of the skin incision – either S-linear or a horseshoe flap – has not only to allow survive of the depressed zone completely but also to obtain pericranium for enough for dural grafting, enlargement of the bony defect by craniectomy, and finally debriding of lacerated scalp.

The depressed bony fragment may be elevated directly assuming they (the bony fragments) are not wedged and do not lay over a venous sinus: The lacerated pericranium is incised circularly around the depressed zone allowing to mobilize the dural adhesion to the bony fragments and to extract them separate when completely loose (Fig. 1.12).

Depressed skull fracture: Elevation of depressed bony fragments

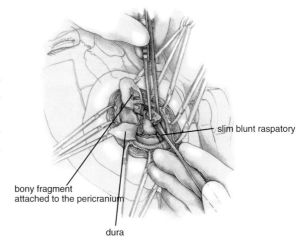

slim blunt raspatory

bony fragment attached to the pericranium

dura

Fig. 1.12 Depressed skull fracture: Elevation of depressed bony fragments

However, if the fragments are firmly impact, a burr-hole is placed at the margin of the fracture to allow identification of the regular dura before touching the fragments. With a rongeur, small amounts of bone are removed then to get access to the bony fragments. Mobilization has to be done very carefully to prevent additional damage to the underlying structures by the very sharp edges of the inner table of the fragments (Fig. 1.13).

Overlying the depressed zone of a sinus, the procedure must allow to expose the region of the sinus quickly: Several burr-holes are placed along the depressed zone on both sides of the sinus, the normal dura is identified. Next, the fragments are isolated from the surrounding intact bone using punches and rongeurs. Bone is removed laterally until intact dura is reached circumferential.

Controlling dural venous sinus injury: Head elevation helps to reduce or stop the bleeding but on the other hand may cause air embolism. Bleeding from a minor tear of the sinus wall may be stopped by direct suturing or oversewing with muscle stamps. Mayor tears or avulsed sections of sinus wall may need pericranium patch or fold over leaf of dura sutured on to the leak. If the sinus is

Depressed skull fracture: Elevation of depressed bony fragments starting from a burr hole

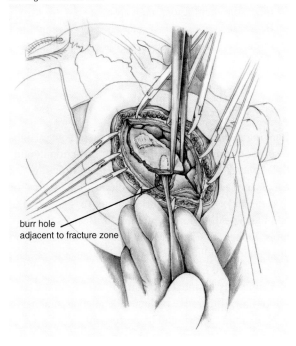

burr hole
adjacent to fracture zone

Fig. 1.13 Depressed skull fracture: Elevation of depressed bony fragments starting from a burr-hole

destroyed over too great a distance to be repaired conventionally, the anterior half of the SSS may be ligated with minor risk, the posterior half of the sagittal sinus should not be permanently ligated – high likelihood of precipitating hemispheric venous infarction – but rather should be repaired by interposing a venous graft [374].

The same advice applies when one of the transverse sinuses is lacerated. Thereby, it is mandatory to know if the SSS drains unilaterally, because ligature of draining transverse sinus would not be tolerated. Also it should be known if one of the sinuses is hypoplastic.

Water-tight closure of the debrided dura (patch graft) is mandatory. At the end of the procedure, the fractured area should be covered with a full thickness of scalp. Intraoperative complications (see Sect. 1.7.1.4):

- Severe bleeding from a lacerated venous sinus
- Brain swelling subsequently to obstruction of a venous sinus

Postoperative complications: (see Sect. 1.7.1.4):

- Delayed hemorrhage
- Venous sinus thrombosis
- Infection/disturbance of wound healing
- Posttraumatic epilepsy

Special Remarks

Type of anesthesia

Depressed skull fractures are approached in general anesthesia. When a fracture of the skull base is suspected, insertion of a nasogastric tube should be avoided to prevent intracranial placement of a nasogastric tube.

1.7.2.2.2 Fractures of the Skullbase

Definition

Fractures of the skull base include: *Frontobasal skull fractures* including fractures of the upper third of the face and anterior skull base (frontal bone with frontal sinus, the cribriform plate of the ethmoid bone, the sphenoid bone (wings)). Closed depressed fractures that involve the paranasal sinuses should be regarded as open (compound). Frontal sinus fractures (linear, depressed, compound, comminuted) may involve the anterior or the posterior wall or both, and the frontonasal duct.

Fracture of the temporal bone (the squamous, petrous, mastoid, and tympanic portions, styloid process)

Fracture of the occipital bone (squama occipitalis, separated from its basal portion (lower clivus) by the foramen magnum on either side of which are the occipital condyles) [186].

Etiology/epidemiology

Fractures of the frontal bone and the anterior skull base are caused mainly by high-speed motor vehicle and industrial accidents delivering a large amount of frontal impact force. They are frequently associated with significant orbital, ethmoidal (lamina cribrosa), nasal, and midface fractures, with soft tissue injury and with brain injuries (contusions and hemorrhage/hematomas). Being firmly attached to the skull base, the dura is easily torn bringing brain tissue in contact with the potentially contaminated paranasal sinuses (open fracture), and contaminated material may be introduced through the wound into the cranial cavity. A cerebrospinal fluid leak may be the result of injury to the posterior frontal sinus wall and subsequent disruption of the attached dura and/or the result of a disruption of the anterior cranial fossa floor at the level of the cribriform plate, the fovea ethmoidalis, or the sphenoid sinus. A CSF leak can be combined with a pneumacephalon [236].

The most severe form of frontal bone fractures result in open cerebral injuries (penetrating injury; brain wound; through-and-through fracture).

Temporal bone fracture is diagnosed in up to 75% of patients with a skull base fracture. Longitudinal fracture occurs in the temporoparietal region and involves the squamous portion of the temporal bone, the superior wall of the external auditory canal, and the tegmen tympani. These fractures may run either anterior or posterior to the cochlea and labyrinthine capsule, ending in the middle cranial fossa near the foramen spinosum or in the mastoid air cells, respectively. Transverse fractures begin at the foramen magnum and extend through the cochlea and labyrinth, ending in the middle cranial fossa [133]. They may cause facial palsy, deafness, and CSF leakage with otorrhoea or paradoxal rhinoliquorrhoea. Injury to middle (temporal) fossa may affect the carotid canal, injure the internal carotid artery, and result in carotid-cavernous fistula. With a *crushing injury* (progressive compression to the head), bilateral temporal bone fractures may result [393].

Fracture of the occipital bone may lacerate the major venous sinuses (see Sect. 1.7.2.7), and affect the cranio-cervical stability [259, 392, 407].

Clinical presentation/symptoms [189, 339]. The condition of the patient parallels the severity of the concomitant brain injury. Anterior skull base: Besides unilateral or bilateral (raccoon eyes) monocle hematoma, the patient may present CSF leakage, anosmia (I), diplopia (III, IV), and blindness (II), additionally maxillo-facial injuries and signs and symptoms of brain injury.

Temporal skull base: Patients may present with "battle sign," hearing loss (VIII), vestibular dysfunction (VIII), and facial nerve injury (VII). CSF leakage may be noted both from the ear and/or nose.

Posterior skull base: Patients may present with difficulty in phonation and aspiration and ipsilateral motor paralysis of the vocal cord (X), soft palate (IX, curtain sign), superior pharyngeal constrictor (X), sternocleidomastoid (XI), and trapezius (XI).

Occipital condylar fracture: patient may present with lower cranial nerve injuries and hemiplegia or quadriplegia (associated cervical spinal injuries).

Complications

- Vessel damage: bleeding (hematoma), ischemia (encephalomalacy)
- CSF-leak (otorrhoe; rhinorrhoe)
- Herniation of brain tissue
- (Tension-)Pneumocephalon
- Infection: meningitis, brain abscess
- Recurrence of previously ceased cerebrospinal fluid rhinorrhea and delayed onset of cerebrospinal fluid rhinorrhea [394].

Diagnostic Procedures

Imaging: Computed tomography is first choice. High-resolution computed tomography of the region in multiple planes (completed by 3-D reconstructions as necessary) is essential for predicting the degree of osseous and associated injuries (brain, vessels, nerves), and the type of procedure indicated. Besides the fractures looked for, hematosinus and pneumocephalon are frequent findings.

Recommended European Standard

Clinical assessment according to ATLS. In the conscious and cooperative patient, a detailed cranial nerve (CN) examination should be performed.

Imaging: High-resolution computed tomography of the region in multiple planes (completed by 3-D reconstructions eventually) [401]. Both patients presenting with a GCS score of 14 points or less and patients presenting with a GCS score of 15 in the presence of risk factors are to be scanned.

Angiography has to be preformed when vessel injury is suspected (fracture involving carotid channel, occipital condyles, or clivus).

Additional/useful diagnostic procedures

Metrizamid CT can help to localize the CSF leak. If the site of the leak is not apparent on CT scan, a high-resolution T2-weighted MRI may allow visualization of fluid within sinus(es) or the actual site if leakage occurs at the time of scanning. CSF leakage may be proven by testing of the leaking fluid for beta-2-transferrin an localized by intrathecal application of fluorescein.

Therapy

Conservative therapy
Recommended European Standard

- Frontal sinus fracture: With closed fracture of the anterior wall, surgery is needed only because of aesthetic considerations. If posterior wall fracture displacement appears to be only a few millimeters and the resultant sinus contour is generally smooth, and there is no apparent CSF leak, the dura usually is intact and exploration unnecessary. The majority of CSF leaks resolve spontaneously (within 1 week) without intervention – if going on a lumbar drain (or daily spinal taps) can be placed. Operation should be considered if the fistula persists 10–14 days after injury. Frontobasal, temporal, and posterior skull base fracture: Patients suffering from a simple fracture are observed several days, dismissed if no complications occur and followed the as outpatients.
Useful additional therapeutic strategies

- Repeat head CT after neurologic deterioration or inexplainable rise of ICP.
- Antibiotic prophylaxis: Actually, the effectiveness of antibiotics in patients with basal skull fracture cannot be determined, but currently available evidence from RCTs does not support prophylactic antibiotic use in patients with BSF, whether there is evidence of CSF leakage or not [288, 319].
Surgical treatment
Recommended European Standard

- Frontal sinus fracture: With the skin lacerated over the fractured anterior wall, debridement is mandatory. If the posterior sinus wall is jagged or a comminuted fragment protrudes intracranially, more by more than the thickness of the posterior wall or if

CSF rhinorrhea or pneumocephalus or accompanies a disrupted posterior frontal sinus wall, then exploration and repair is warranted [388].

- If surgical intervention is required emergently for the evacuation of an epidural or subdural hematoma, the frontal sinus could be managed concurrently with the neurologic injury. Frontobasal fractures: Fractures of the frontal skull base combined with a intracranial mass lesion or a massive bleeding are managed as emergencies, as are through-and-through fractures with escape of CSF and/or brain tissue and severe frontobasal injuries involving tissue loss. Comminuted fractures of the frontal bone and the frontal skull base are treated within 24 h, if combined with severe parenchymal brain injury (radiographic evidence of multiple small intraparenchymal hematomas not acting as a mass lesion) revision is postponed unless they contribute to the neurologic morbidity. Bone reconstruction of calvarial defects can be managed at a second stage when the patient is stable neurologically.
- Temporal and posterior skull base fracture: mass lesions or massive bleedings are managed as emergencies, as are through-and-through fractures with escape of CSF and/or brain tissue and severe injuries involving tissue loss. These procedures are done in collaboration with neurosurgeons, ENT-surgeons, and maxillofacial surgeons.
- CSF leak: Operation is performed
- Without delay: when there is radiographic evidence of elevation of a spicule of bone with brain penetration or there is a large defect in the floor of the frontal fossa with hemiation of brain into one of the paranasal sinuses later on:
- If CSF leakage does not stop within 2 weeks or occurs late in the postinjury course - in any patient who develops meningitis (after the meningitis is controlled).

Remark: Indication concerning surgical decompression of cranial nerves (for example optic nerve [216], facial nerve [82]) are scope of the ENT department and the ophthalmologic department, respectively.

Differential Diagnosis

By computed tomography, the presumed diagnosis of a depressed skull fracture is to be validated without any doubt.

Prognosis/Outcome

Outcome depends predominantly on the severity of the accompanying brain injuries and the occurrence of infectious complications. CSF leaks may appear even years after the initial injury.

Surgical Principles

Surgery is an interdisciplinary procedure performed in close collaboration with neurosurgeons – the cranial procedures are performed first – maxillofacial surgeons and ENT surgeons, respectively. Reconstruction is focused on maintaining a durable water-tight closure separating the nasal cavity from cranial contents as well as the restoration of lost volume. Reestablishing aesthetic integrity to the region is also vitally important [270]. The type and the extent of the surgical approach is to be chosen according to the actual lesion [209, 241, 320].

Technique

Frontal sinus fracture: Fractures of the frontal sinus and nasofrontal-ethmoidal complex are managed by ENT surgeons/maxillofacial surgeons, joined by a neurosurgeon in "through-and-through fracture" (external laceration, a fracture of both the anterior and posterior sinus walls, and usually dural lacerations and contusion of the adjacent frontal lobes fracture) [236]. CSF-fistula: An extradural search for the site of the tear/fistula is avoided because the technique may create additional dural tears indistinguishable from the initial traumatic tears (see below: "Fractures of the anterior skull base"). One of the main causes of continued leakage is a bony spicule in the fracture. This should be sought and removed at the time of surgery.

When the CSF fistula is in the region of the cribriform plate or the sphenoid sinus a transethmoidal repair is to be preferred minimizing the loss of sense of smell and the risk of intracerebral hemorrhage, cerebral edema, seizures, frontal lobe dysfunction with, osteomyelitis of the frontal bone [245].

Anterior skull base fracture

Craniotomy: With the patient under general anesthesia and in prone position, the head positioned maneuverable on donut or on a horseshoe a headrest.

A coronal skin flap incision (the incision starts anterior to the tragus just flush with the zygomatic arch preauricularly, ending at the identical point contralaterally) is performed. A large based pericranium flap is prepared. To prevent injury to the supraorbital nerves,

Frontal craniotomy

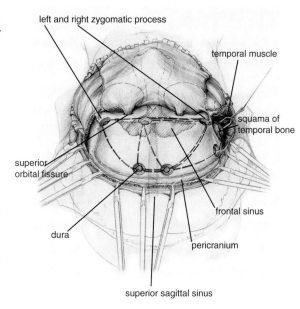

Fig. 1.14 Frontal craniotomy

the galea is separated from the pericranium down to a line 3 cm over the superior orbital rims only, further mobilization of the flap is done subperiosal. A bifrontal craniotomy is performed then (unilateral if applicable). The craniotomy can be modified by placing additional burr-holes in the squama temporal squama and on the linea temporalis superior, respectively (Fig. 1.14), allowing complete exploration of the basal cortex of the frontal lobe, of the optic nerve, the intradural segment of the carotid artery, the basal cisterns, the proximal sylvian fissure, and the temporal pole. The SSS is ligated in its most anterior part and dissected.

If no intradural lesions requiring exploration are present, the fractures are approached extradurally (Fig. 1.15). Otherwise, the dura is opened according as the position of the intradural lesions. The depressed bone fragments are elevated, hematoma and contusions are evacuated.

Exenteration of the frontal sinus mucosa, cranialization of the sinus, and packing of the nasofrontal ducts bilaterally is accomplished. Thereafter, the dural lacerations are repaired, attempting primary closure with sutures if feasible. For larger dural tears, the pericranium flap is placed either intra- or extradurally (Fig. 1.16a, b) combined eventually with a temporalis muscle or fascial variants of this flap.

Transfrontal extradura revision of the frontal skull base.

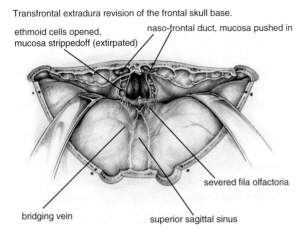

ethmoid cells opened,
mucosa strippedoff (extirpated)

naso-frontal duct, mucosa pushed in

severed fila olfactoria

bridging vein

superior sagittal sinus

Fig. 1.15 Transfrontal extradura revision of the frontal skull base

If postoperative cerebrospinal fluid (CSF) leak is expected (large dural or basal bony defects), a lumbar drain is inserted providing there is no risk of rising ICP postoperatively. Patients with a ventricular drain for intracranial pressure monitoring do not need lumbar drainage. The calvarium is reconstructed and the skin closed in layers.

Postoperative computed tomographic (CT) scans were obtained to assess bony reconstruction and follow-up intracranial injuries.

Remark: The use of free tissue transfer can provide dependable, vascularized tissue to fill volume defects as well as reinforce dural closures to prevent cerebrospinal fluid leaks and meningitis. Local flaps are a powerful adjunct to free tissue reconstruction and in

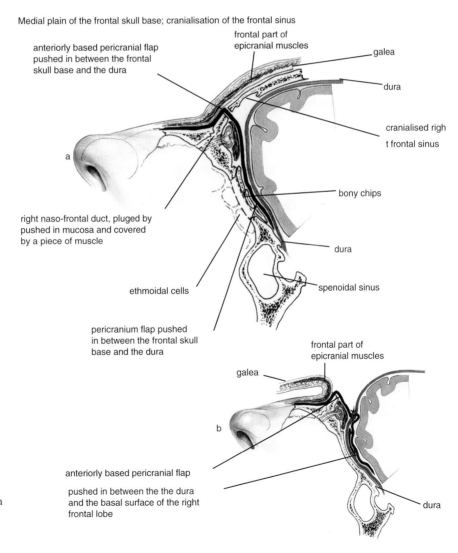

Medial plain of the frontal skull base; cranialisation of the frontal sinus

anteriorly based pericranial flap pushed in between the frontal skull base and the dura

frontal part of epicranial muscles

galea

dura

cranialised right frontal sinus

a

bony chips

right naso-frontal duct, pluged by pushed in mucosa and covered by a piece of muscle

dura

ethmoidal cells

spenoidal sinus

pericranium flap pushed in between the frontal skull base and the dura

frontal part of epicranial muscles

galea

b

anteriorly based pericranial flap

pushed in between the the dura and the basal surface of the right frontal lobe

dura

Fig. 1.16 (**a**, **b**) Medial plain of the frontal skull base; cranialization of the frontal sinus

select cases may be sufficient alone for skull base reconstruction [169, 270].

Temporal and posterior skull base fracture

Contrary to the frontal base, the middle and occipital skull base do not imply air-filled sinuses and are underlaid well. In the acute stage, surgical interventions are mandatory first and foremost with mass lesions and penetrating injuries [169].

CSF leaks (rhino- and otorrhoe) are handled according to the principles mentioned before.

Intraoperative complications (see Sect. 1.7.1.4)

- Severe bleeding (venous sinus; dural/cerebral arteries)
- Brain swelling

Postoperative complications (see Sect. 1.7.1.4)

- Delayed hemorrhage
- Venous sinus thrombosis: Interruption of flow through the sinus along its most caudal third segment carries a several-fold higher likelihood of precipitating hemispheric venous infarction than it does in the anterior most two.
- Infection
- Posttraumatic seizures

Special Remarks

When a fracture of the skull base is suspected, insertion of a nasogastric tube should be avoided to prevent intracranial placement of a nasogastric tube. On patients with accompanying severe maxillofacial trauma, a tracheostomy is performed.

1.7.2.3 Diffuse Traumatic Brain Injury (DTBI)

Synonym: Shearing injury, diffuse white matter shearing injury

Definition

Microscopic structural damage throughout the brain.
Concussion: Mild form of diffuse TBI

- Mild concussion: no loss of consciousness
- Classical cerebral concussion: loss of consciousness for less than 6 h

Diffuse axonal injury (DAI): More severe form of diffuse TBI (microscopical structural damage throughout the brain), loss of consciousness for 6 h or longer. DIA is classified as

- Mild DIA: Posttraumatic coma lasting 6–24 h
- Moderate DIA: Prolonged coma lasting longer than 24 h without brain stem signs
- Severe DIA: Prolonged coma lasting longer than 24 h and brain stem signs (decerebrate or decorticate posturing) [122]

Etiology/epidemiology

Diffuse traumatic brain injury is a consequence of indirect transmission of energy (impulsive loading) to the head resulting in a rotational motion of the brain, which causes shear, tensile, and compression strains. As an effect of the tissue shearing many nerve fibers are torn at the moment of injury.

Axonal damage may occur

- In isolation or
- In conjunction with actual tissue tears, where both axons and small vessels are torn.

The degree of this disruption marks the severity of injury, as indicated by measures of coma depth and duration, or duration of posttraumatic amnesia. The following stages of involvement have been described by Adams and colleagues according to the anatomic location of the lesions:

Stage I: This involves the parasagittal regions of the frontal lobes, the periventricular temporal lobes, and, less likely, the parietal and occipital lobes, internal and external capsules, and cerebellum.

Stage II: This involves the corpus callosum in addition to the white-matter areas of stage I. Stage II is observed in approximately 20% of patients. Most commonly, the posterior body and splenium are involved; however, the process is believed to advance anteriorly with increasing severity of disease. Both sides of the corpus callosum may be involved; however, involvement more frequently is unilateral and may be hemorrhagic. The involvement of the corpus callosum carries a poorer prognosis.

Stage III: This involves the areas associated with stage II, with the addition of brainstem involvement. A predilection exists for the superior cerebellar peduncles, medial lemnisci, and corticospinal tracts [4].

DIA is the most frequent brain injury occurring in about 40% of comatose patients (loss of consciousness for more than 6 h) and is the result of accidents occurring at relatively high velocities, i.e., in vehicular traumas (passengers or pedestrians). Falls produce a higher incidence of focal lesions and affect the elderly and the very young while vehicular traumas tend to involve young adults [38].

Young children have the highest rates of concussion. Sports [251] and bicycle accidents account for the majority of cases among 5- to 14-year-olds, whereas falls and vehicular accidents are the most common causes of concussion in adults [332].

Very often indirect transmission of energy to the head is combined with the much more frequent direct transmission, for example in a fall with subsequent dashing of the head against the ground. [123, 140]. Therefore, DIA (posttraumatic coma lasting at least 6–24 h) is seldom "pure" but mostly combined with focal lesions (contusions, extracerebral hematomas, and intraparenchymal hemorrhage).

Clinical presentation/symptoms

Concussion: The disturbance of neuronal function is temporary. Mostly, patients complain of headache, dizziness, or nausea, and are recording confusion, eventually a temporary loss of consciousness (LOC) or a loss of memory concerning the actual impact (amnesia). When awake some mental confusion may persist for a short time. Patients do not present localized neurological signs.

Diffuse axonal injury: DAI may cause - according to amount and localization of the wide spread axonal injury – moderate or severe neurologic signs (e.g., decerebrate (extensor posturing) or decorticate (flexor posturing), or deficits, either prolonged or permanent [5].

Complications

Postconcussion syndrome [137, 281] consisting of a constellation of mainly headache, dizziness, and trouble concentrating, in the days and weeks following concussion.

Misdiagnosis: Missing additional lesions such as traumatic parenchymal hemorrhage (see Sect. 1.7.2.8) and mass lesions: Progressive drowsiness or focal neurologic deficits (as hemiplegia or aphasia) after concussion may point to the possibility of a delayed subdural or epidural hematoma or vascular damage and call for additional imaging studies.

Massive brain swelling caused by hyperemia, occurring minutes or hours after head injury, rather in children than in adults, causing a rise of the intracranial pressure, which can add deleterious effects to the primary injury by causing increased ICP→brain shift→herniation [45, 227, 262]. Therapy: see Sect. 1.1.7. Moderate and severe traumatic brain injury: Surgical management; Chap. 2.

NICU-management. *Refractory intracranial pressure*: Following diffuse TBI, raised intracranial pressure refractory to standard treatment measures (sedation, ventricular CSF drainage, mild hyperventilation, mannitol) is a common problem [379]. The importance of intracranial hypertension in determining the outcome of head-injured patients is well known [61, 263] and has been confirmed by Juul [187] in a large clinical trial.

Posttraumatic seizures: The risk of posttraumatic seizures corresponds with the severity of the DTBI. Patients with MTBI have only a slightly increased risk of developing posttraumatic seizures [19, 342].

Diagnostic Procedures

Recommended European Standard

Both in adults and in children, CT is recommended as diagnostic tool.

Especially in children, the risk of missing a relevant intracranial lesion has to be weighed against the risk to radiation exposure of the CNS. The classification of the findings of a CT scan performed within 24 h after the impact, proposed by Marshall [243] and colleagues (1991) is useful in identifying patients at risk for developing intracranial hypertension (see Sect. 1.1.4.2), and thereby identifying the need for continuous monitoring of the intracranial pressure (ICP).

Indication: Criteria for use of CT as set forth by the United Kingdom National Institute for Clinical Excellence [401] relevant in children and adults (see Sect. 1.1.4.2).

Computed tomography findings: Among patients eventually proven to have DAI, 50–80% demonstrate a normal CT scan on presentation.

Emergency CT scan shows no mass lesion, but eventually small hemorrhages at the gray–white matter junction and/or cerebral swelling (superimposed with hypoxia or ischemia) combined with eccentric callosal hemorrhage. Traumatic subarachnoid hemorrhage (tSAH) in the basilar cisterns and adjacent to the falx are often visible. Small focal areas of low density on CT scans; these correspond to areas of edema occurring where shearing injury took place.

The following CT-scan criteria have been suggested by Wang [421] and colleagues: One or more small intra-parenchymal hemorrhages less than 2 cm in diameter, located in the cerebral hemispheres, intraventricular hemorrhage, hemorrhage in the corpus callosum, small focal areas of hemorrhage less than 2 cm in diameter, adjacent to the third ventricle and brainstem hemorrhage.

The classification of the findings of a CT scan performed within 24 h after the impact, proposed by Marshall [243]and colleagues (1991) is useful in identifying patients at risk for developing intracranial hypertension (see Sect. 1.1.4.2), and thereby identifying the need for continuous monitoring of the intracranial pressure (ICP).

Additional/useful diagnostic procedures

MRI is more sensitive in the detection of subtle soft-tissue abnormalities. Magnetic resonance tomography may demonstrate focal and diffuse lesions within the white matter and the brain stem, proofing the existents of DIA [166, 341] and may be in children an alternative to CT scanning (see Sect. 1.4.3).

Therapy

Conservative therapy
Recommended European Standard

Pure diffuse axonal injury does not produce mass lesions. Therefore, the therapy is conservative, consisting of neuromonitoring and treatment in the ICU aiming at the prevention of secondary damage to the brain (see Sect. 1.6).

Indications for conservative treatment: No concomitant mass lesions.

Useful additional therapeutic strategies

Repeat head CT after neurologic deterioration or inexplicable rise of ICP.

Prophylactic antiepileptic treatment is not warranted. There is insufficient proof for prophylactic antiepileptic treatment after an early seizure [420].

Surgical treatment
Recommended European Standard

Decompressive procedures, including subtemporal decompression, temporal lobectomy, and hemispheric decompressive craniectomy, are treatment options for patients with refractory intracranial hypertension and diffuse parenchymal injury with clinical and radiographic evidence for impending transtentorial herniation [50].

Differential Diagnosis

With concussion and ambiguous history any cause of loss of consciousness has to be considered.

Prognosis/Outcome

The prognosis of diffuse brain injury is dependent on the amount of anatomical tissue disruption:

- With concussion the prognosis is favorable,
- With severe DIA most patients either die or remain in a vegetative state.

The concern that decompressive craniectomy (DCE) may save life at the expense of increasing the number of patients in vegetative state and severe disability appears not to be founded by the literature [1, 305].

Surgical Principles

Decompressive craniectomy: An obvious way to convert the closed box surrounding the brain into an open box is to open the skull by a decompressive craniectomy (DCE), which has been performed for decades [139, 195, 201, 318]. Muench and colleagues [272] found that the mean volume gained by surgical decompression ranged from 15.9 to 348.4 cm^3 with a median volume of 73.6 cm^3. In subtemporal craniectomy without opening the dura Alexander [11] measured a gain of 30 cm^3 in volume. Examining the effects of the procedure on CT appearance, a decrease in midline shift and improved visibility of the mesencephalic cisterns was observed as a result of decompression [272].

The effect of DCE on outcome has not been established. There is, however, evidence that the operation does favorably influence intracranial pressure, intracranial volume, and midline shift and basal cisterns as a surrogate endpoint [168, 272, 424]. The guidelines established by the AANS [50] name DCE as the last of the second-tier therapeutic options. However, among second-tier measures, DCE leads to the fastest relief by immediate reduction of intracranial hypertension and has the lowest rate of complications (systemic side-effects) when compared with other medical options, notably barbiturates and hypothermia [74, 328, 329].

When discussing DCE, two entirely different situations have to be distinguished [411]:

- The *prophylactic* DCE during evacuation of a mass lesion, based on clinical signs (neurologic state, CT-scan, intraoperative swelling) instead of physiologic parameters.
- The *therapeutic* DCE
- When in patients not suffering from an evacuable mass lesion fatal pontine damage is already primarily present or
- When with protocol-driven management ICP becomes intractable.

Typically, therapeutic DCE is considered a last resort when staged application of medical interventions (including hypothermia and barbiturates) and ventricular CSF drainage have failed to control posttraumatic intracranial hypertension [145, 257, 276, 344] of over 30 mmHg when associated with a CPP of less than 70 mmHg, or when the ICP exceeded 35 mmHg irrespective of CPP [424].

Polin [87] and colleagues argue that once the ICP reaches a sustained level above 40 mmHg, the chance for intervention before permanent neurological devastation has passed.

Technique

The most favorable effect seems to result from large fronto-subtemporo-parieto-occipital craniectomies combined with enlargement of the dura (see Sect. 1.7.1.1). It is essential that the craniotomy extends down to the floor of the of middle cranial fossa. Canioplasty should be performed as earlier as edema has resolved [13, 202].

The removed bone flap can be frozen (Hutchinson 2004) or placed in the abdominal or thigh subcutaneous tissues [364] and put back as early as 5–8 weeks later [217].

The need for subsequent surgical bone replacement otherwise introduced by traditional decompressive craniectomy can be prevented by the hinge technique [134].

Intraoperative complications (see Sect. 1.7.1.4):

- Intraparenchymal hemorrhage
- Injury to the cerebral cortex, reactive cerebral edema, and brain herniation through the defect [114, 141]
- Injury to the sigmoid and/or superior sagittal sinuses (thrombosis).
- Severe bleeding (venous sinus; dural/cerebral arteries)
- Brain swelling

Postoperative complications (see Sect. 1.7.1.4):

- Delayed hemorrhage
- Venous sinus thrombosis
- Infection
- Hygroma; hydrocephalus [145, 312]
- Sinking scalp flap syndrome may develop, in which there is neurologic deterioration, thought to be related to the concavity of the skin flap and underlying brain tissue secondary to atmospheric pressure and also to the in-and-out displacement of the brain through the skull defect [343].
- Skull reconstruction itself is associated with infections and bone flap resorption after cranioplasty.

Special Remarks (see Sect. 1.1.2.6)

See Chap. 2.

1.7.2.4 Acute Epidural Hematoma (AEDH) (Fig. 1.CT-2)

Synonym: Extradural hematoma

Definition

An epidural hematoma (EDH), a type of intracranial hematoma, is a blood clot that develops between the skull and the dura.

Usually, EDH are classified based on the period that has elapsed from the inciting event (if known) to the diagnosis. When the inciting event is unknown, the appearance of the hematoma on CT scan or MRI can help determine when the hematoma occurred.

- Acute EDH (AEDH): exist since less than 72 h
- Subacute EDH (SEDH): exist since up to 2 to 3 weeks [304, 316]
- Chronic EDH/CEDH: exist longer than 3 weeks [46, 73, 421]

Epidemiology/Etiology

An epidural hematoma (EDH) usually develops after trauma – frequently after a blunt impact to the head from a fall, an assault or a traffic accident and is often

Fig. 1.CT-2 Typical CT appearance (native) of a left-sided temporoparietal located acute epidural hematoma: biconvex hyperdense extra-axial fluid collection with less dense parts indicating active hemorrhage and severe midline shift from left to right (subfalcial herniation)

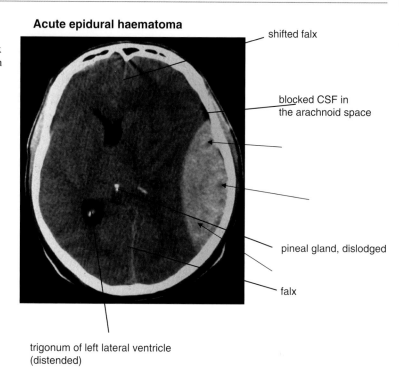

Acute epidural haematoma

shifted falx

blocked CSF in the arachnoid space

pineal gland, dislodged

falx

trigonum of left lateral ventricle (distended)

associated with an overlying skull fracture. In newborns forceps delivery and excessive skull molding through the birth canal have been implicated in EDH [304].

EDH is mainly caused by structural disruption of the dural and skull vessels. Laceration of the middle meningeal artery and its accompanying dural sinuses (diploic veins, middle meningeal veins) is the most common etiology [432]. As evidenced by radiologic examinations or by direct visualization at surgery [206], more than 90% of patients have at least one apparent skull bone fracture, whereas the fracture extremely seldom is localized contralateral to the AEDH.

In the posterior fossa, disruption of dural venous sinuses (such as transverse or sigmoid sinus) by fracture may lead to EDH. Disruption of the superior sagittal sinus may cause vertex EDH [316]. Other nonarterial sources of epidural hemorrhage include venous lakes (parasagittal, temporobasal), diploic veins, arachnoid granulations, and the petrosal sinuses (see Sect. 1.6.2.7).

More than 90% of epidural hematomas are unilateral and supratentorial, commonly occurring in the temporoparietal area. In the posterior fossa, epidural hematoma (PFEDH) are uncommon, but are the most common type of hematoma in this region [155] (see Sect. 1.7.2.7).

In severely injured or comatose patients, the incidence of AEDH may be as high as 9% [349]. Epidural

hematomas may be seen in any age group, least often in elderly where the adherence of the dura to the tabula interna is very strong [115].

Epidural hematomas are less likely to be associated with severe underlying brain injury than subdural hematomas: In about 25% of patients presenting EDH concomitant subdural hematomas, hemorrhagic contusions and hemisphere swelling [174] are diagnosed. Especially at risk are victims of a high-speed trauma [147].

Extradural hematoma is considered to be an acute complication of head injury whose maximum development takes place in the minutes following trauma. Delayed extradural hematoma - defined as an epidural hematoma that is not present in the first neuroradiologic examination made after trauma but that appears in sequential neuroradiologic examinations several hours later – is an infrequent complication that usually appears in hypotensive multiple trauma patients or is related to severe head injury with other intracranial lesions [89, 323].

Nontraumatic epidural hematoma is an extremely rare finding. The etiologies include infectious diseases of the skull, vascular malformations of the dura mater, and metastasis to the skull. Spontaneous EDH can also develop in patients with coagulopathies associated with other primary medical problems (such as end-stage liver disease, chronic alcoholism, other disease states associated with dysfunctional platelets) [33, 142].

Clinical Presentation/Symptoms

The clinical presentation depends on the amount of time elapsed since the injury, the rapidity of hematoma growth, and the presence of intradural lesions.

Some patients lose consciousness during the injury, regain it, and have a period of unimpaired mental function (lucid interval) before consciousness begins to deteriorate again when the mass effect of the hemorrhage itself results in increased intracranial pressure, a decreased level of consciousness, hemiparesis, and finally a herniation syndrome. This classic "lucid interval" occurs in 20–50% of patients with a EDH. Patients showing the classic "lucid interval" usually have "pure" EDH's with higher hematoma volumes and CT signs of active bleeding [206].

During the lucid interval, a scalp bruise or laceration may be the only but unmistakable hint at the suffered head injury. A severe headache may develop immediately or after several hours. The headache sometimes disappears but returns several hours later, worse than before. Deterioration in consciousness, including increasing confusion, sleepiness, paralysis, collapse, and a deep coma, can quickly follow.

Patients with direct onset of coma may present associated signs of diffuse axonal injury [174] due to high-speed trauma [352] and a significant proportion will have associated intradural lesions (subdural hematoma, intracerebral posttraumatic damage, and hemispheric swelling). In the comatose patient, the acute traumatic EDH is often lethal [349].

Complications

Missed or delayed diagnosis: Failure to diagnose an epidural hematoma is the single most disastrous complication leading to brainstem compression and even death. Allowing asymptomatic patients to become symptomatic: Mild head injury patients are at risk for poor outcome because of observed waiting for clinical deterioration before appropriate CT examination and referral to neurosurgical centers [222, 352]. Even when correctly detected, the volume and the mass effect may easily be underestimated: *Missed associated intracranial pathology* such as subdural hematomas and cortical lesions.

Seizures, metabolic derangement: In a series comprising 95 patients suffering from traumatic epidural hematoma, the overall incidence of late epilepsy was found to be 6%, but in group A (extradural hematoma with no evidence of intradural damage), the incidence was 2% and 17% in group B (an intradural abnormality in addition to the extradural hematoma [175]).

Children (aged <15 years) have a higher incidence of early posttraumatic epilepsy but a significantly lower incidence of late epilepsy than adults [18].

Diagnostic Procedures

Imaging: Computed tomography is the first choice. CT scan shows that EDH usually appears as a biconvex mass lesion with a higher density than the brain tissue adjacent to often visible fracture. The so-called "hyperacute" extradural hematoma displays "bubbles" iso- or hypodense within the hyperdense mass. The identification of lucent areas within the epidural hematoma suggests active bleeding [150]. This combination of different densities has been attributed to the coexistence of fresh blood, which has a low attenuation capacity, with clotted blood, a decrease in hematocrit, a mixture of blood with CSF due to dural tears, or a coagulation disorder [20]. Vertex epidural hematomas can be mistaken as artifact in traditional axial CT scan sections and is to be confirmed best by coronar and/or sagittal sections. In a patient with an evolving acute epidural hematoma, an ultra-early CT may be missed [365].
Recommended European Standard
Clinical assessment according to ATLS.

Imaging [401]: Both patients presenting with a GCS score of 14 points or less and patients presenting with a GCS score of 15 in the presence of risk factors are to be scanned. Helical computed tomography (three window-level settings without the use of intravenous iodinated contrast agents, reconstructions in three planes) should be obtained immediately after the patient is stabilized using standard advanced trauma life support (ATLS) guidelines (see Sect. 1.4.2).
Additional/useful diagnostic procedures

If a CT scanner is not available, skull roentgenograms are justified. If EDH is present, it is located practically always ipsilateral to the skull fracture.

Burr-hole exploration: Patients with early tentorial herniation or upper brain stem compression have a high incidence of immediate extraaxial hematomas and a low incidence of intracerebral hematomas. This is particularly true with patients over 30 years of age and those who suffer low-speed trauma, such as falls. Therefore, burr-hole exploration for the diagnosis of EDH (as SDH) should be done if CT scan is not readily available [15, 222, 279].

EDH enlargement occurs frequently, but early. When AEDH are managed conservatively, repeat imaging (CT) is most appropriate within 36 h after injury [385].

Therapy

Conservative treatment

Nonoperative management of lesions <1 cm thick appears to be a safe treatment option provided that there is close monitoring with immediate availability of repeat CT and neurosurgeons for emergent operation [87, 297].

Recommended European Standard

An EDH less than 30 cm³ *and* with less than a 15-mm thickness *and* with less than a 5-mm midline shift (MLS) in patients with a GCS score greater than 8 *without* focal deficit can be managed nonoperatively with serial computed tomographic (CT) scanning and close neurological observation in a neurosurgical center [48].

Useful additional therapeutic strategies

Repeat head CT after neurologic deterioration or inexplainable rise of ICP.

Surgical treatment

Recommended European Standard

An epidural hematoma (EDH) greater than 30 cm³ should be surgically evacuated regardless of the patient's Glasgow Coma Scale (GCS) score. It is strongly recommended that patients with an acute EDH in coma (GCS score <9) with anisocoria undergo surgical evacuation as soon as possible.

Perioperative antibiotic prophylaxis starts 60 min prior to incision. During prolonged procedures, antibiotic prophylaxis should be readministered every 3 h [292].

In patients who are not in coma at the time of hematoma removal, the degree of tightness or slackness of the brain serves as an index as to whether or not ICP monitoring is advisable [48].

Differential Diagnosis

Imaging features are characteristic.

Prognosis/Outcome

Prognosis is related to degree and duration of brain compression and consequently entirely depends on early diagnosis and subsequent hematoma evacuation. Mortality and morbidity could potentially approach zero if the patient is treated in a noncomatose condition. In patients unconscious at the time of operation, the mortality may be as high as 27% [43, 226, 327, 352]. In patients with an acute EDH, clot thickness, hematoma volume, and midline shift on the preoperative CT scan are related to outcome. In influencing outcome time from neurological deterioration, as defined by onset of coma, pupillary abnormalities, or neurological deterioration to surgery is more important than the time between trauma and surgery [48].

Surgical Principles

Adequate exposure to the hematoma and its bleeding source is paramount to successful evacuation. Basically are evacuated according the principles described with "Standard craniotomy." However, the procedure can be modified according to the actual condition of the patient (herniating, see below) and the location and dimension of the hematoma (see below AEDH parieto-occipital). As a rule, the size of the bone flap is slightly larger than dimension of the hematoma. The rare chronic EDH is evacuates as a chronic SDH (see Sect. 1.7.2.6)

Technique

The patient is placed supine on the operation table. The head – slightly elevated and slightly rotated to the contralateral side – is fixed in a rigid skull fixation device.

In a patient deteriorating rapidly or demonstrating evidence of brain stem compression, a subtemporal craniectomy is performed through a low temporal burr-hole allowing a rapid partial evacuation of the clot (See Sect. 1.7.1.1 Standard Craniotomy – *Immediate subtemporal decompression*). Coagula gushing out of the craniectomy are aspirated. This will alleviate some of the pressure on the brain stem.

Acute epidural haematoma: evacuation of coagula

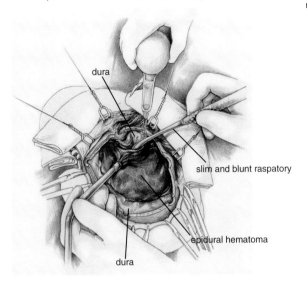

Fig. 1.17 Acute epidural hematoma: evacuation of coagula

Epidural haematoma: coagula evacuated, situation before replacement of the bone flap

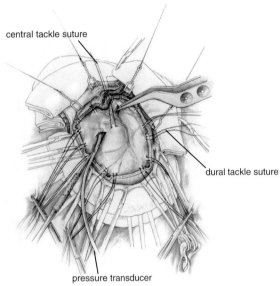

Fig. 1.18 Epidural hematoma: coagula evacuated, situation before replacement of the bone flap

Afterwards, a regular craniotomy is performed that will expose the entire extradural hematoma. The remaining epidural clots are mobilized gently with the help of a blunt small raspatory and removed then by suction and irrigation with a bulb syringe (Fig. 1.17). The dural bleeding sites are secured by bipolar coagulation. If the hematoma spread out widely and if there is a bleeding from underneath the adjacent bony rim, the craniotomy must be extended. Eventually, the middle meningeal artery has to be coagulated at its exit from the foramen spinosum at the bottom of the middle fossa or the foramen spinosum is packed with bone wax. Complete hemostasis is mandatory even if a suction drain is used to obliterate the epidural space. Packing with hemostatic material is insufficient.

Dural tenting sutures are placed in short intervals along the bony edges. Special attention is to give not to damage the underlying cortex, especially in the region of the pterion/spenoid ridge.

Before securing the bone flap in place, the dura can be opened for about 1 cm to rule out the existence of a concomitant subdural hematoma. This opening is mandatory, if the dura appears tight, blue, and without pulsation. When an acute SDH or severe contusions are detected, the procedure continues according to "Subdural Hematoma" and "Intraparenchymal hemorrhage," respectively. With regular findings, this incision is to be

closed in a water-tight fashion to prevent CSF leaking and a central dural tacking suture is placed (Fig. 1.18).

The decision to install an ICP probe depends on both the preoperative condition of the patient/preoperative CT findings and the intraoperative findings.

After bone is fixed, the central tack-suture and the temporal muscle are attached to the bone and a subgaleal suction drain is inserted before galea and skin is closed in anatomic layers.

Acute Epidural hematoma parieto-occipital

With an AEDH in the parieto-occipital region, the patient is placed in prone position or in reclining park bench position. The head is fixed as shown in Fig. 1.19, the external occipital protuberance being the highest point or is positioned on the donut or the horseshoe (allowing lifting and rotating of the head during the procedure). If face down position is for any reason impossible, the extreme three quarter lateral variant of the lateral orientation is useful. If the hematoma lies over the superior sagittal sinus (SSS), the craniotomy crosses the sagittal suture (Fig. 1.20): two burr-holes should be placed within 1 cm on either side of the midline. Following careful separation of the underlying dura, the craniotome can be used to cut across the midline with minimal risk. Frequently, the SSS and the confluens sinuum are located out of the midline as

Fig. 1.19 Parieto-occipital craniotomy: prone position, fixation of the head

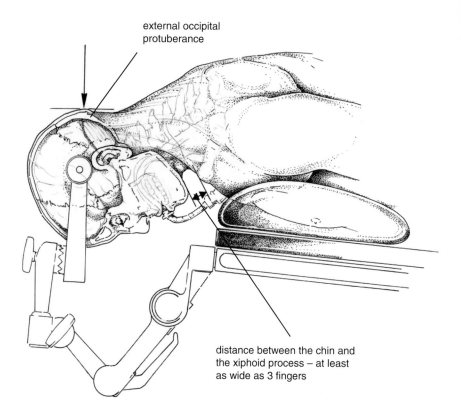

Parieto-occipital craniotomy: prone position, fixation of the head.

external occipital protuberance

distance between the chin and the xiphoid process – at least as wide as 3 fingers

may be realized by assessing the preoperative CT scans. The burr-holes are to be placed accordingly (Fig. 1.20).

The dura overlaying the SSS (or transverse sinus) is freed only when the sew cuts not crossing the sinus are done. The bone over the sinus is cut as the final step. This allows rapid removal of the bone flap and control of venous bleeding should the sinus be lacerated.

In the parasagittal region, the coagula are freed from the dura gently to avoid laceration of the SSS or the venous lacunas lateral of the SSS.

Venous bleeding from a sinus is difficult to control. To prevent widening of the bleeding source, bipolar coagulation is not used. Instead, the leak is covered with a piece of muscle that will be sutured or stricken to the dura (Fig. 1.21) before the head is elevated slightly to lower the pressure within the sinus (risk of air embolism). Not all the SSS should be occluded in its posterior two thirds. In contrast, one of the transverse sinuses can be ligated if not the main drainage of the SSS.

If the subdural space has to be explored, the dura is opened by creating a flap based on the SSS. When closing the dura, no tack-sutures are applied in the parasagittal region.

Installing an ICP probe and closing the wound is done according to "Standard Craniotomy."

Intraoperative complications (see Sect. 1.7.1.4):

- Acute swelling of the brain
- Acute bleeding (arterial or venous), provoked by decompression or coagulopathy.
- Increase in volume of an additional traumatic intracranial (ipsi- or contralateral) hematoma.
- Air embolism

Postoperative complications (see Sect. 1.7.1.4):

- Elevated intracranial pressure (mostly in compound brain injuries, seldom in pure EDH only)
- Delayed appearance of intracranial hematoma [113]
- Reaccumulation of blood in the epidural space
- Central nervous system infection

Fig. 1.20 Occipital craniotomy (prone position)

Occipital craniotomy (prone position)

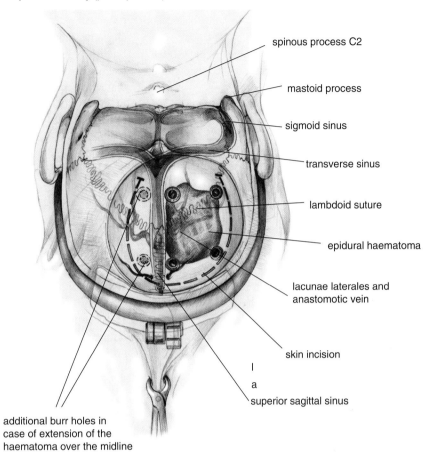

- spinous process C2
- mastoid process
- sigmoid sinus
- transverse sinus
- lambdoid suture
- epidural haematoma
- lacunae laterales and anastomotic vein
- skin incision
- l
- a
- superior sagittal sinus

additional burr holes in case of extension of the haematoma over the midline

Special Remarks

Type of anesthesia

Acute epidural hematomas are evacuated in inhalation/intravenous anesthesia. In patients experiencing rapid deterioration, operation can be begun with local anesthesia and completed using general anesthesia.

1.7.2.5 Acute Subdural Hematoma (aSDH) (Fig. 1.CT-3)

Synonym: Subdural hematoma, Subdural hemorrhage
Definition

Subdural hematoma (SDH), a type of intracranial hematoma, is a blood clot that develops between the dura and the brain.

Usually, SDHs are classified based on the period that has elapsed from the inciting event (if known) to the diagnosis. When the inciting event is unknown, the appearance of the hematoma on CT scan or MRI can help determine when the hematoma occurred.

- Acute SDH: exists less than 72 h
- Subacute SDH: exists since up to 2 weeks
- Chronic SDH: exists longer than 2 to 3 weeks (see Sect. Chronic Subdural Hematoma)

These three types of SDH are not only different in time course, but also in pathogenesis, epidemiology, clinical presentation, and outcome [255].
Etiology/epidemiology

ASDH are of the most lethal of all intracranial injuries. Combining several publications, acute SDH was diagnosed in 11% of patients suffering mild, moderate, and severe head injuries TBI, in patients suffering severe TBI in 21%. The mean age for this combined group is between 31 and 47 years, with the vast majority of patients being men [49].

Mostly, ASDH is caused by motor vehicle-related accidents (MVA), falls, and assaults. In the younger age group (18–40 year), ASDH are caused by MVA 56%, in the older groups (>65 year) the identical percentage by falls [164]. In the pediatric group, child abuse or shaken baby syndrome has to be considered. Studies with comatose patients describe MVA as the mechanism of injury in 53–75% of SDH, indicating that MVA causes more severe injury, possibly because of high-velocity accidents and diffuse axonal injury [199, 348, 428]. Very often, ASDHs are associated by traumatic subarachnoidal hemorrhage (tSAH), ipsi- or contralateral contusions and intracerebral hemorrhage.

The hematoma develops either from damaged cortical vessels located in a contusioned territory or from torn veins that bridge from the brain surface to the dura. The same forces that act to shear the bridging veins also may act to shear underlying nerves within the brain. Therefore, acute SDH is often a marker of diffuse TBI. Usually, ASDH are located over the convexity, less often underneath the frontal and temporal lobe, and seldom interhemispheric. Interhemispheric SDHs compress the ipsilateral lateral ventricle and are frequently associated with adjacent parenchymal lesions [225].

The sequelae of ASDH are caused mostly by ischemic damage to the brain. Rather than a direct effect of the hematoma on the underlying brain, ischemia is the consequence of arterial compression secondary to brain shift and brain herniation. Major vascular impairment occur with herniation across the falx compromising flow within one or both anterior cerebral

Occipital craniotomy: Torn superior sagittal sinus: haemostasis

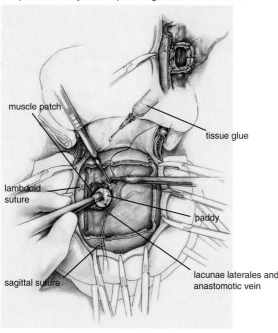

Fig. 1.21 Occipital craniotomy: Torn superior sagittal sinus: hemostasis

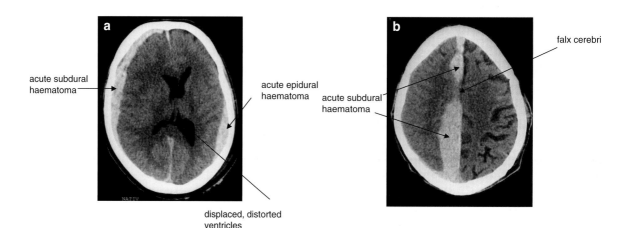

Fig. 1.CT-3 (**a**) Typical CT appearance (native) of a right-sided acute subdural hematoma: hyperintense crescent-shaped collection along the convexity with a sharp margin between the collection and adjacent brain. Acute epidural hematoma on the opposite side. Midline shift from right to left. (**b**) Acute interhemispheric subdural hematoma on the left side, marked compression in the left hemisphere

vessels and across the tentorium compromising flow within one or both posterior cerebral arteries. Other common injury sites occur where the blood supply from perforating vessels is compromised by brain shifting [2, 184].

More benign forms of SDH may result as the brain atrophies with age. The bridging veins become significantly stretched and shear with a very minor force. These types of hematomas are known as subacute and chronic SDH, respectively (see Sect. Chronic SDH). Traumatic chronic SDH in younger people are seldom, except with coagulopathy or medical anticoagulation.

Nontraumatic intradural hemorrhages may arise related to coagulopathies, cerebral aneurysm, arteriovenous malformation, hemodialysis, or tumor (meningioma or dural metastases).

Clinical presentation/symptoms

The clinical course is determined by the severity of the lesions and the rate of the extension of the hematoma, while the actual clinical presentation depends on the localization and size of the hematoma and on the degree of any associated parenchymal brain injury. Any patient suffering from acute SDH may present with a coma or with severe confusion. Some patients remain conscious before then deterring as the hematoma expands.

Neurological findings associated with acute SDH may include the following:

- Altered level of consciousness
- A dilated or nonreactive pupil ipsilateral to the hematoma (or earlier: a pupil with a more limited range of reaction)
- Hemiparesis, mostly contralateral to the site of the hematoma.
- Coma with a dilated fixed pupil usually indicates unilateral transtentorial herniation.

Less commonly, the hemiparesis may be ipsilateral to the hematoma and to the dilated pupil (the "Kernohan's notch phenomenon") [434]. This is possibly due to direct parenchymal injury or compression of the cerebral peduncle contralateral to the hematoma against the edge of the tentorium cerebelli during transtentorial herniation. Therefore, if the findings are conflicting, the most reliable indicator (by examination) of the side of the hematoma is a dilated or nonreactive pupil, which appears on the same side as the hematoma.

Subacute SDHs may present by simple headache or mild confusion often combined with a hemiparesis.

Complications

- Delay of surgery: Haselsberger et al. [13] studied the time interval from onset of coma to surgery in 111 patients with SDH. Thirty-four patients were operated on within 2 h after the onset of coma. Of those patients, 47% died and 32% recovered with good outcome or moderate disability. However, 54 patients who underwent surgery longer than 2 h after the onset of coma had a mortality of 80% and only 4% had a favorable outcome [153].
- Cerebral swelling: Acute SDHs are commonly associated with parenchymal brain injury. The consequence is cerebral swelling causing rise in ICP and ischemic damage of the brain, respectively. Arterial compression secondary to the brain shift and brain herniation is one of the most important factors determining the outcome with ASDH [2].
- Evolving contusions: Patients with traumatic subarachnoid hemorrhage (tSAH) on early CT are those at the highest risk for associated evolving contusions [355].
- Posttraumatic seizures: The amount of focal tissue destruction visible on CT is the most important factor in predicting the development of late posttraumatic seizure [98, 398].

Diagnostic Procedures

Imaging: Computed tomography is the first choice.

An ASDH appears on the noncontrast head CT scan as a crescent-shaped hyperdense (with the brain tissue) area between the inner table of the skull and the surface of the cerebral hemisphere, usually unilateral [314]. An ASDH may also be located along the falx (interhemispheric). Lens-shaped ASDH are rare findings. All or part of an ASDH may appear hypodense or isodense to brain if the patient's hematocrit is low, if the clot is hyperacute (e.g., <1-h old), if the subdural space contains active bleeding, if coagulopathy is present, or if the CSF if creating a dilutional effect.

Early (within 3 h from injury) CT underestimates the ultimate size of parenchymal contusions: associated parenchymal damage is demonstrated in about 25% while CT scans repeated in the following day showed additional parenchymal lesions in 50%[355].

Subacute SDHs are isodense or hypodense compared with the brain. Detection of an isodense SDH may require a high index of suspicion; subtle changes in the appearance or position of the cortical sulci may be found. A small ASDH may be difficult to appreciate because of the appearance of the overlying skull. Use of the bone window setting may aid in discrimination [347, 406].

Recommended European Standard

Clinical assessment according to ATLS. Imaging: Acute stage – Both patients presenting with a GCS score of 14 points or less and patients presenting with a GCS score of 15 in the presence of risk factors are to be scanned (see Sect. Computed tomography, [401]). The CT scan – in three window-level settings without the use of intravenous iodinated contrast agents – should be obtained immediately after the patient is stabilized using standard advanced trauma life-support (ATLS) guidelines.

Imaging follow-up: If elevated ICP is an issue postoperatively, an urgent CT scan should be obtained to look for a new intracranial mass lesion or reaccumulation of the SDH. Hematoma resolution should be documented with serial imaging because an acute SDH that is treated conservatively can evolve into a chronic SDH. For serial imaging, MRI may be more sensitive.

Additional/useful diagnostic procedures

MRI may help to better define isodense lesion. These may be either hypointense or hyperintense on T2-weighted MRI [429].

Therapy

Conservative treatment

Interhemispheric subdural hematomas often resolve without surgery [225].

Recommended European Standard [49]

Patients who present in a coma (GCS > 9) but with an SDH with a thickness less than 10 mm and an MLS less than 5 mm be treated conservatively, provided that they undergo ICP monitoring, they are neurologically stable since the injury, they have no pupillary abnormalities, and they have no intracranial hypertension (ICP < 20 mmHg).

Useful additional therapeutic strategies

Repeat head CT after neurologic deterioration or inexplainable rise of ICP.

Surgical treatment

Recommended European Standard [49]

An acute SDH with a thickness greater than 10 mm *or* a midline shift greater than 5 mm on computed tomo-

graphic (CT) scan should be surgically evacuated, regardless of the patient's Glasgow Coma Scale (GCS) score.

A comatose patient (GCS score less than 9) with an ASDH less than 10-mm thick and a midline shift less than 5 mm should undergo surgical evacuation of the lesion if the GCS score decreased between the time of injury and hospital admission by 2 or more points in the GCS and/or the patient presents with asymmetric or fixed and dilated pupils and/or the ICP exceeds 20 mmHg.

In patients with ASDH and indications for surgery, surgical evacuation should be performed as soon as possible.

Perioperative antibiotic prophylaxis starts 60 min prior to incision. During prolonged procedures, antibiotic prophylaxis should be readministered every 3 h [292]. All patients with ASDH in coma (GCS score less than 9) should undergo intracranial pressure (ICP) monitoring.

Differential Diagnosis

Acute epidural hematoma

Prognosis/Outcome

Clinical factors related to prognosis are age, presence of hypoxia/hypotension, presenting neurologic condition (GCS motor score and pupillary abnormalities), and elevated postoperative ICP greater than 45 mmHg [199, 355, 426]. The length of the time interval from onset of coma to surgery is strongly related to outcome [153].

Individuals with SDH that required evacuation showed a 27.8% cumulative probability of developing late posttraumatic seizure within 24 months after injury. Those individuals with nonevacuated SDH had a cumulative probability of 15.3%, whereas those with no SDH had a cumulative probability of 9.5% of developing late posttraumatic seizure [98].

Besides GCS, the most important factor affecting outcome seems to be the extent of primary brain injury underlying the subdural hematoma. CT findings on admission that correlated with outcome were hematoma thickness (>10 mm), midline shift (>5 mm), and status of the basal cisterns (absent). Prognosis was also worsened by the presence of associated lesions; brain contusion is the single most powerful predictor of worse outcome [164, 247, 355, 436].

Surgical Principles

If surgical evacuation of an acute SDH in a comatose patient (GCS < 9) is indicated, it should be performed using a craniotomy with or without bone flap removal and duraplasty [49].

In patients presenting a very tight brain after the standard craniotomy exposure, the dura may be opened in a mesh-like fashion rather than opening regularly. The clot can then be removed through the small dural openings [146].

Subacute SDH may be evacuated often via a limited craniotomy centered over the hematoma.

Technique

Acute SDH are evacuated in general anesthesia. Positioning, fixation of the head, and craniotomy is described in "Standard craniotomy." It is important to perform a large craniotomy providing exposure to view both the parasagittal area with the bridging veins and the floor of the frontal and middle fossa. The procedure is performed using an operating microscope or surgical loopes combined with a head lamp.

With signs of an impending herniation, the procedure is started with a small temporal osteoclastic craniectomy (Fig. 1.23). While the dura is opened, coagula are gushing out of the subdural space. With help of a suction device and gentle irrigation with a bulb syringe, the clots are lifted off the pial surface and then aspirated. Thereby, attention is given not to injure an already compromised cerebral cortex.

The procedure is continued then according to Sect. 1.7.1.1.

The frontal lobe is carefully lifted with a broad brain spatula (fixed on a retractor) allowing both controlled removal of frontobasal coagula and inspection of the frontobasal cortex, which is contusioned often. Thereafter, the temporal lobe is cleared in the same way whereby taking care of the basal bridging veins (Fig. 1.22). The temporal and frontal tips often contain contusions that should be resected (see Sect. 1.7.2.8).

Solid portions of the clot can be lifted with round broad grasping cup forceps. Small remnants of hematoma under the parasagittal dura should not be pursued at the expense of additional damaging of the brain. During the surgical evacuation, the sites of bleeding

Acute subdural haematoma: evacuation

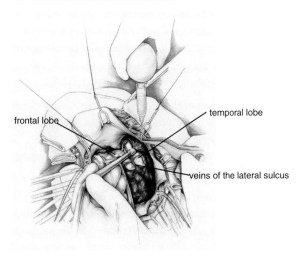

Fig. 1.22 Acute subdural hematoma: evacuation

Temporal burr hole enlarged osteoclastically

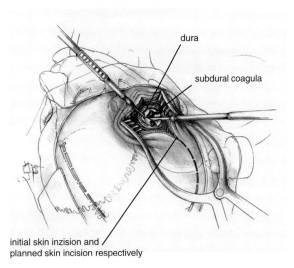

Fig. 1.23 Temporal burr-hole enlarged osteoclastically

are to be identified and controlled by cautiously used bipolar tangential coagulation of bleeding points on injured vessels, at most by covering with absorbable cellulose (e.g., Surgicel). Bridging veins torn and bleeding into the subdural space can be identified close to the midline or at the base. A leak in a sinus (superior sagittal sinus, sphenoparietal sinus) can be controlled by placing a piece of beaten temporalis muscle on the wall of the sinus. Surgicel should be used sparingly.

A ventricular catheter or a parenchymal ICP monitor strain gauge is installed, then the dura is tacked and closed water-tight using grafts. Usually, the bone flap is not replaced in acute SDH. Closure of soft tissues is according to "Standard Craniotomy."

Remark: CT within 24 h following the craniotomy is mandatory

Intraoperative complications (see Sect. 1.7.1.4):

- Acute swelling of the brain
- Acute bleeding (arterial or venous), provoked by decompression or coagulopathy
- Increase in volume of an additional traumatic intracranial (ipsi- or contralateral) hematoma [250]

Postoperative complications (see Sect. 1.7.1.4):

Cerebral edema; Evolving contusion/delayed intracranial hematoma [355]. Recurrence of SDH; intracranial hypertension; CSDH; hygroma; posttraumatic hydrocephalus; postoperative central nervous system infection; posttraumatic traumatic seizures (see Sect. 1.7.1.4)

Special Remarks

Type of anesthesia

Acute subdural hematomas are evacuated in inhalation/intravenous anesthesia. In patients experiencing rapid deterioration, operation can be begun with local anesthesia and completed using general anesthesia.

1.7.2.6 Chronic Subdural Hematoma (CSDH) (Fig. 1.CT-5)

Synonym: Subdural hemorrhage – chronic; Subdural hematoma – chronic; Pachymeningitis haemorrhagica interna

Definition

Traumatic chronic subdural hematoma (CSDH) applies to those subdural hematomas that present over 20 days after injury. As acute SDH, CSDH are positioned in the virtual space between the dura mater and the arachnoidea over the cortex. Contrary to ASDH, CSDHs are surrounded by a (neo)membrane.

Etiology/epidemiology

Chronic subdural hematoma is one of the most common types of intracranial hemorrhage and is a typical disease of elderly patients, predominately men. In this age group, brain atrophy and decreasing brain volume allow greater movements of the brain and causes stretching of veins, bridging between dural venous sinuses and cerebral cortex. Additionally, older people are predisposed to trivial trauma [21, 24, 207, 268].

In the absence of risk factors as alcoholism, chronic substance abuse, anticoagulant or antithrombotic medications, and middle fossa cysts [424], CSDH are uncommon in patients younger than 40 years.

CSDH result mostly from a relatively mild head trauma (often a consequence of falls or a bump against the head) causing tear and rupture of bridging veins. As a rule, this trivial trauma happened some weeks ago and is often not long remembered by the patient. CSDH probably start out as small traumatic subdural effusion. Contrary to acute SDH, CSDH are seldom associated with relevant underlying parenchymal injury. With time, these small hematomas will be encapsulated in neomembranes of which the membrane adjacent to the dura contains strong sinusoidal capillary channels and sticks together with the dura. In contrast, the membrane abutting the arachnoidea is scarcely vascularized. Exudation from the macrocapillaries in the outer membrane of chronic SDH plays an important role in their enlargement [405]. Long-lasting CSDH may be partitioned and contain liquid blood in different grades of degradation or may be organized (granulation tissue gradually replaces the clot) hematomas. Very seldom CSDHs calcify [101, 228, 268]. Mostly, CSDH extend over the whole hemisphere with the mass center frontoparietal, in about 14% bilateral [203].

Clinical presentation/symptoms

Generally, CSDH evolve slowly causing symptoms starting several weeks after an initial minor head injury: Gait disturbance, headache, dementia, incontinence, slowing of cognitive processing, disturbance of memory, and mild to moderate focal signs such as hemiparesis. Mostly, the hemiparesis arises contralaterally to the location of the CSDH; however, ipsilateral symptoms may arise (see Sect. 1.7.2.4, *Kernohan sign*). More significant disorders emerge with increase in size caused by recurrent hemorrhages into the encapsulated hematoma. Thereby, an unexpected sudden deterioration with signs of impending transtentorial herniation may arrive [268].

Complications

Repeated hemorrhage. Herniation, causing sudden deterioration, especially in bilateral CSDH [203].

Epileptic seizures: Seldom patients present with epileptic fits before surgery. The overall incidence of

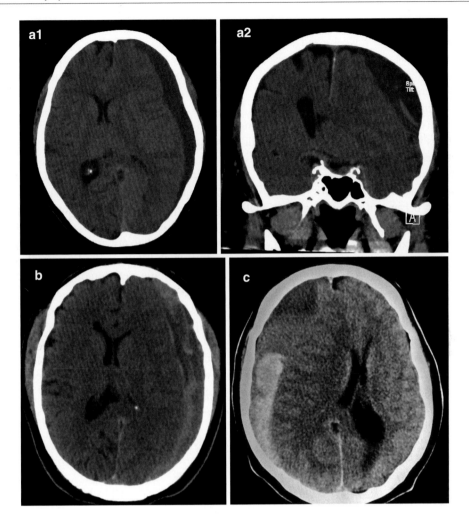

Fig. 1.CT-5 (**a**) Typical chronic SDH (**a1** axial, **a2** coronar) appearing homogeneously hypodense relative to gray matter; ventricular displacement and distortion. (**b**) Left-sided chronic SDH with membranes producing multiple compartments having different attenuation characteristics, marked ventricular displacement. (**c**) Right-sided chronic SDH after repeated hemorrhages, marked ventricular displacement, and distortion (left ventricle compressed, right ventricle distended) (left foramen of Munro blocked). *1*, hypodense layer in the less dependent position; *2*, hyperdense component in the dependent position; *3*, fresh hemorrhage

postoperative epilepsy amounts to about 7% [198, 336].

Diagnostic Procedures

Imaging: Computed tomography is the first choice. Imaging in three planes facilitates appropriate positioning of burr-holes (see Sect. 1.4.2).

CT demonstrates chronic SDH mostly as [347] a crescent-shaped and hypodense formation between the inner table of the skull and the surface of the cerebral hemisphere. Typical signs of mass effect, such as midline shift and ventricular compression, may be observed. On a contrast-enhanced CT scan, the chronic SDH membrane enhances to varying degrees, depending on numerous factors. In an early stage, CT demonstrates CSDH as isodense, which may relay on its mass effect (compression of ventricular system, midline shift) only. Bilateral isodense CSDH may be misdiagnosed easily. With recurrent bleeding, CSDH appears as a heterogeneously dense lesion with a fluid level between the acute (hyperdense) and chronic (hypodense) components of the hematoma.

Postoperatively, CT may not show resolution of a subdural hematoma before 3 weeks and sometimes collections may persist even long before resolving completely.

Recommended European Standard

Clinical assessment according to ATLS.

Imaging: Helical computed tomography (three window-level settings without the use of intravenous iodinated contrast agents, reconstructions in three planes) is the method of choice.

Additional/useful diagnostic procedures

When CT scans because of isodensity of the CSDH are difficult to interpret, magnetic resonance imaging is especially useful [94].

Therapy

Conservative Treatment

Recommended European Standard

In patients with significant brain atrophy, it has to be decided whether or not the fluid collection is causing the patient's symptoms. In patients who have no significant mass effect on imaging studies and no neurological symptoms or signs except mild headache, the follow-up may be observed with serial scans.

Useful additional therapeutic strategies

Whenever possible, iatrogenic anticoagulation should be reversed. However, hematoma resolution cannot be reliably predicted, and no medical therapy (say steroids) has been shown to be effective in expediting the resolution of acute or chronic SDHs [28, 386].

Surgical treatment

Recommended European Standard

The prevailing neurosurgical opinion is that symptomatic patients are best managed with operation, common procedure is burr-hole evacuation followed by drainage. This surgical procedure can be carried out safely, also under local anesthesia [423]. However, in confused patients, general anesthesia is preferable.

Evacuation of CSDH is indicated in patients showing

- Symptoms as focal deficits and/or mental changes
- CT: maximal thickness >10 mm, especially with bilateral CSDH [203].

Signs of beginning herniation indicate an emergency procedure. Perioperative antibiotic prophylaxis starts 60 min prior to incision. During prolonged procedures, antibiotic prophylaxis should be readministered every 3 h [292].

Differential Diagnosis

CSDH are to be differentiated from brain atrophy, and from traumatic subdural hygroma, respectively [207], and from arachnoid cyst, respectively [431].

Prognosis/Outcome

About 90% of patients with CSDH (89%) recover after burr-hole craniostomy with closed system drainage. Age, systemic complications as cardiovascular disease in elderly patients, coagulopathy, and poor preoperative state are contributory causes of postoperative death [268]. Early diagnosis before a significant neurologic deterioration may correlate with a more favorable prognosis [99, 237]. After reaccumulation, a secondary evacuation is successful in about 95% [372].

If the patient was on anticoagulation therapy preoperatively, the risks and benefits of anticoagulation must be weighed against the risks of rebleeding to determine when to restart therapy.

Surgical Principles

Technique

The three principal techniques - twist drill craniostomy, burr-hole craniostomy, and craniotomy – used in contemporary neurosurgery for chronic subdural hematoma have different profiles for morbidity, mortality, recurrence rate, and cure rate. Twist drill and burr-hole craniostomy can be considered as first-tier treatment [423]. In adults, CSDHs are evacuated and flushed via a single- or two burr-hole craniostomy frequently followed by closed-system drainage. The choice of technique, either burr-hole or twist drill, is largely a matter of preference. Craniotomy may be used as a second-tier treatment [423].

Surgery

Burr-hole craniostomy followed by closed-system drainage: Positioning, accomplishment of burr–holes, and opening of the dura is done as described related to "1.7.1.2 Burr-hole exploration." With bilateral cSDHs and when local anesthesia is used, skull will not be fixed.

The number of burr-holes depends of the CT findings. With two or more burr-holes evacuation, irrigation and inspection of the cavity is facilitated, especially if the cavity is loculated. The primary burr-hole is positioned over the thickest portion of the hematoma or slightly posterior, the second burr-hole in the midpupillary line anterior to the coronal suture. Scalp incisions are positioned best on an imaginative (Fig. 1.24) question mark incision required for a craniotomy.

The dura and the outer membrane are opened with a small incision. To prevent a rapid decrease of the ICP provoking intraparenchymal hemorrhage eventually, the outflow rate of the auburn chronic subdural fluid has to be done with the help of a small cotton pad. As soon as spontaneous outflow has stopped, the edges of the dura and membrane are coagulated for hemostasis and to shrink them back in order to widen the exposure (Fig. 1.25). Then, the subdural cavity is irrigated with large amounts of isotonic saline as long as the irrigation return is clear. The need of opening the inner membrane is judged inconsistent, with underlying

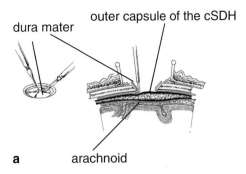

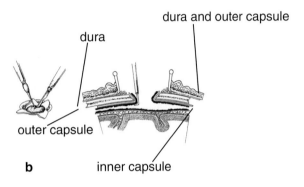

Fig. 1.25 (**a, b**) Chronic subdural hematoma: schematical illustration of the meningeal layers and the membranes

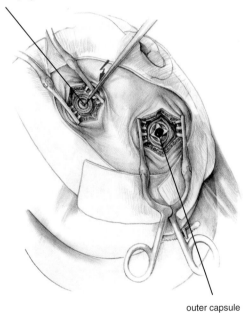

Chronic subdural haematoma: evacuation: incision of the dura

dura mater discoloured bluely as a consequence of the underlying cSDH

outer capsule of the cSDH

Fig. 1.24 Chronic subdural hematoma: evacuation: incision of the dura

fluid collection the internal capsule of the hematoma may be sharply fissured [118].

Provided that the brain does not expand rapidly, the tip of a pediatric feeding tube or a ventriculostomy catheter, controlled by means of forceps, is pushed gently forward into the cavity, less than 5 cm is sufficient. To minimize the risk of penetrating the cerebral cortex by the tip of the tube, a small portion of the outer lip of the burr-hole has been is drilled away. By this, the curve of the drain is less acute where it enters the burr-hole. The proximal drain is brought out through a separate incision and sutured to the skin before the incisions are closed in two layers and the drain is connected to a urine collection bag.

The drainage bag is placed about 20 cm below the level of the burr-hole (on the mattress) monitored along with the patient's neurological condition.

The patient has to stay in the supine position (even while being nursed) until the drain is removed on the second or third day. A CT scan is performed routinely before moving the drain, of course earlier if the patient deteriorates.

Intraoperative complications (see Sect. 1.7.1.4):

The worst complications is to trigger

- An acute intraparenchymal hemorrhage, possibly a consequence of re-expansion or arterial hypertension [267, 268] or intraparenchymal penetration of the drain.
- An acute SDH caused by bleeding from injury to bridging veins or from the scalp into the evacuated subdural space.

Postoperative complications (see Sect. 1.7.1.4):

- Reaccumulation and residual hematoma, respectively, has been found on 92% of postoperative CT scans within 4 days of operation; however, clinical improvement may proceed regardless of the size of this collection [278]. The lack of expansion of the brain may correspond with the peculiarity of the subdural neomembranes [237].
- The rate of recurrence of CSDH demanding re-evacuation is about 15%, whereby cranial base CSDHs have a higher rate than convexity CSDH [99, 278, 372]. In contrast, postoperative tension pneumocephalon [171] is a rare complication. Air under tension is released by needle puncture of the subdural space through the frontal burr-hole.
- After operative drainage of a chronic SDH, the rate of infection – empyema, brain abscess, and meningitis – is reported to be up to 2% [237].
- Postoperative seizures have been reported in 4–18% of patients (Chen Sabo). Whether prophylactic anticonvulsants therapy can decrease this risk is debatable. In these patients (60, 198), as with acute SDH,

serial neurological examinations are used and coagulation parameters may need to be followed. Serial CT scans are used to document the resolution of the chronic SDH.

Special Remarks

If the patient is either oriented clearly or comatose, the procedure can be done with local anesthesia, with poorly cooperative patients monitored sedation by an anesthesiologist is recommended strongly.

1.7.2.7 Traumatic Hematomas of the Posterior Fossa (Fig. 1.CT-4)

Synonym: None
Definition

Posterior fossa traumatic hematoma – epidural (PFEDH), subdural (PFSDH), and intracerebral (PFICH) – are hematomas within the narrow subtentorial space.
Etiology/epidemiology

In the posterior fossa, traumatically induced hematomas are considerably less frequent than in the supratentorial space and commonly unilateral.

The most common type [30, 34] are extradural hematomas, more often in children [157] than in adults (mostly males). The majority of posterior fossa epidural hematomas (PFEDH) is combined with a skull fracture

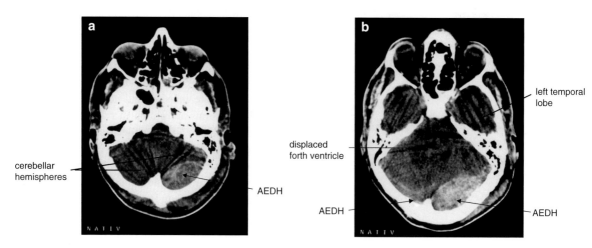

Fig. 1.CT-4 Axial computed tomography, native. (**a**, **b**) Acute bilateral epidural hematoma (AEDH) of the posterior fossa. As a consequence of a coagulation disorder, the hematoma shows hypo- and hyperdense segments. The fourth ventricle is displaced. The hematoma extends to the opposite side (b).

and is often associated with supratentorial lesions. Often, PFEDHs reach across the transverse or sigmoid sinus up over the occipital pole (as parieto-occipital hematomas may spread out over the cerebellum). Source of bleeding are tears of the outer wall of the transverse or sigmoid sinus and torcular herophili, respectively, or hemorrhage from the fractured bone (diploic bleeding). Acute course (signs of medullary compression within 24 h) occurs in about 50% of PFEDH affected people, subacute course (symptoms and signs within 2–7 days of injury) in about 40% [30].

Both subdural hematoma and intracerebellar (d'Avella) hemorrhagic contusions/hematomas are not frequent in the posterior fossa [35, 84, 163].

Patients with midline hemorrhage tend to have a rapid course because of earlier ventricular obstruction and brain stem compression. Traumatic hemorrhagic cerebellar contusions are prone to increase in size and evolve into intraparenchymal hematomas.

Clinical presentation/symptoms

Inspection reveals scalp hematomas, abrasions, lacerations, or an open skull fracture.

Clinical manifestations (signs and symptoms) were frequently nonspecific [34]. Cerebellar signs and the palsy of one or several cranial nerves (VII, IX, X, XI, XII) seldom are prominent [30]. If typical, occipital trauma is associated with severe nuchal and/or occipital pain, marked alteration in the state of consciousness, and, occasionally, a lucid interval. This is followed within hours of injury by rapid brainstem compression, with respiratory depression and death if not treated promptly. Ipsilateral mydriasis is frequent and may be explained by the upward herniation of the cerebellum through the tentorial hiatus deforming and compressing the oculomotor nerve.

Delayed PFEDH often gives rise to headache and neck pain as well as symptoms of a posterior fossa lesion, including lower cranial nerve dysfunction and cerebellar signs. Concurrent systemic traumatic lesions leading to a hypotensive state and intracranial traumatic lesions with associated increased ICP have been classically identified as mechanisms responsible for the development of delayed PFEDH.

On clinical grounds alone PFSDH cannot be distinguished from PFEDH or PFICH.

Complications

Patient suffering from posterior fossa hematoma often present contrecoup lesions in the frontal or temporal region. Progressive enlargement of traumatic intracerebellar hemorrhagic contusions may develop in previously contused areas, but hematomas also may develop in brain areas that appear normal on first CT scans [84].

Mass lesions within the narrow subtentorial space are prone

- To compress the brainstem, the fourth ventricle, and the aqueduct causing obstruction of CSF circulation and hydrocephalus, respectively,
- To displace cerebellar tissue resulting in upward herniation (clinically midbrain syndrome) and/or downward (tonsillary)
- Herniation (clinically: bulbar syndrome). Besides venous structures, the vertebral arteries and the basal artery may be torn when involved in a basal skull fracture.

Diagnostic Procedures

Imaging: Computed tomography is the first choice. The typical PFEDH appears as a hyperdense biconvex extraaxial lesion. Contrarily to subdural or intracerebellar PFH (which are not seldom combined), PFEDH may extend above the tentorium to the occipital region.

Mass effect on CT scan is defined as distortion, dislocation, or obliteration of the fourth ventricle; compression or loss of visualization of the basal cisterns, or the presence of obstructive hydrocephalus.

Recommended European Standard

Clinical assessment according to ATLS.

Imaging: Both patients presenting with a GCS score of 14 points or less and patients presenting with a GCS score of 15 in the presence of risk factors are to be scanned. [401] (see Sect. 1.4.2).

Helical computed tomography (three window-level settings without the use of intravenous iodinated contrast agents, reconstructions in three planes – see Sect. 1.4.2) should be obtained immediately after the patient is stabilized using standard advanced trauma life support (ATLS) guidelines. For severe brain injury where the patient is intubated, the upper whole cervical spine should be included in the scan.

Additional/useful diagnostic procedures

Cervical spine X-ray and/or CT scan: While computed tomography (CT) is the appropriate technique for the urgent detection of hematomas and contusions, MRI is much more effective at documenting diffuse injury and brain stem lesions [235]. When supposing vessel injury, angiography (CT-Angiography or iaDSA) is mandatory. Intracerebellar clots may increase in size until day 4 after injury, which implies that these patients need to be rescanned at least daily until the lesion stabilizes.

Therapy

Conservative treatment

A conservative approach can be considered a viable, safe treatment option for noncomatose patients with intracerebellar clots measuring less than or equal to 3 cm, except when associated with other extradural or subdural posterior fossa focal lesions [84].
Recommended European Standard
Patients with lesions and no significant mass effect on CT scan and without signs of neurological dysfunction may be managed by close observation and serial imaging [51].
Useful additional therapeutic strategies
Repeat head CT after neurologic deterioration or inexplainable rise of ICP (continuous monitoring of ICP).

Surgical treatment
Surgery is aimed

- To evacuate clots completely, thereby preventing or ending herniation,
- To decompress the cerebellum and the brainstem, thereby preventing evolution of occlusive hydrocephalus
- To avoid development of perifocal edema

Recommended European Standard
Surgery should be recommended for all patients with clots larger than 3 cm, for patients with mass effect on CT-scan *or* with neurological dysfunction *or* deterioration referable to the lesion [51, 84]. In patients with indications for surgical intervention, evacuation should be performed as soon as possible because these patients can deteriorate rapidly, thus worsening their prognosis considerably. Suboccipital craniectomy is the predominant method [51].

Surgery may be withheld from patients unconscious since the injury and presenting with bilateral maximally dilated pupils without reaction during more than 2 h as from patients suffering from CT-proofed severe brain stem lesions.

Perioperative antibiotic prophylaxis starts 60 min prior to incision. During prolonged procedures, antibiotic prophylaxis should be readministered every 3 h [292].

Differential Diagnosis

Imaging features are characteristic.
Posterior fossa hematoma may be a result of a spontaneous hemorrhage (for example with rupture of an aneurysm of the posterior inferior cerebellar artery (PICA) or bleeding from a cerebellar arteriovenous malformation (AVM), provoking then an accident.

Prognosis/Outcome

With PFEDH, outcome correlates with the patient's neurologic status. High GCS score (of 8 or higher; 84) at the time of operation, which, to a certain extent, is also related to the rapidity of the course and the size of the lesion, has a good prognosis. Children have better outcomes than do adults. The presence of hydrocephalus on CT scan is an ominous sign. Sudden-onset symptomatology, associated intracranial injuries, bilateral PFEDH, acute hydrocephalus; effaced fourth ventricle, and posterior fossa cisterns have turned out as bad prognostic factors [233].

With acute PFSDH, comatose patients present usually with signs of posterior fossa mass effect and have a high percentage of bad outcomes. On the contrary, patients admitted with a GCS of 8 or higher are expected to recover [233].

Surgical Principles

Mass lesions in the posterior fossa are evacuated with the patient in prone position and the table in slight anti-Trendelenburg position. The head with the face down rests on the donut or in a rigid fixation, the external occipital protuberance being the highest point of the operation field. Park bench position is an alternative; sitting position is not to be recommended.

In patients deteriorating rapidly and CT showing large ventricles, cannulation (ventricular catheter) of lateral ventricles is mandatory (see Fig. 1.11). To prevent transtentorial (upward) herniation, CSF is drained not until the craniectomy is completed.

Technique

Lateral Suboccipital Craniectomy

When operating on a lateral lesion – mostly AEDH or less often cerebellar contusions/parenchymal hematomas - the skin incision starts on the appropriate side 1–2 cm beyond and 4–5 cm lateral of the external occipital protuberance reaching down to the level of the processus spinosus C2 (Fig. 1.26). The paravertebral muscles and fascia are divided and the occiput exposed. A burr-hole is placed over the point where the fracture crosses the transverse or sigmoid sinus and enlarged (according to the dimension of the hematoma) to a craniectomy after as much of the hematoma as possible has been removed. Alternatively, several burr-holes are applied and a bone flap is sawed out. The risk of damaging the underlying sinus or dura with the craniotome is minimal in the face of a large epidural clot. After completion of the removal of the hematoma (see Sect. Acute epidural hematoma), injury to the sinus is closed primarily, dural bleeders are cauterized. The subdural space is inspected through a small dural incision, which is closed then water-tight. Closure see below.

Medial suboccipital craniectomy

With a more widespread hematoma of the posterior fossa as an SDH over the cerebellar hemispheres and the vermis, a medial suboccipital craniotomy with removal of the posterior rim of the foramen magnum and the posterior arch of C1 via a midline incision may be indicated to gain access to the cervicomedullary junction (Fig. 1.27). To allow cannulation of the lateral ventricle, a hockey stick extension may be added to its superior aspect (see Sect. 1.7.1.3).

The incision is deepened stepwise down to the occipital bone and to the spinous process of C2, staying in white fibrous tissue between the muscles of both sides. The superior extent of the craniectomy should expose at least the inferior half of transverse sinus. Evacuation of the hematoma is according to evacuation of ASDH and intraparenchymal hemorrhage, respectively.

Closure: The dura is closed water-tight. Epidural tack-up sutures are placed at the edges and fixed at the bone (small holes) or at the at the pericranium or muscles. Either the bone flap is replaced or a cranioplasty is performed as a subsequent procedure. A subgaleal drain-

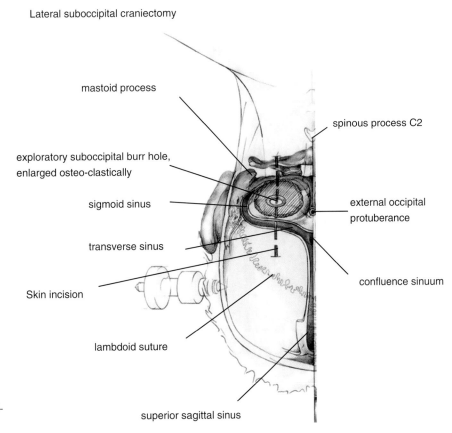

Lateral suboccipital craniectomy

mastoid process

spinous process C2

exploratory suboccipital burr hole, enlarged osteo-clastically

sigmoid sinus

external occipital protuberance

transverse sinus

confluence sinuum

Skin incision

lambdoid suture

superior sagittal sinus

Fig. 1.26 Lateral suboccipital craniectomy

Medial suboccipital craniotomy

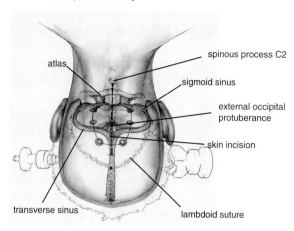

Fig. 1.27 Medial suboccipital craniotomy

age is positioned and the wound is closed in layers.
Intraoperative complications (see Sect. 1.7.1.4):

- Acute swelling of the brain
- Acute bleeding (arterial or venous (dural sinus injury))
- Increase in volume of an additional traumatic intracranial (ipsi- or contralateral) hematoma
- Tonsillar herniation
- Tension pneumoencephalon
- Air embolism

Postoperative complications (see Sect. 1.7.1.4):

- Delayed appearance of intracranial hematoma
- Reaccumulation of blood at the operation site
- Brain edema (intracranial hypertension)
- Posttraumatic hydrocephalus
- Central nervous system infection

Special Remarks

Type of anesthesia

Inhalation/intravenous anesthesia: In patients experiencing rapid deterioration, operation can be begun with local anesthesia and completed using general anesthesia. With the patient in prone position and the table in slight anti-Trendelenburg position, intraoperative air embolism is to be expected.

1.7.2.8 Traumatic Intraparenchymal Hemorrhage (Fig. 1.CT-6)

Synonym: Intraparenchymal hemorrhage/intraparenchymal hemorrhagic lesion/intraaxial hemorrhage/intracerebral hemorrhage/intracerebral hematoma

Definition [333]

Traumatic intraparenchymal cerebral hemorrhage (tIPH): A collective term covering

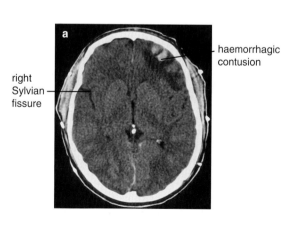

Fig. 1.CT-6 (**a**) Hemorrhagic cortical contusion (axial computed tomography, native, brain window): area of high density interspersed with areas of low density in the left frontal region. (**b**) Frontal contusions in the right frontal lobe. Widespread intraparenchymal hematoma (axial computed tomography, native, brain window), hemorrhagic cortical contusions, strait subdural hematoma, air within the subdural space as a result of a (not depicted) open fracture with laceration of the dura

- Traumatic cerebral contusion:
- Cortical contusion: An almost always hemorrhagic, wedge-shaped lesion with its base on the cortical surface and its tip pointed toward the center of the brain, when reaching the ventricular system producing a ventricular hemorrhage. The gyral crest is maximally involved, and the subjacent white matter is affected to a more variable extent. Cortical contusions are often associated with an overlying subdural hematoma.
- Laceration: tear in the parenchyma.
- Traumatic intracerebral contusion: a heterogeneous area of necrosis, hemorrhage, and infarction as well as edema within the brain.
- Traumatic intracerebral hematoma: a homogeneous blood clot that develops after trauma within the brain substance. The hemorrhage itself is free of brain tissue, having pushed this tissue aside. The brain around the hematoma may be necrotic or edematous.
- Traumatic subarachnoidal hemorrhage (tSAH): a consequence either of ventricular hemorrhage or an admixture of blood to the cerebrospinal fluid (CSF) caused by a bleeding of cortical arteries, veins, and capillaries from brain surface cerebral contusions.
- "Burst lobe" describes the appearance of intracerebral hematoma mixed with necrotic brain tissue, rupturing out into the subdural space into a subdural hematoma.

Etiology/epidemiology

The commonest mechanism causing tIPH is an impact of the moving head against a fixed object as this arrives in falls and vehicle (traffic) accidents. A blow to the posterior part of the vault results in (contrecoup) contusions frontobasal and in temporal contusions and hematomas, respectively. The hemorrhage starts in the cortex and may then spread deep into the white matter eventually into the ventricles. Cerebral contusions are the commonest traumatic lesion visualized on CT scan.

Traumatic tIPH may occur at any age, most in men 30–40 years old caused in more than 50% by traffic accidents, less by falls. Intraventricular hemorrhage is diagnosed in about 1–5% of TBI victims and is practically always combined with intraparenchymal lesions [211]. Moreover, by direct impact to the head, tIPH are caused by pure acceleration/deceleration of the head and by penetrating injuries.

Traumatic IPH can occur almost everywhere within the brain. However, 80–90% are located in the frontal and temporal regions - on the basal surfaces and tips [83, 208, 326]. Bilateral ICH are very common [56]. Occipital and cerebellar contusions and intracerebral hematomas are rare. Probably induced by shear stress, small hemorrhages occur in the corpus callosum, in the deep gray matter of the centrum semiovale, and in the brainstem.

Most patients present with two or more tIPH. In a series of more than 200 patients, 77% of lesions were 1 cc or less in volume, another 15% between 2 and 5 cc, and the remaining 8% greater than 5 cc. With respect to pattern type, 159 (70%) were petechial-appearing contusions, and 70 (30%) were solid-appearing hematomas. Many patients exhibited additional non-IPH intracranial pathology, most common tSAH (84%) usually located around the hemispheric convexities and often bilateral, followed by ASDH (48%) and AEDHs (8%), intraventricular hemorrhage occurred in 17% of patients [58]. A lower frequency of SAH was observed among patients whose CT scans either did not exhibit other parenchymal damage or demonstrated only an epidural hematoma and a higher frequency of SAH among patients with subdural hematomas, parenchymal damage, or multiple lesions [357]. Linear skull fractures are a frequent accompaniment of tIPH also [326].

Patients suffering from tIPH are often "coagulopathic" [58].

Clinical presentation/symptoms

The clinical presentation is a function of the severity of the immediate impact injury and the size, location, and subsequent growth of the intraparenchymal hematoma and any extraparenchymal hematoma that may be present. Therefore, these lesions may present with a simple, severe headache or with seizures. In severe cases, a patient may lapse immediately into a coma [58, 369].

Complications

- Progression of intraparenchymal hemorrhage: Delayed enlargement of traumatic intraparenchymal contusions and hematomas is the most common cause of clinical deterioration and death in patients who have experienced a lucid interval after traumatic brain injury [330]. Important predictors of enlargement of the parenchymal clot are the presence of subarachnoid hemorrhage and subdural hematomas and the size of the clot on initial computed tomography [58].

Intraparenchymal lesions in the frontal, orbitofrontal, and temporal regions [208] accounted for 85% of all enlarging parenchymal lesions [296].

- Occlusive hydrocephalus, caused by extension of parenchymal bleeding into the ventricles.
- Herniation brainstem compression: Patients with temporal or temporoparietal hematomas appear to be at greater risk of brain-stem compression, especially if the lesion is larger than 30 cc and caused by head injury, than are those with hematomas in other sites [16].

Diagnostic Procedures

Imaging: Computed tomography is the first choice. By resolving differences in density, CT scan allows to distinguish intracerebral hematomas from cerebral contusions or posttraumatic edema readily. Additionally, CT scanning allows quantification of tIPH with relation to outcome [108, 244]. Follow-up CT scans in patients with intraparenchymal clots on their initial CT are justified by the high risk of enlargement of tIPH, at least as long as the patients are not awake and stable.

Recommended European Standard

Clinical assessment according to ATLS. Imaging [401]: Both patients presenting with a GCS score of 14 points or less and patients presenting with a GCS score of 15 in the presence of risk factors are to be scanned. Helical computed tomography (three window-level settings without the use of intravenous iodinated contrast agents, reconstructions in three planes) should be obtained immediately after the patient is stabilized using standard advanced trauma life support (ATLS) guidelines (see Sect. 1.4.2).

Additional/useful diagnostic procedures

With suspicion of a spontaneous intraparenchymal hemorrhage, an angiography (CTA, MRA, or iaDSA) is performed to evaluate possible presence of causative lesions. Those patients with subdural hematoma, subarachnoid hemorrhage, large-sized intraparenchymal lesions, and mass effect should undergo ICP monitoring ("Guidelines for Management of Severe TBI").

Therapy

Aggressive medical management (early intubation, ventriculostomy, ICP monitoring (see Chap. 2)) may avoid the need for removing large portions of the frontal and possibly temporal lobes [208].

Traumatic IPH are very often accompanied by additional intracranial lesions. Their management should be guided by the predominant pathology. It is therefore mandatory to ascertain priority of therapy concerning the different lesions [56].

The presence of subdural hematoma, subarachnoid hemorrhage, or an initial intraparenchymal lesion with a size >5 cm³) or mass effect are causes of concern.

Aggressive correction of any coagulation disturbances is indispensable [426].

Conservative therapy

Recommended European Standard

Patients with parenchymal mass lesions who do not show evidence for neurological compromise have controlled intracranial pressure (ICP) and no significant signs of mass effect on CT scan may be managed nonoperatively with intensive monitoring on serial imaging [50].

Useful additional therapeutic strategies

Repeat head CT after neurologic deterioration or inexplainable rise of ICP.

Surgical therapy

Recommended European Standard

Patients with parenchymal mass lesions and signs of progressive neurological deterioration referable to the lesion, medically refractory intracranial hypertension, or signs of mass effect on computed tomography scan should be treated operatively.

Patients with Glasgow Coma Scale scores (GCS) of 6–8 with frontal or temporal contusions greater than 20 cm³ with midline shift of at least 5 mm and/or cisternal compression on CT scan, and patients with any lesions greater than 50 cm³ in volume should be treated operatively [50].

Decompressive procedures, including subtemporal decompression, temporal lobectomy, and hemispheric or bihemispheric decompressive craniectomy (Fig. 1. CT-7) are treatment options for patients with refractory intracranial hypertension and diffuse parenchymal injury with clinical and radiographic evidence of impending transtentorial herniation [50].

Bilateral ICH decompressive craniectomy (even without treatment of the lesion itself) should be considered as a useful means to lower ICP and to reduce mortality [354].

Perioperative antibiotic prophylaxis starts 60 min [292].

ventricular catheter

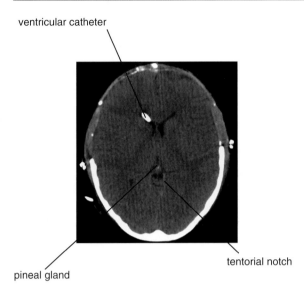

pineal gland

tentorial notch

Fig. 1.CT-7 (Axial, native): Postoperative condition after extensive bifrontal decompressive craniotomy; right frontal horn drained

Differential Diagnosis

Intraparenchymal hemorrhage may also develop spontaneously, thereby being the source of an accident. Causes of spontaneous hemorrhages are arteriovenous malformations, tumors, or anticoagulants. Spontaneous subarachnoid hemorrhage (SAH) may occur with rupture of a cerebral aneurysm as the primary event, with the trauma resulting from SAH-associated incapacity. However, if a saccular cerebral aneurysm is found on angiogram after a patient has been injured, it is often difficult to know if the aneurysm is incidental, caused the SAH and trauma, or bled as a result [81].

Prognosis/Outcome

Patients with a temporal or temporoparietal hematoma tend to a worse outcome than patients suffering from hematomas in other sites. Patient with signs of tentorial herniation have a high probability of a bad outcome [16]. Multiple lesions have the same prognosis as the corresponding single lesions; ASDH combined with ICH is a predictor of a bad outcome (dead or vegetative state) [56]. Traumatic SAH has an adverse prognostic significance. Poor outcomes among patients with tSAH at admission are related to age, GCS score, CT classification, amount of subarachnoid blood, and presence of

contusions. The CT classification, amount of subarachnoid blood, and presence of contusions also predict significant lesion progression, thus linking poor outcomes with CT changes [70]. Death among patients with tSAH seems related to the severity of the initial mechanical damage, rather than to the effects of delayed vasospasm and secondary ischemic brain damage.

Surgical Principles

Subcortical IPH are reached by a direct approach, especially when in continuity with an overlaying ASDH. Deeper sitting hematomas are reached by entering through a "silent zone" eventually supported by intraoperative ultrasonography. A corticotomy or a corticectomy is necessary to evacuate intracerebral hematomas that do not come to the surface.
Technique
   The intraoperative position of the patient and the localization of the craniotomy is dependent on the site of the hematoma, but mostly a modified "Standard craniotomy" is performed. Occipital and cerebellar hematomas are evacuated in prone or park bench position.
   Whenever possible, the cortex is opened in the overlaying contusioned area by gently bipolar coagulation and subsequent incision, followed then by stepwise progressing down to the hematoma using bipolar forceps, paddys, and suctioning. A pure hematoma often is pressed out then.
   A slender brain retractor is advanced in the cavity before the evacuation is completed by gentle aspiration and instilling Ringer solution (Fig. 1.28). Thereby, the walls of the cavity should not be touched with the sucker, the tip of which has to be visible throughout this action. On the contrary, by removing the blood clot mixed with contused nonviable brain tissue, the contused tissue is aspirated, as far as regular brain tissue is reached. Major cortical contusions are resected in an analogous manner. Bleeding points in the wall of the cavity are controlled by bipolar cauterization on covering with hemostatic gauze as are pial bleedings. Because of strong tendency of postoperative brain swelling in these type of TBI, usually an ICP monitor (device) is employed and not seldom the bone flap is replaced.
   Closure is performed as delineated in "1.7.1.1 Standard craniotomy"

Intraparenchymal temporal haematoma: evacuation

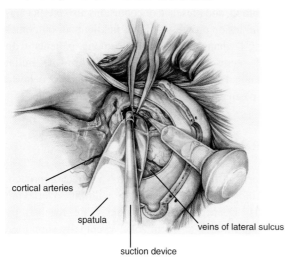

Fig. 1.28 Intraparenchymal temporal hematoma: evacuation

Intraoperative complications (see Sect. 1.7.1.4):

- Intraoperative bleeding as a consequence of reduced tamponade or injury to cerebral vessels
- Diffuse brain swelling

Postoperative complications (see Sect. 1.7.1.4):

- Delayed cerebral hemorrhage
- Progressing cerebral edema
- Disturbance of CSF circulation
- Infection

Special Remarks

Type of anesthesia

Intracerebral hematomas are evacuated in inhalation/intravenous anesthesia.

1.7.2.9 Penetrating Brain Injury (PBI)

Synonym: Penetrating head trauma, penetrating cranial injury, penetrating injury of head, open intracranial injury.

Definition

Penetrating brain injury (PBI) is an open traumatic brain injury in which the dura mater is breached, i.e., there is a direct communication from the environment to the intradural compartment, cerebrospinal fluid

(CSF), and brain tissue may escape. *Penetrating* head injuries can be the result of numerous intentional or unintentional events, including missile wounds, stab wounds, and motor vehicle or occupational accidents.

Perforating brain injury is a "through-and-through" injury, characterized by entry and exit wounds, mostly caused by a gunshot.

1.7.2.9.1 Stab Wounds to the Head (Fig. 1.CT-8)

Definition

A cranial stab wound is a wound caused by an object (e.g., knife [212], screwdriver [368], nail gun [221]) with a small impact area and wielded at low velocity. The most common, a knife injury, produces a classic slot fracture of the skull with an underlying tract hematoma [91].

Etiology/epidemiology

The majority of cranial stab wounds are as a consequence of an assault, although some are accidental and even self-inflicted. Most stab wounds to the cranium occur to the left parietal region, which is a reflection of the high incidence of right-handedness among the population. Other frequent stab wound sites are the orbital and temporal areas (thin bone). Transcranial (penetrating) stab wounds are uncommon.

Stab wounds typically result in a localized zone of hemorrhage and necrosis only around the injury tract.

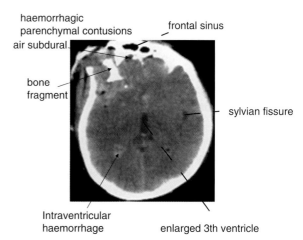

Fig. 1.CT-8 Penetrating head injury (computed tomography axial, native): stab wound producing large compound fracture frontal right with laceration of the dura. Hemorrhagic parenchymal contusions, intraventricular hemorrhage, indriven bone fragments, air intraparenchymal

Stab wound cause no diffuse shearing injury. Hematoma occur in about half of the patients with penetrating stab wounds to the brain. Other injuries that can be seen on computed tomography include cerebral contusion (31%), subdural hematoma (9%), cerebral infarction (5%), and, rarely, extradural hematoma. Resulting vascular lesions have been reported such as carotid-cavernous or arteriovenous fistula, arterial occlusions, arterial transections, delayed vasospasm, and traumatic aneurysms. Unlike missile injuries, no concentric zone of coagulative necrosis caused by dissipated energy is present. Unlike motor vehicle accidents, no diffuse shearing injury to the brain occurs [54, 416].

Clinical presentation/symptoms

Usually, the scalp wound is not ostentatious; besides bleeding, exit of CSF or brain tissue may be noticed. Patients who present after sustaining stab wounds to the skull may or may not have normal findings on neurologic examination. In a review of 330 stab wounds to the head, du Trevou and van Dellen [92] reported a mean GCS score of 11 with 25% of patients presenting with a GCS score less than 8 and 75% of patients presenting fully conscious. In the latter, neurologic deficits are a manifestation of the localized brain injury. Loss of consciousness is the consequence of a focal injury, not of a diffuse shearing injury.

Complications

- Missing the diagnosis: Stab wounds to the head are to be missed easily, especially in the neurologically intact patient. Diagnosis relies heavily on a high level of clinical suspicion [93, 212].
- Vascular problems: Approximately 30% of patients with transcranial stab wounds will have vascular lesions (laceration, transsection, traumatic aneurysm, arterio-venous fistula). Transorbital and temporal injuries tend to have a higher incidence of hemorrhage. Vascular injury may present at the outset with intracranial bleeding; however, delayed hemorrhage can also occur, especially if a false aneurysm develops and then ruptures. Traumatic subarachnoid hemorrhage (tSAH) may initiate vasospasm [53].
- Subarachnoid hemorrhage and intraventricular bleeding may cause *obstructive hydrocephalus* [280].
- *Infectious complications* can result when the knife wound traverses mucosal surfaces – therefore often in transorbital stabbing.
- CSF fistula

- *Posttraumatic seizures* are common in patients following all brain injury. Factors associated with increased risk of seizure include intracerebral hemorrhage, subdural hematoma, depressed skull fractures, prolonged amnesia, and focal neurological deficits.

Diagnostic Procedures

If transcranial stab wounds are not suspected based on history and mechanism of injury, the diagnosis can be easily missed especially when palpation of the characteristic "slot" fracture by examination of the wound through the small stab laceration is not possible and/or with massive swelling of the soft tissue in the orbital or temporal entry zone.

Imaging: Computed tomography is the first choice. Skull X-ray films often fail to show fractures.

Recommended European Standard

Clinical assessment according to ATLS. Computed tomography should be obtained as soon as possible. Helical computed tomography is ideally suited to demonstrate the fracture and accompanying contusions, hematomas, and foreign material (see Sect. 1.4.2). Once intracranial penetration has been diagnosed, cerebral angiography (CTA or iaDSA, see Sect. 4.4) – preferably performed in a center where interventional neuroradiology is available – should be scheduled to the earliest possible to exclude vascular injury, and whenever possible performed before starting craniotomy [54].

Additional/useful diagnostic procedures

Wooden foreign body is best diagnosed by magnetic resonance imaging. By computed tomography, dry wood can be isodense with air and orbital fat [370].

Because of vasospasm or "cut-off" of a vessel, a second angiogram may be necessary to further elucidate a vascular abnormality that might not have been evident originally [92, 182].

Repeat head CT after neurologic deterioration or inexplainable rise of ICP.

Therapy

Because of the risk of provoking a massive bleeding, no attempt to remove the wounding object should be made outside the operation theater – ideally the object is not removed before the craniotomy is done [416].

Conservative treatment

None

Useful additional therapeutic strategies

Use of prophylactic broad-spectrum antibiotics is recommended for patients with PBI [288] as is antiseizure medications in the first week after PBI [289]. Prophylactic treatment with anticonvulsants beyond the first week after PBI has not been shown to prevent the development of new seizures, and is not recommended.

Surgical treatment

Recommended European Standard

In the absence of significant mass effect, surgical debridement of the track in the brain and routine surgical removal of fragments lodged distant from the entry site and reoperation solely to remove fragments are not recommended. However, where feasible, wooden objects should be removed as completely as possible, to avoid long-term infective complications such as abscess formation [260]. Accompanying traumatic vascular lesions are to be assessed concerning endovascular/neurosurgical treatment. Repair of an open-air sinus injury with water-tight closure of the dura is recommended (see Sect. 1.7.2.2.2). Clinical circumstances dictate the timing of the repair. Transorbital stab injuries may require additional ophthalmological surgery. The entry wound has to be debrided and closed [290].

Differential Diagnosis

Simple laceration of the scalp.

Prognosis/Outcome

Patients in whom the penetrating object is left in place have a significantly lower mortality than those in whom the objects are inserted and then removed (26% vs. 11%, respectively) [416].

Outcomes generally depend on the site of the injury and the depth of penetration. Stab wounds to the temporal fossa are more likely to result in major neurological deficits because of the thinness of the temporal squama and the shorter distance to the deep brain stem and vascular structures. Transcranial brainstem stabs are very often fatal injuries. Transorbital injuries tend to have a high incidence of hemorrhage and infection [54]. For neurologically intact patient, the outcome is generally good

Surgical Principles

Because of the risk of provoking a massive bleeding, no attempt to remove the wounding object should be made outside the operation theater – ideally the object is not removed before the craniotomy is done [416].

Technique

See Sect. 1.7.2.9.2

Intraoperative/postoperative complication (see Sects. 1.7.2.9.2 and 1.7.1.4, respectively):

- Massive bleeding
- Brain swelling
- Infection (wound infection, osteomyelitis, meningitis, cerebral abscess)

Special Remarks

None

1.7.2.9.2 Civilian Gunshot Wounds (GSW) (Fig. 1. CT-9)

Definition [415]

- Penetrating gunshot wounds:
- Penetrating: The missile penetrates skull and dura and remains lodged within the intracranial cavity.
- Perforating: The missile passes "through-and-through," characterized by entry and exit wounds.

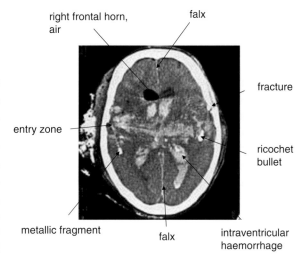

Fig. 1.CT-9 Self-inflicted gunshot wound: bullet entering the right temporal region, crossing the midline, and ricocheting at the left-lateral bone

Debris and bone fragments commonly are present within the brain in this type of injury.

- Tangential gunshot wound: The missile glances off the skull, often driving bone fragments into the brain

Etiology/epidemiology

Gunshot wounds to the head account for the majority of penetrating brain injuries. Civilian gunshot wounds occur through accidents with firearms but more often results from intentional injury caused by singular acts of self-destruction. Accordingly, the PBI is caused mainly by low-caliber (.22 to.38) missiles used in handguns or shotguns (low velocity) [193, 246].

Damage to brain parenchyma is the consequence of laceration and crushing, cavitation, and shock waves. The intensity of the resulting damage depends on projectile mass, projectile velocity, projectile construction, and the characteristics of the tissue penetrated. Depending on the velocity of the bullet, it may have insufficient energy to exit the cranial vault and may ricochet off the inner table opposite the entry site or off a dural structure, thereby creating several tracts [105]. In a *"through-and through"* pass, usually the exit wound is more extended than the entry wound. While the entry wound may be contaminated by indriven material - skin, hair, and bone fragments - the exit wound is characterized by a more widespread destruction of brain tissue, dura, bone, and scalp.

A *tangential gunshot wound* (see below) may cause contusion of the brain, dural tears, and indriving of fragments of the inner table of the calvaria.

Suicide is a major cause of gunshot injuries among civilians, predominantly because of gunshot wounds to the head. Suicide is associated with higher mortality than other causes of PBI, because with the muzzle close to the head the missile has still a high velocity and thereby a high kinetic energy. The age distribution in those series that include patients dead at the scene of accident or dead on arrival have many more patients over the age of 50. Another cause is urban violence, the cranial lesions secondary to penetrating missile injuries have become a very important cause of death or permanent neurologic deficits, which affect mainly young males

Penetrating craniocerebral missile injuries in civilians have a very high rate of early mortality [190, 359] and are the most lethal type of head injury. Outcomes tend to be very polarized: the majority of patients die, and those who survive usually have little or no disability.

Clinical presentation/symptoms

The pathological consequences of gunshot head wounds depend on the circumstances of the injury, including the properties of the weapon or missile, the energy of the impact, and the location and characteristics of the intracranial trajectory. The injury may range from a depressed fracture of the skull resulting in a focal hemorrhage to devastating diffuse damage to the brain. With tangential wound to the head, the patient may be normal.

Accordingly, the patient may lapse immediately into a coma and die on the scene or may present with none or minor neurologic symptoms.

Complications

- Missing diagnosis: As in a stab wound, the scalp wound resulting from a low-caliber missile may be small, especially small with direct contact of the muzzle to the head. A tangential gunshot wound is apt to misinterpretation.
- Vascular injury [286] causing:

  - Traumatic subarachnoid hemorrhage, extraaxial and/or intraparenchymal acute or delayed hematoma.
  - Traumatic intracranial aneurysms [149, 162]
  - Traumatic arteriovenous fistula as carotid-cavernous sinus fistula [59]
  - Occlusive dissection

- *Disturbance of the "milieu interne"* (endocrine disturbance and/or water–electrolyte imbalance)
- Migrating of the missile within the ventricular system, causing *obstructive hydrocephalus*
- CSF leak [287]
- Infection (meningitis; cerebral abscess): The risk of intracranial infection among patients with PBI is high because of the presence of contaminated foreign objects driven into the brain along the missile track. The presence of air sinus wounds or cerebrospinal fluid (CSF) fistulae may further increase the risk of infection [288].
- Posttraumatic seizures/posttraumatic epilepsy: Seizures – Patients with bone and metal fragments have increased seizure risk compared with those without, but minimally increased risk with metal alone and none with only bony fragments [98, 289].

Diagnostic Procedures

Imaging: CT scanning is the procedure of choice to evaluate the patient with penetrating brain injury. It allows to identify the lesion extension, to determine the missile track, to identify hematoma and other associated lesions, provides useful information for the planning of the surgical procedure, and usually defines the prognosis.

Recommended European Standard

Clinical assessment according to ATLS. In addition to the standard axial views, coronal sections may be helpful for patients with skull base involvement or high convexity injuries [246, 284] (see Sect. 1.4.2). Angiography is recommended in PBI where a vascular injury is suspected [182]. Patients with an increased risk of vascular injury include cases in which the wound's trajectory passes through or near the

- Sylvian fissure,
- Supraclinoid carotid,
- Cavernous sinus, or
- A major venous sinus.

The development of substantial and otherwise unexplained subarachnoid hemorrhage or delayed hematoma should also prompt consideration of a vascular injury and of angiography.

Additional/useful diagnostic procedures

Because of a concern for retained ferromagnetic fragments, routine magnetic resonance imaging (MRI) is not generally recommended for use in the acute management of missile-induced PBI [284]. Repeat head CT after neurologic deterioration or inexplainable rise of ICP.

Therapy

Vigorous resuscitation and early surgery often resulted in useful survivals and occasionally in spectacular recoveries. However, the high mortality rate on the scene or soon after the injury restricts the possibility of effective management to a minority of cases. [359]. However, supportive measures should be considered in most cases (for possibility of organ donation, opportunity for family to adjust to situation, and requirements for observation period to determine actual brain death).

Conservative treatment

None

Recommended European Standard

There is no indication for conservative treatment except in those patients who are at the highest risk of death secondary to a craniocerebral gunshot wound: patients with penetrating wounds and GCS score of 3–5 in the absence of hematoma causing a mass effect [246] and for patients with evidence of likelihood of brain death within 24 h [399]. However, at least local wound care (closure) is mandatory.

Useful additional therapeutic strategies

Use of prophylactic broad-spectrum antibiotics is recommended for patients with PBI [288] as is antiseizure medications in the first week after PBI [289]. Prophylactic treatment with anticonvulsants beyond the first week after PBI has not been shown to prevent the development of new seizures, and is not recommended.

Surgical treatment

Currently, surgical management of PBI clearly tends toward minimizing the degree of debridement. There are no controlled studies that have examined the relative efficacy of various degrees of debridement to prevent infection and minimize the development of seizure disorders.

In cases that maintain extremely high mortality, aggressive treatment such as surgical debridement may not be indicated. Basis for extended surgery is stable vital signs and GCS > 3

Recommended European Standard

Recommended procedures [285]

- Treatment of small-entrance bullet wounds to the head with local wound care and closure in patients whose scalp is not devitalized and have no "significant" intracranial pathologic findings. (The volume and location of the brain injury, evidence of mass effect, e.g., displacement of the midline > 5 mm or compression of basilar cisterns from edema or hematoma, and the patient's clinical condition all pertain to significance.
- Treatment of more extensive wounds with nonviable scalp, bone, or dura with more extensive debridement before primary closure or grafting to secure a water-tight wound
- Treatment of more extensive wounds with nonviable scalp, bone, or dura with more extensive debridement before primary closure or grafting to secure a water-tight wound
- With significant fragmentation of the skull: Debridement of the cranial wound with either craniectomy or craniotomy
- In the presence of significant mass effect: Debridement of necrotic brain tissue and safely accessible bone fragments

- Evacuation of intracranial hematomas with significant mass effect
- Repair of an open-air sinus injury with water-tight closure of the dura is recommended.

Not recommended procedures (BTF):

- Surgical debridement of the missile track in the brain in the absence of significant mass effect.
- Routine surgical removal of fragments lodged distant from the entry site and reoperation was solely to remove retained bone or missile fragments. Clinical circumstances dictate the timing of the repair. Any repairs requiring duraplasty can be at the discretion of the surgeon as to material used for closure.

Differential Diagnosis

Clinical and imaging features are characteristic in penetrating injuries/gunshot injuries.

Prognosis/Outcome

Gunshot wounds to the head have a high morbidity and early mortality. The mortality rates in the literature range from 23% to 92% and are considerably higher (87–100%) in patients admitted in a poor neurologic state. Outcomes tend to be very polarized: the majority of patients die, and those who survive usually have little or no disability. The initial GCS is a very powerful predictor of outcome. Respiratory arrest on admission, hypotension on admission, a low GCS score at admission, unilateral dilated pupil or medium fixed pupil, transventricular or bihemispheric central type trajectory, and bilobar or multilobar wounds noted through CT scan are predictive factors of high morbidity and mortality [10, 246, 273, 290, 312, 359].

Evidence of likelihood of brain death within 24 h: GCS 5 in the emergency department and CT scan showing at least one of the following findings: Mass lesion with transtentorial or falcine herniation/subarachnoid hemorrhage/penetrating wound to brain with path of projectile crossing midline [399].

Surgical Principles

The objective in operating on gunshot wounds to the head is to close the dura, to remove indriven foreign material and bone fragments, which can act as nidus of infection, and to evacuate possible mass lesions. Bullets are removed, when accessible without causing additional damage to the brain [130, 131].

Surgical management of penetrating and perforating missile injuries is a variation of those for open-depressed skull fracture.

Technique

The patient has to be positioned and draped in such a way that access to both the entry site and the exit site is given, that metal fragment resting near the opposite inner table or distant from the entry site are accessible, and that extension of the scalp incisions is possible.

The generous skin incision – S-shaped (in the direction of the underlying fracture) comprising the entry wound – has to consider blood supply to the skin. With concomitant brain injury, a large skin flap centered over the wound of entrance is preferred.

The entry site is excised, removing all devitalized and avascular scalp. For legal purposes, excised areas of powder burn are taken as evidence.

Craniectomy begins when meticulous debridement of pericranium and temporalis or suboccipital muscle is completed, starting with a burr-hole away from entry site. The dura is exposed in a circular fashion over intact dura, staying away from the entry site, resulting in an opening of about 5×5 cm. Alternatively, a suitable craniotomy can be performed.

Beginning at the penetration site, the dura mater is debrided, then incised in stellate fashion.

Brain debridement is done analogous to the removal of a contusion/parenchymal hemorrhage (see Sect. 1.7.2.8). It begins at the boundary of normal and damaged brain where the arachnoid is coagulated and incised circumferentially. Proceeding to the depth, the devitalized and hemorrhagic tissue together with bony fragments and foreign tissue is removed with help of a small sucker and irrigation. Meticulous debridement is possible without additional injury as long as the sucker is moved forward within the necrotic tract without entering intact brain tissue (Fig. 1.29).

Bony fragments are to be removed as completely as possible as long as not underlying eloquent cortex or lodged at a distance from the entry site or in proximity of a potentially lacerated venous sinus. The risk of adverse effects on the neurological function is judged higher than the risk of developing a cerebral abscess.

If an ICP device is inserted, it is away from the craniotomy and the corresponding skin incision.

Tacking sutures are placed before the dura is patched (pericranium) and closed water-tight (without tension)

Gunshot wound: debridement of brain tissue

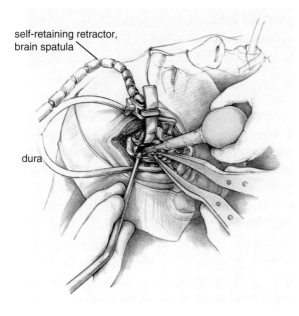

self-retaining retractor, brain spatula

dura

Fig. 1.29 Gunshot wound: debridement of brain tissue

to prevent CSF leak. The use of artificial synthetic or biological dural substitutes should be avoided.

The bone flap may be replaced after drilling back the missile entry site. The scalp is closed in layers without tension.

If a metal fragment or a bullet contralateral to the entry site is easily accessible, it should be removed at the primary operation. This applies especially for large intact bullets, which tend to migrate.

When present, the exit wound is treated in the same way. Contrary to the entry wound, there are fewer bone fragments, but injury to the dura and the skin is more complex.

Intraoperative complication (see Sect. 1.7.1.4):

• Massive bleeding [286]
• Brain swelling

Postoperative complication (see Sect. 1.7.1.4):

• Brain swelling/brain edema
• Delayed hematoma
• CSF leak [287]
• Infection (late abscess or early or late hematoma formation about the metal will necessitate its removal)

Special Remarks

Type of anesthesia

When a fracture of the floor of the frontal fossa is suspected or demonstrated radiographically, a naso-gastric must not be used. If suspicion of injury to cerebral vessels is confirmed, the anesthetist has to be oriented about the impending risk of massive intraoperative bleeding. If the skull base and/or the viscerocranium is involved, the management has to be agreed in advance with ENT maxillo-facial surgeons.

Civilian Tangential Gunshot Wound

Synonym: Graze wound; Grazing shot
Definition

A missile passing through the soft tissues of the skull without penetrating the bone causes a tangential injury.
Etiology/epidemiology

Civilian tangential gunshot wound (TGSW) occurs when a missile fired at close range strikes the skull in a very oblique angle, causing eventually fractures (compound), possibly only as a fragmentation of the inner table leaving the outer table intact. The momentarily displaced bone strikes the brain to cause a localized injury. TGSW can result in cerebral damage with or without the presence of a skull fracture. In a large series, 18% of all patients showed pathologic CT scans and major operative procedures were required in 9% of the patients [381, 382].
Clinical presentation/symptoms

The wound may be rather inconspicuous. Besides the entry wound, there may be an exit wound, assuming the bullet did not get stuck underneath the scalp. Loss of consciousness is seldom. In civilian practice, most of the patients with TGSW are presenting with a GCS of 15, and most of the patients have no neurologic deficit. Possibly, neurologic deficits are focal corresponding to the point of impact such as visual field defects, speech disorder, or hemiparesis.
Complications

• Misinterpretation of the clinical situation.
• Early or delayed intracranial hemorrhage, mostly contusions/ICH; fracture is not a prerequisite [381]
• Seizures as a consequence of a cerebral contusion.
• Infection of soft tissue and/or bone with possible spread of infection into the intracranial compartment causing epidural abscess, meningitis, subdural

empyema or brain abscess, or septic thrombosis of a venous sinus.

Diagnostic Procedures

Imaging: Computed tomography is the first choice. Besides an osseous lesion (linear skull fracture, a depressed fracture, or fragmentation of the inner table leaving the outer table relatively or completely intact), CT scan may demonstrate extracranial metallic fragments, cortical contusions, traumatic SAHe, intrusion of bony fragments, and extra- or intra-axial hematomas.
Recommended European Standard
Clinical assessment according to ATLS. CT scan is warranted in all cases of tangential gunshot wounds to the head [382]. If the history is unknown, performing computed tomography follows the recommendations of guidelines (see Sect. 1.4.2).
Additional/useful diagnostic procedures
Repeat head CT after neurologic deterioration or inexplainable rise of ICP.

Therapy

Wound revision with debridement is mandatory to prevent infections.
Conservative treatment
Recommended European Standard
Patients with less significant intraparenchymal hemorrhage or contusion should be observed carefully with follow-up CT scans and clinical examination to monitor changes in neurologic status.
Useful additional therapeutic strategies
Antibiotic prophylaxis/Seizure prophylaxis: Both prophylactic medication of antibiotics and prophylactic medication of antiepileptic medication are discussed controversially. The author group [52] recommends that all management strategies for open (compound) depressed fractures should include antibiotics.
Surgical treatment
Additional to the through debridement of the laceration of the scalp and removal of retained missiles overlying intact calvarium, patients have to be treated according to the intracranial injuries: Patients with depressed skull fractures should be debrided, the fracture has to be handled according to the BTF Guidelines (see Sect. 1.7.2.2.1). Patients with compressive extra-

axial hemorrhage or large intraparenchymal hemorrhage should undergo evacuation of clots (see Sect. 1.7).

Differential Diagnosis

Simple wound of the scalp; tangential stab wound

Prognosis/Outcome

According to the mostly minor severity of the brain lesion, the prognosis is generally good.

Surgical Principles

Technique
See Sect. 1.7.2.2.1.

Special Remarks

None

References

1. Aarabi B, Hesdorffer DC, Ahn ES (2006) Outcome following decompressive craniectomy for malignant swelling due to severe head injury. J Neurosurg 104:469–479
2. Abe M, Udono H, Tabuchi K et al (2003) Analysis of ischemic brain damage in cases of acute subdural hematomas. Surg Neurol 59:464–472, discussion 472
3. Acosta J, Yang J, Winchell R et al (1998) Lethal injuries and time to death in a Level I trauma center. J Am Coll Surg 186:528–533
4. Adams JH, Doyle D, Ford I et al (1989) Diffuse axonal injury in head injury: definition, diagnosis and grading. Histopathology 15:49–59
5. Adams JH, Jennett B, McLellan DR et al (1999) The neuropathology of the vegetative state after head injury. J Clin Pathol 52:804–806
6. af Geijerstam JL, Britton M (2003) Mild head injury – mortality and complication rate: meta-analysis of findings in a systematic literature review. Acta Neurochir (Wien) 145:843–850, discussion 850. Review
7. af Geijerstam JL, Britton M (2005) Mild head injury: reliability of early computed tomographic findings in triage for admission. Emerg Med J 22:103–107
8. af Geijerstam JL, Oredsson S, Britton M et al (2006) Medical outcome after immediate computed tomography or admission for observation in patients with mild head injury: randomised controlled trial. BMJ 333(7566):465
9. Akopian G, Gaspard DJ, Alexander M (2007) Outcomes of blunt head trauma without intracranial pressure monitoring. Am Surg 73:447–450

10. Aldrich EF, Eisenberg HM, Saydjari C et al (1992) Predictors of mortality in severely head-injured patients with civilian gunshot wounds: A report from the NIH Traumatic Coma Data Bank. Surg Neurol 38:418–423

11. Alexander E, Ball MR, Laster DW (1987) Subtemporal decompression: radiological observations and current surgical experience. Br J Neurosurg 1:427–1433

12. Al-Haddad SA, Kirollos R (2002) A 5-year study of the outcome of surgically treated depressed skull fractures. Ann R Coll Surg Engl 84:196–200

13. Alves OL, Bullock R (2003) "Basal durotomy" to prevent massive intra-operative traumatic brain swelling. Acta Neurochir (Wien) 145:583–586, discussion 586. Review

14. American college of Surgeons Committee on Trauma (2004) Advanced Trauma Life support for doctors, 7th edn. American College of Surgeons, Chicago, pp 1–391

15. Andrews BT, Pitts LH, Lovely MP et al (1986) Is computed tomographic scanning necessary in patients with tentorial herniation? Results of immediate surgical exploration without computed tomography in 100 patients. Neurosurgery 19: 408–414

16. Andrews BT, Chiles BW 3rd, Olsen WL et al (1988) The effect of intracerebral hematoma location on the risk of brainstem compression and on clinical outcome. J Neurosurg 69: 518–522

17. Andrews BT, Mampalam TJ, Omsberg E et al (1990) Intraoperative ultrasound imaging of the entire brain through unilateralexploratory burr holes after severe head injury: technical note. Surg Neurol 33:291–294

18. Annegers JF, Grabow JD, Groover RV et al (1980) Seizures after head trauma in population study. Neurology 30:683–689

19. Annegers JF, Hauser WA, Coan SP et al (1998) A population-based study of seizures after traumatic brain injuries. N Engl J Med 338:20–24

20. Arrese I, Lobato RD, Gomez PA et al (2004) Hyperacute epidural haematoma isodense with the brain on computed tomography. Acta Neurochir (Wien) 146:193–194

21. Asghar M, Adhiyaman V, Greenway MW et al (2002) Chronic subdural haematoma in the elderly – a North Wales experience. J R Soc Med 95:290–292

22. Atzema C, Mower WR, Hoffman JR et al (2004) Defining "therapeutically inconsequential" head computed tomographic findings in patients with blunt head trauma. Ann Emerg Med 44:47–56

23. Badjatia N, Carney N, Crocco TJ et al (2008) Guidelines for prehospital management of traumatic brain injury 2nd edition. Prehosp Emerg Care 12(Suppl 1):S1–S52

24. Baechli H, Nordmann A, Bucher HC et al (2004) Demographics and prevalent risk factors of chronic subdural haematoma: results of a large single-center cohort study. Neurosurg Rev 27:263–266

25. Baker SP, O'Neill B (1976) The injury severity score: an update. J Trauma 16:882–885

26. Baker SP, O'Neill B, Haddon W Jr (1974) The injury severity score: a method for describing patients with multiple injuries and evaluating emergency care. J Trauma 14:187–196

27. Balki M, Manninen PH, McGuire GP et al (2003) Venous air embolism during awake craniotomy in a supine patient. Can J Anaesth 50:835–838

28. Bender MB, Christoff N (1974) Non-surgical treatment of subdural hermatomas. Arch Neurol (Chicago) 31:73–79

29. Berne JD, Norwood SH, McAuley CE et al (2004) J Trauma 57:11–17, discussion 17–9

30. Besson G, Leguyader J, Bagot d'Arc M et al (1978) Extradural hematoma of the posterior fossa. Neurochirurgie 24: 53–63 [Article in French]

31. Blaha M, Lazar D (2005) Traumatic brain injury and haemorrhagic complications after intracranial pressure. J Neurol Neurosurg Psychiatry 76:147

32. Blumenfeld H An interactive online guide to neurologic examination. http://www.neuroexam.com/

33. Bolliger SA, Thali MJ, Zollinger U (2007) Nontraumatic intracranial epidural hematoma: a case report. Am J Forensic Med Pathol 28:227–229

34. Bor-Seng-Shu E, Aguiar PH, de Almeida Leme RJ, et al (2004) Epidural hematomas of the posterior cranial fossa. Neurosurg Focus 16:ECP1

35. Borzone M, Rivano C, Altomonte M et al (1995) Acute traumatic posterior fossa subdural haematomas. Acta Neurochir (Wien) 135:32–37, Review

36. Bouillon B, Kanz KG, Lackner CK et al (2004) The importance of Advanced Trauma Life Support (ATLS) in the emergency room. Unfallchirurg 107:844–850, German

37. Bouras T, Stranjalis G, Korfias S et al (2007) Head injury mortality in a geriatric population: differentiating an "edge" age group with better potential for benefit than older poor-prognosis patients. J Neurotrauma 24:355–1361

38. Bowers SA, Marshall LF (1980) Outcome in 200 consecutive cases of severe head injury treated in San Diego County: a prospective analysis. Neurosurgery 6:237–242

39. Braakman R (1972) Depressed skull fracture: Data, treatment, and follow-up in 225 consecutive cases. J Neurol Neurosurg Psychiatry 35:395–402

40. Braakman R, Avezaat CJJ, Maas AIR et al (1977) Interobserver agreement in the assessment of the motor response Glasgow coma scale. Clin Neurol Neurosurg 80: 100–106

41. Foundation BT (2007) American Association of Neurological Surgeons; Congress of Neurological Surgeons; Joint Section on Neurotrauma and Critical Care. AANS/CNS. Guidelines for the management of severe traumatic brain injury. VI. Indications for intracranial pressure monitoring. J Neurotrauma 24(Suppl 1):S37–S44

42. Bratton SL, Chestnut R, Ghajar J, et al (2007) IV infection prophylaxis. J Neurotrauma 24(Suppl 1):S-26–S-31

43. Bricolo AP, Pasut ML (1984) Extradural hematoma: Toward zero mortality. A prospective study. Neurosurgery 14:8–11

44. Brown CV, Zada G, Salim A et al (2007) Indications for routine repeat head computed tomography (CT) stratified by severity of traumatic brain injury. J Trauma 62:1339–1344, discussion 1344–1345

45. Bruce DA, Alavi A, Bilaniuk L et al (1981) Diffuse cerebral swelling following head injuries in children: the syndrome of 'malignant brain edema. J Neurosurg 54:170–178

46. Bullock R, Van Dellen JR (1982) Chronic extradural hematoma. Surg Neurol 18:300–302

47. Bullock R, Hanemann CO, Murray L et al (1990) Recurrent hematomas following craniotomy for traumatic intracranial mass. J Neurosurg 72:9–14

48. Bullock MR, Chesnut R, Ghajar J (2006) Surgical management of acute epidural hematomas. Neurosurgery 58(3 Suppl): S7–S15

49. Bullock MR, Chesnut R, Ghajar J et al (2006) Surgical management of acute subdural hematomas. Neurosurgery 58(3): 16–24, discussion Si-iv. Review

50. Bullock MR, Chesnut R, Ghajar J et al (2006) Surgical management of traumatic parenchymal lesions. 3 58(3):25–46, discussion Si-iv. Review

51. Bullock MR, Chesnut R, Ghajar J et al (2006) Surgical management of posterior fossa mass lesions. Neurosurgery 58(3):47–55, discussion Si-iv. Review

52. Bullock MR, Chesnut R, Ghajar J et al (2006) Surgical management of depressed cranial fractures. Neurosurgery 58(3):56–60, discussion Si-iv. Review

53. Butcher I, McHugh GS, Lu J et al (2007) Prognostic value of cause of injury in traumatic brain injury: results from the IMPACT study. J Neurotrauma 24:281–286

54. Caldicott DG, Pearce A, Price R et al (2004) Not just another 'head lac'… low-velocity, penetrating intra-cranial injuries: a case report and review of the literature. Injury 35:1044–1054, Review

55. Cardoso ER, Galbraith S (1985) Posttraumatic hydrocephalus – a retrospective review. Surg Neurol 23:261–264

56. Caroli M, Locatelli M, Campanella R et al (2001) Multiple intracranial lesions in head injury: clinical considerations, prognostic factors, management, and results in 95 patients. Surg Neurol 56:82–88

57. Chan KH, Mann KS, Yue CP et al (1990) The significance of skull fracture in acute traumatic intracranial hematomas in adolescents: A prospective study. J Neurosurg 72:189–194

58. Chang EF, Meeker M, Holland MC (2006) Acute traumatic intraparenchymal hemorrhage: risk factors for progression in the early post-injury period. Neurosurgery 58:647–656, discussion 647–656

59. Chedid MK, Vender JR, Harrison SJ et al (2001) Delayed appearance of a traumatic intracranial a et al (2001) neurysm. Case report and review of the literature. J Neurosurg 94:637–641, Review

60. Chen CW, Kuo JR, Lin HJ et al (2004) Early post-operative seizures after burr-hole drainage for chronic subdural hematoma: correlation with brain CT findings. Clin Neurosci 11:706–709

61. Chesnut RM, Marshall LF (1991) Management of head injury. Treatment of abnormal intracranial pressure. Neurosurg Clin North Am 2:267–284

62. Chesnut RH, Ghajar J, Maas AIR, et al Early indicators of prognosis in severe traumatic brain injury. III. Glasgow coma scale score.http://www.braintrauma.org/site/PageServer?pagename=Guidelines

63. Chesnut RH, Ghajar J, Maas AIR, et al: Early indicators of prognosis in severe traumatic brain injury. IV. Age. http://www.braintrauma.org/site/PageServer?pagename=Guidelines

64. Chesnut RH, Ghajar J, Maas AIR, et al: Early indicators of prognosis in severe traumatic brain injury. VI. Hypotension. http://www.braintrauma.org/site/PageServer?pagename=Guidelines

65. Chesnut RH, Ghajar J, Maas AIR, et al: Early indicators of prognosis in severe traumatic brain injury. V. Pupillary Diameter & Light Reflex. http://www.braintrauma.org/site/PageServer?pagename=Guidelines

66. Chesnut RH, Ghajar J, Maas AIR, et al: Early indicators of prognosis in severe traumatic brain injury. VII. CT scan features.http://www.braintrauma.org/site/PageServer?pagename=Guidelines

67. Chesnut RM, Marshall LF, Klauber MR et al (1993) The role of secondary brain injury in determining outcome from severe head injury. J Trauma 34:216–222

68. Chesnut RM, Marshall SB, Piek J et al (1993) Early and late systemic hypotension as a frequent and fundamental source of cerebral ischemia following severe brain injury in the Traumatic Coma Data Bank. Acta Neurochir Suppl Wien 59:21–125

69. Chesnut RM, Gautille T, Blunt BA et al (1994) The localizing value of asymmetry in pupillary size in severe head injury. Neurosurgery 34:840–845, discussion 845–846

70. Chieregato A, Fainardi E, Morselli-Labate AM et al (2005) Factors associated with neurological outcome and lesion progression in traumatic subarachnoid hemorrhage patients. Neurosurgery 56:671–680, discussion 671–680

71. Chim H, Schantz JT (2005) New frontiers in calvarial reconstruction: integrating computer-assisted design and tissue engineering in cranioplasty. Plast Reconstr Surg 116:1726–1741, Review

72. Choi SC, Muizelaar JP, Barnes TY et al (1991) Prediction tree for severely head-injured patients. J Neurosurg 75:251–255, Comment in: J Neurosurg, 76: 561–562

73. Clavel M, Onzain I, Gutierrez F (1982) Chronic epidural haematomas. Acta Neurochir (Wien) 66:71–81

74. Clifton GL, Miller ER, Choi SC et al (2001) Lack of effect of induction of hypothermia after acute brain injury. N Engl J Med 344:556–563

75. Cohen JE, Montero A, Israel ZH (1996) Prognosis and clinical relevance of anisocoria-craniotomy latency for epidural hematoma in comatose patients. J Trauma 41: 120–122

76. Coles JP (2007) Imaging after brain injury. Br J Anaesth 99:49–60, Review

77. Cooper PR (1992) Delayed traumatic intracerebral hemorrhage. Neurosurg Clin North Am 3:659–665

78. CRASH head-injury prognostic models. http://www.crash2.lshtm.ac.uk/Risk%20calculator/index.html

79. Cremer OL, Moons KG, van Dijk GW et al (2006) Prognosis following severe head injury: Development and validation of a model for prediction of death, disability, and functional recovery. J Trauma 61:1484–1491

80. Culotta VP, Sementilli ME, Gerold K et al (1996) Clinicopathological heterogeneity in the classification of mild head injury. Neurosurgery 38:245–250

81. Cummings TJ, Johnson RR, Diaz FG et al (2000) The relationship of blunt head trauma, subarachnoid hemorrhage, and rupture of pre-existing intracranial saccular aneurysms. Neurol Res 22:165–170

82. Darrouzet V, Duclos JY, Liguoro D et al (2001) Management of facial paralysis resulting from temporal bone fractures: Our experience in 115 cases. Otolaryngol Head Neck Surg 125:77–84

83. D'Avella D, Cacciola F, Angileri FF et al (2001) Traumatic intracerebellar hemorrhagic contusions and hematomas. J Neurosurg Sci 45:29–37

84. D'Avella D, Servadei F, Scerrati M et al (2003) Traumatic acute subdural haematomas of the posterior fossa: clinicoradiological analysis of 24 patients. Acta Neurochir (Wien) 145:1037–1044, discussion 1044

85. Davis PC (2007) Expert Panel on Neurologic Imaging. Head trauma. Am J Neuroradiol 28:1619–1621, Review

86. Dawson SL, Hirsch CS, Lucas FV et al (1980) The contrecoup phenomenon. Reappraisal of a classic problem. Hum Pathol 11:155–166

87. De Souza M, Moncure M, Lansford T et al (2007) Nonoperative management of epidural hematomas and subdural hematomas: is it safe in lesions measuring one centimeter or less? J Trauma 63:370–372

88. Deutsche Gesellschaft für Neurologie, Leitlinien (2004) Diagnostische Liquorpunktion. http://www.uni-duesseldorf.de/AWMF/ll/030–107.htm

89. Domenicucci M, Signorini P, Strzelecki J et al (1995) Delayed post-traumatic epidural hematoma. A review. Neurosurg Rev 18:109–122, Review

90. Donovan DJ, Moquin RR, Ecklund JM (2006) Cranial burr holes and emergency craniotomy: review of indications and technique. Mil Med 171:12–19

91. du Plessis JJ (1993) Depressed skull fracture involving the superior sagittal sinus as a cause of persistent raised intracranial pressure: a case report. J Trauma 34:290–292

92. du Trevou MD, van Dellen JR (1992) Penetrating stab wounds to the brain: the timing of angiography in patients presenting with the weapon already removed. Neurosurgery 31:905–911

93. du Trevou M, Bullock R, Teasdale E et al (1991) False aneurysms of the carotid tree due to unsuspected penetrating injury of the head and neck. Injury 22:237–239

94. Duhem R, Vinchon M, Tonnelle V et al (2006) Main temporal aspects of the MRI signal of subdural hematomas and practical contribution to dating head injury. Neurochirurgie 52:93–104, French

95. Dupuis O, Silveira R, Dupont C et al (2005) Comparison of "instrument-associated" and "spontaneous" obstetric depressed skull fractures in a cohort of 68 neonates. Am J Obstet Gynecol 192:165–170

96. Ellis TS, Vezina LG, Donahue DJ (2000) Acute identification of cranial burst fracture: comparison between CT and MR imaging findings. Am J Neuroradiol 21:795–801

97. Engberg A, Teasdale T (2001) Traumatic brain injury in Denmark 1979–1996. A national study of incidence and mortality. Eur J Epidemiol 17:437–442

98. Englander J, Bushnik T, Duong TT et al (2003) Analyzing risk factors for late posttraumatic seizures: a prospective, multicenter investigation. Arch Phys Med Rehabil 84:365–373

99. Ernestus RI, Beldzinski P, Lanfermann H et al (1997) Chronic subdural hematoma: surgical treatment and outcome in 104 patients. Surg Neurol 48:220–225

100. Evans RW (1992) The postconcussion syndrome and the sequelae of mild head injury. Neurol Clin 10:815–847, Review

101. Evans SJ (2007) Armored brain. Neurology 68:1954

102. Eyes B, Evans AF (1978) Post-traumatic skull radiographs. Time for a reappraisal. Lancet 2(8080):85–86

103. Fabbri A, Servadei F, Marchesini G et al (2004) Prospective validation of a proposal for diagnosis and management of patients attending the emergency department for mild head injury. J Neurol Neurosurg Psychiatry 75:410–416

104. Fabbri A, Servadei F, Marchesini G et al (2005) Clinical performance of NICE recommendations versus NCWFNS proposal in patients with mild head injury. J Neurotrauma 22:1419–1427

105. Fackler ML (1988) Wound ballistics: a review of common misconceptions. JAMA 259:2730–2736

106. Fakhry SM, Trask AL, Waller MA et al (2004) Management of brain-injured patients by an evidence-based medicine protocol improves outcomes and decreases hospital charges. J Trauma 56:492–499, discussion 499–500

107. Feiz-Erfan I, Horn EM, Theodore N et al (2007) Incidence and pattern of direct blunt neurovascular injury associated with trauma to the skull base. J Neurosurg 107:364–369

108. Fisher CM, Kistler JP, Davis JM (1980) Relation of cerebral vasospasm to subarachnoid hemorrhage visualized by computerized tomographic scanning. Neurosurgery 6:1–9

109. Flaada JT, Leibson CL, Mandrekar JN et al (2007) Relative risk of mortality after traumatic brain injury: a population-based study of the role of age and injury severity. J Neurotrauma 24:435–445

110. Flibotte JL, Lee KE, Koroshetz WJ (2004) Continuous antibiotic prophylaxis and cerebral spinal fluid infection in patients with intracranial pressure monitors. Neurocritical Care 1:61–68

111. Fodstad H, Love JA, Ekstedt J et al (1984) Effect of cranioplasty on cerebrospinal fluid hydrodynamics in patients with the syndrome of the trephined. Acta Neurochir (Wien) 70:21–30

112. Foreman BP, Caesar RR, Parks J et al (2007) Usefulness of the abbreviated injury score and the injury severity score in comparison to the Glasgow Coma Scale in predicting outcome after traumatic brain injury. J Trauma 62:946–950

113. Fukamachi A, Koizumi H, Nukui H (1985) Postoperative intracerebral hemorrhages: a survey of computed tomographic findings after 1074 intracranial operations. Surg Neurol 23:575–580

114. Gaab M, Knoblich OE, Fuhrmeister U et al (1979) Comparison of the effects of surgical decompression and resection of local edema in the therapy of experimental brain trauma. Child's Brain 5:484–498

115. Galbraith SL (1973) Age-distribution of extradural haemorrhage without skull fracture. Lancet 1(7814):1217–1218

116. Gale T, Leslie K (2004) Anaesthesia for neurosurgery in the sitting position. J Clin Neurosci 11:693–696, Review

117. Gallagher CN, Hutchinson PJ, Pickard JD (2007) Neuroimaging in trauma. Curr Opin Neurol 20:403–409

118. Gastone P, Fabrizia C, Homere M et al (2004) Chronic subdural hematoma: Results of a homogeneous series of 159 patients operated on by residents. Neurol India 52:475–477

119. Gatscher S, Brew S, Banks T et al (2007) Multislice spiral computed tomography for pediatric intracranial vascular pathophysiologies. J Neurosurg 107(3 Suppl):203–208

120. Gelabert-González M, Ginesta-Galan V, Sernamito-García R et al (2006) The Camino intracranial pressure device in clinical practice. Assessment in a 1000 cases. Acta Neurochir (Wien) 148:435–441

121. Gennarelli TA (1983) Head injury in man and experimental animals: clinical aspects. Acta Neurochir Suppl (Wien) 32:1–13

122. Gennarelli TA (1987) Cerebral concussion and diffuse brain injuries. In: Cooper PR (ed) Head Injury. Williams & Wilkins, Baltimore

123. Gennarelli TA (1993) Mechanisms of brain injury. J Emerg Med 11:5–11

722

736

73678636636

124. Gennarelli TA, Thibault LE (1982) Biomechanics of acute subdural hematoma. J Trauma 22:680–686

125. Gennarelli TA, Thibault LE, Adams JH et al (1982) Diffuse axonal injury and traumatic coma in the primate. Ann Neurol 12:564–574

126. Gennarelli TA, Champion HR, Sacco WJ et al (1989) Mortality of patients with head injury and extracranial injury treated in trauma centers. J Trauma 29:1193–1201

127. Gennarelli TA, Champion HR, Copes WS et al (1994) Comparison of mortality, morbidity, and severity of 59,713 head injured patients with 114,447 patients with extracranial injuries. J Trauma 37:62–968

128. Gentleman D, Nath F, Macpherson P (1989) Diagnosis and management of delayed traumatic intracerebral haematomas. Br J Neurosurg 3:367–372

129. Gentry LR, Godersky JC, Thompson B et al (1988) Prospective comparative study of intermediate-field MR and CT in the evaluation of closed head trauma. Am J Roentgenol 150:673–682

130. George ED, Bland LI (1993) Missiles injuries. In: Apuzzo MLJ (ed) Brain surgery. complication avoidance and management. Churchill Livingstone, New York, Edinburgh, London, Melbourne, Tokyo, pp 1953–1965

131. George ED, Rusyniak WG (1993) Missile injuries of the frontal and middle fossa. In: Apuzzo MLJ (ed) Brain surgery. complication avoidance and management. Churchill Livingstone, New York, Edinburgh, London, Melbourne, Tokyo, pp 1335–1350

132. Ghajar JB, Hairiri RJ, Paterson RH (1993) Improved outcome from traumatic coma using only ventricular CSF drainage for ICP control. Adv Neurosurg 21:173–177

133. Gladwell M, Viozzi C (2008) Temporal bone fractures: a review for the oral and maxillofacial surgeon. J Oral Maxillofac Surg 66:513–522, Review

134. Goettler CE, Tucci K (2007) Decreasing the morbidity of decompressive craniectomy: the Tucci flap. Trauma 62:777–778

135. Gómez PA, Lobato RD, Ortega JM et al (1996) Mild head injury: differences in prognosis among patients with a Glasgow Coma Scale score of 13 to 15 and analysis of factors associated with abnormal CT findings. Br J Neurosurg 10:453–460

136. Gonzalez Tortosa J, Martínez-Lage JF, Poza M (2004) Bitemporal head crush injuries: clinical and radiological features of a distinctive type of head injury. Neurosurg 100:645–651

137. Goodman H, Brundage SI, Diaz-Marchan PJ (2005) Diagnostic criteria for postconcussional syndrome after mild to moderate traumatic brain injury. J Neuropsychiatry Clin Neurosci 17:350–356

138. Goodman SJ, Cahan L, Chow AW (1977) Subgaleal abscess-A preventable complication of scalp trauma (Medical Information). West J Med 127:169–172

139. Gower DJ, Lee KS, McWhorter JM (1988) Role of subtemporal decompression in severe closed head injury. Neurosurgery 23:417–422

140. Graham DI, Adams JH, Gennarelli TA (1988) Mechanisms of non-penetrating head injury. Prog Clin Biol Res 264:159–168

141. Grande PO, Asgeirsson B, Nordstrom CH (2002) Volume-targeted therapy of increased intracranial pressure: the Lund concept unifies surgical and non-surgical treatments. Acta Anaesthesiol Scand 46:929–941

142. Griffiths SJ, Jatavallabhula NS, Mitchell RD (2002) Spontaneous extradural haematoma associated with craniofacial infections: case report and review of the literature. Br J Neurosurg 16:188–191

143. Gudeman SK, Young HF, Miller JD et al (1989) Indications for operative treatment and operative technique in closed head injury. In: Becker DP, Gudeman SK (eds) Textbook of head injury. WB Saunders, Philadelphia

144. Guérit JM (2005) Evoked potentials in severe brain injury. Prog Brain Res 150:415–426, Review

145. Guerra WK, Gaab MR, Dietz H et al (1999) Surgical decompression for traumatic brain swelling: indications and results. J Neurosurg 90:187–196

146. Guilburd JN, Sviri GE (2001) Role of dural fenestrations in acute subdural hematoma. J Neurosurg 95:263–267

147. Gusmão SN, Pittella J (1998) Extradural haematoma and diffuse axonal injury in victims of fatal road traffic accidents. Br J Neurosurg 12:123–126

148. Gutman MB, Moulton RJ, Sullivan I et al (1992) Risk factors predicting operable intracranial hematomas in head injury. J Neurosurg 77:9–14

149. Haddad FS, Haddad GFF, Taha J (1991) Traumatic intracranial aneurysms caused by missiles: their presentation and management. Neurosurgery 28:1–7

150. Hamilton MG, Wallace C (1992) Nonoperative management of acute epidural hematoma diagnosed by CT: The neuroradiologist's role. AJNR 13:853–859

151. Harhangi BS, Kompanje EJ, Leebeek FW et al (2008) Coagulation disorders after traumatic brain injury. Acta Neurochir (Wien) 150:165–175, discussion 175. Review

152. Harris MB, Kronlage SC, Carboni PA et al (2000) Evaluation of the cervical spine in the polytrauma patient. Spine 25:2884–2891, discussion 2892

153. Haselsberger K, Pucher R, Auer L (1988) Prognosis after acute subdural or epidural haemorrhage. Acta Neurochir (Wien) 90:111–116

154. Hawley CA, Ward AB, Long J et al (2003) Prevalence of traumatic brain injury amongst children admitted to hospital in one health district: a population-based study. Injury 34:256–260

155. Hayashi T, Kameyama M, Imaizumi S et al (2007) Acute epidural hematoma of the posterior fossa - cases of acute clinical deterioration. Am J Emerg Med 25:989–995

156. Haydel MJ, Preston CA, Mills TJ et al (2000) Indications for computed tomography in patients with minor head injury. N Engl J Med 343:100–105

157. Herrera EJ, Viano JC, Aznar IL et al (2000) Posttraumatic intracranial hematomas in infancy. a 16-year experience. Childs Nerv Syst 16:585–589

158. Hierner R, van Loon J, Goffin J et al (2007) Free latissimus dorsi flap transfer for subtotal scalp and cranium defect reconstruction: report of 7 cases. Microsurgery 27:425–428

159. Hofman PA, Nelemans P, Kemerink GJ et al (2000) Value of radiological diagnosis of skull fracture in the management of mild head injury: metaanalysis. J Neurol Neurosurg Psychiatry 68:416–422

160. Holloway KL, Barnes T, Choi S et al (1996) Ventriculostomy infections: the effect of monitoring duration and catheter exchange in 584 patients. J Neurosurg 85:419–424

161. Holly LT, Kelly DF, Counelis GJ et al (2002) Cervical spine trauma associated with moderate and severe head injury: incidence, risk factors, and injury characteristics. J Neurosurg 96(Suppl):285–291

162. Holmes B, Harbaugh RE (1993) Traumatic intracranial aneurysms: a contemporary review. J Trauma 35:855–860

163. Holzschuh M, Schuknecht B (1998) Traumatic epidural haematomas of the posterior fossa: 20 new cases and a review of the literature since 1961. Br J Neurosurg 3:171–180, Review

164. Howard MA 3rd, Gross AS, Dacey RJ Jr et al (1989) Acute subdural hematomas: An age-dependent clinical entity. J Neurosurg 1:858–863

165. Hughes DG, Jackson A, Mason DL et al (2004) Abnormalities on magnetic resonance imaging seen acutely following mild traumatic brain injury: correlation with neuropsychological tests and delayed recovery. Neuroradiology 46:550–558

166. Huisman TA, Sorensen AG, Hergan K (2003) Diffusion weighted imaging for the evaluation of diffuse axonal injury in closed head injury. J Comput Assist Tomogr 27: 5–11

167. Hukkelhoven CW, Steyerberg EW, Farace E et al (2002) Regional differences in patient characteristics, case management, and outcomes in traumatic brain injury: experience from the tirilazad trials. J Neurosurg 97:549–557

168. Hutchinson PJ, Kirkpatrick PJ (2004) Decompressive craniectomy in head injury. Curr Opin Crit Care 10:101–104, Review

169. Imola MJ, Schramm V (2006) Skull base: reconstruction. http://www.emedicine.com/ent/topic703.htm

170. Ingebrigtsen T, Romner B, Kock-Jensen C (2000) Scandinavian guidelines for initial management of minimal, mild, and moderate head injuries. J Trauma 48:760–766

171. Ishiwata Y, Fujitsu K, Sekino T et al (1988) Subdural tension pneumocephalus following surgery for chronic subdural hematoma. J Neurosurg 68:58–61

172. Iwabuchi T, Sobata E, Ebina K et al (1986) Dural sinus pressure: various aspects in human brain surgery in children and adults. Am J Physiol 250:H389–H396

173. Jagger J, Jane JA, Rimel R (1983) The Glasgow coma scale: to sum or not to sum? Lancet 2(8341):97

174. Jamjoom A (1992) The influence of concomitant intradural pathology on the presentation and outcome of patients with acute traumatic extradural haematoma. Acta Neurochir (Wien) 115:86–89

175. Jamjoom AB, Kane N, Sandeman D et al (1991) Epilepsy related to traumatic extradural haematomas. BMJ 302(6774): 448

176. Jend HH, Helkenberg G (1995) Über den Wert der konventionellen Schädelaufnahmen nach Kopfverletzungen. Rofo Fortschr Geb Rontgenstr Neuen Bildgeb Verfahr 162:7–12

177. Jennett B (1996) Epidemiology of head injury. J Neurol Neurosurg Psychiatry 60:362–369

178. Jennett B, Miller J (1972) Infection after depressed fracture of skull Implications for management of nonmissile injuries. Neurosurg 36:333–339

179. Jennett B, Bond M (1975) Assessment of outcome after severe brain damage. Lancet 1(7905):480–484

180. Jennett B, Miller J, Braakman R (1974) Epilepsy after nonmissile depressed skull fracture. J Neurosurg 41:208–216

181. Jiang JY, Xu W, Li WP et al (2005) Efficacy of standard trauma craniectomy for refractory intracranial hypertension with severe traumatic brain injury: a multicenter, prospective, randomized controlled study. J Neurotrauma 22:623–628

182. Jinkins JR, Dadsetan MR, Sener RN et al (1992) Value of acute-phase angiography in the detection of vascular injuries caused by gunshot wounds to the head: analysis of 12 cases. Am J Roentgenol 159:365–368

183. Joffe AR (2007) Lumbar puncture and brain herniation in acute bacterial meningitis: a review. J Intensive Care Med 22:194–207

184. Jonas H (2003) Commentary to: Abe M, Udono H, Tabuchi K et al (2003) Analysis of ischemic brain damage in cases of acute subdural hematomas. Surg Neurol 59:464–472, discussion 472

185. Jones PA, Andrews PJ, Midgley S et al (1994) Measuring the burden of secondary insults in head-injured patients during intensive care. J Neurosurg Anesthesiol 6:4–14

186. Joshi AS (2007) Skull base: anatomy. http://www.emedicine.com/ent/TOPIC237.HTM

187. Juul N, Morris GF, Marshall SB et al (2000) Intracranial hypertension hypertension and cerebral perfusion pressure: influence on neurological deterioration and outcome in severe head injury – The Executive Committee of the International Selfotel Trial L. J Neurosurg 92:1–6

188. Kaplan JL, Roesler DM, (2008) Critical care considerations in trauma. http://www.emedicine.com/med/topic3218.htm

189. Katzen JT, Jarrahy R, Eby JB et al (2003) Craniofacial and skull base trauma. J Trauma 54:1026–1034, Review

190. Kaufman HH (1993) Civilian gunshot wounds to the head. Neurosurgery 32:962–964

191. Kaufmann MA, Buchmann B, Scheidegger D et al (1992) Severe head injury: should expected outcome influence resuscitation and first day decisions? Resuscitation 23: 99–206

192. Kerner T, Fritz G, Unterberg A et al (2003) Pulmonary air embolism in severe head injury. Resuscitation 56:111–115

193. Kim TW, Lee JK, Moon KS et al (2007) Penetrating gunshot injuries to the brain. J Trauma 62:1446–1451

194. King N (1997) Mild head injury: neuro-pathology, sequelae, measurement and recovery. Br J Clin Psychol 36:161–184

195. Kjellberg RN, Prieto AJ (1971) Bifrontal decompressive craniotomy for massive cerebral edema. J Neurosurg 34: 488–493

196. Klauber MR, Marshall LF, Luerssen TG et al (1989) Determinants of head injury mortality: Importance of the low risk patient. Neurosurgery 24:31–36

197. Korinek AM, Golmard JL, Elcheick A et al (2005) Risk factors for neurosurgical site infections after craniotomy: a critical reappraisal of antibiotic prophylaxis on 4,578 patients. Br J Neurosurg 19:155–162

198. Kotwica Z, Brzeiński J (1991) Epilepsy in chronic subdural haematoma. Acta Neurochir (Wien) 113:118–120

199. Kotwica Z, Brzeiński J (1993) Acute subdural haematoma in adults: An analysis of outcome in comatose patients. Acta Neurochir (Wien) 121:95–99

200. Kraus JF, McArthur DL (1996) Epidemiologic aspects of brain injury. Neurol Clin 14:435–450

201. Kunze E, Meixensberger J, Janka M et al (1998) Decompressive craniectomy in patients with uncontrollable intracranial hypertension. Acta Neurochir Suppl 71:16–18

202. Kuo JR, Wang CC, Chio CC et al (2004) Neurological improvement after cranioplasty - analysis by transcranial Doppler ultrasonography. J Clin Neurosci 11:486–489

203. Kurokawa Y, Ishizaki E, Inaba K (2005) Bilateral chronic subdural hematoma cases showing rapid and progressive aggravation. Surg Neurol 64:444–449, discussion 449

204. Lang EW, Chesnut RM (1995) Intracranial pressure and cerebral perfusion pressure in severe head injury. New Horizons 3:400–409

205. Lee AC, Ou Y, Fong D (2003) Depressed skull fractures: a pattern of abusive head injury in three older children. Child Abuse Negl 27:1323–1329

206. Lee E, Hung Y, Wang L et al (1998) Factors influencing the functional outcome of patients with acute epidural hematomas: analysis of 200 patients undergoing surgery. J Trauma 45:946–952

207. Lee KS (1998) The pathogenesis and clinical significance of traumatic subdural hygroma. Brain Inj 12:595–603

208. Lee TT, Villanueva PA (1997) Orbital-frontal delayed hemorrhagic contusions: clinical course and neurosurgical treatment protocol. Surg Neurol 48:333

209. Lee TT, Ratzker PA, Galarza M et al (1998) Early Combined Management of Frontal Sinus and Orbital and Facial Fractures. J Trauma 44:665–669

210. Leedy JE, Janis JE, Rohrich RJ (2005) Reconstruction of acquired scalp defects: an algorithmic approach. Plast Reconstr Surg 116:54e–72e

211. LeRoux PD, Haglund MM, Newell DW et al (1992) Intraventricular hemorrhage in blunt head trauma: an analysis of 43 cases. Neurosurgery 31:678–684

212. Lesieur O, Verrier V, Lequeux B et al (2006) Retained knife blade: an unusual cause for headache following massive alcohol intake. Emerg Med J 23:e13

213. Levin HS, Mattis S, Ruff RM et al (1987) Neurobehavioral outcome following minor head injury: a three-center study. J Neurosurg 66((2):234–243

214. Levin HS, Williams D, Crofford MJ et al (1988) Relationship of depth of brain lesions to consciousness and outcome after closed head injury. J Neurosurg 69:861–866

215. Levin HS, Aldrich EF, Saydjari C et al (1992) Severe head injury in children: experience of the Traumatic Coma Data Bank. Neurosurgery 31:435–443, discussion 443–444

216. Levin LA, Beck RW, Joseph MP et al (1999) The treatment of traumatic optic neuropathy: the International Optic Nerve Trauma Study. Ophthalmology 106:1268–1277

217. Liang W, Xiaofeng Y, Weiguo L et al (2007) Cranioplasty of large cranial defect at an early stage after decompressive craniectomy performed for severe head trauma. J Craniofac Surg 18:526–532

218. Licata C, Cristofori L, Gambin R et al (2001) Post-traumatic hydrocephalus. J Neurosurg Sci 45:141–149

219. Lietard C, Thébaud V, Besson G et al (2008) Risk factors for neurosurgical site infections: an 18-month prospective survey. J Neurosurg 109:729–734

220. Lin S, Levi L, Grunau PD et al (2007) Effect measure modification and confounding of severe head injury mortality by age and multiple organ injury severity. Ann Epidemiol 17:142–147

221. Litvack ZN, Hunt MA, Weinstein JS et al (2006) Self-inflicted nail-gun injury with 12 cranial penetrations and associated cerebral trauma. Case report and review of the literature. J Neurosurg 104:828–834, Review

222. Liu JT, Tyan YS, Lee YK et al (2006) Emergency management of epidural haematoma through burr hole evacuation and drainage. A preliminary report. Acta Neurochir (Wien) 148:313–317, discussion 317

223. Livingston DH, Lavery RF, Passannante MR et al (2000) Emergency department discharge of patients with a negative cranial computed tomography scan after minimal head injury. Ann Surg 232:126–132

224. Livingston DH, Lavery RF, Mosenthal AC et al (2005) Recovery at one year following isolated traumatic brain injury: a Western Trauma Association prospective multicenter trial. J Trauma 59:1298–1304, discussion 1304

225. Llamas L, Ramos-Zúñiga R, Sandoval L (2002) Acute interhemispheric subdural hematoma: two case reports and analysis of the literature. Minim Invasive. Neurosurg 45:55–58, Review

226. Lobato RD, Rivas JJ, Cordobes F et al (1988) Acute epidural hematoma: an analysis of factors influencing the outcome of patients undergoing surgery in coma. J Neursosurg 68:48–57

227. Lobato RD, Sarabia R, Cordobes F et al (1988) Post-traumatic cerebral hemispheric swelling. Analysis of 55 cases studied with computerized tomography. J Neurosurg 68:417–423

228. Ludwig B, Nix W, Lanksch W (1983) Computed tomography of the "armored brain". Neuroradiology 25:39–43

229. Maas AI, Dearden M, Teasdale GM et al (1997) EBIC-guidelines for management of severe head injury in adults. European Brain Injury Consortium. Acta Neurochir (Wien) 139:286–294

230. Maas AI, Dearden M, Servadei F et al (2000) Current recommendations for neurotrauma. Curr Opin Crit Care 6:281–292

231. Maas AI, Hukkelhoven CW, Marshall LF et al (2005) Prediction of outcome in traumatic brain injury with computed tomographic characteristics: a comparison between the computed tomographic classification and combinations of computed tomographic predictors. Neurosurgery 57:1173–1182, discussion 1173–1182

232. Maas AI, Steyerberg EW, Butcher I et al (2007) Prognostic value of computerized tomography scan characteristics in traumatic brain injury: results from the IMPACT study. J Neurotrauma 24:303–314

233. Malik NK, Makhdoomi R, Indira B et al (2007) Posterior fossa extradural hematoma: our experience and review of the literature. Surg Neurol 68:155–158, discussion 158

234. Malohtra AK, Camacho M, Ivatury RR et al (2007) Computed tomographic angiography for the diagnosis of blunt carotid/vertebral artery injury: a note of caution. Ann Surg 246:632–642, discussion 642–643

235. Mannion RJ, Cross J, Bradley P et al (2007) Mechanism-based MRI classification of traumatic brainstem injury and its relationship to outcome. J Neurotrauma 24:128–135

236. Manolidis S, Hollier LH Jr (2007) Management of frontal sinus fractures. Plast Reconstr Surg 120(7 Suppl 2): 32S–48S

237. Markwalder TM, Reulen HJ (1986) Influence of neomembranous organisation, cortical expansion and subdural pressure on the post-operative course of chronic subdural

haematoma – an analysis of 201 cases. Acta Neurochir (Wien) 79:100–106

238. Marmarou A, Anderson RL, Ward JD et al (1991) NINDS traumatic coma data bank: intracranial pressure monitoring methodology. J Neurosurg 75:s21-s27

239. Marmarou A, Anderson RL, Ward JD et al (1991) Impact of ICP instability and hypotension on outcome in patients with severe head trauma. J Neurosurg 75:s59-s66

240. Marmarou A, Foda MA, Bandoh K et al (1996) Posttraumatic ventriculomegaly: hydrocephalus or atrophy? A new approach for diagnosis using CSF dynamics. J Neurosurg 85:1026–1035

241. Marmarou A, Lu J, Butcher I, McHugh GS et al (2007) Prognostic value of the Glasgow Coma Scale and pupil reactivity in traumatic brain injury assessed pre-hospital and on enrollment: an IMPACT analysis. J Neurotrauma 24:270–280

242. Marshall AH, Jones NS, Robertson IJA (2001) CSF rhinorrhea: the place of endoscopic sinus surgery. Br J Neurosurg 15:8–12

243. Marshall LF, Gautille T, Klauber RM, et al (1991) The outcome of severe closed head injury. J Neurosurg 75(Suppl): S28–S36

244. Marshall LF, Marshall SB, Klauber MR et al (1991) A new classification of head injury based on computerized tomography. J Neurosurg 75(5S):S14–S20

245. Marshall LF, Marshall SB, Klauber MR et al (1992) The diagnosis of head injury requires a classification based on computed axial tomography. J Neurotrauma 1:S287–S292

246. Martin TJ, Loehrl TA (2007) Endoscopic CSF leak repair. Curr Opin Otolaryngol Head Neck Surg 15:35–39, Review

247. Martins RS, Siqueira MG, Santos MT et al (2003) Prognostic factors and treatment of penetrating gunshot wounds to the head. Surg Neurol 60:98–104, discussion 104

248. Massaro F, Lanotte M, Faccani G et al (1996) One hundred and twenty-seven cases of acute subdural haematoma operated on. Correlation between CT scan findings and outcome. Acta Neurochir (Wien) 138:185–191

249. Masters SJ (1980) Evaluation of head trauma: efficacy of skull films. AJR Am J Roentgenol 135:539–547

250. Masters SJ, McClean PM, Arcarese JS et al (1987) Skull x-ray examinations after head trauma. Recommendations by a multidisciplinary panel and validation study. Engl J Med 316:84–91

251. Matsuno A, Katayama H, Wada H et al (2003) Significance of consecutive bilateral surgeries for patients with acute subdural hematoma who develop contralateral acute epi- or subdural hematoma. Surg Neurol 60:23–30, discussion 30

252. McCrory P, Johnston K, Meeuwisse W et al (2005) International Symposium on Concussion in Sport. Summary and agreement statement of the 2nd International Conference on Concussion in Sport, Prague 2004. Clin J Sport Med 15:48–55, Review

253. McElhaney JH, Hopper RH Jr, Nightingale RW et al (1995) Mechanisms of basilar skull fracture. J Neurotrauma 12: 669–678

254. McHugh GS, Engel DC, Butcher I et al (2007) Prognostic value of secondary insults in traumatic brain injury: results from the IMPACT study. J Neurotrauma 24:287–293

255. McKinney A, Ott F, Short J et al (2007) Angiographic frequency of blunt cerebrovascular injury in patients with carotid canal or vertebral foramen fractures on multidetector CT. Eur J Radiol 62:385–393

256. Meagher RJ, Young WF (2006) Subdural hematoma. http//www.emedicine.com/NEURO/topic575.htm

257. Meerhoff SR, de Kruijk JR, Rutten J et al (2000) Incidence of traumatic head or brain injuries in catchment area of Academic Hospital Maastricht in 1997. Ned Tijdschr Geneeskd 144:1915–1918, Dutch

258. Meier U, Grawe A (2003) The importance of decompressive craniectomy for the management of severe head injuries. Acta Neurochir Suppl 86:367–371

259. Meixensberger J, Roosen K (1998) Clinical and pathophysiological significance of severe neurotrauma in polytraumatized patients. Langenbecks Arch Surg 383:214–219, Review

260. Menkü A, Koç RK, Tucer B et al (2004) Clivus fractures: clinical presentations and courses. Neurosurg Rev 27: 194–198

261. Miller CF, Brodkey JS, Colombi BJ (1977) The danger of intracranial wood. Surg Neurol 7:95–103

262. Miller JD, Becker DP (1982) Secondary insults to the injured brain. J R Coll Surg Edinb 27:292–298

263. Miller JD, Becker DP, Ward JD et al (1977) Significance of intracranial hypertension in severe head injury. J Neurosurg 47:503–516

264. Miller JD, Butterworth JF, Gudeman SK et al (1981) Further experience in the management of severe head injury. J Neurosurg 54:289–299

265. Miller JD, Murray LS, Teasdale GM (1990) Development of a traumatic intracranial hematoma after a "minor" head injury. Neurosurgery 27:669–673

266. Miller JD, Dearden NM, Piper IR et al (1992) Control of intracranial pressure in patients with severe head injury. J Neurotrauma 9(Suppl 1):S317–S326

267. Miller PR, Fabian TC, Croce MA et al (2002) Prospective screening for blunt cerebrovascular injuries: analysis of diagnostic modalities and outcomes. Ann Surg 236:386–395

268. Missori P, Salvati M, Polli FM et al (2002) Intraparenchymal haemorrhage after evacuation of chronic subdural haematoma. Report of three cases and review of the literature. Br J Neurosurg 16:63–66, Review

269. Mori K, Maeda M (2001) Surgical treatment of chronic subdural hematoma in 500 consecutive cases: clinical characteristics, surgical outcome, complications, and recurrence rate. Neurol Med Chir (Tokyo) 41:371–381

270. Moulton RJ, Shedden PM, Tucker WS et al (1994) Somatosensory evoked potential monitoring following severe closed head injury. Clin Invest Med 17:87–195

271. Moyer JS, Chepeha DB, Teknos TN (2004) Contemporary skull base reconstruction. Curr Opin Otolaryngol Head Neck Surg 12:294–299

272. Muchow RD, Resnick DK, Abdel MP et al (2008) Magnetic resonance imaging (MRI) in the clearance of the cervical spine in blunt trauma: a meta analysis. J Trauma 64: 179–189

273. Muench E, Horn P, Schürer L et al (2000) Management of severe traumatic brain injury by decompressive craniectomy. Neurosurger 47:315–323

274. Murano T, Mohr AM, Lavery RF et al (2005) Civilian craniocerebral gunshot wounds: an update in predicting outcomes. Am Surg 71:1009–1014

275. Murray GD, Butcher I, McHugh GS et al (2007) Multivariable prognostic analysis in traumatic brain injury: results from the IMPACT study. J Neurotrauma 24: 329–337

276. Mushkudiani NA, Engel DC, Steyerberg EW et al (2007) Prognostic value of demographic characteristics in traumatic brain injury: results from the IMPACT study. J Neurotrauma 24:259–269

277. Mussack T, Wiedemann E, Hummel T et al (2003) Secondary decompression trepanation in progressive post-traumatic brain edema after primary decompressive craniotomy. Unfallchirurg 106:815–825

278. Muth CM, Shank ES (2000) Gas embolism. Engl J Med 342:476–482

279. Nakaguchi H, Tanishima T, Yoshimasu N (2001) Factors in the natural history of chronic subdural hematomas that influence their postoperative recurrence. J Neurosurg 95: 256–262

280. Natarajan M, Asok Kumar N et al (1989) Usefulness of exploratory burr holes in the management of severe head injury. J Indian Med Assoc 87:256–258

281. Nathoo N, Boodhoo H, Nadvi SS et al (2000) Transcranial brainstem stab injuries: a retrospective analysis of 17 patients. Neurosurgery 47:1117–1122

282. Necajauskaite O, Endziniene M, Jureniene K (2005) The prevalence, course and clinical features of post-concussion syndrome in children. Medicina (Kaunas) 41:457–464

283. Nee PA, Hadfield JM, Faragher EB (1999) Significance of vomiting after head injury. J Neurol Neurosurg Psychiatry 66:470–473

284. No authors listed: Early Indicators of Prognosis in Severe Traumatic Brain Injury. http://www.braintrauma.org/site/DocServer/Prognosis_Guidelines_for_web.pdf?docID=241

285. No authors listed (2001) Neuroimaging in the management of penetrating brain injury. J Trauma 51:S7–S11 http://www.neurosurgery.org/sections/Section.aspx?Section=TR&Page=guidelines/home.asp

286. No authors listed (2001) Surgical management of penetrating brain injury. J Trauma 51(2 Suppl) S16–S25; http://www.neurosurgery.org/sections/Section.aspx?Section=TR&Page=guidelines/home.asp

287. No authors listed (2001) Vascular complications of penetrating brain injury. J Trauma 51(2 Suppl) S26-S28; http://www.neurosurgery.org/sections/Section.aspx?Section=TR&Page=guidelines/home.asp

288. No authors listed (2001) Management of cerebrospinal fluid leaks. J Trauma 51(2 Suppl) S29–S33; http://www.neurosurgery.org/sections/Section.aspx?Section=TR&Page=guidelines/home.asp

289. No authors listed (2001) Antibiotic prophylaxis for penetrating brain injury. J Trauma 51(2 Suppl) S34–S40; http://www.neurosurgery.org/sections/Section.aspx?Section=TR&Page=guidelines/home.asp

290. No authors listed (2001) Antiseizure prophylaxis for penetrating brain injury. J Trauma 51(2 Suppl) S41–S43; http://www.neurosurgery.org/sections/Section.aspx?Section=TR&Page=guidelines/home.asp

291. No authors listed (2001) Part 2: Prognosis in penetrating brain injury. J Trauma 51(2 Suppl) S44–S86; http://www.neurosurgery.org/sections/Section.aspx?Section=TR&Page=guidelines/home.asp

292. No author (2004) Overview of adult traumatic brain injuries http://www.orlandoregional.org/pdf%20folder/overview%20adult%20brain%20injury.pdf

293. No author (2006) Antibiotic prophylaxis in surgery. http://www.surgicalcriticalcare.net/Guidelines/antibiotic_prophylaxis.pdf

294. No authors listed (2006) Appendix I: post-traumatic mass volume measurement in traumatic brain injury patients. Guidelines for the Surgical Management of Traumatic Brain Injury. Neurosurgery 58(Suppl 3):S2–S61

295. No authors listed (2006) Appendix II: evaluation of relevant computed tomographic scan findings. Guidelines for the surgical management of traumatic brain injury. Neurosurgery 58(Suppl 3):S2–62

296. Nortje J, Menon DK (2004) Traumatic brain injury: physiology, mechanisms, and outcome. Curr Opin Neurol 7: 711–718

297. Oertel M, Kelly DF, McArthur D et al (2002) Progressive hemorrhage after head trauma: predictors and consequences of the evolving injury. J Neurosurg 96:109–116

298. Offner PJ, Pham B, Hawkes A (2006) Nonoperative management of acute epidural hematomas: a "no-brainer". Am J Surg 192:801–805

299. Ommaya AK, Gennarelli TA (1974) Cerebral concussion and traumatic unconsciousness. Correlation of experimental and clinical observations of blunt head injuries. Brain 97:633–654

300. O'Neill BR, Velez DA, Braxton EE et al (2008) A survey of ventriculostomy and intracranial pressure monitor placement practices. Surg Neurol 70:268–273

301. Osterwalder J, Riederer M (2000) Quality assessment of multiple trauma management bu ISS, TRISS or ASCOT? Schweiz Med Wochenschr 130:499–504

302. Paci GM, Sise MJ, Sise CB et al (2008) The need for immediate computed tomography scan after emergency craniotomy for head injury. J Trauma 64:326–333

303. Palmer S, Bader MK, Qureshi A et al (2001) The impact on outcomes in a community hospital setting of using the AANS traumatic brain injury guidelines. Americans Associations for Neurologic Surgeons. J Trauma 50: 657–664

304. Parizel PM, Van Goethem JW, Ozsarlak O et al (2005) New developments in the neuroradiological diagnosis of craniocerebral trauma. Eur Radiol 15:569–581

305. Park SH, Hwang SK (2008) Surgical treatment of subacute epidural hematoma caused by a vacuum extraction with skull fracture and cephalohematoma in a neonate. Pediatr Neurosurg 42:270–272

306. Patel HC, Menon DK, Tebbs S et al (2002) Specialist neurocritical care and outcome from head injury. Intensive Care Med 28:547–553

307. Piatt JH Jr (2006) Detected and overlooked cervical spine injury in comatose victims of trauma: report from the

Pennsylvania Trauma Outcomes Study. J Neurosurg Spine 5:210–216

308. Pickard JD, Coleman MR, Czosnyka M (2005) Hydrocephalus, ventriculomegaly and the vegetative state: a review. Neuropsychol Rehabil 15:224–236

309. Piek J (1995) Medical complications in severe head injury. New Horiz 3:534–538

310. Platzer P, Jaindl M, Thalhammer G et al (2006) Clearing the cervical spine in critically injured patients: a comprehensive C-spine protocol to avoid unnecessary delays in diagnosis. Eur Spine J 15:1801–1810

311. Poca MA, Sahuquillo J, Báguena M et al (1998) Incidence of intracranial hypertension after severe head injury: a prospective study using the Traumatic Coma Data Bank classification. Acta Neurochir Suppl 71:27–30

312. Pohlman TH, BjerkeHS, Offner P (2007) Trauma scoring systems. www.emedicine.com/med/topic3214.htm

313. Polin RS, Shaffrey ME, Bogaev CA et al (1997) Decompressive bifrontal craniectomy in the treatment of severe refractory posttraumatic cerebral edema. Neurosurgery 41:84–92

314. Prabhu VC, Kaufman HH, Voelker JL et al (1999) Prophylactic antibiotics with intracranial pressure monitors and external ventricular drains: a review of the evidence. Surg Neurol 52:226–236, discussion 236–237

315. Provenzale J (2007) CT and MR imaging of acute cranial trauma. Emerg Radiol 14:1, Review

316. Quereshi NH, Harsh IVG (2008) Skull fracture. http://www.emedicine.com/med/TOPIC2894.HTM

317. Ramesh VG, Sivakumar S (1995) Extradural hematoma at the vertex: a case report. Surg Neurol 43:138–139

318. Rankin J (1957) Cerebral vascular accidents in patients over the age of 60. Scott Med J 2:200–215

319. Ransohoff J, Benjamin MV, Gage EL et al (1971) Hemicraniectomy in the management of acute subdural hematoma. J Neurosurg 34:70–76

320. Ratilal B, Costa J, Sampaio C (2006) Antibiotic prophylaxis for preventing meningitis in patients with basilar skull fractures. Cochrane Database Syst Rev. 2006 Jan 25;(1): CD004884

321. Raveh J, Laedrach K, Vuillemin T et al (1992) Management of combined frontonaso-orbital/skull base fractures and telecanthus in 355 cases. Arch Otolaryngol Head Neck Surg 118:605–614

322. Reed D (2007) Adult trauma clinical guidelines, initial management of closed head injury in adults. NSW institute of trauma and injury management. http://www.itim.nsw.gov.au/download.cfm?DownloadFile=1F04C4DE-1321-1C29-704622360C25D479

323. Reilly PL, Simpson DA, Sprod R et al (1988) Assessing the conscious level in infants and young children: a paediatric version of the Glasgow Coma Scale. Childs Nerv Syst 4: 30–33

324. Riesgo P, Piquer J, Botella C et al (1997) Delayed extradural hematoma after mild head injury: report of three cases. Surg Neurol 48:226–231

325. Rimel RW, Giordani B, Barth JT et al (1981) Disability caused by minor head injury. Neurosurgery 9:221–228

326. Rinker CF, McMurry FG, Groeneweg VR et al (1998) Emergency craniotomy performed in a rural level III trauma center. J Trauma 44:984–990

327. Rivano C, Borzone M, Carta F et al (1980) Traumatic intracerebral hematomas. 72 cases surgically treated. J Neurosurg Sci 24:77–84

328. Rivas JJ, Lobato RD, Sarabia R et al (1988) Extradural hematoma: analysis of factors influencing the courses of 161 patients. Neurosurgery 23:44–51

329. Roberts I (2000) Barbiturates for acute traumatic brain injury. Cochrane Database 2000; Syst Rev 2: CD000033

330. Robertson CS, Valadka AB, Hannay HJ et al (2004) Prevention of secondary ischaemic insults after severe head injury. Crit Care Med 27:2086–2095

331. Rockswold GL, Leonard PR, Nagib MG (1987) Analysis of management in thirty-three closed head injury patients who talked and deteriorated. Neurosurgery 21:51–55

332. Roos KL (2003) Lumbar puncture. Semin Neurol 23:105–114, Review

333. Ropper AH, Gorson KC (2007) Concussion. N Engl J Med 356:166–172

334. Rosenblum W (1989) Pathophysiology of human head injury. In: Becker D, Gudeman SK (eds) Head injuries. WB Saunders, Philadelphia

335. Rosenfeld JV (2004) Damage control neurosurgery injury. Injury 35:655–660, Review

336. Royal College of Surgeons of England. A working party on the management of the head injured patient. Holborn, London: RCS England, Lincoln's Inn Fields, 1999. http://www.rcseng.ac.uk/publications/docs/report_head_injuries.html/attachment_download/pdffile

337. Rubin G, Rappaport ZH (1993) Epilepsy in chronic subdural haematoma. Acta Neurochir (Wien) 123:39–42, Review

338. Ruff RM, Marshall LF, Crouch J et al (1993) Predictors of outcome following severe head trauma: follow-up data from the Traumatic Coma Data Bank. Brain Inj 7:101–111; Comment in: Brain Inj (1993), 7:99–100

339. Sakas DE, Bullock MR, Teasdale GM (1995) One-year outcome following craniotomy for traumatic hematoma in patients with fixed dilated pupils. J Neurosurg 82:961–965

340. Samii M, Tatagiba M (2002) Skull base trauma: diagnosis and management. Neurol Res 24:147–156, Review

341. Schaefer PW, Huisman TA, Sorensen AG et al (2004) Diffusion-weighted MR imaging in closed head injury: high correlation with initial glasgow coma scale score and score on modified Rankin scale at discharge. Radiology 233:58–66

342. Schierhout G, Roberts I (1998) Prophylactic antiepileptic agents after head injury: a systematic review. J Neurol Neurosurg Psychiatry 64:108–112

343. Schiffer J, Gur R, Nisim U et al (1997) Symptomatic patients after craniectomy. Surg Neurol 47:231–237, Review

344. Schneider GH, Bardt T, Lanksch WR et al (2002) Decompressive craniectomy following traumatic brain injury: ICP, CPP and neurological outcome. Acta Neurochir Suppl 81: 77–79

345. Schüttler J, Schmitz B, Bartsch AC et al (1995) The efficiency of emergency therapy in patients with head-brain, multiple injury. Quality assurance in emergency medicine. Anaesthesist 44:850–858, German

346. Scolozzi P, Martinez A, Jaques B (2007) Complex orbito-fronto-temporal reconstruction using computer-designed PEEK implant. J Craniofac Surg 18:224–228

347. Scotti G, Terbrugge K, Melançon D et al (1977) Evaluation of the age of subdural hematomas by computerized tomography. J Neurosurg 47:311–315

348. Seelig J, Becker D, Miller J et al (1981) Traumatic acute subdural hematoma: Major mortality reduction in comatose patients treated within four hours. N Engl J Med 304:1511–1518, 1981

349. Seelig JM, Marshall LF, Toutant SM et al (1984) Traumatic acute epidural hematoma: unrecognized high lethality in comatose patients. Neurosurg 15:617–620

350. Selhorst B (1989) Neurological examination of head injured patients. In: Becker DP, Gudeman SK (eds) Textbook of head injury. Saunders WB, Philadelphia, pp 82–101

351. Servadei F (1995) Extradural haematomas: how many deaths can be avoided? Protocol for early detection of haematoma in minor head injuries. Acta Neurochir (Wien) 133:50–55

352. Servadei F (1997) Prognostic factors in severely head injured adult patients with epidural haematomas. Acta Neurochir (Wien) 139:273–278

353. Servadei F, Ciucci G, Pagano F et al (1988) Skull fracture as a risk factor of intracranial complications in minor head injuries: A prospective CT study in a series of 98 adult patients. J Neurol Neurosurg Psychiatry 51:526–528

354. Servadei F, Nanni A, Nasi MT et al (1995) Evolving brain lesions in the first 12 h after head injury: Analysis of 37 comatose patients. Neurosurgery 37:899–907

355. Servadei F, Nasi MT, Giuliani G et al (2000) CT prognostic factors in acute subdural haematomas: the value of the 'worst' CT scan. Br J Neurosurg 14:110–116

356. Servadei F, Teasdale G, Merry G et al (2001) Defining acute mild head injury in adults: a proposal based on prognostic factors, diagnosis, and management. J Neurotrauma 18:657–664

357. Servadei F, Murray GD, Teasdale GM et al (2002) Traumatic subarachnoid hemorrhage: demographic and clinical study of 750 patients from the European Brain Injury consortium survey of head injuries. Neurosurgery 50:261–269

358. Shafi S, Diaz-Arrastia R, Madden C et al (2008) Intracranial pressure monitoring in brain-injured patients is associated with worsening of survival. J Trauma 64:335–340

359. Siccardi D, Cavaliere R, Pau A et al (1991) Penetrating craniocerebral missile injuries in civilians: a retrospective analysis of 314 cases. Surg Neurol 35:455–460

360. Siegel JH (1995) The effect of associated injuries, blood loss, and oxygen debt on death and disability in blunt traumatic brain injury: the need for early physiologic predictors of severity. J Neurotrauma 12:579–590

361. Sifri ZC, Homnick AT, Vaynman A et al (2006) A prospective evaluation of the value of repeat cranial computed tomography in patients with minimal head injury and an intracranial bleed. J Trauma 61:862–867

362. Simon B, Letourneau P, Vitorino E et al (2001) Pediatric minor head trauma: indications for computed tomographic scanning revisited. J Trauma 51:231–237, discussion 237–238

363. Skandsen T, Ivar Lund T, Fredriksli O et al (2008) Global outcome, productivity and epilepsy 3–8 years after severe head injury. The impact of injury severity. Clin Rehabil 22: 653–662

364. Smith ER, Carter BS, Ogilvy CS (2002) Proposed use of prophylactic decompressive craniectomy in poor-grade aneurysmal subarachnoid hemorrhage patients presenting with associated large sylvian hematomas. Neurosurgery 51: 117–124

365. Smith HK, Miller JD (1991) The danger of an ultra-early computed tomographic scan in a patient with an evolving acute epidural hematoma. Neurosurgery 29:258–260

366. Smits M, Dippel DW, de Haan GG et al (2007) Minor head injury: guidelines for the use of CT- a multicenter validation study. Radiology 245:831–838

367. Smits M, Hunink MG, van Rijssel DA et al (2008) Outcome after complicated minor head injury. AJNR Am J Neuroradiol 29:506–513

368. Smrkolj V, Balazic J, Princic J (1995) Intracranial injuries by a screwdriver. Forensic Sci Int 76:211–216

369. Soloniuk D, Pitts LH, Lovely M et al (1986) Traumatic intracerebral hematomas: timing of appearance and indications for operative removal. J Trauma 26:787–794

370. Specht CS, Varga JH, Jalali MM et al (1992) Orbitocranial wooden foreign body diagnosed by magnetic resonance imaging. Dry wood can be isodense with air and orbital fat by computed tomography. Surv Ophthalmol 36:341–344

371. Sperry JL, Gentilello LM, Minei JP (2006) Waiting for the patient to "sober up": effect of alcohol intoxication on glasgow coma scale score of brain injured patients. J Trauma 61: 1305–1311

372. Stanisic M, Lund-Johansen M et al (2005) Treatment of chronic subdural hematoma by burr-hole craniostomy in adults: influence of some factors on postoperative recurrence. Acta Neurochir (Wien) 147:1249–1256, discussion 1256–1257

373. Stegemann T, Heimann M, Düsterhus P et al (2006) Diffusion tensor imaging (DTI) and its importance for exploration of normal or pathological brain development. Fortschr Neurol Psychiatr 74:136–148

374. Steiger HJ, Reulen HJ, Huber P et al (1989) Radical resection of superior sagittal sinus meningioma with venous interposition graft and reimplantation of the rolandic veins. Case report. Acta Neurochir 100:108–111

375. Steigerwald C, Draf W, Hofmann E et al (2005) Angiography of the carotid artery in centro-lateral skull base fractures? Laryngorhinootologie 84:910–914, German

376. Stein SC (2001) Minor head injury: 13 is an unlucky number. J Trauma 50:759–760

377. Stiell IG, Clement CM, Rowe BH et al (2005) Comparison of the Canadian CT head rule and the New Orleans criteria in patients with minor head injury. JAMA 294:1511–1518

378. Stocchetti N, Longhi L, Magnoni S et al (1999) Cranial trauma and multiple trauma: from the street to the operating room. Minerva Anestesiol 65:353–356, Review. Italian

379. Stocchetti N, Rossi S, Buzzi F et al (1999) Intracranial hypertension in head injury: management and results. Intensive Care Med 25:371–376

380. Stocchetti N, Colombo A, Ortolano F et al (2007) Time course of intracranial hypertension after traumatic brain injury. J Neurotrauma 24:1339–1346

381. Stone JL, Ladenheim E, Wilkinson SB et al (1991) Hematoma in the posterior fossa secondary to a tangential gunshot wound of the occiput: case report and discussion. Neurosurgery 28:603–605, discussion 605–606

382. Stone JL, Lichtor T, Fitzgerald LF et al (1996) Civilian cases of tangential gunshot wounds to the head. J Trauma 40:57–60

383. Stranjalis G, Bouras T, Korfias S et al (2008) Outcome in 1,000 head injury hospital admissions: the Athens head trauma registry. J Trauma 65:789–793

384. Stuke L, Diaz-Arrastia R, Gentilello LM et al (2007) Effect of alcohol on Glasgow Coma Scale in head-injured patients. Ann Surg 245:651–655

385. Sullivan TP, Jarvik JG, Cohen WA (1999) Follow-up of conservatively managed epidural hematomas: implications for timing of repeat CT. Am J Neurorad 20:107–113

386. Sun TF, Boet R, Poon WS (2005) Non-surgical primary treatment of chronic subdural haematoma: preliminary results of using dexamethasone. Br J Neurosurg 19:327–333

387. Sundstrøm T, Sollid S, Wentzel-Larsen T (2007) Head injury mortality in the Nordic countries. J Neurotrauma 24: 147–153

388. Swinson BD, Jerjes W, Thompson G (2004) Current practice in the management of frontal sinus fractures. J Laryngol Otol 118:927–932, Review

389. Sykes LN Jr, Cowgill F (1989) Management of hemorrhage from severe scalp lacerations with Raney clips. Ann Emerg Med 18:995–996

390. Synek VM (1988) EEG abnormality grades and subdivisions of prognostic importance in traumatic and anoxic coma in adults. Clin Electroencephalogr 19:160–166

391. Tagliaferri F, Compagnone C, Korsic M et al (2006) A systematic review of brain injury epidemiology in Europe. Acta Neurochir (Wien) 148:255–268, discussion 268

392. Taguchi Y, Matsuzawa M, Morishima H et al (2000) Incarceration of the basilar artery in a longitudinal fracture of the clivus: case report and literature review. J Trauma 48:1148–1152, Review

393. Takeshi M, Okuchi K, Nishiguchi T et al (2006) Clinical analysis of seven patients of crushing head injury. J Trauma 60:1245–1249

394. Talamonti G, Fontana RA, Versari PP et al (1995) Delayed complications of ethmoid fractures: a "growing fracture" phenomenon. Acta Neurochir (Wien) 137:164–173

395. Teasdale G, Jennett B (1974) Assessment of coma and impaired consciousness. A practical scale. Lancet 2:81–84

396. Teasdale G, Skene A, Parker L et al (1979) Age and outcome of severe head injury. Acta Neurochir Suppl (Wien) 28: 140–143

397. Teasdale GM, Pettigrew LE, Wilson JT et al (1998) Analyzing outcome of treatment of severe head injury: a review and update on advancing the use of the Glasgow Outcome Scale. J Neurotrauma 15:587–597

398. Temkin NR (2003) Risk factors for posttraumatic seizures in adults. Epilepsia 44(Suppl 10):18–20

399. Tenn-Lyn NA, Doig CJ, Shemie SD et al (2006) Potential organ donors referred to Ontario neurosurgical centres. Can J Anaesth 53:732–736

400. Thamburaj V Intracranial pressure http://thamburaj.com/ intracranial_pressure.htm

401. The National Collaborative Centre for Acute Care, (2007) Head injury. Triage, assessment, investigation and early management of head injury in infants, children and adults. Selecting patients for CT imaging of the head (Partial update of NICE clinical guideline 4) http://www.nice.org. uk/nicemedia/pdf/CG56NICEGuideline.pdf

402. Thillainayagam K, MacMillan R, Mendelow AD et al (1987) How accurately are fractures of the skull diagnosed? Injury 18:319–321

403. Thiruppathy SP, Muthukumar N (2004) Mild head injury: revisited. Acta Neurochir (Wien) 146:1075–1082, discussion 1082–1083

404. Tisdall M, Smith M (2007) Multimodal monitoring in traumatic brain injury: current status and future directions. Br J Anaesth 99:61–67

405. Tokmak M, Iplikcioglu AC, Bek S et al (2007) The role of exudation in chronic subdural hematomas. J Neurosurg 107:290–295

406. Tsai FY, Huprich JE, Segall HD et al (1979) The contrast-enhanced CT scan in the diagnosis of isodense subdural hematoma. J Neurosurg 50:64–69

407. Tuli S, Tator CH, Fehlings MG et al (1997) Occipital condyle fractures. Neurosurgery 41:368–376, discussion 376–377

408. Turetschek K, Wunderbaldinger P, Zontsich T (1998) Trauma des Gesichtsschädels und der Schädelkalotte. Radiologe 38:645–658

409. Turnage B, Maull KI (2000) Scalp laceration: an obvious 'occult' cause of shock. South Med J 93:265–266

410. Twijnstra A, Brouwer O, Keyser A, et al (2001) Richtlijnen voor diagnostiek en behandeling van patiënten met een licht schedel-hersenletsel (Guidelines for diagnosis and management of patients with minor head injury). Dutch Association of Neurology. http://www.neurologie.nl/ uploads/136/78/richtlijnen_-_LSHL.doc

411. Ucar T, Akyuz M (2001) Management of severe traumatic brain injury by decompressive craniectomy. Neurosurgery 49:1022

412. Van Beek JG, Mushkudiani NA, Steyerberg EW et al (2007) Prognostic value of admission laboratory parameters in traumatic brain injury: results from the IMPACT study. J Neurotrauma 24:315–328

413. van den Heever CM, van der Merwe DJ (1989) Management of depressed skull fractures. Selective conservative management of nonmissile injuries. J Neurosurg 71:186–190

414. van Olden GD, Meeuwis JD, Bolhuis HW et al (2004) Clinical impact of advanced trauma life support. Am J Emerg Med 22:522–525

415. Vik A, Nag T, Fredriksli OA et al (2008) Relationship of "dose" of intracranial hypertension to outcome in severe traumatic brain injury. J Neurosurg 109:678–684

416. Vinas FC, Pilitsis J, Penetrating head trauma. http://www. emedicine.com/MED/topic2888.htm

417. Vitaz TW, Jenks J, Raque GH et al (2003) Outcome following moderate traumatic brain injury. Surg Neurol 60:285–291, discussion 291

418. Vollmer DG, Torner J, Jane JA et al (1991) Age and outcome following traumatic coma; why do older patients worse? J Neurosurg 75 Suppl:S37–S49

419. von Wild KR, Hannover, Münster TBI, Study Council (2008) Posttraumatic rehabilitation and one year outcome following acute traumatic brain injury (TBI): data from the well defined population based German Prospective Study 2000–2002. Acta Neurochir Suppl 101:55–60

420. Vos PE, Battistin L, Birbamer G (2002) EFNS guideline on mild traumatic brain injury: report of an EFNS task force. Eur J Neurol 9:207–219, Review

421. Wang H, Duan G, Zhang J et al (1998) Clinical studies on diffuse axonal injury in patients with severe closed head injury. Chin Med J (Engl) 111:59–62

422. Watanabe T, Nakahara K, Miki Y et al (1995) Chronic expanding epidural haematoma. Case report. Acta Neurochir (Wien) 132:150–153

423. Weigel R, Schmiedek P, Krauss JK (2003) Outcome of contemporary surgery for chronic subdural haematoma: evidence based review. J Neurol Neurosurg Psychiatry 74:937–943

424. Wester K, Helland CA (2008) How often do chronic extracerebral haematomas occur in patients with intracranial arachnoid cysts? J Neurol Neurosurg Psychiatry 79: 72–75

425. Whitfield PC, Patel H, Hutchinson PJ et al (2001) Bifrontal decompressive craniectomy in the management of posttraumatic intracranial hypertension. Br J Neurosurg 15: 500–507

426. Wilberger JE (2006) Discussion: Chang EF, Meeker M, Holland MC, (2006) Acute traumatic intraparenchymal hemorrhage: risk factors for progression in the early post-injury period. Neurosurgery 58:647–656

427. Wilberger JE Jr, Harris M, Diamond DL (1990) Acute subdural hematoma: morbidity and mortality related to timing of operative intervention. J Trauma 30:733–736

428. Wilberger JJ, Harris M, Diamond D (1991) Acute subdural hematoma: morbidity, mortality, and operative timing. J Neurosurg 74:212–218

429. Wilms G, Marchal G, Geusens E et al (1992) Isodense subdural haematomas on CT: MRI findings. Neuroradiology 34:497–499

430. Wylen EL, Willis BK, Nanda A (1999) Infection rate with replacement of bone fragment in compound depressed skull fractures. Surg Neurol 51:452–457

431. Yamakawa H, Ohkuma A, Hattori T et al (1991) Primary intracranial arachnoid cyst in the elderly: a survey on 39 cases. Acta Neurochir (Wien) 113:42–47

432. Yilmazlar S, Kocaeli H, Dogan S et al (2005) Traumatic epidural haematomas of nonarterial origin: analysis of 30 consecutive cases. Acta Neurochir (Wien) 147:1241–1248, discussion 1248

433. Yokota H, Eguchi T, Nobayashi M et al (2006) Persistent intracranial hypertension caused by superior sagittal sinus stenosis following depressed skull fracture. Case report and review of the literature. J Neurosurg 104:849–852, Revie

434. York G, Barboriak D, Petrella J et al (2005) Association of internal carotid artery injury with carotid canal fractures in patients with head trauma. Am J Roentgenol 184:1672–1678

435. Zafonte RD, Lee CY (1997) Kernohan-Woltman notch phenomenon: an unusual cause of ipsilateral motor deficit. Arch Phys Med Rehabil 78:543–545

436. Zanini MA, de Lima Resende LA et al (2008) Traumatic subdural hygromas: proposed pathogenesis based classification. J Trauma 64:705–713

437. Zumkeller M, Behrmann R, Heissler H et al (1996) Computed tomographic criteria and survival rate for patients with acute subdural hematoma. Neurosurgery 39: 708–712

Intensive Care Treatment Options of Elevated Intracranial Pressure Following Severe Traumatic Brain Injury

2

John F. Stover and Reto Stocker

Abbreviations

ADH	Antidiuretic hormone
ADP	Adenosine diphosphate
AEP	Acoustic evoked potentials
ALI	Acute lung injury
APOE	Apolipoprotein E
ARDS	Adult respiratory distress syndrome
ATP	Adenosine triphopshate
BGA	Blood gas analysis
BIS	Bispectral index
CPP	Cerebral perfusion pressure
CSD	Cortical spreading depression
CSF	Cerebrospinal fluid
CSW	Cerebral salt wasting
CT	Computerized tomography
CYP	Cytochrome P
DIC	Disseminated intravascular coagulopathy
ECG	Electrocardiogram
EEG	Electroencephalogram
EVD	External venrtricular drainage
GABA	gamma aminobutyric acid
GCS	Glasgow Coma Scale
GFAP	Glial fibrillary acidic protein
ICP	Intracranial pressure
I/ E	Inspiratory to expiratory ratio
LGI	Lactate-to-glucose index
LOI	Lactate-to-oxygen index
MABP	Mean arterial blood pressure
MRI	Magnetic resonance imaging
NaCl	sodium chloride

NSE	Neuron specific enolase
OER	Oxygen extraction ratio
OGI	Oxygen-to-glucose index
paO2	Partial arterial oxygen pressure
paCO2	Partial arterial carbon dioxide pressure
PARP	Poly ADP ribose polymerase
PET	Positron emission tomography
PEEP	Positive endexpiratory pressure
ptiO2	Partial pressure tissue oxygenation
ScvO2	Central venous oxygen saturation
SEP	Sensory evoked potentials
SIADH	Syndrome of inappropriate antidiuretic hormone secretion
SjvO2	Jugular venous oxygen saturation
SPECT	Single photon emission computed tomography
SVR	Systemic vascular resistance
TCD	Transcranial Doppler sonography

2.1 Summary

The intensive care treatment of patients with severe traumatic brain injury (TBI) must consider local alterations as well as systemic influences. This, in turn, requires broad clinical experience and knowledge to see and comprehend these severely injured patients in their entirety. This not only pertains to patients with additional injuries but is also valid for patients with isolated severe TBI. Only then can we practice a brain-oriented therapy. A merely brain-centered therapy carries the risk of inducing extracerebral organ injuries.

The main focus of our attention is to prevent secondary damage, which implies active search and identification of secondary insults. In addition, this forces us to conduct a preemptive and – if required – aggressive strategy. Apart from our clinical judgment we

J.F. Stover (✉) and R. Stocker
Surgical Intensive Care Medicine, University Hospital Zürich,
Rämistrasse 100, 8091 Zürich, Switzerland
e-mail: john.stover@usz.ch
e-mail: reto.stocker@usz.ch

H.-J. Oestern et al. (eds.), *Head, Thoracic, Abdominal, and Vascular Injuries*,
DOI: 10.1007/978-3-540-88122-3_2, © Springer-Verlag Berlin Heidelberg 2011

must rely on specific cerebral and systemic monitoring tools which allow us to make senseful therapeutic decisions and to also adapt the type and extent of the different therapeutic interventions according to dynamic changes over time. Only then can we reduce the risks of damage induced by the well-meaning therapeutic interventions.

To date we do not possess a simple, easy-to-use, and widely accepted concept with which all patients with their different traumatic lesions and individual courses could be treated identically. Even the classical and much cited works, i.e., the "Rosner concept" and the "Lund concept," can actually only be applied to small proportions of the TBI population as investigated in the original works. These descriptions were never corroborated in prospective, randomized, placebo-controlled trials, which, of course, would subject us to a tremendous ethical burden.

The large mistake lies within the academic attempt of (over)simplifying complex and difficult-to-understand pathophysiologic and pharmacologic interactions with the aim of generating broad knowledge. This, of course, results in a loss of important and decisive pieces of information which falsely declare the "Rosner concept" as a hyperdynamic and hypervolemic treatment option to modulate cerebral perfusion pressure (CPP) and by which the "Lund-concept" is misunderstood as a categoric and inflexible reduction in CPP to 50 mmHg in all TBI patients.

Based on the pathophysiologic changes, the interacting cascades, and the differential pharmacological and therapeutic influences, we are forced to search for individualized treatment options which allow more flexible adaptation of the different treatment options over time. Thus, it is conceivable that we must combine integral parts of different pathophysiologically – and pharmacologically – driven concepts.

In the following chapters we will elaborate on certain principles which allow improving the treatment of patients with severe TBI. Concomitantly certain procedures and interventions must be categorically practiced, e.g., administration of oxygen including safety intubation, controlled ventilation, stabilization of the arterial blood pressure, and adequate analgesia and sedation, to avoid inducing secondary insults at *any* time point.

The reader is reminded that in-depth and specialized clinical experience cannot be substituted by this chapter but it surely can be broadened.

2.2 Introduction

Severe TBI is characterized by its complexity and the difficulty in precisely predicting occult secondary alterations which can lead to a progression of the existing brain damage. In this context, the secondary increase of space-occupying lesions such as extra- and intracranial hemorrhages (epidural, subdural hematomas, and contusions) and the progressive growth of brain edema are mediated by activated cascades and simultaneously promote activation of new destructive cascades. The increase in volume (hemorrhages and edema) induces a local and then a global increase in intracranial pressure (ICP). The resulting local as well as global compression of the brain with subsequent impairment of cerebral microcirculation will involve progression of ischemia to local infarcts and thus aggravate preexisting injury and also induce new structural and functional damage. These additional injuries are subsummarized as secondary brain damage which stereotypically follow the primary injury and determine survival per se and most importantly quality of individual survival (Fig. 2.1).

While the primary damage cannot be influenced any more it is our interdisciplinary duty to prevent secondary growth and aggravation of the present damage

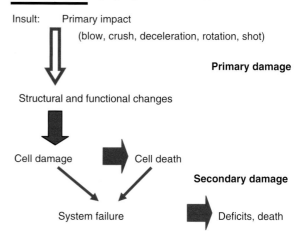

Traumatic brain injury: dynamic continuum

Insult: Primary impact
               (blow, crush, deceleration, rotation, shot)

                                   Primary damage

Structural and functional changes

Cell damage   Cell death

                              Secondary damage

System failure   Deficits, death

Fig. 2.1 Schematic drawing of dynamic cascades activated by a defined primary lesion which can progress to a larger lesion over time. This secondary brain damage can be influenced by other pathologic forces. In the worst case, these alterations can induce irreversible damage and ultimately result in death of these patients

and to avoid induction of new injuries. This, however, requires specialized knowledge, and continuous and active search of different secondary brain insults. These secondary insults, in turn, can only be treated aggressively if they are sought for aggressively in daily clinical routine.

For this we cannot only rely on our theoretical knowledge but we must also incorporate different monitoring techniques to unmask otherwise occult alterations.

While the arising problem of space-occupying and ICP-increasing hematomas is solved relatively easily by surgical evacuation, treatment of vasogenic and cyto-toxic edema is far more cumbersome since all investi-gated anti-edematous drugs which provided promising results in preclinical experimental studies failed in clini-cal investigations. Apart from species- and model-related issues influences of different treatment modalities differing between centers must also be considered. Furthermore, we lack clear evidence-based data regard-ing benefit and potential deleterious effects of contem-porary treatment options and modalities which are strongly influenced by our personal conviction.

Within the scope of this chapter we will characterize different nonsurgical possibilities aimed at treating elevated ICP following severe TBI. In this context, pre-vention and treatment of secondary brain damage are mutually dependent and show a reciprocal influence.

2.3 Pathophysiologic Basis

2.3.1 Local Autodestructive Cascades and Local Secondary Insults

The structural and functional injuries encountered fol-lowing severe TBI are influenced by a plethora of differ-ent pathophysiologic cascades which are activated in parallel and sequentially. In principle, these cascades involve alterations within the extra- and intracellular space: activated enzymes (e.g., caspases, metalloprotei-nases, poly ADP ribose polymerase (PARP)), disturbed perfusion and microcirculation, metabolic impairment due to energetic deficit and mitochondrial dysfunction, excessive and uncontrolled neuronal excitation, exces-sive glial activation, activated inflammatory reactions, production of free oxygen radicals with concomitant

impaired antioxidative compensation. In addition, acti-vation of transcription factors which may aggravate DNA damage (e.g., c-fos, c-jun), reduce DNA injury (e.g., bcl-2, p53), or mediate both beneficial as well as damaging effects (e.g., PARP) have been identified [1]. These different damaging processes are expanded by a certain genetic predisposition (e.g., APOE ε4 associated with posttraumatic dementia) [2, 3]. These activated processes contribute to apoptotic and necrotic altera-tions with their detailed regulatory processes and phar-macologic targets currently being characterized [4]. The different cascades are characterized by a heterogeneous regional and temporal profile and consist of progressive injury of different cellular compartments:

- Endothelial cells with activation of inflammatory cascades, development of local microthrombi, vaso-constriction and vasodilation;
- Cell membrane with transport proteins and distur-bance of electrolyte homeostasis;
- Cytosol with enzymes and production of different pro-inflammatory cyotokines and destructive free oxygen radicals;
- Endoplasmic reticulum with disturbed calcium homeostasis;
- Mitochondria with impaired oxidative phosphory-lation and reduced ATP synthesis.

In addition, different cellular compartments are dis-turbed functionally (neurons ↔ glia ↔ endothelial cells), which results in disturbed autoregulation, a pro-gressive energetic deficit as a harbinger of ensuing ischemia in terms of cortical spreading depression (CSD), as well as a disturbed balance between excit-atory and inhibitory transmitters with subsequent exci-totoxicity and/or prolonged coma (Table 2.1).

As revealed by animal experiments, these signs of secondary functional and structural deterioration develop under otherwise stable conditions with sufficient cere-bral perfusion as well as adequate oxygenation, normo-thermia, and normocapnia. These alterations can be aggravated by systemic secondary insults. This stresses the necessity of preventing additional insults to avoid aggravation of the processes which stereotypically evolve during the early posttraumatic phase.

While processes confined to the intracellular com-partment remain occult at the bedside and can only be determined histologically, changes within the extracel-lular space and later on in the cerebrospinal fluid (CSF)

Table 2.1 Local secondary insults

Secondary insult	Causes	Consequences	Time point	Treatment
EEG activity	Neuronal activation	Energetic deficit Brain edema, ICP⇑	Always	Analgesia, sedation Hypothermia
Ischemia	Microthrombus Compression	Infarct, brain edema, ICP⇑	Always	Increase CPP, administer volume
Hyperemia	Disturbed autoregulation Excessive dilatation Impaired constriction	Brain edema, ICP⇑	Always	Hyperventilation Controlled CPP reduction *CAVE*: increased ICP due to vasodilation resulting from decreased CPP
Vasospasm	Disturbed autoregulation Impaired dilatation Excessive constriction	Brain edema, ICP⇑	Always	Hypoventilation Controlled CPP increase
Cortical spreading depression	Functional impairment: neurons, astrocytes	Ischemia, brain edema, ICP⇑	Always	Maintain blood glucose > 5 mM, upper limit is currently under debate Barbiturates
Coagulopathy	Thrombus formation Fibrinolyse	Ischemia/infarct Hemorrhage	Early phase	Correct systemic coagulation parameters
Inflammation/ infections	Ventriculitis Meningitis Abscess	Hydrocephalus, ICP⇑ Seizures	Late phase	Antibiotics, removal of ventricular drainage/shunt Excision

and blood can unmask previous events. For this, modern intensive care medicine uses different invasive and noninvasive techniques. These are described in detail in (see Sect. 2.4).

2.3.2 Systemic Secondary Insults

Apart from local processes, systemic changes are also of pathophysiologic relevance as they are known to influence brain edema formation (Table 2.2).

The classical secondary insults which increase mortality and morbidity are arterial *hypotension*, *hypoxia* [5], and uncontrolled (prophylactic) *hyperventilation* [6]. Insufficient cerebral perfusion and oxygenation of the already injured brain and excessive vasoconstriction with subsequent local and global perfusion and impaired metabolic supply are the leading characteristics of these secondary insults.

Further secondary insults are *fever* with cerebral vasodilation [7], and systemic inflammation due to infectious processes (e.g., pneumonia) with additional activation of local destructive cascades. Sepsis, in turn,

with its detrimental hypotension and coagulopathy, can induce multiorgan failure, thereby resulting in hypotension and hypoxia, which will increase secondary brain damage. In addition, fast and uncontrolled rewarming of hypothermic patients will induce systemic vasodilation with subsequent impaired cerebral perfusion and disturbed cerebral autoregulation. This, in turn, increases the risk for ICP, raising hyperemia.

Anemia with a hematocrit <24% due to active bleeding, insufficient transfusions, excessive volume administration, and reduced production and effect of erythropoietin will impair cerebral oxygen supply of the injured brain, thereby promoting edema progression and ICP elevation, explaining the increased mortality and rate of complications [8].

Excessive activation of the coagulation cascade with an imbalance between activation and inhibition of activated cascades can result in *coagulopathy*, which unfortunately is not obvious clinically. Excessive fluid administration is feared for inducing *dilution coagulopathy*. Liberation of tissue plasminogen activator (t-PA) highly concentrated within the brain maintains activation of the coagulation cascade resulting in a loss of various coagulation factors, e.g., factor XIII. This,

Table 2.2 Systemic secondary insults

Secondary insult	Causes	Consequences	Time point	Treatment
Hypotension	Hypovolemia Cardiodepression Warming Fever	Reduced perfusion → Ischemia → Infarct Brain edema, ICP⇑	Always	Volume infusion Vasopressors, inotropics Slow warming Treat fever
Hypoxia	Pulmonary pathology	Cell damage Brain edema, ICP⇑	Always	Adapt ventilatory settings (FiO$_2$, PEEP, I/E, Tidal volume)
Fever	Central, infection	Brain edema, ICP⇑	Always	pharmacologic, physical cooling
Hyperglycemia	Stress, nutrition	Brain edema, ICP⇑	Always	Insulin
Hypoglycemia	Nutrition, insulin	Brain edema, ICP⇑	Always	Adapt nutrition, maybe controlled glucose infusion
Hypernatremia	Diabetes insipidus	Brain edema, ICP⇑, Pontine myelinolysis	Early phase	Desmopressin, *CAVE*: long half-life, difficult to guide
	Hyperaldosteronism			Maybe: aldosteron antagonists, *CAVE*: difficult to guide
	Iatrogenic			Volume infusion
Hyponatremia	SIADH, CSW, iatrogenic	Brain edema, ICP⇑	Late phase	Fludrocortison, *CAVE*: difficult to guide
	Hypoaldosteronism, diuretics			Reduce or increase volume infusion
Coagulopathy	Activated coagulation Increased consumption of factors Reduced synthesis Dilution Consumption of platelets	New hemorrhages Increased volume of existing hemorrhages Brain edema, ICP⇑	Early phase	Substitution of factors, including factor XIII and fibrinogen, administration of vitamin K, platelets, and normalize ionized calcium
Anemia	Uncontrolled hemorrhages dilution	Hypoxemia Brain edema Brain edema, ICP⇑	Early phase	Transfusion
Hyperammonemia	Disturbed hepatic function (genetic, pharmacologic: antiepileptics, barbiturates, altered intestinal flora, increased protein administration)	Brain edema, ICP⇑	Late phase	Change nutrition: reduce amount of protein; dialysis, avoid valproic acid

in turn, promotes faster lysis of already formed thrombi. Consequently, an increase in volume of existing hemorrhages or generation of new hemorrhages [9] will increase ICP and promote progression of brain edema. In conjunction with the activated coagulation cascade platelets are used, thereby resulting in *thrombocytopenia* and functional disturbance of circulating platelets [10], which are aggravated by preexisting endocrinologic illnesses and pharmacologic-induced thrombocytopathies (e.g., renal insufficiency, platelet aggregation inhibitors). These alterations support damaging intracranial and intracerebral hemorrhages.

Disseminated intravascular coagulopathy (DIC) as well as platelet loss and platelet dysfunction promote severe blood loss in case of additional injuries, which, in turn, increases the risk of hypotension and ischemia, and hypoxia in all organ systems.

Manifest blood glucose deviations in terms of *hyper- and hypoglycemia* (i.e., above 10 and below 5 mmol/L) as well as strong undulations are of pathophysiologic importance. In this context, hyperglycemia activates local inflammatory processes which are associated with a sustained rate of multiorgan failure and increased mortality [11]. Hypoglycemic episodes aggravate the generation of progredient functional disturbances in terms of CSD [12].

Strong and mainly fast decreases in blood sodium levels are feared for their edema-promoting effect and limited therapeutic options [13]. In this context, *hyponatremia* (<120 mmol/L) due to excessive release of antidiuretic hormone ADH (SIADH, Schwarz-Bartter syndrome) or release of natriuretic peptides (cerebral salt wasting (CSW)) can promote brain edema formation and reduce the threshold for seizures. A relative adrenal insufficiency with subsequent hypoaldosteronism resulting from previous administration of etomidate, usually for intubation [14], deep sedation [15], or within the context of sepsis [16], will induce hyponatremia. Initially *hypernatremia* reduces edema formation. However, within 3 days of constant hypernatremia it automatically induces compensatory uptake of osmotic active substances, so-called osmolytes, i.e., mainly amino acids, to normalize intracellular volume and cell membrane tension [17]. A later decrease in blood sodium will result in a relative increase of the intracellularly trapped osmolytes expanding their osmotic strength. This, in turn, will cause a strong increase in intracellular edema formation with a subsequent potentially lethal increase in ICP. Hypernatremia during the early phase can result from a loss in ADH due to pituitary ischemia, a sign of functional herniation. Hypernatremia developing later on could result from excessive infusion of sodium-containing solutions or liberal administration of diuretics with subsequent hypovolemia. Hormonal changes with typical lab signs of a hyperaldosteronism are also encountered.

Rare cases of *hyperammonemia* must be actively searched for. Due to its high solubility, lipophilicity, and diffusion properties ammonia easily penetrates the brain where it induces intracellular water accumulation related to enzymatic compensatory and detoxification processes mainly involving glutamate and glutamine. Increased neuronal excitation also plays an important role. The evolving brain edema results in an increase in ICP, which in a worst case scenario can end in lethal brain stem herniation [18, 19]. Apart from the real hyperammonemia we must consider a laboratory artifact resulting from concomitantly increased blood gamma-glutamyl transpeptidase (GGT) levels as elevated GGT induces an enzymatic release of ammonium predominantly from glutamate which is measured as ammonia, thus resulting in artificially

elevated blood ammonia concentrations. Apart from a genetic predisposition which is rather rare in adults and predominantly determined in children, pharmacological influences in combination with exhausted enzymes and co-enzymes of the urea cycle and/or excessive uptake of protein stemming from enteral and/or parenteral nutrition are discussed as potential inductors of hyperammonemia. The classical drugs known to induce hyperammonemia are antiepileptics, barbiturates, and volatile anesthetics which can mutually perpetuate their hyperammonemia-inducing properties. In addition, change in intestinal bacteria resulting in increased production of ammonia must be considered.

In general, this hyperammonemia is reversible, provided it is identified in time. However, it is of utmost importance to measure blood ammonia in regular intervals or whenever an increase in ICP cannot be explained otherwise. Only then can we decrease mortality and reduce additional brain damage if adequate interventions are started at blood ammonia levels exceeding 50 μmol/L.

On a therapeutic basis production of ammonia must be reduced and circulating ammonia must be removed. Production of ammonia is decreased by enteral administration of lactulosis or changing nutrition solution to a protein-poor or even protein-free solution. In rare cases, other compounds, such as arginine, sodium benzoate, sodium phenylbutyrate, or L-carnitine, must be tried. In cases of elevated ICP and blood ammonia levels exceeding 100 μmol/L hemodialysis must be begun immediately.

These different systemic secondary insults must be prevented in modern intensive care.

2.3.2.1 Crucial Points and Pearls

- The primary brain damage is followed by a stereotypical increase during the first 24–48 h and is considered as secondary brain damage.
- The different destructive cascades are aggravated by local and systemic secondary insults which enlarge the secondary brain damage.
- Systemic secondary insults can develop at any time and must be corrected to prevent progression of the secondary brain damage.
- Systemic secondary insults, i.e., hypotension, hypoxia, hyperventilation, anemia, fever, hypo-/hyperglycemia,

hypo-/hypernatremia, coagulopathy/thrombocytopenia, hyperammonemia, must be sought for actively so they can be prevented and corrected adequately.

2.3.3 Increase in Intracranial Volume and Intracranial Pressure

As already described in 1823 by Monro and Kelly the simple concept of the pathophysiologic interrelationship of intracranial volume and pressure continues to be of clinical relevance even in contemporary neurotraumatology. The basis for the Monro–Kelly doctrine is formed by the anatomic boundaries consisting of the inflexible skull bones and the different partial volumes defined by the brain: approx. 85%, CSF: approx. 5–15%, and intracranial blood volume: approx. 5–10%. Under normal conditions these different partial volumes result in a total volume which is maintained constant by a compensatory adaption of the different partial volumes. In this context an increase in intracranial blood volume is observed in cases of vasodilation (hyperemia), and CSF is moved from the cranial space to the spinal compartment. In case the total volume cannot me maintained constant or the compensatory mechanisms have been exploited, then any additional increase in volume will elevate ICP. Under pathologic conditions the net volume is increased by various intracranial lesions, which will decrease the compensatory shifts of the physiologic partial volumes (Fig. 2.2). In this context, the age of the patient is decisive. While younger brains nearly completely fill the intracranial space and are limited by a reduced elasticity with an increased resistance, older brains are characterized by the opposite characteristics. This explains why older patients with preexisting global atrophy and reduced resistance can tolerate larger volumes for a longer period of time before they suffer from clinical worsening and require neurosurgery.

Following severe TBI, space-occupying processes (hemorrhages, contusion, brain edema) and their additional increase in volume result in a faster exhaustion of the physiologic compensatory mechanisms. As a consequence an increase in volume which normally is tolerated well results in disproportionately elevated ICP. This increase in pressure, in turn, induces new and progressing secondary damage which can induce and maintain a vicious circle [20].

$$V_{intracranial} = V_{brain} + V_{CSF} + V_{blood} + V_{lesion}$$

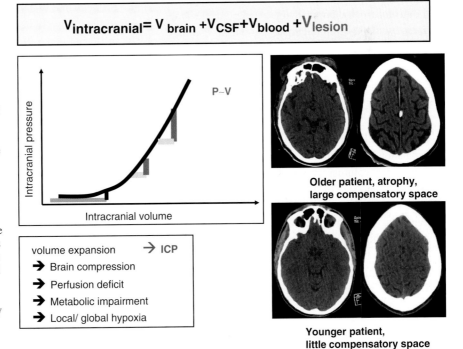

Fig. 2.2 Schematic drawing of the relationship of intracranial volume and intracranial pressure (ICP) (Monroe–Kelly doctrine) and possible pathophysiologic cascades which can result in secondary brain damage. The included computed tomography (CT) pictures illustrate the influence of underlying brain volume on the increase in ICP whenever total intracranial volume cannot be maintained constant. In cases of brain atrophy larger lesion volumes can be compensated longer before ICP increases. In brains with less atrophy, i.e., younger patients, already small lesions can induce a faster and more severe increase in ICP

Older patient, atrophy, large compensatory space

Younger patient, little compensatory space

Progressive increases in volume and pressure result from intracranial hemorrhages, contusions, focal and global brain edema, vasodilation with expansion of the intracranial blood volume, and vasospasm with ischemia-induced brain edema formation. Occasionally, disturbed CSF circulation with resulting hydrocephalus (due to lower herniation and occlusion of the aqueduct) and venous infarcts is caused by sinus vein thrombosis (due to fractures in the vicinity of the jugular venous bulb or skull fractures close to the sigmoid/transverse/confluens sinus). In addition, the rare but important and devastating traumatic lesion to the internal carotid artery including its dissection must be remembered, which can result in a fulminant hemispheric edema formation. An inadequate positioning of the patient (too flat or too steep) can impair the venous outflow, which, in turn, will also increase the ICP. Furthermore, a cervical collar as well as a catheter-related formation of a thrombus within the internal jugular vein can also impair cerebral venous outflow.

Apart from intracranial and intracerebral reasons for elevated ICP, an impaired venous outflow due to thoracic and abdominal compartment syndrome must also be considered [21]. These compartment syndromes can result from uncontrolled volume administration or a combination of gastrointestinal paralysis caused by deep analgesia and sedation, immobilization, enteral/parenteral nutrition, hypothermia, and the generalized edema formation related to inflammatory-induced capillary leakage. Under certain circumstances a laparotomy becomes inevitable.

2.3.3.1 Crucial Points and Pearls

- Elevated ICP depends on the intracranial volume expansion, distribution of different physiologic and pathologic volumes (brain, CSF, blood, lesions), elasticity, and size of the brain.
- The volume-dependent ICP increasing effect is dynamic, i.e., the same volume expansion at different time points will result in different extents of elevated ICP and intracranial hypertension (ICP > 25 mmHg).
- The exact reason for an increase in ICP must be identified. Only then can an adequate treatment be initiated.
- Apart from intracranial and intracerebral causes we must also search for systemic reasons such as

impaired venous outflow in case of thoracic and abdominal compartment syndromes.

2.4 Neuromonitoring

To obtain an in-depth insight in otherwise occult changes and thus guide differentiated therapeutic interventions in an intelligent manner, different and supplementary noninvasive and invasive monitoring methods must be combined and integrated in daily routine (Table 2.3). Based on data obtained from animal experiments and the finding that hemorrhages and contusions exhibit a stereotypic growth pattern during the first days under experimental and clinical conditions (Fig. 2.3) specific neuromonitoring must already be used early after TBI, and also during phases with normal ICP values below 15 mmHg. Only then can we unmask pathologic processes early on. This, in turn, is essential to win time for appropriate and correcting interventions before ICP increases and before secondary brain damage progresses. The difficulty, however, is to identify those patients requiring aggressive and invasive surveillance in whom the initial computed tomography (CT) does not exhibit obvious pathologic findings. It is important to bear in mind that diffuse axonal injuries cannot be seen in the initial CT scan and that certain lesions require at least 2–6 h to develop. This is of importance if the initial CT scan is obtained within 2 h in clinically comatose patients whose coma cannot be explained by other reasons such as alcohol, seizure, or hypothermia. Careful evaluation of their trauma history and consideration of the time point when the initial CT scan was performed must be integrated in our decision making. Especially in cases of high-speed accidents and falls with additional injuries an increased risk for hemorrhages and coagulopathy must be considered. Thus, control CT scans should be performed in tight intervals, especially if the patients require surgical procedures and anesthesia/sedation does not allow adequate neurological evaluation. In the presence of pathologic alterations patients should be submitted to a standardized intensive care treatment protocol for at least the first 24 h aimed at preventing progression of secondary brain damage. This protocol should include insertion of an ICP probe.

Table 2.3 shows different monitoring methods with their implications, advantages, and disadvantages.

Table 2.3 Neuromonitoring: areas of interest, implications, advantages, disadvantages

Monitoring	Area of interest	Implications	Advantages	Disadvantages
ICP	Focal/global	Increase in intracranial volume and pressure	Adapt therapeutic interventions	Normal values [1] physiology
EEG	Global	Guide sedation Assess seizure activity	Topographic analysis	Requires special knowledge
BIS EEG	Frontal/global	Guide sedation	Easy to use	No topographic analysis
$SjvO_2$	Global	Guide CPP, $paCO_2$	Continuous (if oximetry works)	Discontinuous, requires BGA
$ptiO_2$	Focal	Guide CPP, $paCO_2$, transfusion threshold	Continuous	Invasive
Microdialysis	Focal	Guide CPP, $paCO_2$, sedation	Metabolic monitoring	Expensive, difficult to interpret
TCD	Focal	Guide CPP, $paCO_2$	Easy, reproducible	Discontinuous, requires expertise
Imaging	Focal/global	Indication for surgery, guide therapy	Visualization of lesions, metabolic alterations	Time-consuming, difficult to perform in unstable patients, specialized centers
Autoregulation	Focal/global	Guide CPP, $paCO_2$, sedation	Noninvasive (ICP, MABP, TCD)	Specialized software

2.4.1 ICP and Compliance

The continuous measurement of ICP was introduced in clinical routine in the 1970s. Following its initial euphoria, ICP was regarded as the primary parameter to unmask pathologic intracranial processes and to explain the high mortality and morbidity observed 30–50 years ago. The general view that an increased ICP is always pathologic led to the widely distributed misconception that a normal ICP value is equal to absence of pathologic processes. This, however, is a fallacy. New data convincingly show that metabolic alterations precede increases in ICP [22]. This, however, can only be seen if the appropriate monitoring is used.

Apart from assessing an increase in ICP, measured ICP allows to calculate the CPP (CPP = MABP – ICP), which is an indirect measure for global cerebral perfusion and which forms the basis for further therapeutic decisions.

The ICP level of 20–25 mmHg is considered pathologic as mortality was significantly increased at ICP levels exceeding 20 mmHg [23]. However, this threshold stems from a time of insufficient monitoring of parameters which have been integrated in modern intensive care following severe TBI, e.g., jugular venous oxygen saturation ($SjvO_2$), partial pressure tissue oxygenation ($ptiO_2$), microdialysis, or transcranial

Doppler sonography (TCD). Strictly adhering to this threshold implies missing an early start of specific interventions, which confounds neuroprotection of various therapeutic interventions. Already in 1982 Saul and Ducker were able to show a significantly reduced mortality at an ICP threshold of 15 mmHg compared to a historical group of patients in whom ICP was not treated before it had reached 20–25 mmHg: 28% vs. 46% [24]. Unfortunately, the impact of these results is weakened by the use of historic control patients and the fact that there was no follow-up study or a prospective randomized controlled trial. From a methodological and technical point the ICP is influenced by several factors, such as the presence of a craniectomy, the region of insertion, and measurement, which are important when interpreting the obtained values (Table 2.4). Following a craniectomy including dural expansion we regularly measure low and even negative ICP values until the brain has expanded into the newly generated space. A similar finding is encountered in patients with entrapped air in the subdural compartment which hampers the correct transmission of pressure values. Thus, falsely low and even negative ICP values are measured until the air has been absorbed. The same holds true for parenchymal probes which are positioned within the extraparenchymal space.

Under these circumstances these "false" ICP values mimic normality and trick us into missing pathologic

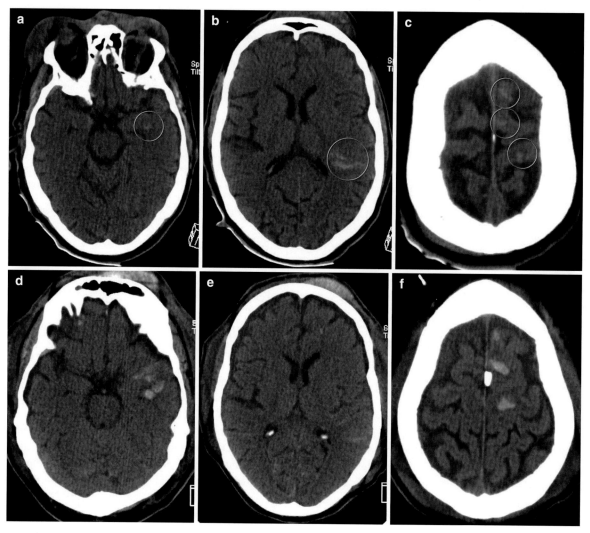

Fig. 2.3 Illustrative example of dynamic changes of different traumatic lesions within the first 24 h. While trying to secure his cat from the roof a patient fell from a height of 7 m. He suffered from severe traumatic brain injury (TBI) and severe abdominal injury and long bone fractures. While only small lesions were seen in the initial computed tomography (CT) scan (marked with red circles) performed 2 h after injury ((**a**) left temporal contusion, (**b**) left parietal traumatic subarachnoid hemorrhage, (**c**) left frontal contusions), the contusions significantly increased (within the first 24 hrs.) in size (**d** and **f**). At the same time, traumatic subarachnoid hemorrhage resolved (**e**). The increase in contusion volume occurred despite intact and normal plasmatic and thrombocytic coagulation

alterations as we do not actively search for otherwise occult signs of evolving brain damage. This enforces the concomitant application of several monitoring methods to allow an internal control and to minimize the risk of missing pathologic changes.

Earlier clinical studies clearly showed that different pressure values and pressure gradients exist within the supratentorial compartment. These pressure gradients are influenced by space-occupying lesions with a lesion >25 mL and a midline shift >3 mm and are only unmasked if several ICP probes are used [25]. Thus,

from a puristic standpoint we must question the validity and correctness of the decisions and therapeutic interventions when only using one ICP probe as we miss the presence of regionally differing pressure values. As a consequence, some areas of the injured brain tend to be over- or undertreated. The complexity of this problem is increased by the regional and temporal heterogeneity of pathologic changes. Based on the presence of these pressure compartments it is recommended to insert the ICP probe on the side with the predominant space-occupying lesion, to obtain a more

Table 2.4 ICP probes, advantages and disadvantages

ICP probe	Area of insertion	Advantages	Disadvantages
Parenchymal probe	Parenchyma	Independent of the ventricular system	Trephination
Ventricular drainage	Ventricular system	Independent of local pressure gradients Release of CSF to decreased ICP	Requires accessible ventricular system Risk of damaging basal ganglia Risk of infections Excessive production of CSF following CSF drainage
Subdural probe	Beneath the dura	No tissue damage	Risk of damaging bridging veins Entrapped subdural air impairs pressure conductance causing strong deviations
Epidural probe obsolete	Outside the dura	No tissue damage	Strong deviations

appropriate CPP. In clinical practice, however, the location and extent of the different lesions are decisive. In this context, some neurosurgeons fear causing severe damage by inserting the ICP probe in the frontal lobe of the left hemisphere assuming this is the dominant hemisphere. Furthermore, insertion of an ICP probe into an existing contusion increases the risk of additional hemorrhage and growth of the contusion. This risk can be minimized by inserting the ICP probe in the contralateral pressure-receiving side.

The least pressure differences are found within the ventricular system, provided the catheters are inserted correctly. To minimize artifacts parenchymal probes are superior to sub-epidural and epidural probes and thus should be favored. Specialized ICP probes inserted in the ventricular system also allow draining of CSF to reduce elevated ICP. CSF drainage, however, is only possible if the ventricular system is accessible and it is not compressed, for example, by progressive generalized brain edema. Thus, external ventricular drainage (EVD) can only be used in a small proportion of patients. Furthermore, the increased risk of ventriculitis compromises the benefit of the EVD.

In an attempt to gain more insight into intracranial pathology, to find an early warning system for ensuing compromised intracranial compensatory mechanisms, and to better unmask dynamic ICP changes, intracranial compliance was investigated. For this, a special catheter equipped with a balloon is inserted in the ventricular system. Standardized volume expansion of the balloon increases ICP, which, in turn, allows calculating resistance and compliance of the intracranial compartment. However, due to poor data quality and the missing predictability of ensuing ICP increases and hypoxic

episodes this technique cannot be recommended for daily clinical routine [26].

A regular ICP curve consists of three peaks which reflect the pressure profile determined in a normal arterial pressure curve. Providing good quality of the ICP curve that changes within the pressure profile allows prediction of disturbance in cerebral autoregulation. While normally the first peak is the highest, the second peak exceeds the first peak in case of disturbed cerebral autoregulation. This results from an absent or inadequate vasoconstriction in response to the arterial pressure wave which expands the diameter of the arteries. This curve pattern can precede the evolving increase in ICP within the following 12 h due to excessive cerebral vasodilation (Fig. 2.4).

Apart from this bedside and simple ICP curve interpretation more refined and mathematically sophisticated analysis of the ICP curve by concomitantly considering changes in arterial blood pressure and continuously assessing changes in flow velocity of the middle cerebral artery (MCA) can be performed. This continuous functional analysis of pressure reactivity reflects pathophysiologic alterations almost in real time and allows differentiating patients with severe functional disturbances and worse outcomes compared to those with reduced mortality and morbidity [27].

As in any neurosurgical procedure insertion of an ICP probe is associated with the risk of inducing additional brain injury. Special care must be taken to limit the penetration depth to a maximum of 3 cm below the skull line and to safely secure the ICP probe to prevent it from accidentally dislocating and penetrating deeper regions of the brain. Thus, special bolts should be used and mere attachment to the skin should be avoided

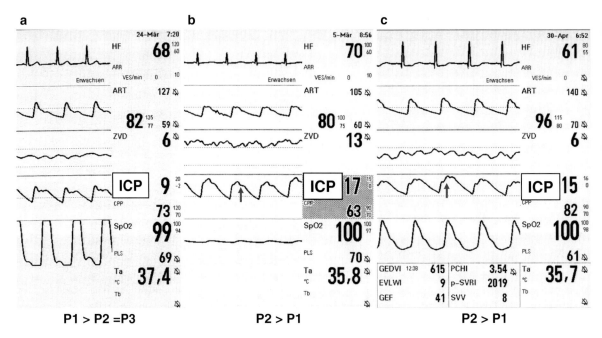

a P1 > P2 =P3   **b** P2 > P1   **c** P2 > P1

Fig. 2.4 Illustrative examples of curve patterns of the intracranial pressure (ICP) curve, which can be analyzed at the bedside. Under normal conditions, i.e., with adequately reacting cerebral arteries, the ICP curve reflects the three pressure peaks of the arterial pressure curve (a). Here, the first peak is the largest and is followed by two smaller peaks. Under pathologic conditions, i.e., whenever cerebral arteries cannot constrict as a response to the first arterial pressure wave that is transmitted to the cerebral arteries, the second peak of the ICP pressure curve will exceed the first peak (b and c). This reflects underlying vasodilation and can be used as an early warning signal for subsequent increases in ICP due to progressive cerebral vasodilation and hyperemia. A further increase in cerebral perfusion pressure (CPP) is then required to force cerebral vasoconstriction, which, in turn, will decrease ICP. Thus, this pattern allows to identify optimal CPP. This pattern reflecting disturbed autoregulation can occur several times per hour per day, and can even persist for 1–2 weeks

(Figs. 2.5 and 2.6). Special care must also be taken in patients with preexisting frontal hygromas since bridging veins are already under strain and thus can be damaged upon introducing an ICP probe or other monitoring catheters (microdialysis, ptiO$_2$, temperature) (Fig. 2.7).

2.4.1.1 Crucial Points and Pearls

- ICP is the primary monitoring parameter following severe TBI.
- A normal ICP <15 mmHg does not guarantee physiologic intracerebral conditions, especially following craniectomy, dura expansion, uncontrolled loss of CSF in case of skull base fractures, or subdural entrapped air, which prevent adequate pressure transmission.
- To date, the general idea is to not escalate therapeutic interventions until ICP exceeds 20 mmHg. This, however, lacks statistically sound evidence. An earlier start, e.g., at 15 mmHg, could reduce stereotypic progression of secondary brain damage.
- With the help of ICP the CPP, an indirect measure of global cerebral perfusion, is calculated.

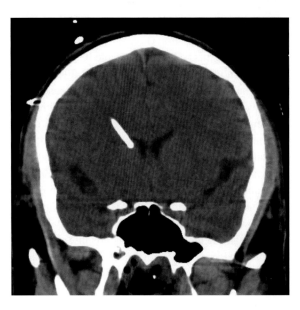

Fig. 2.5 Example of false placement of a parenchymal intracranial pressure (ICP) probe despite using a special bolt: the insertion depth was 6 cm below the skull, nearly penetrating the ventricular system and damaging the caput of the caudate nucleus. The ideal penetration depth is 3 cm below the exterior skull limit

Fig. 2.6 Example of dislocated parenchymal intracranial pressure (ICP) probe which was not fixed with a bolt system but was merely attached to the skin. The ICP probe was accidentally pushed through the brain during transport from a regional hospital (**a**) and nearly touched the basal artery (**b**)

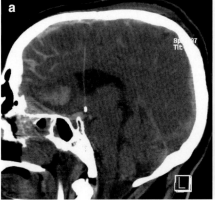
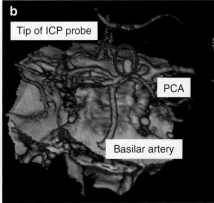

Fig. 2.7 Example of a patient with bifrontal hygroma (**a**) and induction of an acute subdural hematoma by inserting microdialysis, partial pressure tissue oxygenation (ptiO$_2$), and temperature probe (**b**). Special care must be taken in these patients as the bridging veins are under strain due to the existing hygroma. Thus, they can tear easily upon additional manipulation, such as the performed trephination with puncturing of the dura for subsequent insertion of the probes

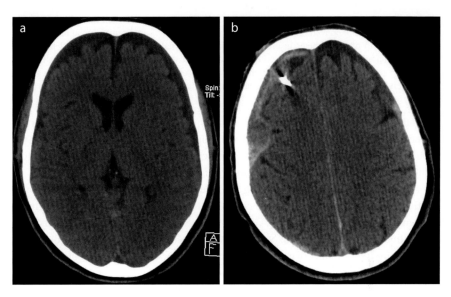

- Locations and extent of brain lesions as well as the surgical window influence the location of the ICP probe.
- Contemporary practice only includes insertion of one ICP probe, thus missing any pressure gradients and different therapeutic requirements.

2.4.2 Jugular Venous Bulb Catheter: SjvO$_2$ and Arterio-Jugular Venous Differences

Guided by ultrasonography to avoid puncturing the carotid artery a single-lumen central venous catheter or alternatively a pediatric pulmonary catheter is inserted in the internal jugular vein. For this, it is of advantage to visualize both internal jugular veins to determine the larger vein. The majority of patients exhibit a dominant right internal jugular vein while approximately 5% present with a dominant left internal jugular vein. Approximately 10% exhibit comparable bilateral vessel diameters. If possible, the jugular venous catheter should be inserted ipsilateral to the predominantly injured hemisphere [28]. To avoid development of a sinus vein thrombosis caused by prolonged disturbance of the cerebral venous outflow the tip of the catheter should project between approximately 1 cm below the mastoid process and the lower rim of the internal acoustic meatus in a conventional lateral skull/cervical spine X-ray (Fig. 2.8a). It is important to verify the position of the catheter rapidly (within 1 h) after its insertion to minimize the risk of a thrombus formation within the sinus. In case the tip of the catheter cannot be adequately visualized the profile of the catheter itself can help in assessing if the catheter has been advanced too far: whenever a bow is seen in the proximal part (close to the skull base) it means

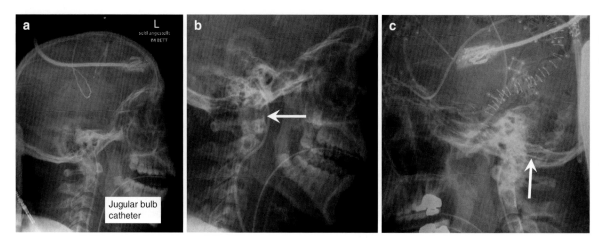

Fig. 2.8 Example of correct placement of a jugular bulb catheter verified in a lateral conventional X-ray of the cervical spine/head (**a**). The tip of the catheter inserted in the larger internal jugular vein should be clearly visible at the height of the mastoid process to approximately 1 cm below the mastoid process. Excessively inserted catheters (**b** and **c**) increased the risk of sinus vein thrombosis. Insufficient depth with the tip of the catheter remaining at the height of the mandible (inflow of the facial vein to the internal jugular vein) will falsely influence jugular venous oxygen saturation (SjvO$_2$) values, resulting in elevated values due to lower oxygen consumption of the facial muscles

the catheter is butting against the skull base and must be retracted by 1–2 cm (Fig. 2.8b). A follow-up X-ray should be performed to document the correct placement following correction of the insertion depth. Cannulation of the sinus vein resulting from deep penetration of the internal jugular vein can be unmasked by conventional X-ray (Fig. 2.8c).

Continuous recording of the SjvO$_2$ allows unmasking the pathologic impact of elevated ICP even in case of "adequate" CPP (Fig. 2.9). However, the employed light cables exhibit a loss in quality within the first 24 h and the diameter of the catheters (especially pediatric pulmonary artery catheters) increases the risk of thrombus formation within the internal jugular vein. The risk of thrombus formation can be minimized by using a single-lumen central venous catheter. This alternative, however, only allows discontinuous investigations based on intermittent arterial and jugular venous blood gas analysis (BGA).

Use of the jugular venous catheters allows to analyze SjvO$_2$, calculate various metabolic indices (e.g., oxygen-glucose index (OGI), lactate-oxygen index (LOI), lactate-glucose index (LGI)) [29], determine the oxygen extraction ratio (OER), and calculate differences

Fig. 2.9 Illustrative example reflecting the necessity of integrating multimodal monitoring in routine intensive care in patients with severe traumatic brain injury (TBI). Intermittent increases in intracranial pressure (ICP) due to disturbed cerebral autoregulation (A-waves) resulted in reduced cerebral perfusion and impaired cerebral oxygen supply despite adequate cerebral perfusion pressure (CPP) (80–90 mmHg). This was only unmasked by concomitant analysis of changes in jugular venous oxygen saturation <50%

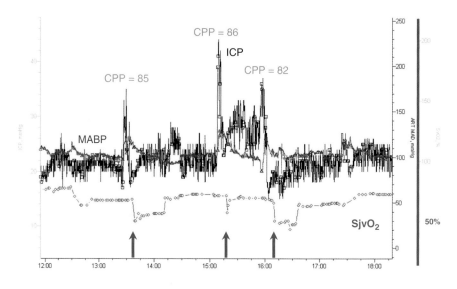

(arterio-jugular venous lactate difference) which together facilitate in-depth assessment of posttraumatic energetic disturbances [30]. Contrary to the microdialysis technique this easy-to-use and inexpensive tool does not require an adaptation period and can be performed on any intensive care unit (ICU) without expensive and difficult analysis and time-consuming upkeep, which also requires substantial experience. However, microdialysis cannot be substituted by the jugular venous blood analyses. This simple technique is excellent to unmask pathologic metabolic alterations within the first hours following severe TBI even under conditions of normal ICP <15 mmHg. In addition, it allows to bridge the time until insertion of microdialysis and ptiO$_2$. Thus, we can attain a semi-continuous monitoring and have the possibility of adapting our therapeutic interventions based on objective parameters and monitoring results. In approximately 70% of our patients we observe signs of early metabolic impairment due to inadequate depth of sedation which is missed when only focusing on ICP values.

The theoretic advantage of continuously assessed SjvO$_2$ using fiber-optic transmission compared to the discontinuous, i.e., intermittent, BGA is limited by the increase in artifacts over time and the higher risk of thrombus formation due to the larger catheters.

The SjvO$_2$ reflects changes in cerebral oxygen supply, cerebral perfusion, and cerebral oxygen consumption as SjvO$_2$ correlates directly with perfusion and correlates inversely with cerebral oxygen consumption. Thus, an increase in MABP with a subsequent amelioration of the CPP as well as reduced hyperventilation to controlled hypoventilation will improve cerebral oxygen supply due to increased perfusion. Reducing cerebral oxygen consumption due to pharmacologic inhibition of neuronal activity by increasing the dose of benzodiazepines, barbiturates, or propofol or by reducing brain temperature will also increase SjvO$_2$ due to metabolic stabilization.

It is important to acknowledge that jugular venous values reflect global changes within the brain which correlate well with local measurements (ptiO$_2$) [31]. In some patients we observe discrepancies between elevated ptiO$_2$ and decreased SjvO$_2$ values following prolonged analgesia and sedation, which suggests regionally heterogeneous functional alterations within the white matter/cortex transition (ptiO$_2$) and basal ganglia (SjvO$_2$). This could result from functional adaptations due to prolonged sedation-induced glutamate receptor downregulation and compensatory increase in adrenergic, dopaminergic, and cholinergic excitation.

Based on the validation studies comparing SjvO$_2$ with ptiO$_2$, Kiening and colleagues [31] demonstrated that SjvO$_2$ £ 50% reflects cerebral ischemia and should be avoided and corrected immediately [32] since this is associated with metabolic perturbation [33] and an increased mortality and morbidity [34] (Table 2.5). In this context, elevated CPP, reduced hyperventilation, induced hypoventilation, decreased temperature, and increased depth of sedation can be used to correct signs of impaired cerebral perfusion. In case of low hemoglobin levels transfusion of red blood cells should be considered. The data concerning changes in arterio-jugular venous lactate differences is less clear and convincing [35, 36]. This could stem from the fact that the brain is capable of consuming lactate and ketone bodies as alternative energetic compounds under

Table 2.5 Jugular venous oxygen saturation (SjvO$_2$), threshold values, and possible therapeutic interventions

SjvO$_2$ values	Meaning	Reasons	Therapy/implications
<55%	Ischemia With increased jugular venous lactate: severe ischemia → fast correction required	Hyperventilation Inadequate analgesia/sedation Insufficient CPP Vasospasmus (TCD) Vasospasm Fever anemia	Normo-/hypoventilation Increase analgesia/sedation Elevate CPP Increase CPP Reduce temperature Transfuse red blood cells
55–75%	Normal values		
>75%	Hyperemia (TCD) = luxury perfusion	Vasodilatation Disturbed autoregulation Elevated CPP Deep analgesia/sedation severe brain damage (>80%)	Hyperventilation Reduce CPP Decrease analgesia/sedation Search for signs of extensive brain damage

pathologic conditions [37]. From an energetic point of view this, however, is less effective than the entire glycolytic pathway including oxidative phosphorylation, which requires intact enzymes and functionally active mitochondria. For the alternative lactate metabolism the glial–neuronal lactate shuttle plays an important role as lactate produced in astrocytes is transported to neurons for subsequent consumption. The glial lactate stems from glutamate which was previously released by neurons and then metabolized to lactate within the astrocytes due to sustained glycolysis [38].

In this context, it is important to acknowledge that cerebral oxygen consumption and thus $SjvO_2$ (as well as $ptiO_2$) and the arterio-jugular venous lactate difference are strongly influenced by brain temperature, depth of sedation, and cerebral perfusion. For example, $SjvO_2$ values >90% are observed in cases of barbiturate-induced suppression of electroencephalogram (EEG) activity (isoelectric line).

$SjvO_2$ values >80% can reflect underlying hyperemia as assessed by TCD, provided the patients' anatomy allows TCD analysis. Such hyperemia or luxury perfusion allows to reduce CPP and to use controlled hyperventilation to decrease pressure, increasing expansion of the intracranial blood volume. Whenever TCD is not available to document hyperemia, $SjvO_2$ > 80% and $ptiO_2$ > 30 mmHg in face of an adequate depth of sedation (e.g., BIS < 40) can be used to unmask hyperemia. In parallel increased $SjvO_2$ values >90% and $ptiO_2$ values >40 mmHg can also reflect extensive brain damage resulting in loss of oxygen consumption due to extensive cell damage and cell loss. To differentiate hyperemia, deep pharmacologic coma, and extensive irreversible brain damage all available monitoring parameters (ICP, temperature, bispectral index EEG (BIS EEG), EEG, somatosensory evoked potential (SEP), $ptiO_2$), including imaging (CT with angiography), must be considered (Table 2.5).

Calculation of different indices, e.g., LOI, LGI, and OGI, has not yet been introduced in daily intensive care routine [30]. These indices allow to determine the different reasons of metabolic perturbation. In this context, the OGI (OGI = $avDO_2$/AJVD glc) at values <6 reflects anaerobic glycolysis while OGI > 6 characterizes cerebral lactate consumption; the LGI (LGI= AJVD lac/AJVD glc) can be used to differ lactate production (negative values) from lactate uptake (positive values). The LOI (LOI = AJVD lac/$avDO_2$) allows to characterize the relationship between anaerobic and oxidative metabolism: while negative LOI values reflect cerebral lactate production positive

values unmask cerebral lactate uptake. The calculated OER (OER = (caO_2 – $cjvO_2$)/caO_2) allows insight into cerebral oxygen consumption.

The analysis of transcerebral gradients of humoral and cellular constituents is still subject to more in-depth analysis and has not yet been integrated in clinical diagnostics and intensive care-related decision making [39].

2.4.2.1 Crucial Points and Pearls

- Insertion of a jugular venous catheter allows in-depth insight into otherwise occult intracerebral pathophysiologic processes.
- Ultrasonographic guidance allows identification of the dominant, i.e., larger, internal jugular vein and minimizes the risk of accidentally puncturing the carotid artery.
- $SjvO_2$ differentiates insufficient oxygen supply due to impaired cerebral perfusion ($SjvO_2$ < 50%) from reduced cerebral oxygen consumption encountered during hyperemia ($SjvO_2$ > 80%), thus allowing to initiate and control different specific therapeutic interventions.
- Unmasking metabolic alterations is the prerequisite to guide the extent and duration of therapeutic interventions such as hyperventilation, CPP level, transfusion of red blood cells, oxygenation, with the aim of avoiding secondary brain damage.

2.4.3 Microdialysis

Cerebral microdialysis with a diameter of 0.3 mm allows detailed insight in otherwise hidden metabolic alterations (Fig. 2.10). Depending on the used size of the pore size of the semipermeable membrane at the tip of the catheter substances with small to large molecular weights can be filtered from the extracellular space according to their existing concentration gradients. In clinical routine, bedside analysis allows enzymatic analysis of glucose, lactate, pyruvate, glycerol, and glutamate (www.microdialysis.se). Calculating various ratios, e.g., lactate/pyruvate, lactate/glucose, lactate/glutamate, allows a more detailed characterization of the underlying metabolic perturbation even at normal ICP levels and at normal concentrations of the different parameters [40]. Furthermore, various proteins can be determined [41] which have not yet been integrated in contemporary clinical decision making.

Fig. 2.10 Overview of the different probes used in specialized centers in intensive care routine: intracranial pressure (ICP), partial pressure tissue oxygenation (ptiO$_2$), temperature, microdialysis. These different probes are much smaller than the diameter of a conventional paper clip, with the ICP probe having the largest diameter

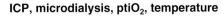

ICP, microdialysis, ptiO$_2$, temperature

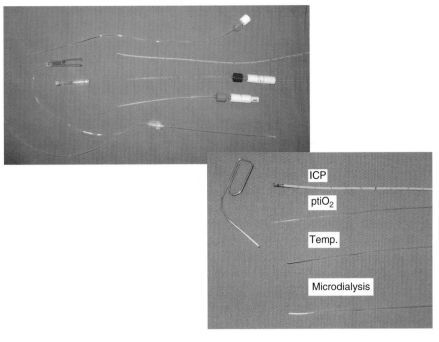

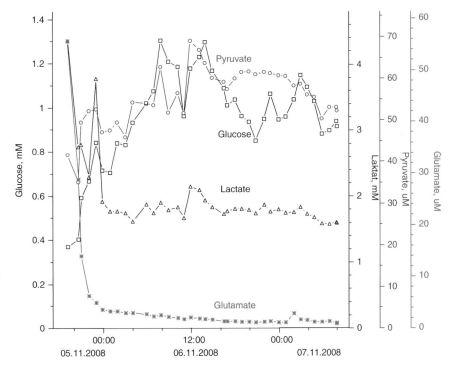

Fig. 2.11 Insertion of the microdialysis catheter induces a local injury reflected by increased extracellular glutamate and lactate levels followed by a steady decrease during the subsequent 2–4 h reaching stable values

Insertion of the microdialysis catheter induces a local tissue trauma which is predominantly reflected by significantly increased glutamate concentrations. Thus, the initial values cannot be used for clinical decision making. By experience metabolic parameters reach stable values within the first 4 h (Fig. 2.11). As a consequence microdialysis cannot be used for clinical decision making during the first hours after TBI, a phase which is characterized by hypotension and hyperventilation during the initial treatment in the emergency and operating rooms.

With microdialysis, both dialysis velocity and investigated time interval are important variables which influence concentration of the different parameters and determine the investigated time frame. In clinical routine, dialysis velocities between 0.3 and 1 μL/min combined with an interval of 60 min are commonly used. This means that clinical decisions are based on metabolic changes which have already occurred in the previously investigated time span. Consequently, the metabolic alterations unmasked by microdialysis should always be judged together with other parameters.

A technical limitation is the in vivo recovery rate which depends on changes within the tissue (hemorrhage, glial scar formation), the used dialysis velocity, and the type of membrane used. In this context, recovery rate correlates inversely to the dialysis velocity [42], which results in lower absolute concentrations of the different parameters at higher velocities and higher concentrations at lower velocities. Consequently, concentrations of the metabolic parameters determined at a dialysis velocity > 0.3 μL/min must be multiplied by

a correction factor, especially if results described in different publications are to be compared and if reference values are to be defined for the clinical routine (Fig. 2.12).

Microdialysis catheters can either be inserted under visual control during neurosurgery (e.g., craniotomy or craniectomy) or be introduced via a burrhole during initial neurosurgery or later on the ICU. For this, a commercially available specialized guiding/bolt system (www.integra-ls.com) is used through which different probes, e.g., microdialysis, ptiO$_2$, temperature probe, and ICP, can be inserted. (Officially, insertion of microdialysis probes is an off-label procedure.) Thus, local changes can be determined at a predefined penetration depth. Reproducibility of the insertion depth and area of interest is strongly influenced by the angle at which the burrhole is drilled (Fig. 2.13). Insertion of microdialysis during neurosurgery also allows strict cortical positioning compared to the white matter/grey matter junction when using the bolt system. Overall, it is of utmost importance not to insert the different probes in the pre- and postcentral gyrus to avoid serious damage resulting in a sensory or motoric hemisyndrome. The exact area of insertion in relation to the

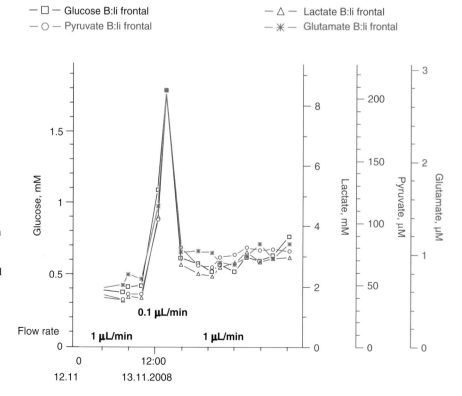

Fig. 2.12 Changing flow velocity from 1 to 0.1 μL/min and back to 1 μL/min significantly increases concentrations of the dialyzed metabolites. This clearly demonstrates the impact of flow velocity on the in vivo recovery rate. This must be considered when comparing data derived in different studies using different flow velocities

Fig. 2.13 Examples of insertion of parenchymal intracranial pressure (ICP) probe (*P*) and microdialysis combined with partial pressure tissue oxygenation (ptiO$_2$) and temperature probe (*M*) (using the same burrhole). Figure 2.13a and b depict projection of probes in axial (**a**) and coronal (**b**) computed tomography (CT) scans. Projection of the inserted probes is also seen in the lateral aspect of a conventional X-ray of the head (**c**)

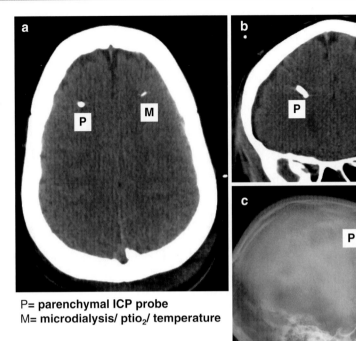

P= **parenchymal ICP probe**
M= **microdialysis/ ptio$_2$/ temperature**

present lesions and the number of catheters which should be used is still discussed controversially.

Similar to the regional heterogeneity of interhemispheric pressure gradients and between the supra- and infratentorial compartments metabolic alterations also show regional differences [43]. Nonetheless, an increase in ICP as well as local and global pathologic influences (e.g., hypotension, hyperemia, vasospasm, hyperventilation, fever, epileptic discharges) induces metabolic alterations. In addition, positive therapeutic effects result in an improvement of signs of metabolic deterioration [44] and integration of microdialysis allows to reduce CPP in a controlled manner to as low as 50 mmHg [45] as practiced within the "Lund-concept." Apart from the absolute values and the relative changes of the different metabolic parameters over time the lactate/pyruvate ratio is routinely used to determine the severity of underlying metabolic impairment. In this context, an increased lactate/pyruvate ratio exceeding 30 which coincides with low cerebral extracellular glucose levels <0.3 mmol/L reflects massive energetic derangement even in face of adequate oxygenation determined by ptiO$_2$ (Fig. 2.14). This pattern is understood as a sign of severe functional mitochondrial disturbance: glucose is excessively metabolized nonoxidatively, which explains the low extracellular glucose levels; concomitantly lactate is produced while pyruvate cannot be regenerated due to

missing oxidative phosphorylation resulting from disturbed mitochondrial respiratory chain accounting for the increased lactate/pyruvate ratio. In addition, other pathophysiologic alterations such as vasospasm, epileptic discharges, and CSD must be actively searched. A pathologic increased lactate/pyruvate ratio is associated with subsequent chronic frontal lobe atrophy and thus deserves intensified consideration [46]. Whether this can be prevented by our present therapeutic interventions warrants further investigation. Combinational investigations using microdialysis and sophisticated imaging such as positron emission tomography (PET) shows that glucose can be metabolized to lactate as well as pyruvate without increasing the lactate/pyruvate ratio [47], suggesting that other pathologic processes must be considered.

Elevated extracellular glutamate levels reflect strong/excessive neuronal excitation or signs of severe cell damage resulting in extrusion of intracellularly stored glutamate in millimolar concentrations compared to micromolar concentrations within the extracellular space. Increased lactate levels exhibit an energetic deficit while decreasing glucose levels can result from increased cellular uptake and metabolism and/or insufficient supply due to systemic hypoglycemia or insufficient expression of glucose transporters. Elevated glycerol values reflect membrane damage.

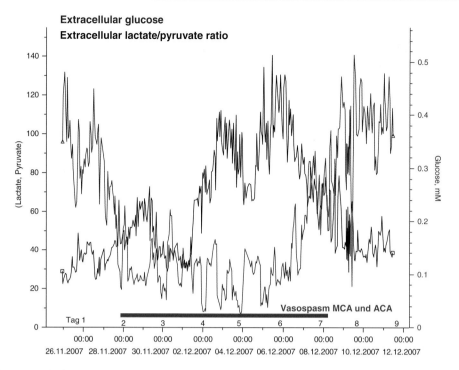

Fig. 2.14 Using cerebral microdialysis allows to differentially search for metabolic disturbances which can be harbingers of additional pathologic alterations. This illustrative case shows an increase in lactate/pyruvate ratio with concomitant decrease in extracellular glucose on the second posttraumatic day in the face of initially normal lactate/pyruvate ratio and normal extracellular glucose levels (CMA 70, flow rate: 1 μL/min, interval: 60 min). Between days 4 and 6 lactate/pyruvate ratio increased further and extracellular brain glucose decreased below 0.2 mM. Thereafter, pathologic values normalized. In this patient, this pathologic metabolic pattern was induced by severe vasospasm in the ipsilateral middle cerebral artery (MCA) and anterior cerebral artery (ACA). In a different patient this pattern coincided with epileptic discharges. Resolution of vasospasm and disappearance of epileptic discharges coincided with resolving pathologic metabolic alterations

Overall, microdialysis can be used to unmask pathologic changes, characterize pathologic relevance of certain alterations, and guide therapeutic interventions (e.g., hyperventilation, oxygenation, sedation, CPP level).

As recently shown by Belli and colleagues the early use of microdialysis corresponds to an early warning system since metabolic alterations unmask pathologic alterations and precede increases in ICP [22].

2.4.3.1 Crucial Points and Pearls

- Microdialysis allows detailed insight into metabolic alterations which otherwise remain hidden in the difficult-to-access brain.
- Local changes can be used to guide therapeutic interventions.

- Due to its time-consuming maintenance and additional costs microdialysis cannot be implemented in all centers yet.

2.4.4 Tissue Oxygenation-ptiO₂

Insertion of ptiO$_2$ probes is performed similar to the technique of implanting a microdialysis catheter [48], which can be performed during neurosurgery or on the ICU via a frontal burrhole and a specialized bolt system (Fig. 2.15). Location of the ptiO$_2$ probe in relation to cerebral lesions and the number of probes are discussed controversially. To minimize the risk for additional injuries, i.e., hemorrhage in edematous frontal lobe, the different probes (ptiO$_2$, microdialysis, temperature, with/without ICP) are usually positioned in the lesser injured hemisphere. The choice of the side of insertion

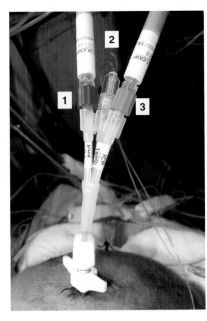

1. **ptiO₂**

2. **Microdialysis**

3. **Temperature**

Fig. 2.15 Picture showing usage of a commercially available bolt system via which a partial pressure tissue oxygenation (ptiO₂) probe (1), a microdialysis catheter (off-label use) (2), and a temperature probe (3) are inserted in the frontal lobe

depends on the predefined interest, i.e., if evolving pathologic alterations are to be unmasked in the more severely injured hemisphere or if new signs of tissue damage are to be diagnosed in the lesser or uninjured hemisphere. In this context it is important to remember that the CT scan does not reveal signs of functional and metabolic damage and that missing structural lesions do not guarantee normal metabolism an function.

The commonly used highly flexible ptiO₂ probe is a so-called Clark-type sensor (www.integra-ls.com) with a diameter of 0.55 mm and with which ptiO₂ is determined polarographically: within the sensor membrane oxygen is reduced at the cathode, thereby changing the polarizing current between anode and cathode. Changes within the electric circuit are proportional to the partial oxygen pressure within the tissue. The measured ptiO₂ depends on the tissue temperature and thus requires correction, which is automatically performed if a specialized temperature sensor is used. Novel probes such as Neurovent PTO® allow simultaneous analysis of ICP, ptiO₂ and temperature, which are combined within one probe (www.raumedic.de).

As determined in validation studies ptiO₂ values <10 mmHg (Licox®) reflect tissue hypoxia which is associated with an increase in extracellular glutamate if not corrected within 30 min [49, 50] and correlates clinically with neuropsychologic deficits in survivors [51].

Although ptiO₂ show local changes these values correlate very well with pathologic SjvO₂ values [31], which reflect global cerebral alterations and thus allow to guide type and extent of therapeutic interventions.

Similar to SjvO₂ ptiO₂ values indirectly reflect cerebral perfusion [52]. In this context, low SjvO₂ and ptiO₂ values unmask reduced cerebral perfusion due to, for example, systemic hypotension or local cerebral vasoconstriction caused by hyperventilation or vasospasm. In parallel, signs of increased oxygen consumption due to increased neuronal activity (insufficient analgesia/sedation, epileptic discharges, systemic hypoglycemia) as well as insufficient oxygen supply (anemia, impaired cardiac output, insufficient oxygenation) must be searched and corrected. Thus, determining SjvO₂ and ptiO₂ allows to perform detailed and controlled therapeutic corrections. In this context, we can decide whether ventilation, hemodynamic support, hematocrit, or blood glucose must be corrected (Table 2.6).

Abnormally elevated ptiO₂ and SjvO₂ values >30 mmHg and ≥80%, respectively, strongly suggest reduced cerebral oxygen consumption most likely due to excessively deep sedation and metabolic uncoupling of cerebral perfusion. This metabolic uncoupling is associated with strong vasodilation, which results in hyperemia and global luxury perfusion. In conjunction with a disturbed autoregulation due to impaired vasoconstriction hyperemia elevates ICP due to an increase in intracranial blood volume [53].

Apart from guiding paCO₂ levels in terms of controlling hyperventilation ptiO₂ values can also be used to individually define adequate CPP and oxygenation limits and targets [54], and also determine the necessity of transfusing red blood cells during otherwise stable intensive care conditions [55]. In this context, transfusion of oxygen carriers in patients with a hematocrit < 30% will only induce a persisting increase in ptiO₂ > 15 mmHg if the ptiO₂ is below 15 mmHg. Thus, patients with a baseline ptiO₂ > 15 mmHg do not profit from red blood cell transfusions. This, in turn, allows to reduce the number of unnecessary red blood cell transfusions.

2.4.4.1 Crucial Points and Pearls

- Measuring tissue oxygenation, i.e., ptiO₂, allows to unmask reduced perfusion and insufficient oxygen supply (<10 mmHg) and also unmasks underlying hyperemia (>30 mmHg).

Table 2.6 Threshold values of partial pressure tissue oxygenation (ptiO$_2$), their meaning and possible therapeutic options

ptiO$_2$ values	Meaning	Reason	Treatment
<10 mmHg	Ischemia With elevated glutamate, lactate, glycerol, L/P ratio: severe ischemia → immediate correction required	Hyperventilation Inadequate analgesia/sedation Insufficient CPP Impaired cardiac output Vasospasmus (TCD) Fever Anemia Hypoxia	Normo- to hypoventilaton Increase analgesia/sedation Elevate CPP Administer volume, inotropics Increase CPP Reduce temperature Transfusion of red blood cells Improve oxygenation
>15 mmHg	Normal values		
>30 mmHg	Hyperemia (TCD) = luxury perfusion	Vasodilatation Disturbed autoregulation CPP too high Cardiac output too high Sedation too deep Oxygenation too severe	Hyperventilation Reduce CPP Decrease CPP Reduce volume and inotropics, search for SIRS, sepsis Reduce sedation Decrease paO$_2$, allow lower hematocrit

- ptiO$_2$ values facilitate controlled adaptation of therapeutic interventions and thus allow to prevent potentially harmful consequences of insufficient or excessive interventions.
- Useful decisions, however, can only be made if these values are considered in conjunction with other metabolic variables and systemic changes.
- Metabolic alterations determined by microdialysis allow to define the individual pathologic ptiO$_2$ threshold.

2.4.5 Analysis of Cerebrospinal Fluid

In patients with a noncollapsed and noncompressed ventricular system an EVD can be inserted which allows therapeutic drainage of CSF with the aim of reducing elevated ICP. In addition, CSF can be used for diagnostic purposes by analyzing different mediators and markers of tissue damage and regeneration processes [56–63]. Moreover, pharmacodynamic as well as pharmacokinetic properties can be characterized [64–67]. Possible methodological difficulties lie within the nature of the EVD itself which need to be considered when interpreting the obtained results. In this context, CSF levels of different parameters are influenced by the presence of intraventricular blood, diffusion of edema from the parenchyma to the ventricular system, and production and absorption of CSF by the choroid plexus. These different influences are usually not

considered in clinical routine. The distance of lesions to the ventricular system is also important [68].

In addition, there is no clear consensus whether one daily measurement is sufficient or whether repetitive or even continuous analysis must be performed. Since EVDs cannot be placed in all patients and since CSF drainage can subside due to evolving edema formation a heterogeneous population of patient is assessed: those with a "less severe" primary injury and those who show tremendous secondary progression of brain edema. Patients with very severe primary damage are "excluded." Thus, general applicability of the obtained data is limited.

Different complications such as iatrogenic injury to basal ganglia or the internal capsule (Fig. 2.16) as well as the increased risk of ventriculitis and meningitis decrease its wide application [69].

2.4.5.1 Crucial Points and Pearls

- Analysis of CSF allows to determine pathophysiologic changes and characterize pharmacologic profiles.
- Since CSF analysis requires introduction of an EVD not all patients can be investigated. Relevant data can only be obtained if the ventricular system is wide enough and if it is not compressed by evolving brain edema.
- To date, therapeutic decisions cannot be based on changes determined in CSF.

Fig. 2.16 Examples showing injuries induced by inserting external ventricular drainage (EVD): internal capsule (**a**), corpus callosum (**b**), corpus callosum and contralateral caudate nucleus (**c**), and thalamus (**d**)

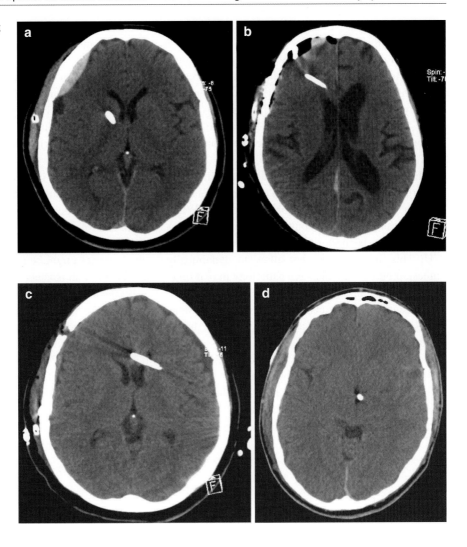

2.4.6 Electrophysiologic Studies: Electroencephalogram, Sensory Evoked Potential, Cortical Spreading Depression

2.4.6.1 EEG and SEP

Functional changes in neuronal activity and axonal information transmission can be assessed by electrophysiologic investigations, e.g., EEG, SEP, or acoustic evoked potential (AEP). These investigations also have a certain prognostic value in severe TBI. This is the case whenever an isoelectric EEG results from severe global brain damage as seen in hypoxia and excluded pharmacologic or toxicologic etiology, and whenever evoked potentials lack appropriate brain stem and cortical responses with missing amplitudes and long latencies at specific anatomic points.

EEG analysis reflects summation potentials generated by excitatory and inhibitory processes within cortical and subcortical areas which are subject to modulatory influences originating within the brain stem and basal ganglia. These processes result in specific frequencies and amplitudes. Simply phrased frequencies and amplitudes correlate inversely: low-frequency bands (delta: δ, tau: τ) exhibit large amplitudes (slow waves) while high-frequency bands (alpha: α, beta: β) show low amplitudes (fast waves). Slow waves/low frequency bands are found in sleep and during pharmacologic coma while fast waves/high frequency bands reflect arousal activity.

Evoked potentials are used to assess intact axonal impulse transmission and adequate central processing within the cortex by analyzing transmission time (latency) and strength of cortical processing (amplitude) at standardized and predefined points in response to exteroceptive tactile, acoustic, and nociceptive stimuli.

EEG and evoked potentials require specialized and well-trained personnel to perform these investigations and to accurately interpret the obtained curves. While the EEG can be recorded continuously, evoked potentials can only be performed discontinuously on the ICU. This, in turn, does not allow to dynamically unmask progressive brain stem pathology in real time.

Changes within the different EEG frequency spectra and amplitudes are also influenced by the lesions themselves, concomitant analgesia/sedation, hypothermia, and hyperventilation.

Pathologic changes in evoked potentials have a very good prognostic potency regarding mortality and morbidity [70]. However, this is not the case for

EEG analysis, which is due to the underlying pharmacologic interference that results in an increase in δ and τ frequency bands. A further difficulty is to interpret shifts within the frequency bands which are not determined in all hospitals. In this context, posttraumatically reduced variability of the alpha frequency gains increasing prognostic importance as this is associated with significantly reduced regeneration [71, 72].

Interpretation of isoelectric line can be very difficult as it could result from the continuous administration of barbiturates and propofol or could reflect brain death. Neurologic examination and imaging including angiography to exclude compression of large intracerebral arteries might be required to differentiate cause and nature of an isoelectric line.

By the use of modern and simplified EEG methods (BIS EEG® – www.aspectmedical.com/Narcotrend® – www.narcotrend.de) changes in neuronal activity – even between the two hemispheres – can be assessed in clinical routine at the bedside without extensive training. These EEG techniques are usually used to guide sedation and barbiturate coma (Fig. 2.17).

a Analgesia, sedation: fentanyl and midazolam

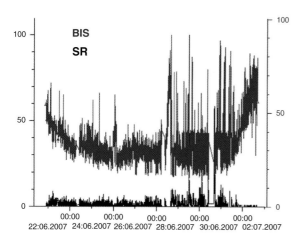

b   Influence of thiopental

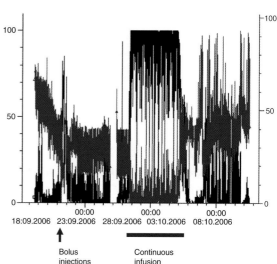

Fig. 2.17 Examples showing changes in neuronal activity determined by bispectral index electroencephalogram (BIS EEG®) (*blue curve* = BIS, *black curve* = suppression rate) in a patient subjected to analgesia and sedation following severe traumatic brain injury (TBI) (a) and a patient requiring continuous thiopental infusion due to increase in intracranial pressure (ICP) > 25 mmHg (b). (a) During continuous infusion of fentanyl and midazolam and corresponding increase in drug doses BIS value reflecting depth of analgesia/sedation was reduced

and maintained between 20 and 40, our target. During controlled dose reduction of fentanyl and midazolam (10% per day) and concomitant infusion of propofol and clonidine to treat vegetative and motoric signs of withdrawal from fentanyl and midazolam BIS slowly increased >60 and the patient awoke slowly. (**b**) Additional thiopental infusion (0.5–3 mg/kg/h) reduced BIS value below 20 and coincided with a corresponding increase in suppression rate >60%, reflecting increased depth of pharmacologic coma

2.4.6.2 CSD (cortical spreading depression)

The phenomenon of CSD initially described in 1944 by Leão [73] results from neuronal and glial depolarization which traverses the cortex in a wave pattern and is associated with energy-consuming processes. These pathologic alterations contribute to the secondary growth of a preexisting lesion which is also observed under clinical conditions [74, 75]. Initiating factors are elevated extracellular potassium concentrations, decreased cerebral NO levels, and reduced blood glucose concentrations [76]. In addition, low cerebral glucose levels appear to induce CSD, which is associated with increased extracellular lactate [77]. To determine these functional disturbances a special sensor with several electrodes must be positioned on the cortical surface under the dura. This requires a neurosurgical intervention and can only be performed by specialized neurosurgeons. With these sensors temporal and regional changes in electric activity occurring between the individual electrodes are visualized.

Ongoing research conducted in different European centers focuses on the pathophysiologic characterization and identification of possible therapeutic interventions (www.cosbid.org).

2.4.6.3 Crucial Points and Pearls

- Electrophysiologic investigations (EEG, SEP) are helpful in assessing functional alterations and also have certain prognostic value.
- Results obtained by EEG and SEP must always be interpreted in the context of the clinical situation and structural lesions unmasked with conventional imaging (CT, magnetic resonance imaging (MRI)) before definite decisions may be drawn.
- Simplified EEG analyses (BIS EEG®, Narcotrend®) are used in the clinical routine to continuously assess and control sedation by the ICU staff.
- Insertion of specialized sensors to assess CSD known to induce evolving tissue damage is currently only performed in specialized centers.

2.4.7 Assessment of Cerebral Perfusion

Since the initial description of extensive cerebral infarctions by Graham and colleagues in the year 1978

in patients who succumbed to their severe TBI, cerebral perfusion deficit has reached strong pathophysiologic importance [78]. Identification of insufficient cerebral perfusion as well as correction of this perfusion deficit is of imminent importance in modern intensive care treatment following severe TBI. While impaired perfusion with ensuing ischemia due to microthrombosis formation and vasospasm is predominantly found early after TBI (hours to days), sustained perfusion, i.e., hyperemia, is encountered days to weeks after TBI. The easiest way to guide cerebral perfusion is to calculate CPP by subtracting ICP from MABP. However, this is only a crude estimation of global cerebral perfusion and does not guarantee adequate cerebral perfusion in all brain regions which requires more sophisticated direct or indirect, invasive or noninvasive methods. For this, special probes such as thermodilution or Laser Doppler probes can be used [79]. While these techniques only show local alterations the transcranial thermodilution method, Xenon-enhanced CT, perfusion CT, single photon emission computed tomography (SPECT), PET, and perfusion-weighted MRI can be used to visualize both local and global changes in cerebral perfusion [79, 80]. Applicability in the daily intensive care routine of these imaging techniques is limited due to logistic, technical, and time-consuming restraints and the fact that the imaging only reflects a snapshot picture of actual alterations at the time point of analysis. Thus, these images can only partially aid in adapting therapeutic interventions. However, they are able to unmask ischemia in brain regions which are routinely not reached by standard monitoring techniques such as the brain stem or basal ganglia and assess concomitant metabolic alterations (SPECT, PET) and presence as well as differentiation of vasogenic/cytotoxic brain edema (CT, MRT) MRI.

To date, we still lack an easy-to-use and safe bedside tool with which cerebral perfusion can be assessed and most importantly quantified under routine intensive care conditions. We still must rely on indirect methods. In this context, $SjvO_2$, $ptiO_2$, and microdialysis play important roles. A further noninvasive tool is the transcranial Doppler/Duplex sonography with which flow velocity is determined in intracranial cerebral arteries and extracranial arteries. The absolute flow velocities in combination with the calculated Lindegaard ratio, the pulsatility, and resistance indices can be used to assess vasospasm and hyperemia, thereby allowing to adapt posttraumatic therapeutic interventions [81]. [Calculation of the Lindegaard ratio, i.e., mean flow velocity in the mean cerebral artery divided by mean flow velocity in the internal carotid artery (ICA), requires adequate identification of the ICA, which is difficult in patients in whom the carotid bifurcation is hidden behind the mandible or cervical injuries preclude adequate positioning of the ultrasound transducer). Detailed investigations of cerebral autoregulation using TCD, assessing ICP and CPP, and considering calculated ICP/MABP ratio allow to unmask disturbances in vascular adaptation processes [84]. This is important whenever cerebral vessels are not able to adequately constrict or dilate. Thus, blood volume passively follows changes in arterial blood pressure, reflecting disturbed cerebral autoregulation. Elevating MABP can increase cerebral blood volume and thus elevate ICP, which in turn can impair cerebral perfusion. This is related to the loss in normal vasoconstriction. A decrease in MABP reduces cerebral perfusion due to absent vasodilation. While this reduces ICP cerebral perfusion is impaired concomitantly. Some patients suffer from a partially disturbed autoregulation as decreasing MABP (or CPP) results in an increase in ICP. This is a normal response as cerebral vessels dilate. However, the subsequent autonomic vasoconstriction reflex is lost. This, however, can be triggered by increasing MABP and CPP to the individually required level at which vasoconstriction occurs. At the bedside this results in a decrease in ICP, thus allowing to define required and individual CPP targets. This changes and normalizes over time, allowing to lower CPP again without increasing ICP.

Furthermore, disturbed cerebral autoregulation is also unmasked by characteristic changes of the ICP curve as the second peak exceeds the first peak, reflecting hampered autonomic vasoconstriction to the travelling arterial pressure wave. This can be simply diagnosed at the bedside on the monitor screen but requires a very good ICP curve. It is important to know that these alterations can occur several times per hour per day, and can persist for 1–2 weeks.

Combining TCD, $ptiO_2$, and $SjvO_2$ allows to control and adapt therapeutic interventions and thus reduce the risk of inducing additional damage. In this context, elevated flow velocities (e.g., mean flow velocity within the MCA > 90 cm/s) together with elevated $SjvO_2$ > 80% and $ptiO_2$ values > 30 mmHg are suggestive of hyperemia. Thus, hyperventilation

and reduction in MABP and CPP to, for example, 50–70 mmHg can be indicated. Extremely elevated mean flow velocities in the MCA exceeding 120 cm/s with concomitantly reduced $SjvO_2$ and $ptiO_2$ are suggestive of vasospasm and requires imaging before hypoventilation and increase in CPP to 80–100 mmHg is performed. It is also important to adapt these interventions according to changes in ICP, especially in the presence of interhemispheric differences, i.e., signs of vasospasm on the one hand and concomitant hyperemia on the other. Correcting vasospasm on the one hand would aggravate hyperemia on the other hand and vice versa. An increase in ICP limits the induced interventions to avoid active induction of secondary brain damage (Fig. 2.18).

2.4.7.1 Crucial Points and Pearls

- Cerebral perfusion deficit induces secondary brain damage and thus must be prevented.
- Direct assessment of cerebral perfusion is still difficult and must be based on indirect measures such as $SjvO_2$, $ptiO_2$, metabolic changes (microdialysis), and TCD.
- Alterations in perfusion result from disturbed vasomotion, leading to hyperemia (maximal vasodilation) and vasospasm (vasoconstriction) with individual temporal profiles.
- These individual profiles afford individually adapted and controlled therapeutic interventions.

2.5 Therapeutic Interventions

Treatment of patients with severe TBI should only be performed in centers with well-trained interdisciplinary working teams experiencing at least 30 patients with severe TBI annually [82]. In addition, internal quality controls should be used to define own treatment protocols considering experiences of others and official guidelines. Main emphasis should be put on dynamic changes of the different pathologic/pathophysiologic changes and deteriorations as well as the pharmacodynamic and therapeutic effects of the induced interventions. It is also important that the standardized treatment concept remains flexible without becoming inconsistent. Rigid and categorical

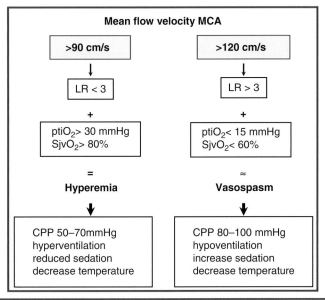

Fig. 2.18 Interplay of different parameters using color-coded duplex sonography of the middle cerebral artery (MCA) and internal carotid artery (ICA) including calculation of the Lindegaard ratio (LR = mean flow velocity MCA/mean flow velocity ipsilateral ICA) and measurement of jugular venous oxygen saturation ($SjvO_2$) and/or tissue oxygenation ($ptiO_2$) allow to differentiate hyperemia and vasospasm. This, in turn, can be used to guide differentiated therapeutic interventions, thereby preventing wrong and possibly damaging interventions. It is important to remember that patients can also suffer from heterogeneous distur-bances. In this context, different flow velocity profiles can be measured on both sides which require diametral treatment: hype-remia versus vasospasm. Here the degree of therapeutic interven-tions must be guided by increases in intracranial pressure (ICP) to avoid iatrogenic secondary brain damage. Should an increase in cerebral perfusion pressure (CPP) be required to treat vasospasm this should not aggravate concomitant hyperemia, which, in turn, would elevate ICP. $SjvO_2$, $ptiO_2$, and microdialysis can be used for subsequent fine-tuning as these methods allow to unmask and define pathologic ICP and CPP values

orders carry the risk of exaggerated treatment which can induce and aggravate secondary brain damage. Furthermore, we must avoid a brain-centered treatment concept which does not consider other organ systems, thereby putting them at stake. A brain-oriented treatment concept considering different effects on all organs is preferred over a brain-centered approach. The different official guidelines – which are not written in rock – [83, 84] provide valuable input regarding how to treat patients with severe TBI. However, local facilities, diagnostic and therapeutic possibilities, as well as the conviction and knowledge of the treating team members are driving forces which strongly impact principal guidelines – influences which cannot be controlled on a broad basis. Principal therapeutic interventions are characterized in detail in the following subchapters.

2.5.1 Crucial Points and Pearls

- Therapeutic interventions must be flexible, and at the same time consistent and not dogmatic.
- A brain-oriented therapy under consideration of potential harm to other organ systems is preferred to a brain-centered treatment concept.
- Official guidelines are recommended and are strongly impacted by local influences and personal knowledge and conviction of the treating physicians.

2.5.2 Positioning

To improve cerebral venous outflow and to reduce increased ICP due to venous congestion it is important to identify optimal positioning of the individual patient. As with many aspects in modern intensive care positioning should not be dealt with categorically since also other organ systems such as lungs and intestines show their own dynamic changes with their individual needs. This must be considered as well. Clinical experience shows that elevating the upper part of the body to 30° as suggested in the guidelines does not always reduce elevated ICP. Thus, the optimal positioning must be searched anew daily and during the individual day. Optimal positioning can range from 0° to 30°, and even more. In addition, patients can profit from positioning themselves on their side and individual side preference must also be remembered. The type of the used pillow or ring can trigger occipital neuralgic points which can increase blood pressure and also elevate ICP.

2.5.2.1 Crucial Points and Pearls

- Optimal positioning (elevation of the upper part of the body, lateral rotation) must be individualized.
- Positioning must be adapted to the clinical situation.

2.5.3 Oxygenation

The metabolically active brain must be supplied with sufficient amounts of oxygen to fuel the oxygen-consuming processes. For this, a sufficient cardiac output with an optimal perfusion and an adequate hemoglobin concentration are required to enable ideal oxygen transport and cerebral oxygen supply. This again requires intact cardiac and pulmonary functions to attain an adequate increase in physically bound and dissolved oxygen in blood. Pulmonary impairment due to atelectasis, pneumonia, and lung failure (acute lung injury (ALI)/acute respiratory distress syndrome (ARDS)) reduces SaO_2 and paO_2. This, in turn, decreases cerebral oxygen supply with the risk of secondary brain damage.

Apart from a direct pulmonary damage which is observed following isolated experimental TBI [85] and in clinical routine [86] exogenous influences due to thoracoabdominal injuries are also discussed as possible reasons for evolving pulmonary impairment and failure. In addition, blood transfusions [87] and excessive infusion of crystalloids and colloids are thought to induce ALI/ARDS following TBI [88].

In lung protective ventilation a peak pressure > 35 mbar and a plateau pressure > 30 mbar must be avoided to prevent volume- and pressure-induced lung damage. Any additional injury leads to progressive damage and forms the basis for facilitated injury such as pneumonia. Ventilatory settings are defined by the predefined paO_2 target. Thus, if the paO_2 target is set too high, then increased positive end-expiratory pressure (PEEP) can induce disadvantageous structural and functional changes in lungs and circulation, especially during hypovolemia as an elevated PEEP will impair venous backflow to the heart and result in secondary reduced pulmonary perfusion with worse blood oxygenation [89, 90].

Cerebral oxygen requirement is reduced by sedation and hypothermia which increases the threshold for hypoxic damage, thereby protecting the brain. Consequently, it is important to monitor cerebral oxygenation by assessing changes in $SjvO_2$ and $ptiO_2$, measuring metabolic changes by microdialysis, and by calculating metabolic indices (see Sect. 2.4.3). This again allows to adapt required paO_2 and actual ventilatory settings, thereby preventing unnecessary and potentially damaging therapeutic interventions. Empirical recommendation is to maintain paO_2 between 11 and 13 kPa, i.e., 83 and 98 mmHg. Using $SjvO_2$ and $ptiO_2$ values even lower paO_2 values can be tolerated under controlled conditions, thereby reducing any ventilatory-induced pulmonary stress and damage.

Increasing paO_2 to elevated levels by normobaric hyperoxygenation improves cerebral oxygen supply [54, 91] and ameliorates aerobic metabolism reflected by reduced lactate production [92]. However, normobaric hyperoxygenation is associated with an increased risk of inducing vasoconstriction [54] and promoting atelectasis [93] with pulmonary shunts. To date, normobaric hyperoxygenation cannot be recommended as a routine therapeutic intervention. The duration and extent of normobaric hyperoxygenation must still be defined.

2.5.3.1 Crucial Points and Pearls

- Cerebral oxygenation is crucial to avoid secondary brain damage.
- The actual and individual oxygen requirement which determines aggressiveness of ventilatory settings and transfusion threshold must be determined by $SjvO_2$ or $ptiO_2$ to prevent any excessive, unnecessary, and damaging therapeutic interventions.

- Normobaric hyperoxygenation is discussed contro- versially. Important details as indication, duration, and extent must still be defined before it can be rec- ommended in clinical routine.

2.5.4 Hyperventilation

Initially, prophylactic hyperventilation was thought to be an elegant way of reducing elevated ICP (Table 2.7). However, experience gained in the past years showed that uncontrolled and prophylactic hyperventilation during the early posttraumatic phase, i.e., the first 5 days induces additional secondary brain damage [94]. In this context, hypocapnia-induced vasoconstriction with impaired perfusion, metabolic and neurochemical alterations [95], and reduced $ptiO_2$ and $SjvO_2$ with ele- vated extracellular glutamate and lactate levels have been documented. Interestingly, even small changes in $paCO_2$ from 38 to 34 mmHg within normal limits is detrimental [96]. According to the official guidelines chronic hyperventilation must be avoided during the first 5 days and most importantly should not be used during the initial 24 h because cerebral perfusion is impaired predominantly during the first 24 h and any further reduction is a secondary insult, thereby aggra- vating underlying structural and functional damage. This, in turn, could increase lesion volume and aggra- vate cerebral edema and impair cerebral vascular reagi- bility, thereby disturbing cerebral autoregulation. In addition, hypocapnia can also induce negative systemic effects such as pulmonary vasodilation with intrapul- monary shunts and vasoconstriction of the coronary arteries with subsequent functional disturbances [6].

Whenever patients are hyperventilated to decrease elevated ICP, hyperventilation must be controlled using appropriate neuromonitoring techniques to unmask signs of cerebral deterioration due to hyperventilation-induced vasoconstriction. For this, changes in $SjvO_2$, $ptiO_2$, or metabolic parameters (microdialysis) are valuable tools with which individually acceptable $paCO_2$ limits can be identified, thereby avoiding induction of secondary brain damage.

2.5.4.1 Crucial Points and Pearls

- Hyperventilation can reduce elevated ICP due to induced vasoconstriction.
- Hypocapnia-induced vasoconstriction can induce cerebral ischemia and mediate secondary brain damage.
- Hyperventilation should always be controlled using $SjvO_2$, $ptiO_2$, or microdialysis; however, these parameters do not offer absolute protection against induced ischemia.
- While controlled hyperventilation can be used to treat underlying hyperemia, hypoventilation with corresponding vasodilation can be performed to treat vasospasm.

2.5.5 Analgesia and Sedation

Following severe TBI the brain is characterized by an increased vulnerability to influences which under nor- mal conditions are not of pathologic importance. In this context, coughing and straining can elevate ICP due to impaired venous outflow and increased oxygen consumption. Uncontrolled hyperventilation due to pain or impaired vigilance can induce vasoconstric- tion, thereby aggravating secondary brain damage. These alterations can be suppressed by administration of analgetics (e.g., fentanyl, sufentanyl), hypnoanalget- ics (e.g., ketamine), sedatives (e.g., benzodiazepines, barbiturates, propofol), and – if necessary – muscle

Table 2.7 Effects of different $paCO_2$ values

$paCO_2$	Indication	Effect	Unwanted cerebral effects
Normocapnia (35–45 mmHg; 4.6–5.9 kPa)			
Hypocapnia (<35 mmHg; <4.6 kPa)	Reduction in ICP	Vasoconstriction	Ischemia, infarct, ICP increase, *CAVE*: vasospasm
Hypercapnia (>45 mmHg; >5.9 kPa)	Improvement of: perfusion, oxygenation, metabolism	Vasodilation	ICP increase Disturbed autoregulation

relaxants (e.g., rocuronium, pancuronium, vecuronium, atracurium). Analgetics and sedatives decrease neuronal activity and thereby reduce cerebral metabolism and oxygen consumption. This, in turn, can reduce cerebral blood volume, thereby decreasing ICP. Consequently, analgetics, sedatives, and muscle relaxants can decrease elevated ICP.

To date, however, it remains elusive which drugs, at which dose, and in which combination are optimal [97]. While administration of single drugs carries an elevated risk of accumulation and prolonged context-sensitive half-life resulting in tolerance with subsequent loss of action, a combination of different drugs with different receptor targets could reduce these unwanted side effects as performed in the "Lund concept." This, in turn, could allow to reduce the dose of the individual drugs.

It also remains unclear whether different traumatic brain lesions influence pharmacodynamic properties of different drugs [98].

Continuous infusion of propofol has the advantage of allowing a faster awakening since its half-life is significantly shorter compared to benzodiazepines and barbiturates (hours vs. days). However, propofol induces more severe hemodynamic instability. In addition, propofol can induce the lethal "propofol-infusion syndrome," characterized by lactic acidosis, rhabdomyolysis, renal insufficiency/failure, arrhythmias, and cardiac failure [99]. Consequently, propofol should be limited to a maximum of 4 mg/kg body weight/h and for a maximum of 4 days; infusion duration, however, is discussed controversially.

In many centers daily wake-up trials are conducted to perform neurological evaluations. For this, analgetics and sedatives are stopped irrespective of the local changes and the overall condition of the patient. Only patients with minor TBI might exhibit normal arousal reaction. Patients with severe TBI will not show an adequate reaction compared to arousal from short anesthesia. Clinically, patients will react with a vegetative storm consisting of hypertension, tachycardia, hyperventilation, hyperhidrosis, hypersalivation, maybe diarrhea, and extreme agitation. These alterations are secondary insults and can induce secondary brain damage. Following such a wake-up trial re-sedation can be very difficult since this excessive excitation observed under conditions of drug withdrawal is associated with functional alterations of various receptor subtypes. According to our experience awakening should only be performed when signs of cerebral edema have completely resolved

on CT scan. As long as brain edema persists, the injured brain is extremely vulnerable to secondary insults. Analgetics and sedatives should be reduced slowly and under controlled conditions to avoid vegetative withdrawal reactions. Withdrawal reactions result from pharmacologic tolerance due to functional alterations of various receptors induced by prolonged sedation and reflects addiction [99]. Vegetative withdrawal symptoms: hyperventilation, tachycardia, hypertension, hypersalivation, hyperhidrosis, and diarrhea can be treated with continuous clonidine infusion. However, clonidine-induced bradycardia and hypotension can limit its administration. Agitation can be treated with continuous infusion of propofol (<4 mg/kg/h). During continuous administration of clonidine/propofol opioids and benzodiazepines can be reduced [100]. With signs of intracranial deterioration reflected by, for example, decreased $SjvO_2$ the wake-up phase must be interrupted by either discontinuing further drug reduction or by increasing the depth of sedation for 12–24 h before continuing controlled drug reduction.

2.5.5.1 Crucial Points and Pearls

- Analgesia, sedation, and cautious administration of muscle relaxants can protect the brain from secondary insults and are important in treating patients with severe TBI.
- To date, it remains elusive which drugs, at which dose, and which duration are optimal.
- Abruptly stopping analgesia and sedation should be avoided as this can induce uncontrollable vegetative reactions (hyperventilation, hypertension) which can additionally damage the brain.
- As long as brain edema persists the brain is vulnerable and secondary insults must be avoided.
- To treat vegetative withdrawal symptoms and motoric agitation resulting from tolerance and addiction due to prolonged administration of analgetics and sedatives, clonidine and propofol can be used; clonidine and propofol do not induce addiction, tolerance, or withdrawal symptoms by themselves.

2.5.6 Optimal Hematocrit and Transfusion Requirements

To prevent posttraumatic ischemic and hypoxic secondary insults adequate perfusion and adequate oxygen supply must be achieved. Oxygen supply is mainly mediated by oxygen bound to hemoglobin and cardiac output. To provide sufficient oxygen to the brain an appropriate number of oxygen carriers, i.e., red blood cells, must be present. However, it remains unclear which red blood cell count, reflected by the hematocrit, is optimal in patients with severe TBI. This is especially difficult since regional as well as temporal heterogeneous pathophysiologic changes have different requirements.

From a physiologic point of view any hematocrit is optimal at which the tissue is sufficiently supplied with oxygen without reducing perfusion due to increased viscosity. According to Gaehtgens and colleagues [101] there is a nearly linear relationship between hematocrit and cerebral perfusion: while decreased hematocrit improves microcirculatory perfusion, microcirculation is impaired at higher hematocrit levels. Concomitantly, however, cerebral oxygen supply shows a U-shaped reduction with a significant worsening at hematocrit <30% and >50%. This janus-faced characteristic profile is explained by the changes in viscosity and the reduction in oxygen carriers. In this context, reduced hematocrit decreases viscosity, which in turn increases blood flow according to the law of Hagen–Poiseulle since viscosity shows an inverse relation to blood flow ($Q = P\pi r^4/8L\eta$, with Q = blood flow, P = pressure gradient, r = vessel radius, L = vessel length, η = viscosity). Increased blood flow, in turn, could induce normal vasoconstriction, which, following severe TBI, however, could impair cerebral perfusion and decrease oxygen supply. Elevated hematocrit, which rarely exceeds 50% under clinical conditions, increases viscosity and thereby decreases blood flow. Thus, the microcirculatory perfusion is slowed and risk of local thrombosis is increased. Vasodilation to overcome decreased blood flow increases ICP, which in turn can aggravate underlying disturbed microcirculation.

Inducing acute hemodilution with a hematocrit < 21% under experimental conditions resulted in damaging effects [102, 103]. In patients with preexisting vasospasm following ruptured aneurysm bleeding, active reduction in hematocrit from 36% to 28% resulted in significantly reduced cerebral oxygen supply [104]. Thus, any form of severe hemodilution should be avoided. However, detailed cerebral effects of slow or fast reduction in hematocrit following severe TBI have not been investigated yet [105].

Overall, it remains unclear which absolute hematocrit value can be considered adequate, and which

relative changes in which time interval and at which time point will induce negative effects. In addition, it remains unclear if reduction in brain temperature, deep sedation, and elevated CPP are neuroprotective in cases of low and high hematocrit levels under clinical conditions. In theory, hypoxic threshold is increased whenever brain metabolism is reduced by hypothermia and deep sedation, thereby allowing a lower hematocrit level and thus decreasing transfusion requirement.

Under stable critical care conditions with stable CPP and stable oxygenation and ventilation it was recently shown that transfusion of red blood cells influences ptiO$_2$ in approximately 75% of the investigated patients [55, 106]. Interestingly patients with a ptiO$_2$ > 15 mmHg do not profit from red blood cell transfusion, suggesting that ptiO$_2$ can be used to continuously assess critical transfusion threshold. Further investigations, especially related to the age of transfused red blood cells, are required [107] as older red blood cells (storage exceeding 2 weeks) show an impaired oxygen-carrying capacity.

The current official recommendation based on a post hoc analysis is that hematocrit values can be maintained at values between 21% and 27%, i.e., during stable critical care conditions [108]. However, only an adequate prospective study will allow to decide whether the suggested hematocrit range of 21–27% can be tolerated in all patients as suggested by the Transfusion Requirements in Critical Care (TRICC) study [109]. In addition, appropriate outcome parameters, such as continuously measured ptiO$_2$, must be included to unmask dynamic changes of the transfusion threshold. This is required to adequately reduce TBI-related mortality and morbidity, to also prevent unnecessary transfusions which contribute to increased mortality and morbidity, and to avoid missing required transfusions.

The search for an optimal hematocrit is also associated with the task of optimizing plasmatic and thrombocytic coagulation parameters since ongoing bleeding will also increase mortality and morbidity. Under stable clinical conditions, platelets > 80,000/μL, INR < 1.4, fibrinogen > 1.5 mg/dL, and ionized calcium > 1.2 mmol/L are required.

2.5.6.1 Crucial Points and Pearls

- Optimal cerebral oxygen supply is essential to avoid secondary brain damage.

- To date, it remains elusive which hematocrit following severe TBI is optimal.
- Further analysis is indispensable to characterize differential needs in different phases and to possibly define phase-specific requirements in cerebral oxygenation and transfusion thresholds. For this, continuous measurement of ptiO$_2$ and metabolic parameters (microdialysis) could be of significant help.
- Regular controls of coagulation parameters are important to unmask and correct disturbed plasmatic and thrombocytic coagulation.

2.5.7 Optimal Blood Glucose Values

Elevated blood glucose levels >9.4 mmol/L (>169 mg/dL) are associated with increased mortality and morbidity [110–114]. During the early phase elevated blood glucose levels reflect the degree of underlying damage and severity of initial stress characterized by corresponding sympathoadrenergic activation. Thus, other pathophysiologically important cascades must also be considered. Hyperglycemia induces mitochondrial damage, aggravates oxidative stress, impairs neutrophil function, reduces phagocytosis, and diminishes intracellular destruction of ingested bacteria. Thus, fast correction of elevated blood glucose levels and normalization should be achieved [115] (Table 2.8). However, it still remains unclear which blood glucose values are optimal. While the group of van den Berghe propagates a protective effect of low normal blood glucose levels between 4.4 and 6.1 mM (80–110 mg/dL) due to reduced morbidity and mortality and decreased hospitalization and its cost effectiveness [116] other groups as well as van den Berghe herself could not reproduce these data in other patients [117–119]. In this context, it is important to acknowledge that the potentially positive effects are not seen until 3–5 days of reduced blood glucose levels. During the first days, however, mortality was even increased upon reducing arterial blood glucose levels [116–118], which is attributed to the increased frequency of hypoglycemia. Despite adhering to a strict protocol which included continuous glucose infusion, hypoglycemic episodes could not be prevented by van den Berghe and colleagues. Absolute and relative hypoglycemic episodes are secondary insults that must be avoided. As shown by Vespa and coworkers reducing blood glucose levels to 4.4–6.1 mmol/L results in significant metabolic and energetic cerebral impairment of the traumatized brain [120]. Apart from elevating extracellular glutamate levels lactate/pyruvate ratio was also significantly increased, reflecting excessive neuronal excitation and metabolic perturbation. In addition, mortality was increased in patients with decreased blood glucose and low cerebral extracellular glucose levels [121]. Under experimental and clinical conditions blood glucose levels <5 mmol/L can induce spontaneous cortical depolarizations (CSD) [12, 76, 122]. Thus any correction to low blood glucose values should be tightly monitored including specific cerebral monitoring such as microdialysis and jugular venous BGA to avoid inducing additional damage and to also

Table 2.8 Effects of reducing blood glucose levels using intensified insulin therapy

Positive effects	Negative effects	Brain-specific effects
Reduce critical illness polyneuropathy	Hypoglycemia	Reduced glucose levels
Attenuate renal injury	Hyperglycemia	Increased glutamate levels
Reduce pneumonia/pulmonary damage	Tight controls, repetitive blood sampling	Elevated lactate/pyruvate ratio
Decrease blood cortisol	Increased insulin requirement	Increased O$_2$ extraction
Reduce morbidity/mortality		
Improved cellular and humoral immunocompetence	Elevated costs	Increased CSD
Improved mitochondrial function		Reduced ICP
Protect endothelial cells		Attenuated norepinephrine requirement
		Reduced seizures
		Diminished diabetes insipidus

facilitate identification of optimal blood glucose values in face of temporal and regional heterogeneous glucose consumption [37, 123–128]. Reducing cerebral glucose supply by decreasing arterial blood glucose can induce secondary brain damage, which is aggravated by concomitantly reduced cerebral perfusion. Induced activation of glucose transporters, e.g., GLUT 1, can provoke additional brain damage as increased activation of these transporters amplifies oxygen deficit created by insufficient blood glucose levels. This, in turn, will increase extracellular glutamate levels, which induces neuronal and glial damage. These cascades can also be provoked by undulating blood glucose levels (Fig. 2.19). Recent data suggest that patients might profit from low blood glucose concentrations in the second posttraumatic week [129]. At present, however, it is unclear whether these beneficial effects are also seen if blood glucose levels are decreased in the second week by intensified insulin administration or whether these effects can only develop over time, thereby requiring early administration during the first and highly vulnerable week.

While the pathologic upper blood glucose limit of 10 mmol/L (180 mg/dL) has been clearly defined, the lower blood glucose limit must still be determined. Based on retrospective analysis arterial blood glucose levels should neither drop below 4 mmol/L (72 mg/dL) nor exceed 9 mmol/L (162 mg/dL) [30]. As a compromise blood glucose values could be maintained between 6 and 8 mmol/L (108 and 144 mg/dL), a range with the highest cerebral metabolic stability.

2.5.7.1 Crucial Points and Pearls

- Persisting hyperglycemia (>10 mmol/L, >180 mg/dL) increases morbidity and mortality.
- Correction and normalization of elevated blood glucose levels is essential.
- Normalization of elevated blood glucose levels to 4.4–6.1 mmol/L (80–110 mg/dL) induces hypoglycemia and undulating blood glucose levels, thus increasing morbidity and mortality.

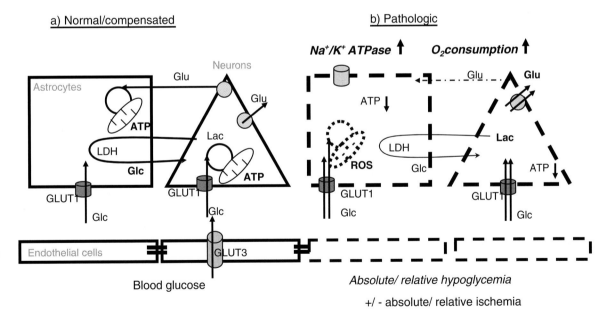

Fig. 2.19 Schematic drawing of physiologic influences of cerebral glucose uptake and intracellular metabolism and glial–neuronal interactions (**a**) and pathophysiologic changes induced by systemic hypoglycemia (**b**). Sustained expression and increased activity of specific glial and neuronal glucose transporters mediate intensified glucose uptake even in the face of low extracellular glucose levels. This compensation, however, only insufficiently satisfies underlying growing energetic requirements. The increased oxygen consumption, in turn, results in an oxygen deficit and insufficient adenosine triphosphate (ATP) production. As a consequence, glutamate uptake is reversed resulting in increased extracellular glutamate. The elevated lactate/pyruvate ratio reflects mitochondrial impairment. Undulating blood glucose levels are feared to aggravate induced cascades

- Those patients must be identified in whom blood glucose levels can be reduced to 4.4–6.1 mmol/L without any additional risks to avoid endangering other patients who will not profit from the intensified insulin treatment.
- A time dependent optimal blood glucose target must still be defined.
- Until new convincing and safe data have been obtained maintaining arterial blood glucose levels between 5 and 8 mmol/L appears to be a safe compromise.
- Improved continuous blood glucose control using a computer-supported automatized insulin administration could facilitate maintenance of stable low blood glucose levels, thereby avoiding damaging hypoglycemic episodes and undulating blood glucose concentrations.

2.5.8 Barbiturate Coma

Barbiturates, depending on concentration, suppress cerebral metabolism and oxygen consumption by activating the neuronal GABA/Cl⁻ receptor channel independently of the inhibitory transmitter GABA. The degree of metabolic suppression strongly depends on the initial level of activation [130]. Overall, reduction in cerebral oxygen consumption decreases intracranial blood volume and improves cerebral autoregulation [131]. In addition, diminished glutamate release and metabolic stabilization were reported [66, 132]. These different effects reduce elevated ICP, which, however, is not observed in all patients to the same extent.

Due to various dose-dependent side effects (hypotension due to cardiac depression, cellular immunosuppression, bone marrow insufficiency, and increased rate of pneumonia) barbiturate coma using a high dose with the induction of 3–6 bursts/min is not seen as a first-tier therapeutic intervention. According to the official guidelines prophylactic barbiturate coma is discouraged as it may increase mortality and morbidity [133]. However, the data were predominantly obtained at a time when intensive care treatment did not meet contemporary standards. One major problem is the barbiturate-induced arterial hypotension due to cardiac depression and barbiturate-induced adrenal insufficiency with consecutive hypotension, which contributed to an increased mortality as shown

in a COCHRANE meta-analysis [134, 135]. In modern intensive care, such barbiturate-induced changes can be corrected easily by infusing appropriate amounts of fluids and by administering vasopressors and inotropics guided by appropriate monitoring tools such as a pulmonary artery catheter or Picco® System. In addition, patients suffering from severe TBI were maintained hypovolemic and received osmotherapeutics on a regular basis and were subjected to prophylactic hyperventilation, which could have provoked deleterious vasospasm that was neither searched for actively nor treated adequately. Furthermore, barbiturate coma induces hypothermia, which per se can induce immunosuppression and coagulopathy, and increase risk for infections. In addition, other important therapeutic and diagnostic interventions have improved in the past decades, which prevents a direct comparison. The official guidelines which propagate a reluctant position in administering barbiturates are challenged by the "Lund-concept" (s. X.Y) (2.5.12.2, p. 39) in which thiopental is infused continuously at a low dose (0.5–3 mg/kg/h compared to the high-dose thiopental as used for barbiturate coma at 6–10 mg/kg/h) in addition to other sedatives and analgetics, e.g., fentanyl, midazolam, clonidine, metoprolol. These different drugs with their different receptor targets are infused in parallel.

Furthermore, the inclusion criteria to begin barbiturate coma if ICP > 30 mmHg for longer than 30 min in addition to a CPP < 60 mmHg or ICP > 40 mmHg despite a CPP > 60 mmHg might be wrong as these indications result in a late start of barbiturate. Thus, secondary brain damage has already occurred which is extremely difficult to treat and manage once it has developed.

2.5.8.1 Crucial Points and Pearls

- Barbiturate coma may reduce therapy-refractory increase in ICP in some patients.
- Barbiturate coma requires detailed invasive hemodynamic monitoring and adequate correction of cardio depression, vasodilation, and adrenal suppression.
- An increased vigilance for infections is also important.
- Contrary to the high dose as used for the conventional barbiturate coma low dose as applied within the "Lund-concept" could be related with less side effects.

2.5.9 Temperature, Fever, Hypothermia, Rewarming

Based on experimental and clinical data increased body temperature exceeding 38.5°C, corresponding to 40–41°C in the brain, induces destructive biochemical cascades leading to structural and functional deficits, which, in turn, aggravate posttraumatic mortality and morbidity [135]. As long as cerebral oxygen supply and cerebral perfusion are optimal fever does not seem to induce metabolic perturbation. Cerebral vasodilation, however, can elevate ICP [136]. Thus, an increase in temperature should be avoided and normo- or even moderate hypothermia should be induced. Reducing temperature by 1°C reduces cerebral oxygen consumption by approximately 5%. To date, it still remains unclear which target temperature should be induced and for how long this temperature should be maintained. While an American multicenter study could not provide convincing evidence of maintaining hypothermia of 32–33°C during the first 24 h [137] other studies were able to demonstrate significant benefits [138, 139]. In children, however, early hypothermia was even associated with increased mortality [140].

To date, target temperature, site of measuring temperature, time point of inducing and duration of maintaining hypothermia, as well as means of cooling and speed of rewarming are discussed controversially.

While some centers primarily target normal body temperature (37–38°C) and only start reducing temperature once ICP increases, other centers initially induce mild hypothermia with a brain temperature of 35–36°C even at normal ICP levels. Moderate hypothermia at 33–35°C is usually accepted as a side effect of barbiturate coma.

The site at which temperature is measured is also discussed controversially. While most centers measure temperature rectally, auricular, in the bladder, in the jugular venous bulb (using a pediatric pulmonary artery catheter), in the artery, or in the pulmonary artery, only few centers determine brain temperature directly. Since brain temperature can exceed temperature determined at other sites by as much as 2°C it is obvious that effects of temperature not determined within the brain will be underestimated. The newer generation of ICP probes possesses an integrated temperature sensor. Alternatively, separate temperature sensors can be inserted in addition to the $ptiO_2$ probe.

The manner in which patients are cooled can range from the conventional, noninvasive, and cheap but difficult-to-control surface cooling using cooling mats to the sophisticated, invasive, and expensive but very easy-to-control intravenous cooling using, for example, Intravascular Temperature Management (IVTM™) (www.alsius.com) [141]. New data propagate noninvasive cooling with the Arctic Sun® 2000 Temperature Management System (www.medivance.com) [142].

Other cooling methods such as selective cooling of the head using a specialized helmet or reducing temperature of the cervical vessels are currently being investigated.

Pharmacologic reduction in temperature using paracetamol and metamizol is widely performed but must be viewed critically and cautiously due to potential severe side effects such as hepatic toxicity and neutropenia.

Rewarming should be performed slowly and controlled by adequate cerebral monitoring. In this context, a speed of rewarming ranging from 1°C/12 h to 1°C/24 h is recommended. Fast rewarming can induce generalized vasodilation with systemic hypotension and disturbed cerebral autoregulation resulting in elevated ICP and metabolic perturbation [143]. Due to individually different responses adequate neuromonitoring is required to control and specifically guide the rewarming process.

2.5.9.1 Crucial Points and Pearls

- Fever induces cerebral secondary damage and must be avoided.
- Reducing brain temperature decreases cerebral metabolism.
- To date, target temperature, duration, and means of reducing temperature remain elusive.
- Early hypothermia with 32–34°C during the first 2 days is associated with an increased mortality and thus cannot be recommended.
- Pharmacologic reduction in temperature must be performed cautiously or even avoided due to possible severe side effects.
- Rewarming must be performed slowly and with appropriate neuromonitoring to avoid inducing secondary brain damage due to systemic hypotension and disturbed cerebral autoregulation with subsequent elevated ICP.

2.5.10 Hemodynamic and Volume Management

Cerebral perfusion as well as perfusion of all organ systems depends on sufficient cardiac output. Nearly all patients with severe TBI exhibit hypotensive blood pressure values even in the absence of hemorrhage, regarded as a side effect of analgesia/sedation and the trauma-induced severe systemic inflammatory response syndrome, which increases endothelial permeability and thus induces volume shift and volume loss into the "third space." To prevent this hypovolemia from becoming a secondary insult and to prevent it from inducing secondary brain damage, volume must be infused for hemodynamic stabilization. Ideally, we should achieve an optimal volume status. In reality, however, it is difficult to reach and maintain euvolemia/normovolemia. The goal is to prevent excessive volume administration, as is discussed, to increase the risk of ARDS [144] and abdominal compartment syndrome [145]. Volume management becomes difficult in septic and bleeding patients in whom prolonged activation of the inflammatory system is associated with an increased volume requirement. In the early phase, a negative fluid balance should be avoided since this is associated with an increased risk of developing cerebral vasospasm and results in an elevated need of catecholamines which will induce organ damage in the face of underlying hypovolemia.

To date, the type of fluid to be administered is discussed controversially. While some countries predominantly use Ringer Lactate or NaCl 0.9%, other countries infuse modern, i.e., balanced crystalloid, solutions in combination with balanced colloid solutions. NaCl as well as glucose solutions should be avoided as severe side effects can induce additional organ damage related to hyperchloremic acidosis (NaCl) and edema promotion and tissue acidosis (glucose solutions). The benefits of the novel balanced solutions must be evaluated in clinical routine.

Apart from volume administration infusion of vasoconstrictors and inotropics are important. In principal, a balance between volume administration and pharmacologic hemodynamic support must be found to prevent excessive administration of catecholamines with the aim of reducing volume load as this can induce organ damage similar to the consequences of volume overload by itself. To date, we are lacking an international consensus regarding which vasoconstrictors are to be used. While many centers use norepinephrine, others administer the synthetic vasopressor phenylephrine and some use ket-

amine, which is known to increase arterial blood pressure due its norepinephrine-releasing effect [146].

Control of hemodynamic and volume management is based on different parameters which can be observed easily, e.g., MABP including the curve form (which requires invasive blood pressure measurement), heart rate, diuresis including color of urine, sodium and osmolality in urine, and to a certain extent central venous pressure. For a more detailed guidance including administration of inotropics (e.g., dobutamine) invasive methods are required such as the Picco® system or a pulmonary artery catheter. As a compromise and until these catheters have been introduced central venous oxygen saturation ($ScvO_2$) can also be used. A $ScvO_2 < 60\%$ suggests a reduced cardiac output resulting in an impaired perfusion of various organs which can be corrected by dobutamine administration and volume infusion. During deep analgesia/sedation, barbiturate coma, and controlled hypothermia $ScvO_2$ can only partially be used due to the generalized decrease in oxygen consumption which increases $ScvO_2$ values.

During hemodynamic management, vasopressor-induced refectory bradycardia can decrease cardiac output and thus impair cerebral perfusion. This can be corrected easily by reducing pharmacologic vasoconstriction and infusing dobutamine. This, however, requires active measurement of cardiac output to differentiate bradycardia. Bradycardia can also result from extensive exercise in athletes, can reflect sick-sinus syndrome, or can result from hypothermia as well as deep analgesia/sedation.

Dysrhythmia can result from hypokalemia, hypophosphatemia, and hypomagnesemia, which must be corrected. Regular electrocardiogram (ECG) controls are indicated for early diagnosis of a prolonged QT-interval which can be corrected by infusing magnesium.

Depending on the severity of the trauma and the trauma-induced extent of sympathoadrenergic activation, signs of subendocardial ischemia can be seen in routine ECG.

2.5.10.1 Crucial Points and Pearls

- For adequate hemodynamic support with the aim of maintaining optimal cerebral perfusion volume, catecholamines, and inotropic agents must be combined. To date, there is no international consensus concerning which drugs are to be used.

- Hemodynamic and volume management must be adjusted to the individual needs to prevent organ damage.
- Periodic ECG controls are important to diagnose cardiac ischemia, arrhythmia, and prolonged QT time, and daily electrolyte controls are essential in preventing arrhythmia and guiding their treatment.

2.5.11 Osmotherapy: Mannitol, Small Volume Resuscitation, Albumin

Concentration-dependent changes predominantly of sodium and alterations in the osmotic gradient across the blood brain barrier contribute to the development and resolution of brain edema. Consequently, influencing the osmotic gradient is a senseful and useful therapeutic option to treat brain edema. In this context, mannitol and hypertonic NaCl solution with and without dextran have been investigated under clinical conditions [147, 148] (Table 2.9).

Due to its strong osmotic effect mannitol expands the blood volume, decreases the hematocrit and reduces blood viscosity. In addition, cerebral perfusion and cerebral oxygen supply are improved rapidly. These effects require a CPP > 70 mmHg and reduced serum osmolality. At an increased serum osmolality above 320 mOsmol/L, which is predominantly induced by elevated sodium levels, mannitol should not be infused. Continuous mannitol infusion is thought to possibly aggravate edema formation and thus increase ICP whenever the blood brain barrier is damaged. A severe and eventually organ-damaging side effect is the induced osmotic diuresis resulting in hypovolemia and electrolyte disturbance. This hypovolemia can increase systemic lactate levels, which is observed in patients who are craniectomized in time due to cerebral herniation who then develop diabetes insipidus resulting from herniation-induced pituitary/hypothalamic ischemic injury. In addition, osmotic nephropathy is feared [149] as recently reported concentration effects resulting from the anti-edematous action could impair cerebral function [150].

As concluded in the recently published COCHRANE analysis, mannitol lacks sufficient evidence to be recommended for routine clinical use [147]. This, however, does not mean there are insufficient indications and does not exclude a search for clear definitions for the controlled application of mannitol such as for therapy-refractory elevations in ICP with herniation signs at normal serum osmolality.

An alternative to mannitol is seen in hypertonic NaCl solutions in terms of small volume resuscitation (SVR). For this, a small volume of usually 4 mL/kg of a 7.2–7.5% NaCl/colloid solution is infused within 5–10 min. Due to the rapid volume expansion related to the osmotic strength of SVR it is mainly the hypotension which is corrected. In a double-blind placebo-controlled trial SVR corrected hypotension without, however, improving mortality and morbidity [151]. Due to the reduced penetration of the blood brain barrier and the anti-edematous action in injured brain regions [152] these osmotherapeutic agents might also qualify as a treatment option for elevated ICP during the ICU phase. Further positive effects are found in improved perfusion at increased vessel diameter resulting from induced tissue dehydration [17]. In addition, hypertonic NaCl solution counteracts glutamate-mediated toxicity by stabilizing cell membranes and reduces infectious complications related to different immunomodulatory effects. Apart from these positive

Table 2.9 Osmotherapy

Compound	Indication	Main effect	Side effects
Albumin (4%, 20%)	Correct plasma albumin, aim > 20 g/dl	Constant colloidosmotic potency, reduce brain edema	Osmotic nephropathy with tubulus injury
Mannitol (20%)	ICP reduction, Serum osmolality <320 mOsmol/kg	Osmotic potency, volume expansion, increase in cerebral perfusion	Osmotic diuresis with electrolyte disturbance Osmotic nephropathy Hypervolemia with pulmonary edema
Hypertonic NaCl-solution (7.2–7.5%) Hypertonic NaCl with dextran	ICP reduction Serum osmolality < 320 mOsmol/kg	Osmotic potency, volume expansion	Hypernatremia, hemorrhage, central pontine myelinolysis Hyperhydration

actions rebound increase in ICP following termination of continuous infusion of hypertonic NaCl solutions must be considered which could induce local and systemic injuries. In this context, central pontine myelinolysis due to rapid changes in sodium, renal failure, dilution coagulopathy, cardiopulmonary failure due to hypervolemia, and hemorrhages induced by hypertension may occur.

Overall, potency of reducing frequency of therapy-refractory increases in ICP due to SVR appears to be superior to mannitol [153]; mortality and morbidity, however, remain uninfluenced. However, the significant difference in osmotic composition of the different solutions (350 vs. 175 mOsmol) reduces the validity of these results. In a recently published study designed to investigate short-term effects within the first 120 min, the actions of equimolar doses of mannitol and 7.45% hypertonic NaCl solution (255 mOsmol each) were compared [154]. Here, mannitol as well as the hypertonic NaCl solution reduced elevated ICP (>20 mmHg) likewise; CPP was significantly increased in the mannitol group due to an increase in MABP.

The importance and position of osmotherapy in the cascade of different therapeutic interventions aimed at decreasing elevated ICP must still be defined. To date, SVR is discussed as a last possibility following unsuccessful administration of mannitol and barbiturates.

The search for the ideal osmotherapeutic continues. Overall, crystalloids [155] and mixed crystalloid/colloid solutions [156] appear to reduce ICP more efficiently than mannitol.

According to the equation developed by Frank Starling describing the intravasal colloid osmotic pressure required to balance the hydrostatic pressure gradient and to reduce development of extravasal edema formation which exceeds lymphatic drainage, it appears useful to maintain plasma albumin levels above 20 g/dL. Albumin substitution is indicated whenever plasma albumin is reduced in critically ill patients. The important role of albumin in the context of reducing brain edema formation is emphasized within the "Lund-concept" [157] (see Sect. 2.5.12.2). In a prospective randomized trial it was shown that administration of albumin 4% increased mortality compared to infusion of NaCl [158]. This increased mortality was caused by an excessive administration of albumin irrespective of plasma albumin concentrations.

2.5.11.1 Crucial Points and Pearls

- Reduction of brain edema can be achieved by infusing osmotically active solutions.
- Rare incidence of side effects, e.g., osmotic diuresis, electrolyte disturbances, osmotic nephropathy, rebound increases in ICP, must be considered.
- Detailed information, i.e., patients, time point, dose, and duration, must be identified to reduce the risk of secondary damage and increase the benefit of osmotherapy.

2.5.12 Controversial Issues Regarding Treatment Concepts: ROSNER vs. LUND

Following severe TBI prevention and reduction of cerebral ischemia is an integral part of modern intensive care treatment. Consequently, cerebral perfusion must be optimized to avoid functional and structural cell damage and to attenuate an increase in mortality and worsened outcome. However, it is difficult to define and assess an optimal cerebral perfusion at the bedside since regional and temporal heterogeneous changes in perfusion ranging from impaired perfusion due to local thrombus formation, tissue compression, and vasoconstriction to vasospasm as well as hyperemia are known to develop with individual profiles. Thus, we must rely on direct and indirect methods which we can use at the bedside to continuously assess pathologic changes and control effects of therapeutic interventions. New data support the concept of individualizing the different treatment options [159].

With the aim of improving cerebral perfusion and thereby protecting the brain two different concepts have been developed: the more senior "Rosner concept" and the younger "Lund concept."

2.5.12.1 Rosner Concept

As described in the original work published by Rosner and colleagues in 1995 [160] CPP was maintained above 70 mmHg. For this, the patients received catecholamines, crystalloid (NaCl, Ringer Lactate), and colloid (albumin, mannitol) solutions and red blood cells (hemoglobin target > 12 g/dL) with the aim of attaining a normovolemic state. CPP was also strongly influenced by the concomitant routine CSF drainage via EVD. Hyperventilation was not controlled. Patients were not given any barbiturates and hypothermia was not induced. Analgesia and sedation were not prioritized. The authors mainly focused on ICP-decreasing measures by CSF drainage and infusing mannitol and albumin. According to the original data, CPP was the main determinant to reduce ICP, suggesting a maintained cerebral autoregulation since an increased CPP will only reduce ICP if the cerebral vessels can respond to this increase in arterial pressure by vasoconstriction, thereby reducing intracranial blood volume. While lowest ICP was measured at a CPP of 123 mmHg in patients not requiring catecholamines, lowest ICP was recorded at a CPP of 90 mmHg in patients in need of catecholamines. Increasing CPP above 113 mmHg resulted in a nonsignificant trend towards elevated ICP. These data clearly demonstrate heterogeneity of functional responses in these patients and consequently question the contemporary opinion of categorically decreasing CPP to 60 mmHg. On average, patients requiring catecholamines had a higher ICP, i.e., 30.4 ± 14.7 vs. 18.1 ± 6.4 mmHg, were more severely injured, and exhibited an increased mortality. Overall mortality was 29%.

Retrospective evaluation of this large patient series does not allow to clearly identify individual treatment requirements since not all patients were treated identically: not all patients received mannitol, albumin, or catecholamines. A statistical subgroup analysis was not performed. In addition, these data were not compared to a historic or subsequently investigated group of patients. Consequently, the drawn conclusions are more suggestions than guidelines. It is important to acknowledge that the "Rosner concept" is not used in its original form and that it has been subject to various modifications, which have also not been investigated in appropriate studies. Nonetheless, it remains unchanged that we have to actively search for those phases in which CPP must be increased. Due to pathophysiologic changes which can occur rapidly and are difficult to predict, a rigid CPP value cannot be recommended as suggested in the current guidelines since impaired perfusion and hyperemia require different CPP targets. Already in their original work Rosner and colleagues clearly concluded that the search for an optimal CPP is dynamic and that the ideal CPP must be viewed in the context of cerebral changes over time. Contrary to the contemporary and insufficiently

documented official recommendation of categorically maintaining CPP around 60 mmHg Rosner and coworkers reported optimal CPP values between 85 and 90 mmHg. Experimental [161] and clinical data [162] show that reducing CPP increases structural damage and impairs cerebral oxygenation. Thus, the oversimplified concept of using a categorically defined CPP value must be considered outdated and wrong. Identification of an optimal CPP is only possible if specific monitoring methods, e.g., cerebral microdialysis, $ptiO_2$ and $SjvO_2$ measurement, local cerebral blood flow assessment using specialized probes [163], and TCD, are integrated in the clinical routine.

2.5.12.2 Lund Concept

The concept which was developed in Lund, Sweden, by pharmacologists, physiologists, and neurosurgeons focuses on pharmacologic modulation of cerebral and systemic targets by which the cerebral ischemic/hypoxic threshold is increased by the employed analgesia/sedation and by which the hydrostatic pressure known to aggravate brain edema formation is reduced [164]. The combination of these central targets allows controlled reduction of CPP. Reduction to low CPP values of 50 mmHg depends on metabolic monitoring of the injured brain using continuous microdialysis. Without metabolic monitoring there is an increased risk of missing pathophysiologic important changes, possibly resulting in secondary brain damage. Thus, metabolic monitoring via microdialysis allows to fine-tune the CPP level and adapt various therapeutic interventions, thereby reducing the risk of damaging potential of excessive therapeutic corrections. It is of high importance not to implement the "Lund concept" within the initial 24 h since any form of hypovolemia and possible coagulopathy must be corrected first.

The therapeutic aims are an ICP < 20 mmHg and a CPP between 50 and 60 mmHg, a $SjvO_2$ 60–70% with an $AJVDO_2$ of 5–6 mL O_2/dL, a serum albumin of 40 g/dL, a hemoglobin between 10 and 13 g/dL, and a daily volume balance of 500 mL. In this context, CPP is not maintained at a rigid and categoric level of 50–60 mmHg, as generally misunderstood. Whenever signs of metabolic impairment unmask potential cerebral ischemia, CPP is increased until the underlying metabolic deterioration has been corrected. Only then can CPP be reduced again.

To achieve these goals cerebral as well as systemic targets are addressed. With the differentiated pharmacologic therapy different receptor subgroups are specifically inhibited or activated as patients receive fentanyl, midazolam, thiopental, or propofol. In addition, metoprolol and clonidine have a cardiodepressive as well as sedative effect. To reduce the hydrostatic pressure with the aim of decreasing the progression of vasogenic edema formation patients receive albumin, red blood cells, and fresh frozen plasma, thereby normalizing blood oncotic pressure. Concomitantly, patients receive a diuretic (furosemid) to promote diuresis and reduce hydrostatic pressure.

Those 53 patients who were investigated in the nonrandomized and uncontrolled original publication showed an otherwise therapy-refractory ICP > 25 mmHg. Thus, these patients do not represent the general TBI population and the success was only compared to a historic group of patients. Consequently, the "Lund concept" cannot be generalized.

Based on heterogeneous lesions and the temporal as well as regional inhomogeneous changes interventions must be considered as being far more dynamic than currently acknowledged.

In principal, it is conceivable that patients could profit more from a fusion of the "Rosner concept" and the "Lund concept" – at least in some parts – than from strictly following rigid predefined values. An individual adaptation of the type and extent of therapeutic intervention, however, is only possible if correct monitoring methods are adequately integrated in daily routine.

2.5.12.3 Crucial Points and Pearls

- Neither the "Rosner concept" nor the "Lund concept" have been validated in prospective randomized clinical trials.
- Both concepts and at least individual parts of these concepts are justified in clinical routine. Criteria to determine which patients profit from which concept must be identified.
- Both concepts are not to be misunderstood as rigid concepts. Signs of deterioration require an adequate adaptation of the induced therapeutic interventions.
- Controlled reduction in CPP to low values of approximately 50 mmHg should only be performed with adequate neuromonitoring including cerebral microdialysis. At present, this is only possible in large centers.

2.5.13 Intraabdominal Compartment

In the past years the abdominal compartment has received increasing attention. Due to impaired gastrointestinal function resulting from hypervolemia-induced edema formation in conjunction with drug-induced gastrointestinal paralysis, the following pathologic changes must be anticipated:

- Increased ICP resulting from reduced venous drainage
- Bacterial translocation with subsequent sepsis
- Pulmonal deterioration with impaired oxygenation and ventilation

These changes, in turn, induce alterations which again activate systemic as well as cerebral destructive cascades, thereby contributing to and inducing secondary brain damage.

In this context, posttraumatic intraabdominal hypertension can increase ICP and reduce CPP, which is detrimental in patients with an impaired intracranial compliance and subsequent elevated ICP [165]. Surgical decompression of an abdominal compartment syndrome [166] can reduce ICP and mortality [167]. To prevent the development of an abdominal compartment syndrome it is important to guarantee regular bowel movements and to avoid hypervolemia.

2.5.13.1 Crucial Points and Pearls

- The abdominal compartment syndrome is also observed in patients with isolated severe TBI and influences the subsequent clinical course.
- Apart from intraabdominal injuries generalized edema can induce an abdominal compartment syndrome.
- Secondary problems are translocation of bacteria as well as impaired oxygenation and ventilation, which, in turn, activate destructive cascades and thereby induce secondary brain damage.
- Sometimes laparotomy must be performed to decrease otherwise therapy-refractory elevated ICP.

2.5.14 Drainage of Cerebrospinal Fluid

According to the Monroe–Kelly doctrine draining of CSF can reduce intracranial volume, thereby decreasing

ICP and supporting tissue viability by improving cerebral perfusion and oxygenation. This, however, requires an accessible ventricular system allowing to adequately position the catheter without injuring important structures such as the internal capsule and basal ganglia, and penetrating the floor of the third ventricle which could result in injury to the basal artery. Inserting a lumbar drainage also allows decreasing elevated ICP [168], which is only possible if patients are not at risk of cerebellar herniation. For this, basal cisterns and the foramen magnum must be clearly visible on routine CT scan.

While CSF drainage is generally recommended since it can positively influence the intracranial volume–pressure relationship there is no clear evidence regarding its general benefit. Proof of its benefit is hampered by the facts that a ventricular drainage can only be inserted in a small group of patients and that progressive brain edema and compression of the ventricular system preclude required CSF drainage. In principal, patients with severe TBI are not at increased risk of developing a hydrocephalus resulting from intraventricular hemorrhage with subsequent congested choroid plexus as found following ruptured aneurysm and spontaneous intracerebral hemorrhage. Thus, there is no forced necessity. Furthermore, repetitive or continuous CSF drainage can result in increased CSF production by the otherwise intact choroid plexus, which, over time, can also contribute to elevated ICP.

Penetration of the ventricular system and the duration of the CSF drain are associated with an increased risk for infections (ventriculitis and meningitis) irrespective of antimicrobial prophylaxis. The different risk factors, e.g., duration, frequency of drainage, type of catheter (i.e., with vs. without antimicrobial sheath), are discussed controversially [169]. Thus, a risk–benefit balance is indispensable to avoid inducing secondary brain damage.

2.5.14.1 Crucial Points and Pearls

- When properly indicated CSF drainage (ventricular or lumbar) can reduce elevated ICP.
- CSF drainage is not indicated in all patients and can only be performed properly in a subset of patients.
- A risk–benefit balance must be evaluated daily since a CSF drain is associated with serious complications such as hemorrhage, structural damage, and infections.

2.5.15 Craniectomy

Surgical treatment of otherwise therapy-refractory intracranial hypertension (>30 mmHg) includes uni- or bilateral decompressive craniectomy. In conjunction with an artificial expansion of the dura the intracranial space is increased, thereby significantly decreasing ICP and improving cerebral perfusion and oxygenation. In addition, therapy intensity can be reduced significantly [170]. However, disturbed autoregulation with an excessive increase in intracranial blood volume has been described following craniectomy [170]. To date, it remains unclear if decompressive craniectomy which is life saving and which facilitates a very good neuropsychological recovery [171, 172] should be performed preemptively in all patients. Whenever a craniectomy is indicated it is important to perform a sufficiently large craniectomy with concomitant expansion of the dura to avoid cerebral herniation with consecutive infarction at the edge of the exposed skull bone. Rigidity of the dura can cause an increase in ICP despite a large craniectomy.

2.5.15.1 Crucial Points and Pearls

- Otherwise therapy-refractory increases in ICP with signs of cerebral and cerebellar herniation are clear indications for uni- or bilateral craniectomy with concomitant expansion of the dura.
- Mortality and morbidity can be reduced.
- The indication of a preemptive craniectomy is currently unclear.

2.5.16 Corticosteroids

Since its identification as a significant inhibitor of phospholipase A_2 and blocking of subsequent activation of destructive prostaglandins and leukotrienes the same anti-edematous effect was searched following TBI as encountered in peri-tumorous vasogenic edema. This, however, was excluded in the study published by Gaab and colleagues in 1994 investigating the effects of high-dose dexamethasone [173] and confirmed in a recently published international multicenter double-blind placebo-controlled trial [174]. In this study, a total of 10,008 patients with mild to severe TBI were randomized in two groups comparing the effects of methylprednisolone (2 g during the first hour, followed by continuous infusion of 0.4 g/h for 48 h) versus placebo. The aim was to determine a potential prophylactic effect of this glucocorticoid with mineralocorticoid action. Due to the significantly increased mortality during the first 2 weeks this trial was terminated prematurely. In addition, there was a trend towards an increased frequency of complications such as seizures, gastrointestinal hemorrhages, wound infections, and pneumonia in the steroid-receiving patients. These complications result from the well-described side effects of high-dose steroid administration: insulin resistance, increased energy consumption with hormonal, inflammatory, and immunologic dysfunction, muscular dysfunction, electrolyte imbalance, disturbance of the hypothalamic–pituitary–adrenal axis, reduced glucose uptake, and decreased cytoprotection. Consequently, based on international consensus prophylactic administration of steroids following TBI is obsolete.

To date, it is unclear if these constraints are also valid for hydrocortison, which is administered in a significantly lower dose to treat septic hypotension and adrenal insufficiency requiring increased administration of vasopressors and volume.

According to recent publications 20–50% of patients with severe TBI show signs of adrenal insufficiency of various degrees [175, 176] which require transient corrective administration of steroids. Apart from the primary brain damage secondary damage as well as pharmacologic side effects of different anesthetic and sedative agents (e.g., etomidate) are discussed as potential triggers [177]. Pituitary and hypothalamic disturbances with subsequent insufficient release of adreno-corticotropic hormone (ACTH) or corticotropin-releasing hormone (CRH) result in insufficient stimulation of adrenal steroid synthesis. Clinically, cortisol deficiency presents with spontaneous hypoglycemia and arterial hypotension with increased catecholamine and volume requirement. In the adrenal cortex the mineralocorticoid aldosteron is also produced which is subject to a different regulatory hormonal circuit (renin–angiotensin–aldosteron system) and which can contribute to hypovolemia, hyponatremia, and hyperkalemia resulting from impaired synthesis.

Depending on the clinical situation these endocrinologic disturbances can be corrected by supporting systemic measures and specific administration of glucocorticoids and mineralocorticoids.

2.5.16.1 Crucial Points and Pearls

- Categorical administration of high-dose steroids following severe TBI is obsolete.
- Administration of low-dose steroids with mineralocorticoid effects can be indicated in patients with clinical signs of adrenal insufficiency (increased catecholamine requirement, hypovolemia, hyponatremia, hyperkalemia, hypoglycemia).

2.5.17 Prophylactic Antiepileptic Therapy

Following severe TBI the threshold for epileptic discharges is significantly decreased by the underlying structural and functional injuries which can trigger seizures at the time of injury, during the first week, and at later time points. In this context, free oxygen radicals which stem from the iron-containing hemoglobin found in hemorrhages are pathophysiologically important mediators that disturb glutamate uptake and different glutamate transporters [178]. This, in turn, aggravates glutamate-mediated excitotoxicity. Analog to animal experiments posttraumatic loss of hippocampal neurons has also been reported in humans and is thought to cause epileptic discharges [179]. In addition, a genetic predisposition in patients expressing the apolipoprotein ε4 allele is discussed [180]. Frequency of posttraumatic seizures is approximately 20–25%. Early after TBI, i.e., within the first 7 posttraumatic days, clinical as well as electrophysiologic signs of epileptic discharges are present [181]. In this context, nonconvulsive discharges and a nonconvulsive status epilepticus must be actively searched [182]. Seizures observed during the early phase appear to be triggered by acute intracerebral and intracranial hemorrhages, especially subdural hematoma, severe injuries, and chronic alcohol intake. Significant risk factors for seizures after the first posttraumatic week are seizures during the first week, intracranial hemorrhages, bitemporal contusions and multiple contusions, age > 65 years, midline shift > 5 mm, open TBI with bone displacement, impaired temporal perfusion, and hydrocephalus [183–185]. Late seizures have also been observed in patients with an initial Glasgow Coma Scale (GCS) 13–15, with the majority of patients exhibiting a GCS < 12 [184]. Long-term seizure activity results from hippocampal sclerosis, excessive neuronal excitation within the dentate gyrus, and uncoordinated neuronal reorganization [186]. These morphological and functional alterations can result in therapy-refractory epilepsia and may even require surgical hippocampectomy [187]. Luckily, these structural and functional changes are not associated with cognitive deficits [185].

As a prophylaxis of possible epileptic discharges, official guidelines suggest administration of phenytoin for the first week which, however, did not prevent the development of seizures at later time points [188]. Whether administration of phenytoin will actually prevent early discharges during the first week is discussed controversially. According to Vespa and colleagues convulsive as well as nonconvulsive discharges could not be prevented by the early administration of phenytoin [182]. Thus, other reasons appear to be important. In this context, type and depth of sedation appears essential. It is conceivable that insufficient analgesia and sedation can promote seizure activity related to alcohol- and drug-related withdrawal after TBI.

Apart from phenytoin other drugs were evaluated, e.g., valproic acid, carbamazepine, barbiturates, levetiracetam [189], which, however, were not superior to phenytoin. In fact, levetiracetam was even associated with an increase in epileptic discharges observed in EEG analysis [190].

Overall, categorical administration of phenytoin with its also serious side effects and narrow therapeutic range must be viewed critically. In this context, phenytoin by itself can induce neuropsychologic impairment and can even induce arterial hypotension and cardiac arrest upon intravenous injection. Co-administration of various antibiotics can inhibit the cytochrome P450 system (CYP 3A4), thereby increasing phenytoin plasma levels, which, in turn, aggravates intended action but also its side effects.

Epileptic discharges must be actively searched for in sedated patients using EEG analysis. Ideal continuous EEG recording, however, requires extensive technical and personal support. Upon identification of typical epileptic discharges administration of antiepileptic drugs is justified. In awake and neuropsychologically adequate patients clinical observation without prophylaxis is possible and acceptable. To date, it remains unclear if these patients really profit from antiepileptic prophylaxis.

2.5.17.1 Crucial Points and Pearls

- Categorical and prophylactic administration of antiepileptic drugs is discussed controversially.

- Potentially damaging side effects must be balanced against unclear benefit.
- Available data do not allow to clearly assess different needs in antiepileptic prophylaxis in sedated and awake patients with significant structural damage.
- To date, a general and valid recommendation cannot be given.

2.6 Treatment Steps

To date, escalation of the different treatment modalities was based on absolute ICP values. Retrospectively, ICP was misinterpreted due to insufficient monitoring and ignorance of important and treatable problems in intensive care. In addition, official guidelines were phrased only for a few specialized centers. These guidelines which suggest starting treatment escalation only at an ICP 20 mmHg implicate a widely encountered fallacy that pathologic intracerebral processes do not exist at ICP values <20 mmHg. According to new experimental and clinical data pathologic changes do occur at ICP values <15 mmHg [22]. Furthermore, data are accumulating which clearly show that pathologic changes do occur despite adherence to the official guidelines [191]. This is best explained by the fact that modern intensive care treatment does not exist of categorical and static concepts as implied by the official guidelines. Pathologic changes characterized by their individual dynamic must be searched for actively. For this, adequate monitoring tools must be used and the search for novel diagnostic methods must continue. It is essential to understand that ICP and CPP – as suggested by the official guidelines – are insufficient when interpreted individually and must be complemented by additional monitoring methods. Furthermore, these patients should be treated in specialized centers with specially trained personnel, sufficient experience, and different monitoring techniques. In this context, mortality can be significantly reduced by experienced teams provided these hospitals treat more than 30 patients annually [82].

The following is an attempt to consider the multifacetted and dynamic changes in face of the official guidelines and contemporary knowledge and experience.

2.6.1 Crucial Points and Pearls

- Categorical treatment is not up to date and must be considered dangerous as it is too rigid and excludes flexible adjustments.
- Starting therapeutic interventions at an ICP > 20 mmHg is too late since many pathologic cascades are active at normal ICP levels (<15 mmHg).
- Only centers with sufficient expertise in surgery, anesthesiology, radiology, and intensive care medicine should treat patients with severe TBI.

2.6.2 Controlled Escalation

2.6.2.1 Basic Measures

The extent of the tiered treatment escalation as suggested in the official guidelines strongly depends on the type and extent of the chosen basic measures (Fig. 2.20). These basic measures, in turn, show large variance between different centers and strongly depend on knowledge, vigilance, attitude, and conviction of the treating physicians and nursing staff [192–194].

Basic measures consist of

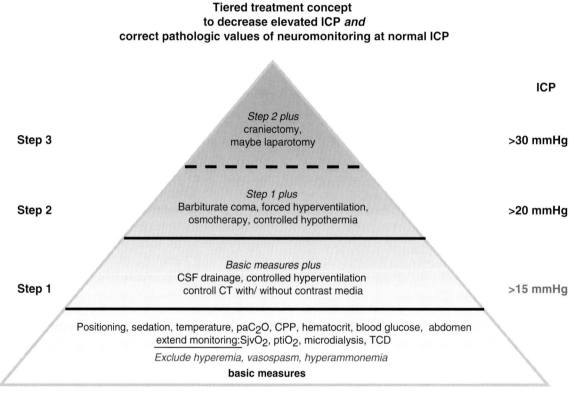

**Tiered treatment concept
to decrease elevated ICP *and*
correct pathologic values of neuromonitoring at normal ICP**

ICP

Step 3 — *Step 2 plus* craniectomy, maybe laparotomy — **>30 mmHg**

Step 2 — *Step 1 plus* Barbiturate coma, forced hyperventilation, osmotherapy, controlled hypothermia — **>20 mmHg**

Step 1 — *Basic measures plus* CSF drainage, controlled hyperventilation controll CT with/ without contrast media — **>15 mmHg**

Positioning, sedation, temperature, paC_2O, CPP, hematocrit, blood glucose, abdomen
extend monitoring:$SjvO_2$, $ptiO_2$, microdialysis, TCD
Exclude hyperemia, vasospasm, hyperammonemia
basic measures

Fig. 2.20 Schematic drawing of tiered treatment consisting of different steps which are strongly influenced by the level of intracranial pressure (ICP). Contrary to the official guidelines which propagate to start escalating treatment at an ICP exceeding 20 mmHg we already search for possibilities to improve therapy as soon as we unmask pathologic alterations ("Stover concept"). These interventions are induced even at an ICP < 15 mmHg, if required, to correct pathologic findings. In this context, we predominantly see pathologically reduced jugular venous oxygen saturation ($SjvO_2$) values in face of elevated bispectral index (BIS) values in the first hours after trauma. This pattern reflects insufficient analgesia and sedation but also prompts the search for impaired perfusion, hypotension, hypoxia, hyperventilation, anemia, fever, and seizure activity. Transient administration of thiopental (200–400 mg/h for 2–6 h) corrects signs of increased cerebral metabolism. Early and specific interventions require adequate monitoring and aggressive vigilance. Integrating the transcranial Doppler to unmask hyperemia or vasospasm guides specific interventions and allows to reduce unnecessary CT scans, especially in case of hyperemia since hyperemia-induced increases in ICP are caused by cerebral vasodilation

- Search for optimal positioning for an improved cerebral venous outflow
- Controlled analgesia and sedation, e.g., BIS EEG 20–40
- Temperature control (35–37°C) and pharmacologic/physical correction of fever
- Volume-controlled ventilation with normoventilation ($paCO_2$ 35–45 mmHg) considering ventilator-induced pulmonary changes (e.g., peak pressure < 35 mbar)
- Sufficient oxygenation, preventing hyperoxygenation (paO_2 > 11–13 kPa)
- Correcting anemia with increasing hematocrit > 28%
- Correcting hypo- and hyperglycemia
- Optimizing CPP through controlled administration of volume and catecholamines (without brain ischemia: 60–70 mmHg, with cerebral ischemia: 70–90 mmHg)
- Active search for hyperemia and vasospasms
- Regular control of blood ammonia levels

The intensive care phase is characterized by different phases in which ICP can remain above 20 mmHg despite maximal exhaustion of all treatment steps. In this context, it is indispensable to consider other important parameters to define the pathologic meaning of the actual ICP value, i.e., an ICP of 20 mmHg is acceptable as long as all other parameters reveal normal values. As long as these parameters, e.g., CPP, $ptiO_2$, $SjvO_2$, microdialysis, TCD, do not reveal any deterioration, controlled de-escalation within and between the different steps can be attempted.

2.6.2.2 Step 1

Whenever ICP > 20 mmHg (actual guidelines) (>15 mmHg at the University Hospital Zürich) a CT is performed to exclude a surgically removable hemorrhage (1) if the reason for this increase in ICP is not obvious at the bedside, and (2) if basic measures (Table 2.10, Fig. 2.20) fail to reduce elevated ICP within 20 min to < 20 mmHg (or <15 mmHg). In this context, it is important to be generous with CT scans since the majority of rebleeding and progression of hemorrhages occur early after TBI. At later time points, especially at the transition of the first to the second week of progression in brain edema, signs of vascular dysfunction (disturbed autoregulation, hyperemia) predominate. In the presence of functional pathologic alterations which cannot be corrected by optimized treatment options a CT should also be performed at normal ICP values since patients with skull base fractures and resulting uncontrolled CSF leakage as well as patients previously craniectomized and those with inadequately inserted ICP probes and infratentorial pathologies are at an increased risk of missing otherwise elevated and pathologic ICP values. Extended neuromonitoring is indicated to define pathogenicity of the actual ICP and to guide subsequent interventions.

In case an EVD is used CSF drainage can be tried to decrease elevated ICP. Controlled hyperventilation ($paCO_2$ 35–45 mmHg) and osmotherapy can also be tried. Depending on the temperature moderate hypothermia (35°C) can be aimed for.

2.6.2.3 Step 2

With progressively increasing ICP > 25 mmHg or proven pathogenicity of any actual ICP even at lower ICP values (≤20 mmHg) controlled hyperventilation ($paCO_2$ >25 and <35 mmHg), barbiturate coma, and increased hypothermia (33–34°C) may be indicated.

2.6.2.4 Step 3

In case of therapy-refractory elevations in ICP (>30 mmHg) uni- or bilateral craniectomy and even laparotomy might be required. In this context, the transition between steps 2 and 3 is fluent.

2.6.2.5 Crucial Points and Pearls

- To guide type and extent of therapeutic interventions monitoring is indispensable.
- Treatment must not be based on ICP or CPP alone.
- A holistic, i.e., brain-oriented, therapy is superior to a brain-centered therapy to avoid inducing organ damage and not to confound anticipated neuroprotection by the induced organ damage.
- Therapeutic interventions should be based on tiered procedures; these tiered procedures, in turn, strongly depend on knowledge, vigilance, attitude, and conviction of the involved team members.
- Without specific knowledge of local and systemic secondary insults senseful therapy of patients with severe TBI is not possible.

Table 2.10 Possible reasons for elevated intracranial pressure (ICP) and potential therapeutic measures

Reasons for increase in ICP	Diagnostics	Possible therapy
Local		
Space occupying lesion: hemorrhage, edema	CT	Surgery: evacuation, craniectomy Pharmacology: barbiturate coma, osmotherapy, hypothermia
Vasodilation, hyperemia	TCD, ptiO$_2$, SjvO$_2$, hematocrit	Controlled hyperventilation, controlled reduction of CPP < 70 mmHg, transfusion
Vasospasm	TCD, imaging (e.g., CT with contrast agent), microdialysis, ptiO$_2$, SjvO$_2$	Controlled hypoventilation, controlled increase of CPP to 110 mmHg
Disturbed autoregulation	ICP curve analysis, PC-guided analysis	Controlled adaption of CPP, slow rewarming
Ischemia	TCD, microdialysis, ptiO$_2$, SjvO$_2$	Controlled hypoventilation, controlled increase of CPP
Insufficient analgesia/sedation	Clinical picture (straining, coughing, hypertension), BIS EEG, SjvO$_2$, ptiO$_2$, microdialysis	Increase dose of analgetics/sedatives, switch to or add more potent drugs
Epileptic discharges	Clinical picture (convulsions), EEG (active search for status epilepticus nonconvulsive), microdialysis, ptiO$_2$, SjvO$_2$	Antiepileptic drugs
Cortical spreading depression	Special electrodes	Increase blood glucose levels (> 5 <10 mM), barbiturate coma, hypothermia
Sinus thrombosis	CT with contrast agent	High dose heparin, barbiturate coma and hypothermia with hemispheric edema
Systemic		
Arterial hypotension	Temperature, blood pressure amplitude, hematocrit/coagulation including factor XIII), electrolytes, sonography/CT Abdomen; Picco® catheter, pulmonary artery catheter Exclusion: Infection/sepsis Adrenal insufficiency	Reduce fever or slow down rewarming, administer volume, correct possible bleeding, treat infection/sepsis, consider glucocorticoids/mineralocorticoids
Intraabdominal hypertension, paralytic ileus, abdominal compartment syndrome	Clinical picture (abdominal pressure, peristaltic sounds, pulmonary function, pulmonary pressure, diuresis), bladder pressure	Aggressive mechanical and pharmacological stimulation, consider laparotomy Change enteral nutrition solution Reduce volume administration
Arterial hypertension	Withdrawal symptom with tachycardia, mydriasis, sweating, diarrhea; Herniation sign with bradycardia Excessive volume infusion	Increase analgesia/sedation Decrease arterial blood pressure; avoid nitrates due to cerebral vasodilation Withdrawal: clonidine plus propofol Administer diuretic ± albumin
Positioning	Clinical picture, change vertical and lateral position	Adapt vertical and lateral position
Hyperammonemia	Analyze blood ammonia level	Change nutrition, reduce protein load, stop antiepileptic drugs, start specific therapy/dialysis

2.6.3 Controlled De-escalation

While escalation of different therapeutic interventions was investigated and is considered in guidelines we are lacking detailed information regarding de-escalation cedures (100). In general, we can advise that de-escalation should be performed slowly and should also be subject to adequate control to avoid any overshooting and thus damaging reactions resulting from an abrupt stop of different interventions. In this context, abruptly stopping analgetics and sedatives will provoke withdrawal symptoms consisting of uncontrolled vegetative alterations, i.e., hyperventilation and hypertension, which, in turn, can induce secondary brain damage. This must be avoided implicitly. In addition, strong variations in blood pressure, CPP, blood glucose, and sodium must be avoided.

Apart from controlling escalation multimodal neuromonitoring allows guiding a controlled de-escalation. In this context, limits of paO_2 and $paCO_2$, CPP, hematocrit, and blood glucose can be corrected dynamically to lower values, thereby reducing the extent of therapeutic interventions. Thus, these new limits are adapted to the actual situation with individual needs. In this context, continuously measured $ptiO_2$ allows to reduce paO_2, decrease $paCO_2$, and adapt CPP to low levels and also reduce hematocrit to, for example, 24% (Fig. 2.21). This, in turn, allows reducing the extent and aggressiveness of therapeutic interventions, thereby diminishing the risk of organ-damaging potential of a too aggressive ventilatory support and a too aggressive volume administration. In addition, transfusion requirement can be attenuated with a good conscience.

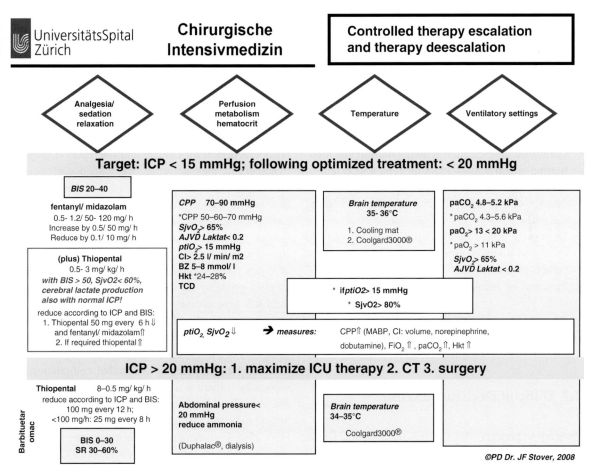

Fig. 2.21 Example of the tiered treatment paradigm involving different therapeutic interventions practiced at the University Hospital Zürich for a controlled escalation and controlled de-escalation ("Stover concept"). Depending on the clinical situation and the nature of the diagnosed pathological findings, therapeutic interventions are adapted dynamically. For this, more than one intervention combined with escalation and de-escalation of different interventions might be required simultaneously

The wake-up period should also be controlled. Here it is essential to base all decisions on the presence of brain edema as seen in control CT scans. As long as signs of hemispheric edema are present analgesia and sedation should not be stopped. However, complete resolution of hemispheric edema does not guarantee a smooth wake-up phase. Even local brain edema can promote an increase in ICP in conjunction with disturbed cerebral autoregulation, which precludes reducing analgesia/sedation. Whenever signs of functional deterioration such as decreased $SjvO_2$ levels develop wake-up should be halted and even a new controlled escalation might become necessary to avoid secondary insults and induction of secondary brain damage. This, in turn, requires adequate monitoring during the vulnerable wake-up phase.

2.6.3.1 Crucial Points and Pearls

- Apart from controlling escalation of different therapeutic interventions, controlled de-escalation is also of imminent importance to avoid missing and actively inducing secondary insults and secondary brain damage.
- Controlled de-escalation requires multimodal monitoring, which allows adapting type and extent of different therapeutic interventions to prevent organ damage of a possibly excessive and overshooting treatment.
- During controlled de-escalation a new controlled escalation might become necessary to correct new pathologic alterations.
- Presence of hemispheric edema forbids wake-up trial.
- Absent signs of hemispheric edema does not guarantee unproblematic wake-up.

2.7 Difficult Decision Making

Contrary to patients with obvious pathologic CT scan and severe obvious neurologic deficits (GCS < 9) patients with an initially unremarkable CT scan with severe neurologic defects and those with a pathologic CT but only marginal or even absent neurologic deterioration (GCS > 13) are very difficult to predict in terms of subsequent deterioration, preemptive neuroprotection

including intubation, controlled ventilation and oxygenation, optimized CPP, analgesia/sedation, and control of ICP and $SjvO_2$. Without signs structural damage in the initial CT neurologic impairment observed at the site of injury can disappear completely or reflect the clinical equivalent of diffuse axonal injury which cannot be determined in the initial CT scan. Neglectful decision making would retrospectively prove wrong if diffuse axonal injury were diagnosed in the control CT scan or MRI. Neglectful decision making, in turn, would imply allowing secondary insults to occur. Patients with clearly pathologic CT findings and stable GCS > 13 would be treated falsely until the secondary neurologic deterioration reflects progression of the structural damage. Again, false decision making will only become obvious retrospectively. Whether this justifies preemptive intubation and positioning of an ICP probe will spur controversial discussions.

2.7.1 Initial GCS

The initial GCS tempts us to inadequately judge intracranial pathology if patients are evaluated too early, they are not recovered for a longer undefined period, they are hypothermic, they are under the influence of alcohol and drugs, they are multiply injured, or if they cannot be assessed adequately due to severe aggressive behavior. Indicated intubation with subsequent sedation renders a further senseful evaluation impossible. Furthermore, stress factor for those who determine the GCS at the site of injury must also be considered. A further misjudgment is given by the imbalance of the three parts of the GCS (eye opening, verbal communication, motor response). A low/bad GCS which is mainly influenced by the motor response must be weighted differently compared to a low GCS which is dictated by the results obtained for eye opening and verbal communication, especially if there is a language barrier or the patients are aphasic. Approximately 20% of all patients are judged to be too severely injured according to the GCS [195, 196]. Furthermore, clinical experience shows that the initial GCS is not a reliable prognostic factor. While mortality is significantly increased at GCS < 8 compared to a GCS > 13, an initial GCS > 13 does not guarantee survival in these patients. Up to 10% of patients with severe TBI succumb due to rapidly progressing intracranial pathologic alterations, which are also influenced by age and further complications such as coagulopathy and severe infections with multiple organ failure. Early signs of beginning herniation are not equal to definite mortality [197].

At a GCS < 8 all therapeutic options should be considered and a definite decision should not be made since not all patients will die and a reluctant attitude might induce preventable secondary insults and thus convey secondary brain damage. At a GCS > 13 we are not allowed to grow negligent as this attitude might also allow many otherwise preventable secondary insults.

2.7.2 First CT Scan Following Severe Trauma and GCS

Depending on the duration between the accident and initial CT scan the resulting time span might be too short to clearly identify intracranial injuries. Hemorrhages, contusions, and edema require time to develop. Usually these lesions will reach their maximal extent during the first 24 h [198]. Unfortunately, in many patients neurologic evaluation insufficiently reflects evolving damage. Any form of neurological deterioration implies an immediate CT scan. Newly diagnosed lesions will then force new decisions. In this context, it is important to realize that GCS shows a strong variability depending on the underlying intracranial compliance which is strongly influenced by age and the corresponding degree of cerebral atrophy. GCS > 13 is not equivalent to small or absent lesions. GCS< 13 does not necessarily imply large lesions with midline shift, as diffuse axonal injuries might be present.

A patient with an initially low GCS > 9 who recover to a GCS of 11–13 must be evaluated neurologically every hour in the emergency room, ICU, and intermediate care, depending on the present infrastructure. When in doubt, repetitive CT scans are required, especially if the patient is under the influence of drugs and alcohol. Whenever, signs of progression and deterioration become evident the patient should be transferred to a specialized center.

Whenever patients remain neurologically stable for at least 24 h (initial GCS > 13) or even improve they can be transferred to a normal ward following control CT scan. With signs of midline shift and progressive brain edema patients should remain in the ICU for a further 24–48 h, even in case of GCS > 13.

Patients with pathologic CT findings and undulating vigilance (GCS 11–13) and even a GCS > 13 must be examined at short intervals and subjected to repetitive CT scans. It is important to actively search for vegetative changes such as tachypnea, hyperventilation, hypertension, and hypotension. Thus, these patients must be controlled on an ICU and require an arterial line to continuously measure mean arterial blood pressure (MABP) and control $paCO_2$. Only then can we unmask and prevent secondary insults. To prevent hyperventilation-induced cerebral vasoconstriction patients with a GCS > 11 might even require preemptive intubation and insertion of an ICP probe. To date, it remains unclear if these patients (GCS > 9) would profit from preemptive intubation and controlled escalation for at least the first 24 h, which is regarded as the most vulnerable phase. Surely, some patients would be intubated in vain and would remain sedated for at least 24 h until the first control CT scan. This could be justified as our main emphasis is to prevent secondary brain damage to increase the regeneration potential of these patients.

In patients who present with an initially unremarkable CT scan following a high-velocity accident or fall (>2 m height) and who must be intubated for surgical stabilization of fractures and additional injuries resulting in impaired neurologic evaluation, a control CT scan should be performed within 6 h. This is indispensable whenever patients develop intraoperative complications including arterial hypotension and coagulopathy. This reduces the risk of missing relevant lesions which develop during the first hours and allows appropriate interventions including insertion of an ICP probe.

2.7.3 Time Point for Surgery

While surgical care of serious and potentially lethal thoracoabdominal and hemorrhagic injuries are treated according to the principle "treat first what kills first," the situation with severe but not immediately life-threatening injuries is less clear and more difficult to evaluate. This mainly pertains to the surgical stabilization of pelvic and long bone fractures in the early phase. Early surgery of these fractures can result in a severe coagulopathy with hemorrhages and arterial hypotension which, in turn, induce autodestructive and difficult-to-manage, and even lethal cascades. It is important to follow the "damage control" principle with initial external fixation since imaging cannot unmask the complete extent of injuries [199]. In this context, clinically based sepsis, which requires experience and differentiated knowledge, is of imminent importance. Trauma mechanism and imagination of possible injuries and deteriorations developing within the first 24 h force us not to underestimate any injury [200]. Only then can we reduce the risk of secondary insults and an increase in secondary brain damage (Figs. 2.22 and 2.23).

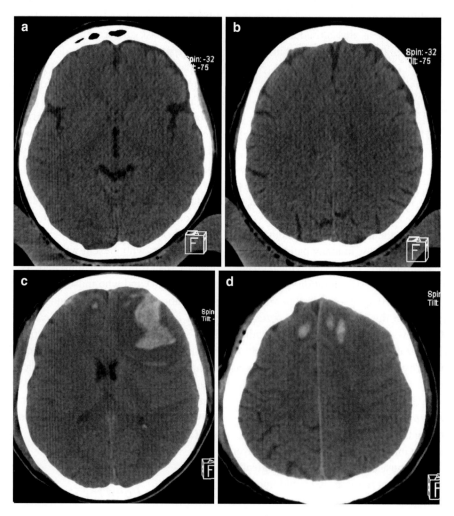

Fig. 2.22 Clinical example of unexpected lesions which determined further clinical course in this patient. Following the crash of a Learjet during landing the patient suffered severe pelvic fractures, and distal fractures to the femur and tibia with a large occipital bleeding scalp lesion. Based on the initial Glasgow Coma Scale (GCS) score of 13 and the unremarkable cerebral computed tomography (CT) which was performed 2 h after trauma (**a, b**) unanimous decision was to operate the long bone fractures in this patient. During surgery the patient developed severe disseminated intravasal coagulopathy inducing anemia and arterial hypotension. Control CT scan performed 12 h after trauma (**c, d**) revealed large bifrontal space-occupying contusions, and contre-coup lesions to the severe bleeding occipital scalp lesion. In addition, left hemispheric edema developed (elapsed sulci and gyri) (**d**). Due to the persisting and difficult-to-correct coagulopathy and abdominal complications the patient succumbed 7 days after trauma. This case impressively and convincingly shows that following high-velocity injuries severe intracranial lesions must be anticipated. In addition, this case clearly demonstrates that CT scans which are performed "too" early cannot reveal cerebral lesions, which in some patients require time to develop. Thus, these patients would be subjected to an increased risk for secondary brain insults. Surgeries with increased risk for hemorrhages and sustained danger of arterial hypotension and coagulopathy should be postponed until after the control CT scan at 24 h, provided these surgeries are not life-saving

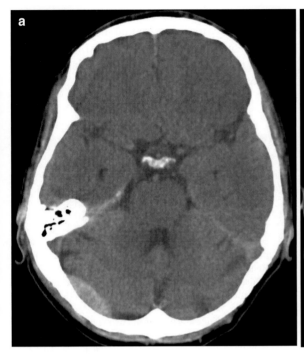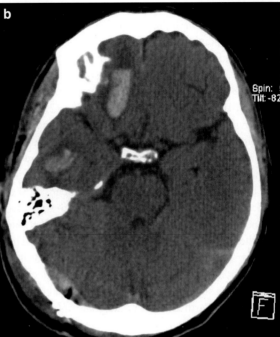

Fig. 2.23 Clinical example of unexpected contre-coup contusions following an initial isolated occipital infra- and supratentorial epidural hematoma (**a** and **b**). Following removal of the epidural hematoma the patient was extubated and constantly had a GCS score of 15. In the CT scan routinely performed 24 h after trauma, frontal and temporal contusions were found (**b**). The epidural hematoma had continued bleeding without clinical relevance

2.7.3.1 Reconstruction of Midfacial Fractures

To optimize conditions for surgical repair of extensive midfacial fractures with and without skull base surgery MABP is reduced intraoperatively pharmacologically using clonidine and nitroglycerin to 60 mmHg with the aim of reducing hemorrhage in the surgically exposed area. Reducing MABP to such low values in combination with nitroglycerine-induced cerebral vasodilation can increase the risk for cerebral secondary brain damage with brain edema formation or aggravation of underlying brain edema. This risk persists for several weeks following severe TBI. It also appears that elevated vulnerability of the injured brain is still present weeks after TBI even after brain edema has resolved.

2.7.4 Influence of Different Factors on Morbidity and Mortality

To identify relevant factors determining subsequent development following severe TBI many clinical and demographic analyses as well as assessment of changes in various parameters in blood and CSF including the individual genetic profile have been considered. These results were then evaluated in the context of mortality and morbidity. Taken together, the following factors were identified to significantly influence mortality and morbidity: age [201], female sex [202], initial GCS and pupil abnormalities [203], type and extent of intracranial damage including brain stem lesion and midline shift [204], presence of secondary insults [205], preexisting alcohol and drug addiction [206, 207], presence of pathologic lab values [110], confirmation of a specific genetic APO-E profile [208], elevated NSE [209], S-100 [210], GFAP [211], IL-10 [212], and troponin values [213].

The inherent problem of these determinant factors is the statistical analysis which allows a certain misinterpretation due to the used probability value ($p < 0.0?$). A $p < 0.05$ corresponds to a probability of 5% of the investigated collective in which an identified parameter is not correctly allocated. This, in turn, means that at a $p < 0.05$ 5 of 100 (i.e., every 20th patient) are misinterpreted. These patients, however, cannot be identified properly. Consequently, none of these factors guarantee an absolute secure and valid predictability. Thus, a generalization in patients without clear signs of brain death is impermissible and results in chaining of incorrect decisions, especially since all identified factors were assessed under the influence of ongoing surgical, anesthesiological, and intensive care interventions with possible complications [214] including inadequate nutrition [215] without having questioned these "basic" influences and without controlling for these influences. The identified factors imply that all therapeutic interventions are correct and that no secondary insults occurred.

These identified influencing factors can only be used to investigate whether adequate and aggressive diagnosis and therapy must be established early to support the regenerative potential in these patients. This, however, requires an adequate professional attitude and conviction as well as the ability to make decisions based on the sum of different parameters and complex interactions. Furthermore, an adequate infrastructure is indispensable to allow maintaining prolonged pharmacologic coma depending on the duration of persisting brain edema.

2.7.4.1 Crucial Points and Pearls

- The initial GCS is insufficient in predicting type and extent of intracranial damage and cannot forecast further development. At a GCS < 8 we are not allowed to give up and at a GCS > 13 we are not allowed to grow neglectful.
- The initial CT does not reveal the full extent of the lesions. According to the clinical picture, an early control CT scan must be performed, especially in intubated patients and those in whom intraoperative complications such as arterial hypotension, hemorrhage, and coagulopathy occurred.
- The initial stabilization of additional injuries must consider the existing leading injuries and possible complications such as hemorrhage and coagulopathy to avoid unnecessary endangerment of these patients. When in doubt, fractures should primarily be stabilized with external fixation and definite stabilization should be performed after control CT scan has excluded or at least unmasked brain lesions. Then, secondary brain damage can be prevented.
- Surgical reconstruction of complex facial fractures should not be performed as long as brain edema persists.

- Prognostic relevance of different factors for the individual patient appears to be of subordinate importance and should not be used to limit treatment prematurely but should rather promote search for optimized treatment.

References

1. Lai Y, Chen Y, Watkins SC, Nathaniel PD, Guo F, Kochanek PM, Jenkins LW, Szabó C, Clark RS (2008) Identification of poly-ADP-ribosylated mitochondrial proteins after traumatic brain injury. J Neurochem 104(6):1700–1711
2. Diaz-Arrastia R, Baxter VK (2006) Genetic factors in outcome after traumatic brain injury: what the human genome project can teach us about brain trauma. J Head Trauma Rehabil 21(4):361–374
3. Jordan BD (2007) Genetic influences on outcome following traumatic brain injury. Neurochem Res 32(4–5):905–915
4. Bayir H, Kagan VE (2008) Bench-to-bedside review: Mitochondrial injury, oxidative stress and apoptosis–there is nothing more practical than a good theory. Crit Care 12(1):206
5. Murray GD, Butcher I, McHugh GS, Lu J, Mushkudiani NA, Maas AI, Marmarou A, Steyerberg EW (2007) Multivariable prognostic analysis in traumatic brain injury: results from the IMPACT study. J Neurotrauma 24(2):329–337
6. Stocchetti N, Maas AI, Chieregato A, van der Plas AA (2005) Hyperventilation in head injury: A review. Chest 127(5):1812–1827
7. Cremer OL, Kalkman CJ (2007) Cerebral pathophysiology and clinical neurology of hyperthermia in humans. Prog Brain Res 162:153–169
8. Salim A, Hadjizacharia P, DuBose J, Brown C, Inaba K, Chan L, Margulies DR (2008) Role of anemia in traumatic brain injury. J Am Coll Surg 207(3):398–406
9. Harhangi BS, Kompanje EJ, Leebeek FW, Maas AI (2008) Coagulation disorders after traumatic brain injury. Acta Neurochir (Wien) 150(2):165–175
10. Nekludov M, Bellander BM, Blombäck M, Wallen HN (2007) Platelet dysfunction in patients with severe traumatic brain injury. J Neurotrauma 24(11):1699–1706
11. Sperry JL, Frankel HL, Vanek SL, Nathens AB, Moore EE, Maier RV, Minei JP (2007) Early hyperglycemia predicts multiple organ failure and mortality but not infection. J Trauma 63(3):487–493
12. Strong AJ, Smith SE, Whittington DJ, Meldrum BS, Parsons AA, Krupinski J, Hunter AJ, Patel S, Robertson C (2000) Factors influencing the frequency of fluorescence transients as markers of peri-infarct depolarizations in focal cerebral ischemia. Stroke 31(1):214–222
13. Powner DJ, Boccalandro C, Alp MS, Vollmer DG (2006) Endocrine failure after traumatic brain injury in adults. Neurocrit Care 5(1):61–70
14. Vinclair M, Broux C, Faure P, Brun J, Genty C, Jacquot C, Chabre O, Payen JF (2008) Duration of adrenal inhibition

following a single dose of etomidate in critically ill patients. Intensive Care Med 34(4):714–719

15. Cohan P, Wang C, McArthur DL, Cook SW, Dusick JR, Armin B, Swerdloff R, Vespa P, Muizelaar JP, Cryer HG, Christenson PD, Kelly DF (2005) Acute secondary adrenal insufficiency after traumatic brain injury: A prospective study. Crit Care Med 33(10):2358–2366

16. Boyer A, Chadda K, Salah A, Annane D (2006) Glucocorticoid treatment in patients with septic shock: Effects on vasopressor use and mortality. Int J Clin Pharmacol Ther 44(7):309–318

17. Tyagi R, Donaldson K, Loftus CM, Jallo J (2007) Hypertonic saline: A clinical review. Neurosurg Rev 30(4): 277–289

18. Lichter-Konecki U (2008) Profiling of astrocyte properties in the hyperammonaemic brain: Shedding new light on the pathophysiology of the brain damage in hyperammonaemia. J Inherit Metab Dis 31(4):492–502

19. Clay AS, Hainline BE (2007) Hyperammonemia in the ICU. Chest 132(4):1368–1378

20. Smith M (2008) Monitoring intracranial pressure in traumatic brain injury. Anesth Analg 106(1):240–248

21. Scalea TM, Bochicchio GV, Habashi N, McCunn M, Shih D, McQuillan K, Aarabi B (2007) Increased intra-abdominal, intrathoracic, and intracranial pressure after severe brain injury: Multiple compartment syndrome. J Trauma 62(3):647–656

22. Belli A, Sen J, Petzold A, Russo S, Kitchen N, Smith M (2008) Metabolic failure precedes intracranial pressure rises in traumatic brain injury: A microdialysis study. Acta Neurochir (Wien) 150(5):461–469

23. Marmarou A, Anderson RL, Ward JD et al (1991) Impact of instability and hypotension in outcome in patients with severe head trauma. J Neurosurg 75:S59–S66

24. Saul TG, Ducker TB (1982) Effect of intracranial pressure monitoring and aggressive treatment on mortality in severe head injury. J Neurosurg 56(4):498–503

25. Sahuquillo J, Poca MA, Arribas M, Garnacho A, Rubio E (1999) Interhemispheric supratentorial intracranial pressure gradients in head-injured patients: are they clinically important? J Neurosurg 90(1):16–26

26. Kiening KL, Schoening WN, Stover JF, Unterberg AW (2003) Continuous monitoring of intracranial compliance after severe head injury: relation to data quality, intracranial pressure and brain tissue PO_2. Br J Neurosurg 17(4):311–318

27. Zweifel C, Lavinio A, Steiner LA, Radolovich D, Smielewski P, Timofeev I, Hiler M, Balestreri M, Kirkpatrick PJ, Pickard JD, Hutchinson P, Czosnyka M (2008) Continuous monitoring of cerebrovascular pressure reactivity in patients with head injury. Neurosurg Focus 25(4):E2

28. Metz C, Holzschuh M, Bein T, Woertgen C, Rothoerl R, Kallenbach B, Taeger K, Brawanski A (1998) Monitoring of cerebral oxygen metabolism in the jugular bulb: reliability of unilateral measurements in severe head injury. J Cereb Blood Flow Metab 18(3):332–343

29. Møller K, Paulson OB, Hornbein TF, Colier WN, Paulson AS, Roach RC, Holm S, Knudsen GM (2002) Unchanged cerebral blood flow and oxidative metabolism after acclimatization to high altitude. J Cereb Blood Flow Metab 22(1):118–126

30. Holbein M, Béchir M, Ludwig S, Sommerfeld J, Cottini SR, Keel M, Stocker R, Stover JF (2009) Differential influence of arterial blood glucose on cerebral metabolism following severe traumatic brain injury. Crit Care 13(1):R13

31. Kiening KL, Unterberg AW, Bardt TF, Schneider GH, Lanksch WR (1996) Monitoring of cerebral oxygenation in patients with severe head injuries: Brain tissue PO_2 versus jugular vein oxygen saturation. J Neurosurg 85(5): 751–757

32. Vigué B, Ract C, Benayed M, Zlotine N, Leblanc PE, Samii K, Bissonnette B (1999) Early SjvO$_2$ monitoring in patients with severe brain trauma. Intensive Care Med 25(5): 445–451

33. Chan MT, Ng SC, Lam JM, Poon WS, Gin T (2005) Re-defining the ischemic threshold for jugular venous oxygen saturation—a microdialysis study in patients with severe head injury. Acta Neurochir Suppl 95:63–66

34. Gopinath SP, Robertson CS, Contant CF, Hayes C, Feldman Z, Narayan RK, Grossman RG (1994) Jugular venous desaturation and outcome after head injury. J Neurol Neurosurg Psychiatry 57(6):717–723

35. Poca MA, Sahuquillo J, Vilalta A, Garnacho A (2007) Lack of utility of arteriojugular venous differences of lactate as a reliable indicator of increased brain anaerobic metabolism in traumatic brain injury. J Neurosurg 106(4):530–537

36. Pérez A, Minces PG, Schnitzler EJ, Agosta GE, Medina SA, Ciraolo CA (2003) Jugular venous oxygen saturation or arteriovenous difference of lactate content and outcome in children with severe traumatic brain injury. Pediatr Crit Care Med 4(1):33–38

37. Glenn TC, Kelly DF, Boscardin WJ, McArthur DL, Vespa P, Oertel M, Hovda DA, Bergsneider M, Hillered L, Martin NA (2003) Energy dysfunction as a predictor of outcome after moderate or severe head injury: indices of oxygen, glucose, and lactate metabolism. J Cereb Blood Flow Metab 23(10):1239–1250

38. Pellerin L, Bouzier-Sore AK, Aubert A, Serres S, Merle M, Costalat R, Magistretti PJ (2007) Activity-dependent regulation of energy metabolism by astrocytes: an update. Glia 55(12):1251–1262

39. Miñambres E, Cemborain A, Sánchez-Velasco P, Gandarillas M, Díaz-Regañón G, Sánchez-González U, Leyva-Cobián F (2003) Correlation between transcranial interleukin-6 gradient and outcome in patients with acute brain injury. Crit Care Med 31(3):933–938

40. Tisdall MM, Smith M (2006) Cerebral microdialysis: Research technique or clinical tool. Br J Anaesth 97(1): 18–25

41. Brody DL, Magnoni S, Schwetye KE, Spinner ML, Esparza TJ, Stocchetti N, Zipfel GJ, Holtzman DM (2008) Amyloid-beta dynamics correlate with neurological status in the injured human brain. Science 321(5893):1221–1224

42. Hutchinson PJ, O'Connell MT, Nortje J, Smith P, Al-Rawi PG, Gupta AK, Menon DK, Pickard JD (2005) Cerebral microdialysis methodology – evaluation of 20 kDa and 100 kDa catheters. Physiol Meas 26(4):423–428

43. Engström M, Polito A, Reinstrup P, Romner B, Ryding E, Ungerstedt U, Nordström CH (2005) Intracerebral microdialysis in severe brain trauma: The importance of catheter location. J Neurosurg 102(3):460–469

44. Reinert M, Barth A, Rothen HU, Schaller B, Takala J, Seiler RW (2003) Effects of cerebral perfusion pressure

and increased fraction of inspired oxygen on brain tissue oxygen, lactate and glucose in patients with severe head injury. Acta Neurochir (Wien) 145(5):341–349

45. Nordström CH, Reinstrup P, Xu W, Gärdenfors A, Ungerstedt U (2003) Assessment of the lower limit for cerebral perfusion pressure in severe head injuries by bedside monitoring of regional energy metabolism. Anesthesiology 98(4):809–814

46. Marcoux J, McArthur DA, Miller C, Glenn TC, Villablanca P, Martin NA, Hovda DA, Alger JR, Vespa PM (2008) Persistent metabolic crisis as measured by elevated cerebral microdialysis lactate-pyruvate ratio predicts chronic frontal lobe brain atrophy after traumatic brain injury. Crit Care Med 36(10):2871–2877

47. Hutchinson PJ, O'Connell MT, Seal A, Nortje J, Timofeev I, Al-Rawi PG, Coles JP, Fryer TD, Menon DK, Pickard JD, Carpenter KL (2009) A combined microdialysis and FDG-PET study of glucose metabolism in head injury. Acta Neurochir (Wien) 151(1):51–61

48. Bhatia A, Gupta AK (2007) Neuromonitoring in the intensive care unit. II. Cerebral oxygenation monitoring and microdialysis. Intensive Care Med 33(8):1322–1328

49. Sarrafzadeh AS, Sakowitz OW, Callsen TA, Lanksch WR, Unterberg AW (2000) Bedside microdialysis for early detection of cerebral hypoxia in traumatic brain injury. Neurosurg Focus 9(5):e2

50. Meixensberger J, Kunze E, Barcsay E, Vaeth A, Roosen K (2001) Clinical cerebral microdialysis: brain metabolism and brain tissue oxygenation after acute brain injury. Neurol Res 23(8):801–806

51. Meixensberger J, Renner C, Simanowski R, Schmidtke A, Dings J, Roosen K (2004) Influence of cerebral oxygenation following severe head injury on neuropsychological testing. Neurol Res 26(4):414–417

52. Jaeger M, Soehle M, Schuhmann MU, Winkler D, Meixensberger J (2005) Correlation of continuously monitored regional cerebral blood flow and brain tissue oxygen. Acta Neurochir (Wien) 147(1):51–56

53. Jaeger M, Schuhmann MU, Soehle M, Meixensberger J (2006) Continuous assessment of cerebrovascular autoregulation after traumatic brain injury using brain tissue oxygen pressure reactivity. Crit Care Med 34(6):1783–1788

54. Rosenthal G, Hemphill JC 3rd, Sorani M, Martin C, Morabito D, Obrist WD, Manley GT (2008) Brain tissue oxygen tension is more indicative of oxygen diffusion than oxygen delivery and metabolism in patients with traumatic brain injury. Crit Care Med 36(6):1917–1924

55. Smith MJ, Stiefel MF, Magge S, Frangos S, Bloom S, Gracias V, Le Roux PD (2005) Packed red blood cell transfusion increases local cerebral oxygenation. Crit Care Med 33(5):1104–1108

56. Kochanek PM, Berger RP, Bayir H, Wagner AK, Jenkins LW, Clark RS (2008) Biomarkers of primary and evolving damage in traumatic and ischemic brain injury: diagnosis, prognosis, probing mechanisms, and therapeutic decision making. Curr Opin Crit Care 14(2):135–141

57. Morel N, Morel O, Petit L, Hugel B, Cochard JF, Freyssinet JM, Sztark F, Dabadie P (2008) Generation of procoagulant microparticles in cerebrospinal fluid and peripheral blood after traumatic brain injury. J Trauma 64(3):698–704

58. Seifman MA, Adamides AA, Nguyen PN, Vallance SA, Cooper DJ, Kossmann T, Rosenfeld JV, Morganti-Kossmann MC (2008) Endogenous melatonin increases in cerebrospinal fluid of patients after severe traumatic brain injury and correlates with oxidative stress and metabolic disarray. J Cereb Blood Flow Metab 28(4):684–696

59. Ottens AK, Golden EC, Bustamante L, Hayes RL, Denslow ND, Wang KK (2008) Proteolysis of multiple myelin basic protein isoforms after neurotrauma: characterization by mass spectrometry. J Neurochem 104(5):1404–1414

60. Takamiya M, Fujita S, Saigusa K, Aoki Y (2007) Simultaneous detections of 27 cytokines during cerebral wound healing by multiplexed bead-based immunoassay for wound age estimation. J Neurotrauma 24(12):1833–1844

61. Chiaretti A, Antonelli A, Riccardi R, Genovese O, Pezzotti P, Di Rocco C, Tortorolo L, Piedimonte G (2008) Nerve growth factor expression correlates with severity and outcome of traumatic brain injury in children. Eur J Paediatr Neurol 12(3):195–204

62. Maier B, Lehnert M, Laurer HL, Marzi I (2007) Biphasic elevation in cerebrospinal fluid and plasma concentrations of endothelin 1 after traumatic brain injury in human patients. Shock 27(6):610–614

63. Pineda JA, Lewis SB, Valadka AB, Papa L, Hannay HJ, Heaton SC, Demery JA, Liu MC, Aikman JM, Akle V, Brophy GM, Tepas JJ, Wang KK, Robertson CS, Hayes RL (2007) Clinical significance of alpha II-spectrin breakdown products in cerebrospinal fluid after severe traumatic brain injury. J Neurotrauma 24(2):354–366

64. Ost M, Nylén K, Csajbok L, Ohrfelt AO, Tullberg M, Wikkelsö C, Nellgård P, Rosengren L, Blennow K, Nellgård B (2006) Initial CSF total tau correlates with 1-year outcome in patients with traumatic brain injury. Neurology 67(9):1600–1604

65. Stover JF, Pleines UE, Morganti-Kossmann MC, Stocker R, Kempski OS, Kossmann T (1999) Thiopental and midazolam do not seem to impede metabolism of glutamate in brain-injured patients. Psychopharmacology (Berl) 141(1):66–70

66. Stover JF, Pleines UE, Morganti-Kossmann MC, Stocker R, Kossmann T (1999) Thiopental attenuates energetic impairment but fails to normalize cerebrospinal fluid glutamate in brain-injured patients. Crit Care Med 27(7):1351–1357

67. Stover JF, Lenzlinger PM, Stocker R, Morganti-Kossmann MC, Imhof HG, Trentz O, Kossmann T (1998) Thiopental in CSF and serum correlates with prolonged loss of cortical activity. Eur Neurol 39(4):223–228

68. Pleines UE, Stover JF, Kossmann T, Trentz O, Morganti-Kossmann MC (1998) Soluble ICAM-1 in CSF coincides with the extent of cerebral damage in patients with severe traumatic brain injury. J Neurotrauma 15(6):399–409

69. Lozier AP, Sciacca RR, Romagnoli MF, Connolly ES Jr (2008) Ventriculostomy-related infections: a critical review of the literature. Neurosurgery 62(Suppl 2):688–700

70. Carter BG, Butt W (2005) Are somatosensory evoked potentials the best predictor of outcome after severe brain injury? A systematic review. Intensive Care Med 31(6):765–775

71. Roche RA, Dockree PM, Garavan H, Foxe JJ, Robertson IH, O'Mara SM (2004) EEG alpha power changes reflect response inhibition deficits after traumatic brain injury (TBI) in humans. Neurosci Lett 362(1):1–5

72. Hebb MO, McArthur DL, Alger J, Etchepare M, Glenn TC, Bergsneider M, Martin N, Vespa PM (2007) Impaired percent alpha variability on continuous electroencephalography is associated with thalamic injury and predicts poor long-term outcome after human traumatic brain injury. J Neurotrauma 24(4):579–590

73. Leao AAP (1944) Spreading depression of activity in cerebral cortex. J Neurophysiol 7:359–390

74. Dreier JP, Woitzik J, Fabricius M, Bhatia R, Major S, Drenckhahn C, Lehmann TN, Sarrafzadeh A, Willumsen L, Hartings JA, Sakowitz OW, Seemann JH, Thieme A, Lauritzen M, Strong AJ (2006) Delayed ischaemic neurological deficits after subarachnoid haemorrhage are associated with clusters of spreading depolarizations. Brain 129(Pt 12):3224–3237

75. Fabricius M, Fuhr S, Bhatia R, Boutelle M, Hashemi P, Strong AJ, Lauritzen M (2006) Cortical spreading depression and peri-infarct depolarization in acutely injured human cerebral cortex. Brain 129(Pt 3):778–790

76. Strong AJ, Hartings JA, Dreier JP (2007) Cortical spreading depression: an adverse but treatable factor in intensive care? Curr Opin Crit Care 13(2):126–133

77. Parkin M, Hopwood S, Jones DA, Hashemi P, Landolt H, Fabricius M, Lauritzen M, Boutelle MG, Strong AJ (2005) Dynamic changes in brain glucose and lactate in pericontusional areas of the human cerebral cortex, monitored with rapid sampling on-line microdialysis: relationship with depolarisation-like events. J Cereb Blood Flow Metab 25(3):402–413

78. Graham DI, Adams JH, Doyle D (1978) Ischaemic brain damage in fatal non-missile head injuries. J Neurol Sci 39(2–3):213–234

79. Bhatia A, Gupta AK (2007) Neuromonitoring in the intensive care unit. I. Intracranial pressure and cerebral blood flow monitoring. Intensive Care Med 33(7):1263–1271

80. Coles JP (2007) Imaging after brain injury. Br J Anaesth 99(1):49–60

81. White H, Venkatesh B (2006) Applications of transcranial Doppler in the ICU: a review. Intensive Care Med 32(7):981–994

82. Mauritz W, Steltzer H, Bauer P, Dolanski-Aghamanoukjan L, Metnitz P (2008) Monitoring of intracranial pressure in patients with severe traumatic brain injury: an Austrian prospective multicenter study. Intensive Care Med 34(7):1208–1215

83. www.guideline.gov

84. www.leitlinien.net

85. Mirzayan MJ, Probst C, Krettek C, Samii M, Pape HC, van Griensven M, Samii A (2008) Systemic effects of isolated brain injury: an experimental animal study. Neurol Res 30(5):457–460

86. Mascia L, Sakr Y, Pasero D, Payen D, Reinhart K, Vincent JL (2008) Sepsis occurrence in acutely ill patients (SOAP) investigators extracranial complications in patients with acute brain injury: a post-hoc analysis of the SOAP study. Intensive Care Med 34(4):720–727

87. Marik PE, Corwin HL (2008) Acute lung injury following blood transfusion: expanding the definition. Crit Care Med 36(11):3080–3084

88. Lewis CA, Martin GS (2004) Understanding and managing fluid balance in patients with acute lung injury. Curr Opin Crit Care 10(1):13–17

89. Feihl F, Broccard AF (2009) Interactions between respiration and systemic hemodynamics. Part I: basic concepts. Intensive Care Med 35(1):45–54

90. Feihl F, Broccard AF (2009) Interactions between respiration and systemic hemodynamics. Part II: practical implications in critical care. Intensive Care Med 35(2):198–205

91. Nortje J, Coles JP, Timofeev I, Fryer TD, Aigbirhio FI, Smielewski P, Outtrim JG, Chatfield DA, Pickard JD, Hutchinson PJ, Gupta AK, Menon DK (2008) Effect of hyperoxia on regional oxygenation and metabolism after severe traumatic brain injury: preliminary findings. Crit Care Med 36(1):273–281

92. Tisdall MM, Tachtsidis I, Leung TS, Elwell CE, Smith M (2008) Increase in cerebral aerobic metabolism by normobaric hyperoxia after traumatic brain injury. J Neurosurg 109(3):424–432

93. Hedenstierna G, Rothen HU (2000) Atelectasis formation during anesthesia: causes and measures to prevent it. J Clin Monit Comput 16(5–6):329–335

94. Muizelaar JP, Marmarou A, Ward JD, Kontos HA, Choi SC, Becker DP, Gruemer H, Young HF (1991) Adverse effects of prolonged hyperventilation in patients with severe head injury: a randomized clinical trial. J Neurosurg 75(5):731–739

95. Davis DP (2008) Early ventilation in traumatic brain injury. Resuscitation 76(3):333–340

96. Hutchinson PJ, Gupta AK, Fryer TF, Al-Rawi PG, Chatfield DA, Coles JP, O'Connell MT, Kett-White R, Minhas PS, Aigbirhio FI, Clark JC, Kirkpatrick PJ, Menon DK, Pickard JD (2002) Correlation between cerebral blood flow, substrate delivery, and metabolism in head injury: a combined microdialysis and triple oxygen positron emission tomography study. J Cereb Blood Flow Metab 22(6):735–745

97. Citerio G, Cormio M (2003) Sedation in neurointensive care: advances in understanding and practice. Curr Opin Crit Care 9(2):120–126

98. Lee JH, Kelly DF, Oertel M, McArthur DL, Glenn TC, Vespa P, Boscardin WJ, Martin NA (2001) Carbon dioxide reactivity, pressure autoregulation, and metabolic suppression reactivity after head injury: a transcranial Doppler study. J Neurosurg 95(2):222–232

99. Otterspoor LC, Kalkman CJ, Cremer OL (2008) Update on the propofol infusion syndrome in ICU management of patients with head injury. Curr Opin Anaesthesiol 21(5):544–551

100. Zapantis A, Leung S (2005) Tolerance and withdrawal issues with sedation. Crit Care Nurs Clin North Am 17(3):211–223

101. Gaehtgens P, Marx P (1987) Hemorheological aspects of the pathophysiology of cerebral ischemia. J Cereb Blood Flow Metab 7(3):259–265

102. Ge YL, Lv R, Zhou W, Ma XX, Zhong TD, Duan ML (2007) Brain damage following severe acute normovolemic hemodilution in combination with controlled hypotension in rats. Acta Anaesthesiol Scand 51(10):1331–1337

103. Hare GM, Mazer CD, Hutchison JS, McLaren AT, Liu E, Rassouli A, Ai J, Shaye RE, Lockwood JA, Hawkins CE, Sikich N, To K, Baker AJ (2007) Severe hemodilutional anemia increases cerebral tissue injury following acute neurotrauma. J Appl Physiol 103(3):1021–1029

104. Ekelund A, Reinstrup P, Ryding E, Andersson AM, Molund T, Kristiansson KA, Romner B, Brandt L, Säveland H (2002) Effects of iso- and hypervolemic hemodilution on regional cerebral blood flow and oxygen delivery for patients with vasospasm after aneurysmal subarachnoid hemorrhage. Acta Neurochir (Wien) 144(7):703–712

105. Pendem S, Rana S, Manno EM, Gajic O (2006) A review of red cell transfusion in the neurological intensive care unit. Neurocrit Care 4(1):63–67

106. Leal-Noval SR, Rincón-Ferrari MD, Marin-Niebla A, Cayuela A, Arellano-Orden V, Marín-Caballos A, Amaya-Villar R, Ferrándiz-Millón C, Murillo-Cabeza F (2006) Transfusion of erythrocyte concentrates produces a variable increment on cerebral oxygenation in patients with severe traumatic brain injury: a preliminary study. Intensive Care Med 32(11):1733–1740

107. Leal-Noval SR, Muñoz-Gómez M, Arellano-Orden V, Marín-Caballos A, Amaya-Villar R, Marín A, Puppo-Moreno A, Ferrándiz-Millón C, Flores-Cordero JM, Murillo-Cabezas F (2008) Impact of age of transfused blood on cerebral oxygenation in male patients with severe traumatic brain injury. Crit Care Med 36(4):1290–1296

108. McIntyre LA, Fergusson DA, Hutchison JS, Pagliarello G, Marshall JC, Yetisir E, Hare GM, Hébert PC (2006) Effect of a liberal versus restrictive transfusion strategy on mortality in patients with moderate to severe head injury. Neurocrit Care 5(1):4–9

109. Hébert PC, Wells G, Blajchman MA, Marshall J, Martin C, Pagliarello G, Tweeddale M, Schweitzer I, Yetisir E (1999) A multicenter, randomized, controlled clinical trial of transfusion requirements in critical care. Transfusion Requirements in Critical Care Investigators, Canadian Critical Care Trials Group. N Engl J Med 340(6):409–417

110. Van Beek JG, Mushkudiani NA, Steyerberg EW, Butcher I, McHugh GS, Lu J, Marmarou A, Murray GD, Maas AI (2007) Prognostic value of admission laboratory parameters in traumatic brain injury: results from the IMPACT study. J Neurotrauma 24:315–328

111. Jeremitsky E, Omert LA, Dunham CM, Wilberger J, Rodriguez A (2005) The impact of hyperglycemia on patients with severe brain injury. J Trauma 58:47–50

112. Gale SC, Sicoutris C, Reilly PM, Schwab CW, Gracias VH (2007) Poor glycemic control is associated with increased mortality in critically ill trauma patients. Am Surg 73: 454–460

113. Longstreth WT Jr, Inui TS (1984) High blood glucose level on hospital admission and poor neurological recovery after cardiac arrest. Ann Neurol 15:59–63

114. Capes SE, Hunt D, Malmberg K, Gerstein HC (2000) Stress hyperglycaemia and increased risk of death after myocardial infarction in patients with and without diabetes: a systematic overview. Lancet 355:773–778

115. Vanhorebeek I, Langouche L, Van den Berghe G (2007) Tight blood glucose control: what is the evidence? Crit Care Med 35:S496–S502

116. van den Berghe G, Wouters P, Weekers F, Verwaest C, Bruyninckx F, Schetz M, Vlasselaers D, Ferdinande P, Lauwers P, Bouillon R (2001) Intensive insulin therapy in the critically ill patients. N Engl J Med 345:1359–1367

117. Van den Berghe G, Wilmer A, Hermans G, Meersseman W, Wouters PJ, Milants I, Van Wijngaerden E, Bobbaers H,

Bouillon R (2006) Intensive insulin therapy in the medical ICU. N Engl J Med 354:449–461

118. Van den Berghe G, Schoonheydt K, Becx P, Bruyninckx F, Wouters PJ (2005) Insulin therapy protects the central and peripheral nervous system of intensive care patients. Neurology 64:1348–1353

119. Bilotta F, Caramia R, Cernak I, Paoloni FP, Doronzio A, Cuzzone V, Santoro A, Rosa G (2008) Intensive insulin therapy after severe traumatic brain injury: a randomized clinical trial. Neurocrit Care 9(2):159–166

120. Vespa P, Boonyaputthikul R, McArthur DL, Miller C, Etchepare M, Bergsneider M, Glenn T, Martin N, Hovda D (2006) Intensive insulin therapy reduces microdialysis glucose values without altering glucose utilization or improving the lactate/pyruvate ratio after traumatic brain injury. Crit Care Med 34:850–856

121. Oddo M, Schmidt JM, Carrera E, Badjatia N, Connolly ES, Presciutti M, Ostapkovich ND, Levine JM, Le Roux P, Mayer SA (2008) Impact of tight glycemic control on cerebral glucose metabolism after severe brain injury: a microdialysis study. Crit Care Med 36(12):3233–3238

122. Hopwood SE, Parkin MC, Bezzina EL, Boutelle MG, Strong AJ (2005) Transient changes in cortical glucose and lactate levels associated with peri-infarct depolarisations, studied with rapid-sampling microdialysis. J Cereb Blood Flow Metab 25:391–401

123. Thomale UW, Griebenow M, Mautes A, Beyer TF, Dohse NK, Stroop R, Sakowitz OW, Unterberg AW, Stover JF (2007) Heterogeneous regional and temporal energetic impairment following controlled cortical impact injury in rats. Neurol Res 29:594–603

124. Nelson DW, Bellander BM, Maccallum RM, Axelsson J, Alm M, Wallin M, Weitzberg E, Rudehill A (2004) Cerebral microdialysis of patients with severe traumatic brain injury exhibits highly individualistic patterns as visualized by cluster analysis with self-organizing maps. Crit Care Med 32:2428–2436

125. Kato T, Nakayama N, Yasokawa Y, Okumura A, Shinoda J, Iwama T (2007) Statistical image analysis of cerebral glucose metabolism in patients with cognitive impairment following diffuse traumatic brain injury. J Neurotrauma 24:919–926

126. Hattori N, Huang SC, Wu HM, Liao W, Glenn TC, Vespa PM, Phelps ME, Hovda DA, Bergsneider M (2004) Acute changes in regional cerebral (18)F-FDG kinetics in patients with traumatic brain injury. J Nucl Med 45:775–783

127. Wu HM, Huang SC, Hattori N, Glenn TC, Vespa PM, Yu CL, Hovda DA, Phelps ME, Bergsneider M (2004) Selective metabolic reduction in gray matter acutely following human traumatic brain injury. J Neurotrauma 21:149–161

128. Bartnik BL, Hovda DA, Lee PW (2007) Glucose metabolism after traumatic brain injury: estimation of pyruvate carboxylase and pyruvate dehydrogenase flux by mass isotopomer analysis. J Neurotrauma 24:181–194

129. Meier R, Béchir M, Ludwig S, Sommerfeld J, Keel M, Steiger P, Stocker R, Stover JF (2008) Differential temporal profile of lowered blood glucose levels (3.5 to 6.5 mmol/l versus 5 to 8 mmol/l) in patients with severe traumatic brain injury. Crit Care 12(4):R98

130. Cormio M, Gopinath SP, Valadka A, Robertson CS (1999) Cerebral hemodynamic effects of pentobarbital coma in head-injured patients. J Neurotrauma 16(10):927–936

131. Thorat JD, Wang EC, Lee KK, Seow WT, Ng I (2008) Barbiturate therapy for patients with refractory intracranial hypertension following severe traumatic brain injury: its effects on tissue oxygenation, brain temperature and auto-regulation. J Clin Neurosci 15(2):143–148

132. Goodman JC, Valadka AB, Gopinath SP, Cormio M, Robertson CS (1996) Lactate and excitatory amino acids measured by microdialysis are decreased by pentobarbital coma in head-injured patients. J Neurotrauma 13(10):549–556

133. Roberts, I.: Barbiturates for acute traumatic brain injury. Cochrane Database Syst. Rev. 2000;(2):CD000033.

134. Llompart-Pou JA, Pérez-Bárcena J, Raurich JM, Burguera B, Ayestarán JI, Abadal JM, Homar J, Ibáñez J (2007) Effect of barbiturate coma on adrenal response in patients with traumatic brain injury. J Endocrinol Invest 30(5):393–398

135. Greer DM, Funk SE, Reaven NL, Ouzounelli M, Uman GC (2008) Impact of fever on outcome in patients with stroke and neurologic injury: a comprehensive meta-analysis. Stroke 39(11):3029–3035

136. Stocchetti N, Protti A, Lattuada M, Magnoni S, Longhi L, Ghisoni L, Egidi M, Zanier ER (2005) Impact of pyrexia on neurochemistry and cerebral oxygenation after acute brain injury. J Neurol Neurosurg Psychiatry 76(8):1135–1139

137. Clifton GL, Miller ER, Choi SC, Levin HS, McCauley S, Smith KR Jr, Muizelaar JP, Wagner FC Jr, Marion DW, Luerssen TG, Chesnut RM, Schwartz M (2001) Lack of effect of induction of hypothermia after acute brain injury. N Engl J Med 344(8):556–563

138. Tokutomi T, Morimoto K, Miyagi T, Yamaguchi S, Ishikawa K, Shigemori M (2007) Optimal temperature for the management of severe traumatic brain injury: effect of hypothermia on intracranial pressure, systemic and intracranial hemodynamics, and metabolism. Neurosurgery 61(1 Suppl):256–265

139. Polderman KH (2008) Induced hypothermia and fever control for prevention and treatment of neurological injuries. Lancet 371(9628):1955–1969

140. Hutchison JS, Ward RE, Lacroix J, Hébert PC, Barnes MA, Bohn DJ, Dirks PB, Doucette S, Fergusson D, Gottesman R, Joffe AR, Kirpalani HM, Meyer PG, Morris KP, Moher D, Singh RN, Skippen PW (2008) Hypothermia Pediatric Head Injury Trial Investigators and the Canadian Critical Care Trials Group. Hypothermia therapy after traumatic brain injury in children. N Engl J Med 358(23):2447–2456

141. Hoedemaekers CW, Ezzahti M, Gerritsen A, van der Hoeven JG (2007) Comparison of cooling methods to induce and maintain normo- and hypothermia in intensive care unit patients: a prospective intervention study. Crit Care 11(4):R91

142. Hata JS, Shelsky CR, Hindman BJ, Smith TC, Simmons JS, Todd MM (2008) A prospective, observational clinical trial of fever reduction to reduce systemic oxygen consumption in the setting of acute brain injury. Neurocrit Care 9(1):37–44

143. Lavinio A, Timofeev I, Nortje J, Outtrim J, Smielewski P, Gupta A, Hutchinson PJ, Matta BF, Pickard JD, Menon D, Czosnyka M (2007) Cerebrovascular reactivity during hypothermia and rewarming. Br J Anaesth 99(2):237–244

144. Robertson CS, Valadka AB, Hannay HJ, Contant CF, Gopinath SP, Cormio M, Uzura M, Grossman RG (1999) Prevention of secondary ischemic insults after severe head injury. Crit Care Med 27(10):2086–2095

145. An G, West MA (2008) Abdominal compartment syndrome: a concise clinical review. Crit Care Med 36(4):1304–1310, Review

146. Schmittner MD, Vajkoczy SL, Horn P, Bertsch T, Quintel M, Vajkoczy P, Muench E (2007) Effects of fentanyl and S(+)-ketamine on cerebral hemodynamics, gastrointestinal motility, and need of vasopressors in patients with intracranial pathologies: a pilot study. J Neurosurg Anesthesiol 19(4):257–262

147. Wakai, A., Roberts, I., Schierhout, G.: Mannitol for acute traumatic brain injury. Cochrane Database Syst. Rev. 2007;(1):CD001049.

148. White H, Cook D, Venkatesh B (2008) The role of hypertonic saline in neurotrauma. Eur J Anaesthesiol Suppl 42:104–109

149. Dickenmann M, Oettl T, Mihatsch MJ (2008) Osmotic nephrosis: acute kidney injury with accumulation of proximal tubular lysosomes due to administration of exogenous solutes. Am J Kidney Dis 51(3):491–503

150. Sakowitz OW, Stover JF, Sarrafzadeh AS, Unterberg AW, Kiening KL (2007) Effects of mannitol bolus administration on intracranial pressure, cerebral extracellular metabolites, and tissue oxygenation in severely head-injured patients. J Trauma 62(2):292–298

151. Cooper DJ, Myles PS, McDermott FT, Murray LJ, Laidlaw J, Cooper G, Tremayne AB, Bernard SS, Ponsford J (2004) HTS Study Investigators. Prehospital hypertonic saline resuscitation of patients with hypotension and severe traumatic brain injury: a randomized controlled trial. JAMA 291(11):1350–1357

152. Munar F, Ferrer AM, de Nadal M, Poca MA, Pedraza S, Sahuquillo J, Garnacho A (2000) Cerebral hemodynamic effects of 7.2% hypertonic saline in patients with head injury and raised intracranial pressure. J Neurotrauma 17(1):41–51

153. Vialet R, Albanèse J, Thomachot L, Antonini F, Bourgouin A, Alliez B, Martin C (2003) Isovolume hypertonic solutes (sodium chloride or mannitol) in the treatment of refractory posttraumatic intracranial hypertension: 2 mL/kg 7.5% saline is more effective than 2 mL/kg 20% mannitol. Crit Care Med 31(6):1683–1687

154. Francony G, Fauvage B, Falcon D, Canet C, Dilou H, Lavagne P, Jacquot C, Payen JF (2008) Equimolar doses of mannitol and hypertonic saline in the treatment of increased intracranial pressure. Crit Care Med 36(3):795–800

155. Ichai C, Armando G, Orban JC, Berthier F, Rami L, Samat-Long C, Grimaud D, Leverve X (2009) Sodium lactate versus mannitol in the treatment of intracranial hypertensive episodes in severe traumatic brain-injured patients. Intensive Care Med 35(3):471–479

156. Battison C, Andrews PJ, Graham C, Petty T (2005) Randomized, controlled trial on the effect of a 20% mannitol solution and a 7.5% saline/6% dextran solution on increased intracranial pressure after brain injury. Crit Care Med 33(1):196–202

157. Rodling Wahlström M, Olivecrona M, Nyström F, Koskinen LO, Naredi S (2009) Fluid therapy and the use of albumin in the treatment of severe traumatic brain injury. Acta Anaesthesiol Scand 53(1):18–25

158. SAFE Study Investigators; Australian and New Zealand Intensive Care Society Clinical Trials Group; Australian

Red Cross Blood Service; George Institute for International Health, Myburgh J, Cooper DJ, Finfer S, Bellomo R, Norton R, Bishop N, Kai Lo S, Vallance S (2007) Saline or albumin for fluid resuscitation in patients with traumatic brain injury. N Engl J Med 357(9):874–884

159. White H, Venkatesh B (2008) Cerebral perfusion pressure in neurotrauma: a review. Anesth Analg 107(3):979–988

160. Rosner MJ, Rosner SD, Johnson AH (1995) Cerebral perfusion pressure: management protocol and clinical results. J Neurosurg 83(6):949–962

161. Kroppenstedt SN, Kern M, Thomale UW, Schneider GH, Lanksch WR, Unterberg AW (1999) Effect of cerebral perfusion pressure on contusion volume following impact injury. J Neurosurg 90(3):520–526

162. Marín-Caballos AJ, Murillo-Cabezas F, Cayuela-Domínguez A, Domínguez-Roldán JM, Rincón-Ferrari MD, Valencia-Anguita J, Flores-Cordero JM, Muñoz-Sánchez MA (2005) Cerebral perfusion pressure and risk of brain hypoxia in severe head injury: a prospective observational study. Crit Care 9(6):670–676

163. Vajkoczy P, Horn P, Thome C, Munch E, Schmiedek P (2003) Regional cerebral blood flow monitoring in the diagnosis of delayed ischemia following aneurysmal subarachnoid hemorrhage. J Neurosurg 98(6):1227–1234

164. Eker C, Àsgeirsson B, Grände PO, Schalèn W, Nordström CH (1998) Improved outcome after severe head injury with a new therapy based on principles for brain volume regulation and preserved microcirculation. Crit Care Med 26(11):1881–1886

165. Citerio G, Vascotto E, Villa F, Celotti S, Pesenti A (2001) Induced abdominal compartment syndrome increases intracranial pressure in neurotrauma patients: a prospective study. Crit Care Med 29(7):1466–1471

166. Malbrain ML, Deeren D, De Potter TJ (2005) Intra-abdominal hypertension in the critically ill: it is time to pay attention. Curr Opin Crit Care 11(2):156–171

167. Joseph DK, Dutton RP, Aarabi B, Scalea TM (2004) Decompressive laparotomy to treat intractable intracranial hypertension after traumatic brain injury. J Trauma 57(4):687–693

168. Abadal-Centellas JM, Llompart-Pou JA, Homar-Ramírez J, Pérez-Bárcena J, Rosselló-Ferrer A, Ibáñez-Juvé J (2007) Neurologic outcome of posttraumatic refractory intracranial hypertension treated with external lumbar drainage. J Trauma 62(2):282–286

169. Beer R, Lackner P, Pfausler B, Schmutzhard E (2008) Nosocomial ventriculitis and meningitis in neurocritical care patients. J Neurol 255(11):1617–1624

170. Timofeev I, Czosnyka M, Nortje J, Smielewski P, Kirkpatrick P, Gupta A, Hutchinson P (2008) Effect of decompressive craniectomy on intracranial pressure and cerebrospinal compensation following traumatic brain injury. J Neurosurg 108(1):66–73

171. Morgalla MH, Will BE, Roser F, Tatagiba M (2008) Do long-term results justify decompressive craniectomy after severe traumatic brain injury? J Neurosurg 109(4): 685–690

172. Howard JL, Cipolle MD, Anderson M, Sabella V, Shollenberger D, Li PM, Pasquale MD (2008) Outcome after decompressive craniectomy for the treatment of severe traumatic brain injury. J Trauma 65(2):380–385

173. Gaab MR, Trost HA, Alcantara A, Karimi-Nejad A, Moskopp D, Schultheiss R, Bock WJ, Piek J, Klinge H, Scheil F et al (1994) "Ultrahigh" dexamethasone in acute brain injury. Results from a prospective randomized double-blind multicenter trial (GUDHIS). German Ultrahigh Dexamethasone Head Injury Study Group. Zentralbl Neurochir 55(3):135–143

174. Edwards P, Arango M, Balica L, Cottingham R, El-Sayed H, Farrell B, Fernandes J, Gogichaisvili T, Golden N, Hartzenberg B, Husain M, Ulloa MI, Jerbi Z, Khamis H, Komolafe E, Laloë V, Lomas G, Ludwig S, Mazairac G, Muñoz Sanchéz Mde L, Nasi L, Olldashi F, Plunkett P, Roberts I, Sandercock P, Shakur H, Soler C, Stocker R, Svoboda P, Trenkler S, Venkataramana NK, Wasserberg J, Yates D, Yutthakasemsunt S, CRASH trial collaborators (2005) Final results of MRC CRASH, a randomised placebo-controlled trial of intravenous corticosteroid in adults with head injury-outcomes at 6 months. Lancet 365(9475):1957–1959

175. Powner DJ, Boccalandro C (2008) Adrenal insufficiency following traumatic brain injury in adults. Curr Opin Crit Care 14(2):163–166

176. Dusick, J.R., Wang, C., Cohan, P., Swerdloff, R., Kelly, D.F.: Chapter 1: pathophysiology of hypopituitarism in the setting of brain injury. Pituitary. 2008 [Epub ahead of print].

177. Hildreth AN, Mejia VA, Maxwell RA, Smith PW, Dart BW, Barker DE (2008) Adrenal suppression following a single dose of etomidate for rapid sequence induction: a prospective randomized study. J Trauma 65(3):573–579

178. Willmore LJ, Ueda Y (2008) Posttraumatic epilepsy: hemorrhage, free radicals and the molecular regulation of glutamate. Neurochem Res 34(4):688–697

179. Swartz BE, Houser CR, Tomiyasu U, Walsh GO, DeSalles A, Rich JR, Delgado-Escueta A (2006) Hippocampal cell loss in posttraumatic human epilepsy. Epilepsia 47(8):1373–1382

180. Diaz-Arrastia R, Gong Y, Fair S, Scott KD, Garcia MC, Carlile MC, Agostini MA, Van Ness PC (2003) Increased risk of late posttraumatic seizures associated with inheritance of APOE ε4 allele. Arch Neurol 60(6):818–822

181. Ronne-Engstrom E, Winkler T (2006) Continuous EEG monitoring in patients with traumatic brain injury reveals a high incidence of epileptiform activity. Acta Neurol Scand 114(1):47–53

182. Vespa PM, Nuwer MR, Nenov V, Ronne-Engstrom E, Hovda DA, Bergsneider M, Kelly DF, Martin NA, Becker DP (1999) Increased incidence and impact of nonconvulsive and convulsive seizures after traumatic brain injury as detected by continuous electroencephalographic monitoring. J Neurosurg 91(5):750–760

183. Frey LC (2003) Epidemiology of posttraumatic epilepsy: a critical review. Epilepsia 44(Suppl 10):11–17

184. Englander J, Bushnik T, Duong TT, Cifu DX, Zafonte R, Wright J, Hughes R, Bergman W (2003) Analyzing risk

factors for late posttraumatic seizures: a prospective, multi-center investigation. Arch Phys Med Rehabil 84(3):365–373

185. Mazzini L, Cossa FM, Angelino E, Campini R, Pastore I, Monaco F (2003) Posttraumatic epilepsy: neuroradiologic and neuropsychological assessment of long-term outcome. Epilepsia 44(4):569–574

186. Golarai G, Greenwood AC, Feeney DM, Connor JA (2001) Physiological and structural evidence for hippocampal involvement in persistent seizure susceptibility after traumatic brain injury. J Neurosci 21(21):8523–8537

187. Diaz-Arrastia R, Agostini MA, Frol AB, Mickey B, Fleckenstein J, Bigio E, Van Ness PC (2000) Neurophysiologic and neuroradiologic features of intractable epilepsy after traumatic brain injury in adults. Arch Neurol 57(11):1611–1616

188. Chang BS, Lowenstein DH (2003) Quality Standards Subcommittee of the American Academy of Neurology Practice parameter: antiepileptic drug prophylaxis in severe traumatic brain injury: report of the Quality Standards Subcommittee of the American Academy of Neurology. Neurology 60(1):10–16

189. Beghi E (2003) Overview of studies to prevent posttraumatic epilepsy. Epilepsia 44(Suppl 10):21–26

190. Jones KE, Puccio AM, Harshman KJ, Falcione B, Benedict N, Jankowitz BT, Stippler M, Fischer M, Sauber-Schatz EK, Fabio A, Darby JM, Okonkwo DO (2008) Levetiracetam versus phenytoin for seizure prophylaxis in severe traumatic brain injury. Neurosurg Focus 25(4):E3

191. Stiefel MF, Udoetuk JD, Spiotta AM, Gracias VH, Goldberg A, Maloney-Wilensky E, Bloom S, Le Roux PD (2006) Conventional neurocritical care and cerebral oxygenation after traumatic brain injury. J Neurosurg 105(4):568–575

192. Compagnone C, Murray GD, Teasdale GM, Maas AI, Esposito D, Princi P, D'Avella D, Servadei F (2007) The management of patients with intradural post-traumatic mass lesions: a multicenter survey of current approaches to surgical management in 729 patients coordinated by the European Brain Injury Consortium. Neurosurgery 61(1 Suppl):232–240

193. Neumann JO, Chambers IR, Citerio G, Enblad P, Gregson BA, Howells T, Mattern J, Nilsson P, Piper I, Ragauskas A, Sahuquillo J, Yau YH, Kiening K, BrainIT Group (2008) The use of hyperventilation therapy after traumatic brain injury in Europe: an analysis of the BrainIT database. Intensive Care Med 34(9):1676–1682

194. Nilsson P, Enblad P, Chambers I, Citerio G, Fiddes H, Howells T, Kiening K, Ragauskas A, Sahuquillo J, Yau YH, Contant C, Piper I, BrainIT Group (2005) Survey of traumatic brain injury management in European Brain-IT centres year 2001. Acta Neurochir Suppl 95:51–53

195. Stocchetti N, Pagan F, Calappi E, Canavesi K, Beretta L, Citerio G, Cormio M, Colombo A (2004) Inaccurate early assessment of neurological severity in head injury. J Neurotrauma 21(9):1131–1140

196. Davis DP, Vadeboncoeur TF, Ochs M, Poste JC, Vilke GM, Hoyt DB (2005) The association between field Glasgow Coma Scale score and outcome in patients undergoing paramedic rapid sequence intubation. J Emerg Med 29(4):391–397

197. Skoglund TS, Nellgård B (2005) Long-time outcome after transient ranstentorial herniation in patients with traumatic brain injury. Acta Anaesthesiol Scand 49(3):337–340

198. Narayan RK, Maas AI, Servadei F, Skolnick BE, Tillinger MN, Marshall LF, Traumatic Intracerebral Hemorrhage Study Group (2008) Progression of traumatic intracerebral hemorrhage: a prospective observational study. J Neurotrauma 25(6):629–639

199. Lescot T, Abdennour L, Boch AL, Puybasset L (2008) Treatment of intracranial hypertension. Curr Opin Crit Care 14(2):129–134

200. Velmahos GC, Jindal A, Chan LS, Murray JA, Vassiliu P, Berne TV, Asensio J, Demetriades D (2001) "Insignificant" mechanism of injury: not to be taken lightly. J Am Coll Surg 192(2):147–152

201. Mushkudiani NA, Engel DC, Steyerberg EW, Butcher I, Lu J, Marmarou A, Slieker F, McHugh GS, Murray GD, Maas AI (2007) Prognostic value of demographic characteristics in traumatic brain injury: results from the IMPACT study. J Neurotrauma 24(2):259–269

202. Ponsford JL, Myles PS, Cooper DJ, Mcdermott FT, Murray LJ, Laidlaw J, Cooper G, Tremayne AB, Bernard SA (2008) Gender differences in outcome in patients with hypotension and severe traumatic brain injury. Injury 39(1):67–76

203. Marmarou A, Lu J, Butcher I, McHugh GS, Murray GD, Steyerberg EW, Mushkudiani NA, Choi S, Maas AI (2007) Prognostic value of the Glasgow Coma Scale and pupil reactivity in traumatic brain injury assessed pre-hospital and on enrollment: an IMPACT analysis. J Neurotrauma 24(2):270–280

204. Maas AI, Steyerberg EW, Butcher I, Dammers R, Lu J, Marmarou A, Mushkudiani NA, McHugh GS, Murray GD (2007) Prognostic value of computerized tomography scan characteristics in traumatic brain injury: results from the IMPACT study. J Neurotrauma 24(2):303–314

205. McHugh GS, Engel DC, Butcher I, Steyerberg EW, Lu J, Mushkudiani N, Hernández AV, Marmarou A, Maas AI, Murray GD (2007) Prognostic value of secondary insults in traumatic brain injury: results from the IMPACT study. J Neurotrauma 24(2):287–293

206. Vickery CD, Sherer M, Nick TG, Nakase-Richardson R, Corrigan JD, Hammond F, Macciocchi S, Ripley DL, Sander A (2008) Relationships among premorbid alcohol use, acute intoxication, and early functional status after traumatic brain injury. Arch Phys Med Rehabil 89(1):48–55

207. O'Phelan K, McArthur DL, Chang CW, Green D, Hovda DA (2008) The impact of substance abuse on mortality in patients with severe traumatic brain injury. J Trauma 65(3):674–677

208. Zhou W, Xu D, Peng X, Zhang Q, Jia J, Crutcher KA (2008) Meta-analysis of APOE4 allele and outcome after traumatic brain injury. J Neurotrauma 25(4):279–290

209. Meric E, Gunduz A, Turedi S, Cakir E, Yandi M (2008) The prognostic value of neuron-specific enolase in head trauma patients. J Emerg Med 38(3):297–301

210. Nylén K, Ost M, Csajbok LZ, Nilsson I, Hall C, Blennow K, Nellgård B, Rosengren L (2008) Serum levels of S100B, S100A1B and S100BB are all related to outcome after

severe traumatic brain injury. Acta Neurochir (Wien) 150(3):221–227

211. Lumpkins KM, Bochicchio GV, Keledjian K, Simard JM, McCunn M, Scalea T (2008) Glial fibrillary acidic protein is highly correlated with brain injury. J Trauma 65(4):778–782

212. Kirchhoff C, Buhmann S, Bogner V, Stegmaier J, Leidel BA, Braunstein V, Mutschler W, Biberthaler P (2008) Cerebrospinal IL-10 concentration is elevated in non-survivors as compared to survivors after severe traumatic brain injury. Eur J Med Res 13(10):464–468

213. Salim A, Hadjizacharia P, Brown C, Inaba K, Teixeira PG, Chan L, Rhee P, Demetriades D (2008) Significance of troponin elevation after severe traumatic brain injury. J Trauma 64(1):46–52

214. Kemp CD, Johnson JC, Riordan WP, Cotton BA (2008) How we die: the impact of nonneurologic organ dysfunction after severe traumatic brain injury. Am Surg 74(9):866–872

215. Härtl R, Gerber LM, Ni Q, Ghajar J (2008) Effect of early nutrition on deaths due to severe traumatic brain injury. J Neurosurg 109(1):50–56

Craniofacial Trauma

3

Marius G. Bredell and Klaus W. Grätz

3.1 Introduction

Craniofacial trauma is treated by a wide spectrum of specialists, including cranio-maxillofacial surgeons, otolaryngologists, plastic surgeons, general surgeons, neurosurgeons, oral surgeons, as well as other dedicated doctors and dentists. Teamwork often leads to the best possible care and outcome. Ultimately, the patient deserves the best possible treatment to ensure the best possible return to functional as well as aesthetic normality. It is a wide field and a chapter will not give full justice to this important part of trauma management.

The emphasis of this chapter is to share the basic principles of emergency diagnosis and management, early treatment goals as well as offering a brief overview of the potential further definitive treatment the patient will receive. We hope that this is done in a practical way, thereby increasing the understanding and treatment goals in facial trauma.

3.2 History

The face is the center of a person's presence and in most cases represents the first impression after contact with another person. Of course, the significant functional aspects like chewing, swallowing, speech, and facial expression are a critical part of a person's existence. It is indeed every patient's expectation to be normal in all aspects of facial aesthetics and function again after a facial fracture.

In earlier times, the management of facial fractures was less than ideal. It was only since the more sophisticated wars came about that there has been significant development in the management of these debilitating injuries. The initial goals were merely to prevent infection and restore some kind of occlusion. Since the development of plates and screws for the fixation of facial fractures, it was for the first time possible to reliably restore the three-dimensional facial structure and not only the occlusion (Figs. 3.1 and 3.2).

3.3 Etiology

For the most part, facial fractures are the result of trauma, which implies higher than normal forces exerted on the facial skeleton. In some cases, these forces have to be significant to cause fractures. This may of course vary from person to person due to individual differences. Young children have very elastic bone and thus more force is required than in adults and persons suffering from osteoporosis. Exceptional circumstances may prevail where even normal forces (like chewing) may result in facial fractures. This may be the case where underlying pathology exists or when surgery has been performed in the lower jaw, for instance the removal of wisdom teeth that required removal of bone (Fig. 3.3).

Depending on the social structure, values, traditions, sports practiced, the availability of weapons, etc., the etiology and thus indeed the profile of facial fractures may vary from country to country. In many countries, person on person violence would dominate, while in others, sport or workplace injuries predominate.

M.G. Bredell (✉) and K.W. Grätz
Department of Cranio-maxillo-facial Surgery, Frauenklinikstr,
24, CH-8091 Zürich, Switzerland
e-mail: marius.bredell@usz.ch
e-mail: klaus.graetz@usz.ch

H.-J. Oestern et al. (eds.), *Head, Thoracic, Abdominal, and Vascular Injuries*,
DOI: 10.1007/978-3-540-88122-3_3, © Springer-Verlag Berlin Heidelberg 2011

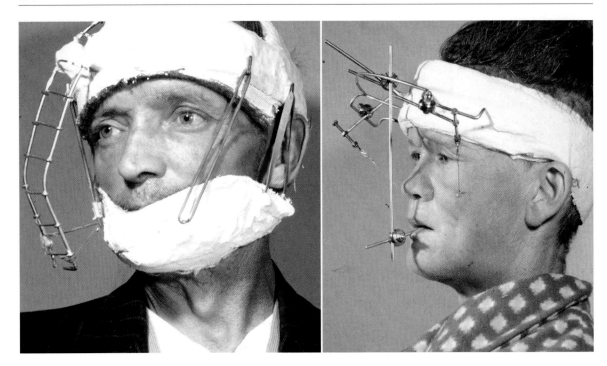

Fig. 3.1 On the *left* merely vertical repositioning and on the *right* an attempt at three-dimensional repositioning of the face by skeletal fixation in the pre-"plate and screw fixation" era

The etiology has a very important role to play in history taking due to the influence it has on the development of characteristic fracture patterns; for instance, cycling injuries often involve condylar combined with symphysis fractures due to direct frontal impact, while a sport like soccer often causes lateral facial fractures like zygoma and mandibular angle fractures.

Important considerations in the etiology of the injury would be:

- The surface area of contact
- The site of contact
- Contact force
- Direction of force (angulation)
- Resistance to the force (movement of the head in the same or opposite direction of the force)

Depending on the above factors and combinations thereof, it would explain the many different fracture patterns and combinations thereof found in the head and neck area.

It is of considerable importance to evaluate the patient's complete body for associated injuries. This is especially important for patients involved in motor vehicle and other diffuse and high force etiologies. Because of the close relationship of the face to the brain and cervical spine, attention to these possible associated injuries as well as routine abdominal and pelvis examination is of paramount importance. A chest as well as a pelvis X-ray or alternatively a CT is important in all multitrauma patients.

Forces needed to generate a facial fracture differ from anatomical area to area and is also dependant on other factors such as age, sex as well as potential underlying pathology.

Broadly, the etiologies could be classified as follows (Figs. 3.4 and 3.5):

Sport
Workplace injuries
Road traffic accidents
Person on person violence

- Blunt injuries
- Sharp injuries
- Bite wounds

War-related injuries or Gunshot wounds (High or low velocity)
Catastrophe injuries like airplane accidents
Activities of daily life (slipping in a bath or on stairs)

- *Sport*: Depending on the type of sport, the injuries could vary considerably. There are, however,

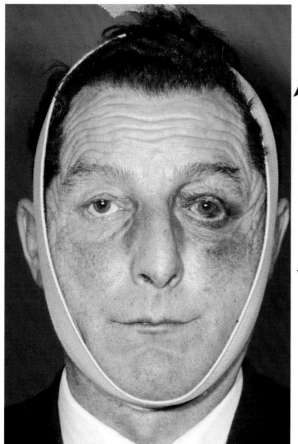

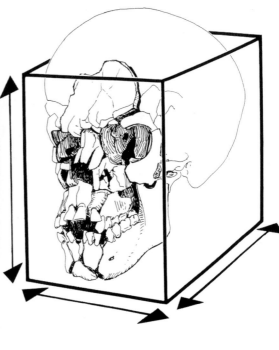

Fig. 3.2 Example of an emergency bandage used for initial stabilization of the facial structures. Modern treatment has the aim not only to correct the vertical height, but restoring the three- dimensional facial complex, which may be challenging in a panfacial fracture as demonstrated on the *right*

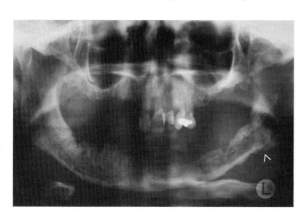

Fig. 3.3 Pathological fracture due to progressive osteoradionecrosis of the mandible

characteristic injuries to be found for certain sports. Since the advent of helmets, there have been considerable changes in the demographics of the injuries. Most noticeable were the decrease in head and midface injuries. This explains why for instance puck injuries in ice hockey now mostly cause fractures in the lower facial third.

- *Workplace injuries*: These may vary greatly, depending on the occupation of the person. Obviously, despite major improvements in safety measures, accidents do happen, especially in the industrial and mining environments.
- *Road traffic accidents*: Some of the worst injuries are seen due to motor vehicle accidents. The use of safety belts as well as air bags has had a major role to play in the reduction in number as well as severity of these injuries. Due to the often, major forces involved, associated injuries are extremely common.
- *Person on person violence*:
  - Blunt injuries (baseball bat, hammer) These objects often cause soft tissue burst injuries and comminuted or impression fractures in the area of impact.

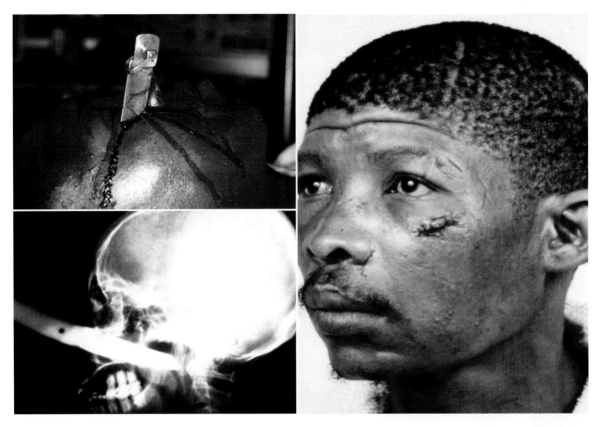

Fig. 3.4 Penetrating knife wound to the face fortunately without damage to any vital structures

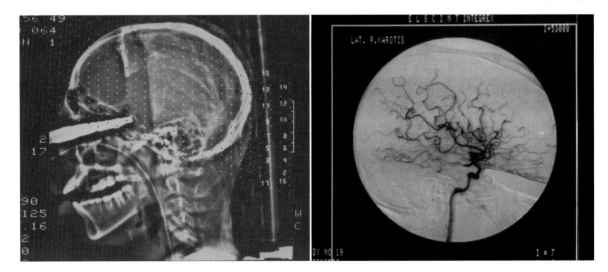

Fig. 3.5 Penetrating injury with close approximation to the internal carotid artery

- Sharp injuries (including knives, mostly low-velocity gunshot injuries in comparison to warfare where high-velocity injuries predominate)
- Bite wounds (may involve loss of tissue and carries a significant risk of infection)

- *War-related injuries or Gunshot wounds*: This makes for a complex group where the possibilities are virtually endless. The major clinical distinction should be if this is a high- or low-velocity injury as it has a major impact on in particular the early as well as early delayed management. (Discussion on this follows later)

- *Catastrophe injuries like airplane accidents*: Here, not only the variety of injuries play a role, but often the sheer volume of workload involved is over-

whelming for a hospital or particular department. Triage and immediate assessment of the need for treatment is of paramount importance. Treatment of the life-threatening problems and injuries take precedence (Fig. 3.6).

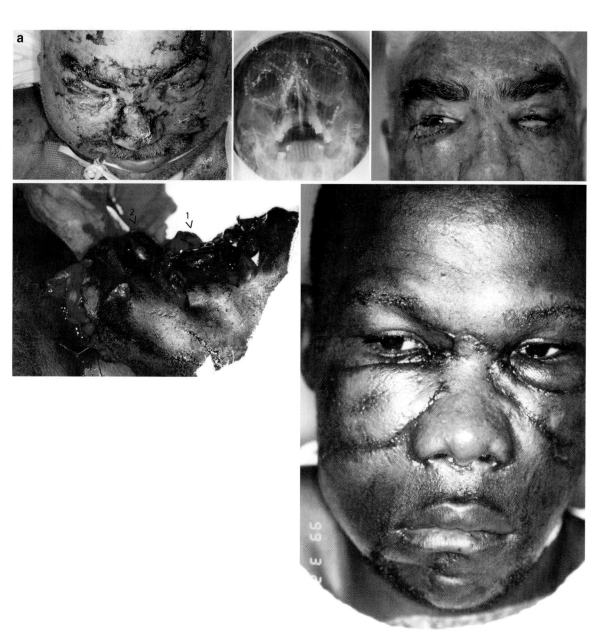

Fig. 3.6 (**a**) Industrial injury resulting from exploding metal causing extensive soft and hard tissue injuries. On the *right*, correction of eyelid competence by means of full thickness skin grafts. (**b**) Another industrial injury with displacement of the whole midface (*1*, indicating normal and *2*, the displaced nasal position), obstructing the oral airway. On the *left*, the preoperative situation and on the *right* the patient 2 months after injury

3.4 Approach to Patient Management

3.4.1 Primary Management

Primary care can be divided into treatment on the accident scene as well as in the hospital.

A systematic approach to the trauma management as propagated by the ATLS - protocol has contributed considerably to the structured management of these patients as well as the survival of patients. The particular influence facial fractures may have on this process is highlighted.

The ATLS - protocol is based on well-established principles and appropriate treatment guidelines.

1. ABCD
2. First do no harm (Primum nil nocere)
3. Treatment of life-threatening injuries within the first hour
4. Constant reassessment for evolving injuries
5. Recognition of the importance of the mechanism of injuries and anticipating the potential evolvement of direct as well as associated injuries.

The presence of facial fractures often complicates the immediate management of a patient with multiple injuries and of course in itself may contribute to life-threatening situations like compromising the airway. It is also important to note that the commonly used GCS is often difficult to judge in the facial trauma patient due to the influence facial injuries may have on both the eye response as well as the verbal response. Facial fractures may thus compromise the whole well-designed pattern of thought and action. Most important in the resuscitation process is the assessment of priorities and being flexible enough to adapt the resuscitation process to the particular situation (Fig. 3.7).

The Glasgow Coma Score (GCS) and Glasgow Paediatric Coma Score (GPCS) are simple and common methods for quantifying the level of consciousness and potential underlying brain injury.

The scale is the sum of three parameters:

- Best eye response
- Best verbal response
- Best motor response

Scales are based on values ranging between 3 (worst) and 15 (best). All these parameters may be influenced by the presence of facial fractures leading to a lower score or difficult assessment.

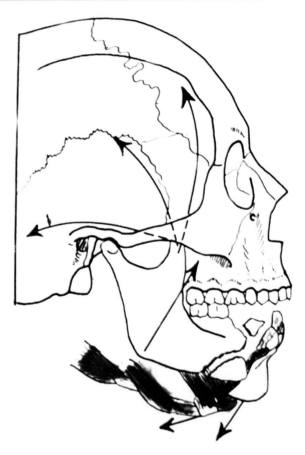

Fig. 3.7 Posterior pull of the suprahyoid musculature may displace mandibular fragments with resultant obstruction of the airway

Table 3.1 The three parameters of the Revised Trauma Score (RTS) are: the Glasgow Coma Scale (GCS), systemic blood pressure (SBP), and the respiratory rate (RR)

Glasgow Coma Scale	Systolic blood pressure	Respiratory rate	Value
13–15	>89	10–29	4
9–12	76–89	>29	3
6–8	50–75	6–9	2
4–5	1–49	1–5	1
3	0	0	0

RTS is equal to 0.9368 GCS plus 0.7326 systolic blood pressure plus 0.2908 respiratory rate
Range is 0–7.8408 and correlates with survival, e.g., a score of 4 indicates 40% mortality

The revised trauma score (Table 3.1) is used as a triage tool in a prehospital setting and also functions as a common physiological scoring system based on the first data sets of three specific physiological parameters obtained from the patient.

Central to all the resuscitation efforts would be to maintain the basic life-support mechanisms.

A. Airway and cervical spine control
B. Breathing and ventilation
C. Circulation and hemorrhage control
D. Disability due to neurological deficit and potential drugs
E. Exposure and environmental control

3.4.2 Secondary Survey

For the secondary survey, the acronym below is often used.

• A M P L E

Allergies Medication Past illness/Pregnant Last meal Events/Environment related to injury (Fig. 3.8).

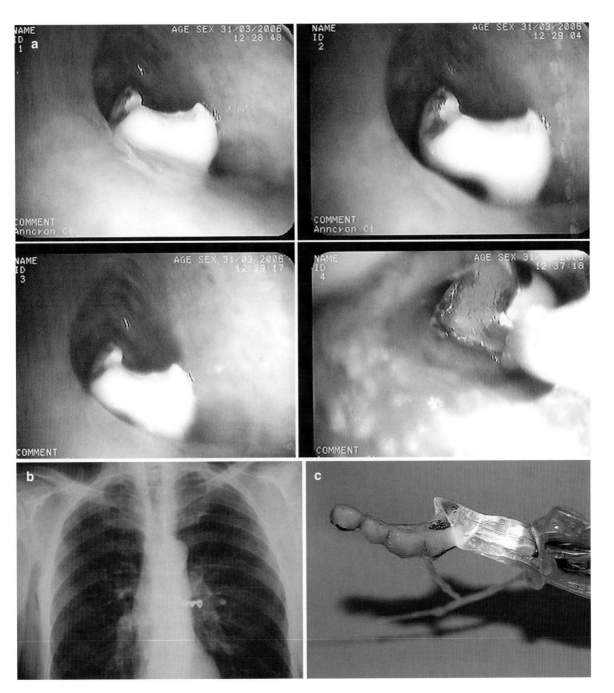

Fig. 3.8 (**a–c**) Aspiration of a dental bridge in the left lung with endoscopic retrieval

Further discussion on this topic is not in the scope of this chapter.

3.5 Facial Examination

As previously noted, it is of paramount importance to assess the face as part of a resuscitation process and not as a separate entity giving it more or less priority than the rest of the body.

Asking the patient regarding his symptoms is vitally important and often a working diagnosis can be made merely after history taking. Patients will often lead one to a more detailed examination of a specific area; however, this should not preclude one from doing a thorough examination of the whole facial skeleton.

When examining the face, it is prudent to divide the evaluation into extraoral and intraoral components.

3.5.1 Extraoral

3.5.1.1 One Should Note by Only Visually Examining the Patient

- Facial asymmetry or swelling
- Abnormal head position or restricted head movement
- Ecchymoses or hematomas (including subconjunctival ecchymosis)
- Eye position and movement
- Symmetric and adequate movement of the musculature of facial expression
- Note abnormal features like increased intercanthal distance (in canthal disruption or naso-ethmoidal fractures) as well as upturned nasal tip (also often seen in naso-ethmoidal fractures).
- Bleeding from nose and ears (rhino- or otorhea).
- Restricted nasal breathing

3.5.1.2 Physical Examination (Noting Steps, Pain, Crepitation, Sensory Disturbance, Surgical Emphysema, Soft Tissue Injuries)

- Start by palpating the neck and cervical spine and note all swellings and areas of tenderness.
- Palpation of the facial bones and the facial contours:

Start from the lower and outer border of the mandible and include the palpation of the condyles with their associated normal movement of rotation and progression to translation.

Frontal and temporal palpation with progression to the scalp, observing for soft or hard tissue defects revealing areas of potential blood loss due to obscured lacerations.

Progress to the prominence of the maxilla as well as the body of the zygoma and zygomatic arch.

Palpate the frontal area, supraorbital, lateral, as well as infraorbital rim. Where swelling is present, constant light finger pressure is often sufficient to enable underlying bony palpation.

Progress to nasal and medial orbital palpation with specific assessment of the medial and lateral canthal position. Both the medial and lateral canthal angles should be sharp and symmetrical and rigidly fixed to the underlying bone. The latter can be confirmed by exerting lateral pull on the medial canthal area and observing that the medial canthal angle stays sharp and well defined.

A blunted medial eye angle is a sign of medial canthal (medial angle of the palpebral fissure) damage. Epiphora is also to be noted. The normal intercanthal distance in the Caucasian population may vary from 32 ± 3 mm to slightly wider in the black population.

During the examination evaluate the following:

- Pupil shape, transparency, size as well as direct and indirect light reflexes and signs of hyphema, lens dislocation as well as iris tear at least should be noted. Note subconjunctival bleeding and swelling.
- Eye movement or the restriction thereof should be noted. Simultaneously, the presence of diplopia in any visual field should be recorded. Important is to differentiate between monocular diplopia (often due to retinal detachment or lens dislocation) and biocular diplopia (due to a difference in focal points of the individual eyes as a result of incoherent eye movement or a change of the eye position).
- Eye position is important. This may either be enophthalmos (posterior positioning of the globe) or hypoglobus (inferior positioning of the globe) or exophthalmos (protrusion of the globe).
- Look for characteristic signs of skull base fractures: Anterior cranial base (biocular periorbital hematoma, nasal cerebrospinal fluid leak), middle cranial fossa (ecchymosis over the mastoid process commonly called Battle's sign, hemotympanum, or cerebrospinal fluid drainage from the external acoustic meatus)

- Examine the external acoustic meatus for lacerations and foreign material and signs of a middle cranial fossa fracture as above. Using a nasal speculum and good lighting will enable one to assess the nasal septum for fractures, deviation, hematomas, and foreign objects obstructing the nasal airway. Septum hematomas have to be drained and a compressive packing applied as soon as possible to prevent potential local septum necrosis due to decreased vascularity (Figs. 3.9 and 3.10).

3.5.2 Intraoral

- Note swelling, ecchymosis, and/or lacerations as well as areas of tenderness in all areas of the oral cavity including the oropharynx.
- Observe the symmetry of mouth opening and measure the distance between the incisors or alveolar ridges in edentulous patients. Mouth opening often deviates to the affected side (Fig. 3.9 i-k).
- Occlusion (Do the teeth fit together in the former position and without premature contact left or right, anterior or posterior?)
- Look for missing, fractured, or mobile teeth or mobile mandibular or maxillary segments (fragments may be loose in the mouth, intruded in soft tissue, aspirated, or swallowed)
- Using finger palpation and direct observation follow the alveolar ridge and vestibulum of the upper and lower jaw and note tenderness, movement, crepitation, or the presence of hematomas.
- Examine the soft palate as well as the pharynx for lacerations or foreign objects.
- Examine the floor of the mouth and tongue for lacerations and hematomas.
- Grasp the maxilla with one hand and stabilize the head with the other hand on the forehead and physically try and move the maxilla from side to side as well as up and down. In Le Fort fractures, the maxilla is usually mobile and bone on bone crepitations can be felt. Even when the maxilla is very mobile, patients experience very little pain as the superior alveolar sensory nerves are often severed.
- Further examine the mandible by grasping it with the index finger below the chin and the thumb on the lower front teeth and gently pull it forward. Look for opening spaces and observe where patients indicate discomfort, particularly feel for normal rotational and translational movement of the condyles (Figs. 3.11 and 3.12).

3.5.3 Special Investigations

Blood examinations as per normal indications are required. Of special importance is a baseline hematokrit or hemoglobin value.

Once a clinical examination has been done and a clinical diagnosis has been established, one can progress to confirmation by radiological diagnosis. In many emergency situations, a computer tomography (CT) is the examination of choice in a polytrauma patient or where severe fractures are suspected. At least two perpendicular planes should be available, namely axial and coronal. In some cases, a sagittal view may be of assistance in accessing the skull base or orbit. A 3D reconstruction may be of assistance, but should only be used as an overview assessment and not as a substitute for careful judgment of individual planes.

In centers where a CT is not available or in patients with less serious injuries, conventional radiographs often are performed before progression to a CT. The following radiographs with alternatives are most commonly requested with the general rule of always requesting views in two perpendicular planes.

Mandible: (Follow the cortical outline of the mandible in the two perpendicular planes that may indicate a fracture; look for absent, displaced, or fractured teeth)

- Orthopantomogram (OPT) and PA Mandible or alternatively an AP Mandible (Fig. 3.13).
- As an alternative to the OPT, an oblique mandible left and right for good visualization of the condyles as well as the mandibular angle and posterior part of the body (Fig 3.14).
- Town's view for condylar fractures as an alternative to the PA where the condyles are not easily identified.
- Lateral transcranial views of the condyles can be an alternative for visualization of the upper part of the condyle.

Midface: Follow the lines known as the McGregor Campbell lines (cortical outlines of the orbits, nose

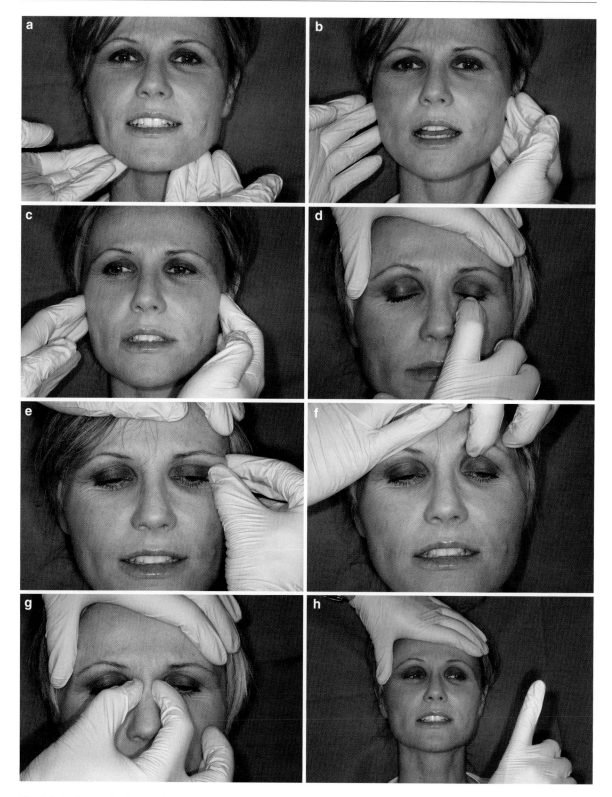

Fig. 3.9 Basic steps in the examination of the traumatized face. A pattern of examination should be developed by each practitioner to cover all aspects described in the text

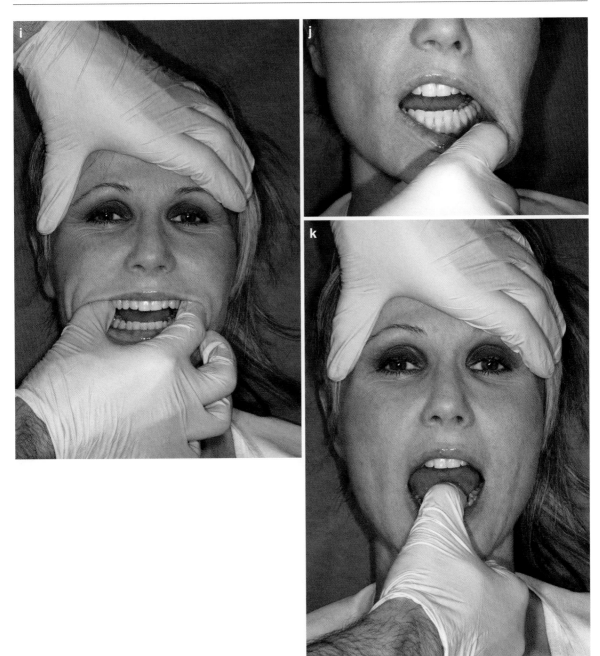

Fig. 3.9 (continued)

maxillary sinuses, maxilla, and mandible), observe for partial or total obliteration of the paranasal sinuses as well as fluid-air levels.

- Occipitomental views (also called Waters view) angulated at 15° and 30° reduces overlap of the skull base with the fields of interest. In this view,

the skull base is moved to overlap the mandibular region.

- For nasal fractures, additional lateral views are indicated (in addition to the occipitomental view).

- For frontal fractures, a lateral skull view is additionally indicated.

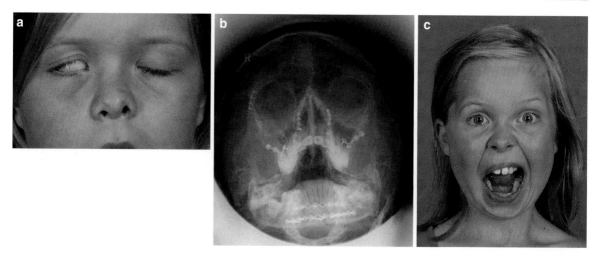

Fig. 3.10 A 9-year-old child with facial nerve paralysis after multiple facial fractures, including a skull base fracture with the postoperative picture in the *middle* and two years post injury on the *right*, showing good recovery

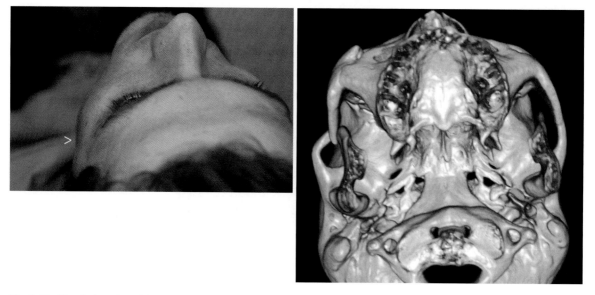

Fig. 3.11 Clear indentation of the *left* zygomatic arch area with on the *right* a 3D reconstruction demonstrating the fracture that also extends well into the body of the zygoma

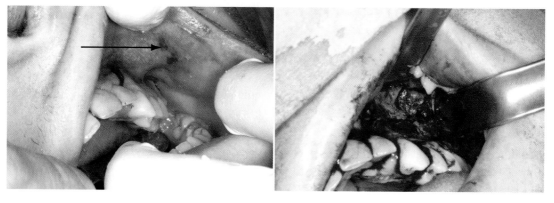

Fig. 3.12 A laceration in the left upper vestibule with slight ecchymosis shown on the *left* and displacement of the dental segment including the canine medially. The intraoperative picture of this large dentoalveolar segment on the *right*

Fig. 3.13 (**a**)
Orthopantomogram with
fracture lines indicated
and (**b**) PA mandible
(remnont of previous internal
wire fixation visible)

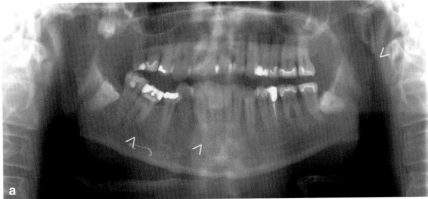

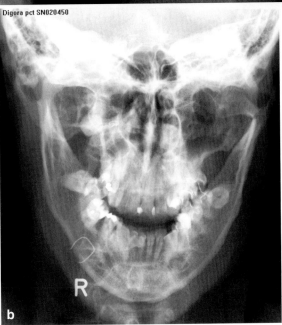

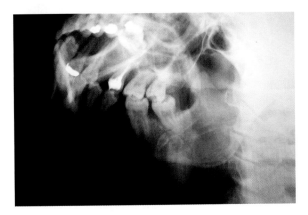

Fig. 3.14 Oblique lateral view of the mandible as an alternative
to the orthopantomogram in demonstrating a mandibular angle
fracture

3.6 Mandibular Fractures

Mandibular fractures can be classified according to the
anatomical site, fracture pattern, fracture displacement, involvement of teeth, and whether it is an open
or closed fracture.

3.6.1 Classification

The classification of fractures has the purpose of communication as well as being a guide to treatment and is
of special value in fractures of the mandible. As a general rule, usually two or more fractures of the mandible
are present.

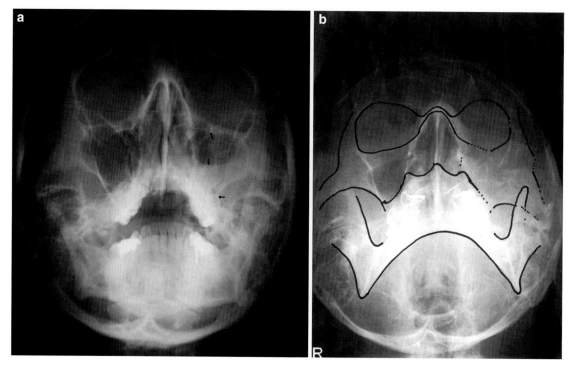

Fig. 3.15 (a) Waters view with fractures of a fractured left zygoma fracture and air–fluid meniscus visible. (b) Cortical lines to be followed when examining an occipitomental view of the midface. Any interruption of these lines represents a fracture, except where the normal sutures are found. Widening of a suture may also represent a fracture

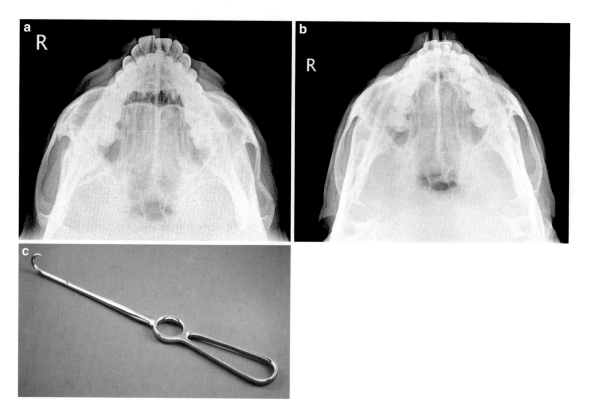

Fig. 3.16 Submento-vertex view demonstrating an isolated zygomatic arch fracture (a) pre and (b) post reduction with (c) a percutaneous hook

I. Anatomical area (site):

• Condylar (Fig. 3.22 and 3.23).

The head may be fractured on a intracapsular or extra-capsular level. Condylar neck fractures may be high, intermediate, or low condylar fractures (above, on the same level, or below the sigmoid notch)

• Symphyseal (segment including the incisal teeth)
• Parasymphyseal (segment from the canine tooth to the mental foramen)
• Body (segment from the mental foramen to the second molar)
• Angle (segment from the second molar to the angle)
• Ramus (sigmoid notch to the inferior border of the mandible) (Figs. 3.17 and 3.18)

II. Pattern

• Simple
• Comminuted (Fig. 3.19)
• Greenstick
• Tissue loss
• Open (all fractures involving full or partial erupted teeth are regarded as open) or closed.
• Pathologic

III. Fracture displacement

Favorable or unfavorable, depending on the fracture line, and resultant possible muscular displacement of fragments may be present. In a favorable fracture, the muscles of mastication would pull the posterior fragment into contact with the opposite, mostly the anterior fragment and thus preventing significant displacement. In an unfavorable fracture, the muscles of mastication would displace the posterior fragment past the anterior segment due to the unfavorable fracture line. This can be evident in the horizontal (Masseter and Temporalis muscle pull) as well as the vertical planes (Medial Pterygoid muscle) (Fig. 3.20).

IV. Involvement of teeth

• Teeth usable (stable with a usable amount of crown left) for reduction or stabilization on both sides of fracture (Class I).
• Teeth usable for reduction or stabilization on one side of the fracture (Class II).
• No teeth or unusable teeth for reduction or stabilization on either side of the fracture (Class III).
• Impacted or unerupted teeth may be in the fracture line, and may sometimes require removal. Impacted

third molars or the recent removal thereof adds to the risk of developing an angular fracture.

• In the mid mixed dentition state (age range 8–13), there may be unerupted, developing teeth in the fracture line. These teeth should be left undisturbed if they do not complicate fracture reduction.

V. Open or closed

• All fractures involving full or partial erupted teeth should be considered as open.
• An open fracture does not, unless it is severely soiled, necessarily lead to a higher incidence of infection if adequately treated from the start. This is mainly due to the excellent direct as well as collateral blood supply in the head and neck area, compared to the extremities.

3.6.2 Symptoms

• Patients may complain that their teeth do not fit as before and that they sense loose teeth.
• They often note numbness of the lower lip, chin, teeth, and gum area as well as bleeding.
• Pain on mouth opening, closing, eating, or clenching.
• Crepitations felt when moving the lower jaw or attempting to chew something.

3.6.3 Signs: (Discussed Before, but Summarized Here as Well)

• Teeth do not fit into their normal position (malocclusion). With unilateral condylar fractures, premature occlusion (contact) due to loss of vertical height as well as a deviation on mouth opening is to be found towards the side of the fracture (Fig. 3.21).
• Bleeding from fracture line that may be excessive if the inferior alveolar artery that accompanies the namesake nerve is severed.
• Spaces between teeth representing the fracture line but may also be misinterpreted as a missing tooth or teeth.
• Mobile segments with possible crepitation.
• Pain on palpation over the fracture line.

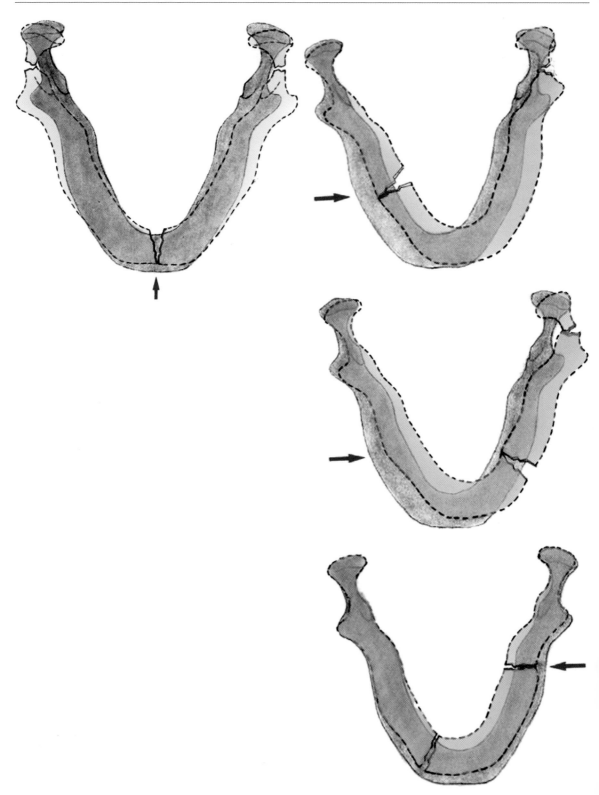

Fig. 3.17 *Left*: Symphysis fracture (coup injury) at point of impact combined with condylar neck fractures due to the "contre-coup" phenomenon. *Right*: Different fracture patterns due to forces from a variety of angles

Fig. 3.18 Emergency loops serving as initial stabilization until a more permanent stabilization can be performed. Preferably, the loop should be around more than one tooth from the fracture in order to prevent undue force on the teeth adjacent to the fracture line

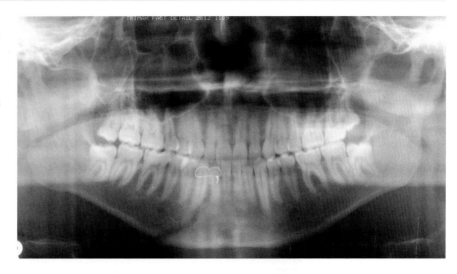

- Hypo- or anesthesia of the lower lip, chin, gingival area. Teeth on the affected side may test negative to cold or electrical stimulation.

3.6.4 Treatment

3.6.4.1 Emergency Treatment

Aim: Ensuring a patent airway, controlling bleeding, stabilizing fragments.

- Secure the airway if compromised by manually retracting the fragments or by performing an endotracheal intubation. This is mostly evident in fractures involving both sides of the mandible and with significant posterior displacement of the fragments. Ensure that there are no loose fragments or teeth that may be dislodged or aspirated.
- Excessive bleeding can often be controlled by repositioning the fragments with a wire loop around stable teeth, alternatively by clamping, bipolar cauterization, or plugging with bone wax.
- Stabilization of very mobile fractures using a wire loop around two teeth on either side of the fracture line and lightly compressing the fragments after reduction. This may significantly add to the patient's comfort.
- Temporary intermaxillary fixation (IMF) or alternatively called maxillo-mandibular fixation by IMF screws, eyelet wires, or arch bars in unstable fractures may ease the patient's discomfort (Figs. 3.24 and 3.25).

- Prescribe a broad-spectrum antibiotic, pain killers, as well as chlorhexidine mouth rinse and instruct the patient only to consume clear fluids where open fractures are present.

3.6.4.2 Definitive Treatment

Aim: Restoring full structural integrity by repositioning and stabilization of the fragments. Function includes a stable occlusion, adequate mouth opening, as well as protecting the neural integrity of the inferior alveolar nerve.

- Definitive treatment may comprise of intermaxillary fixation (if the dentition allows it) in suitable and uncomplicated cases for a period as long as six weeks in adults and as short as 2–3 weeks in children. Open reduction and internal fixation with plates and screws can however be regarded as the current standard of care in all suitable cases (Figs. 3.26 – 3.29).
- Impressions of the upper and lower jaw dentition often assist in determining the correct occlusion in complicated cases and may also be performed for medicolegal reasons.
- Surgical treatment involves the following:
- Surgical exposure of the fractures.
- Intermaxillary (maxillo-mandibular) fixation to aid in the reduction of the fractures as well as restoring the occlusion. In edentulous or partially edentulous patients, the prostheses may be used and should always accompany the patient, even if they are fractured.

Fig. 3.19 Comminuted fracture of the mandible (**a** and **b**) pre- and postconservative treatment with circum mandibular wiring and intermaxillary fixation (**c**). This fracture could be classified as closed, unfavorable, class I, comminuted in the region of the mandibular body. (**d**) Good healing 8 weeks post trauma

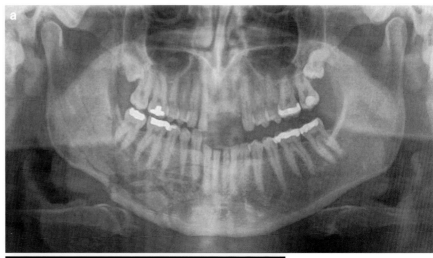

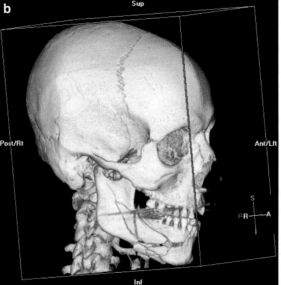

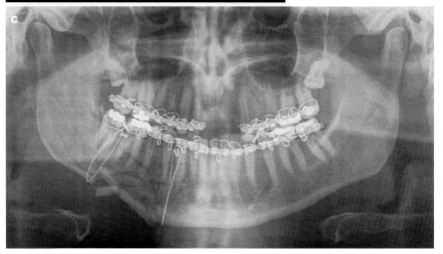

Fig. 3.19 (continued)

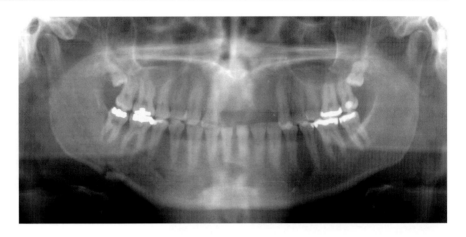

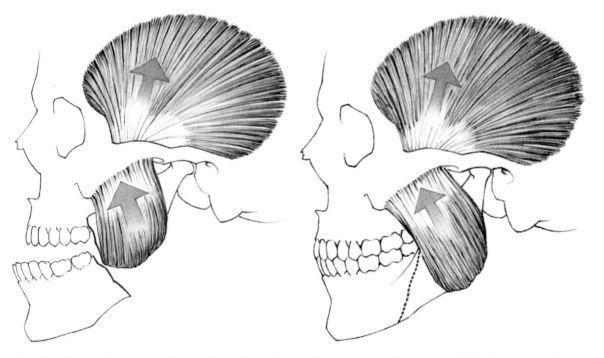

Fig. 3.20 Diagram demonstrating forces and mandibular fracture characteristics on displacement with the fracture allowing displacement on the *left* (unfavorable), but not on the *right* (favorable)

- Reduction of the fracture with repositioning clamps.
- Fixating the fractures with plates and screws or in appropriate cases with lag screws in a rigid or semi-rigid manner.
- Controlling the occlusion
- Soft tissue repositioning and suturing.

3.6.5 Exceptions and Controversies

- How soon should a fracture be treated? As a golden rule, as soon as possible, but fractures accompanied by significant soft tissue damage needs treatment more urgently than undisplaced fractures that may wait for up to a few days. Meticulous oral hygiene

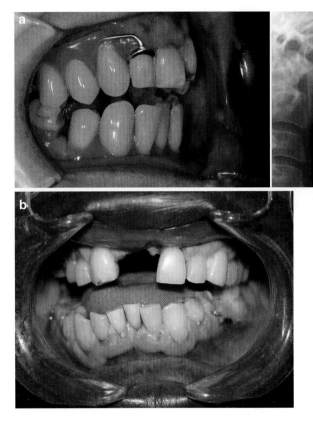

Fig. 3.21 (**a**) Disturbed occlusion on the *left* due a symphysis and bilateral condylar fractures with subsequent loss of posterior vertical height leading to an anterior open bite. The radiograph on the *right* indicating the correction by a Le Fort I osteotomy with posterior impaction. Note the large plate in the symphyseal area to control the lateral forces widening the mandible (**b**) Disturbed occlusion due to unfavorable upward rotation of the posterior mandibular segment creating a premature occlusion on the left. Note the wear facets on the mandibular incisors indicating that the mandibular teeth previously had a good working contact with the upper incisors. These facets are of great assistance for the accurate repositioning of the mandible

and antibiotic coverage is indicated in all patients with open or suspected open fractures.

- Intracapsular fractures of the condyles are important to diagnose as they may lead to ankylosis, especially in children. These fractures require no active treatment (except for a soft diet for 2–6 weeks) if the occlusion is unaffected; but when disturbed, intermaxillary fixation is required for a period of not more than 2 weeks followed by active mobilization to prevent this debilitating complication.

- Significant controversy exists regarding the treatment of condylar neck fractures. Treatment protocols range from intermaxillary fixation for 4–6 weeks in cases of disturbed occlusion to open reduction and internal fixation on virtually all cases. Access for open reduction can be either via an extraoral or intraoral or a combined route. Endoscopic assisted surgery is becoming more popular in this area. Open reduction has the benefits of restoring the patient's occlusion by correcting the vertical height and mostly eliminating intermaxillary fixation.

- Removal of teeth in the fracture line? Severely damaged teeth as well as those with root apex exposure and very mobile teeth that cannot be stabilized should be removed after the fixation as they may lead to infection.

- Immediate reconstruction of continuity defects is often recommended when feasible. The exceptions would be highly contaminated wounds and wounds holding the promise of potential vascular problems like high-velocity gunshot wounds.

- Antibiotics should be prescribed, broad-spectrum penicillin like amoxicillin or, in case of penicillin allergy, clindamycin in all open fractures, and for 24 h after surgical fixation. In contaminated wounds or where comminution is evident, a longer postoperative treatment may be indicated.

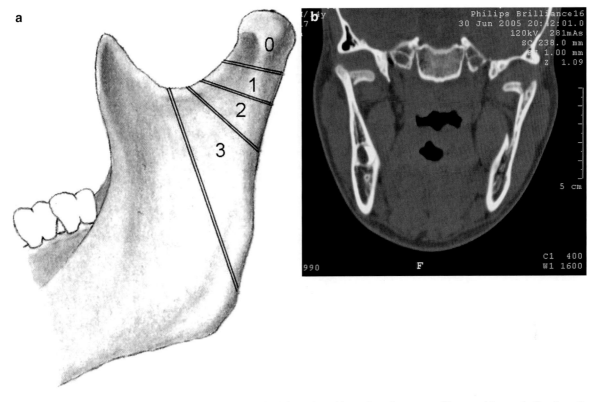

Fig. 3.22 (**a**) Different levels of condylar fractures on the left Area 0: Regarded as condylar head and is often intracapsular, Area 1: Fracture line still above the level of the sigmoid notch and difficult to treat surgically, with bilateral intracapsular fractures seen in the coronal CT picture, Area 2: Fracture line below sigmoid notch and more readily treatable surgically, Area 3: Low subcondylar fracture that is often not displaced due to the stabilizing effect of the medial pterigoid and lateral masseter musculature.(**b**) Coronal CT demonstrating bilateral intracapsular condylar fractures

3.6.6 Complications

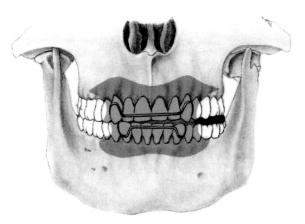

Fig. 3.23 Occlusal disturbance due to condylar fracture and vertical loss on the side of the fracture. As demonstrated, the vertical loss is overcorrected with a splint and gradually ground away to ensure a correct occlusion. This is almost exclusively performed if patients present late with a significantly disturbed occlusion and maxillo-mandibular fixation or open reduction with internal fixation will be difficult or impossible

- Infection
- Nonunion, malunion or fractured plates (Fig. 3.31).
- Disturbed occlusion
- Tooth ache or tooth loss
- Aspiration in patients with intermaxillary fixation. All patients with intermaxillary fixation should receive a wire cutter and should be instructed to cut the fixation wires as soon as they feel nauseous.
- Inferior alveolar nerve damage (hypo-, dys-, or anesthesia of the lower lip and chin area)
- Ankylosis due to prolonged immobilization especially of intracapsular condylar fractures (Fig. 3.30). Active mobilization after the chosen immobilization period is of vital importance. This may be challenging in children.

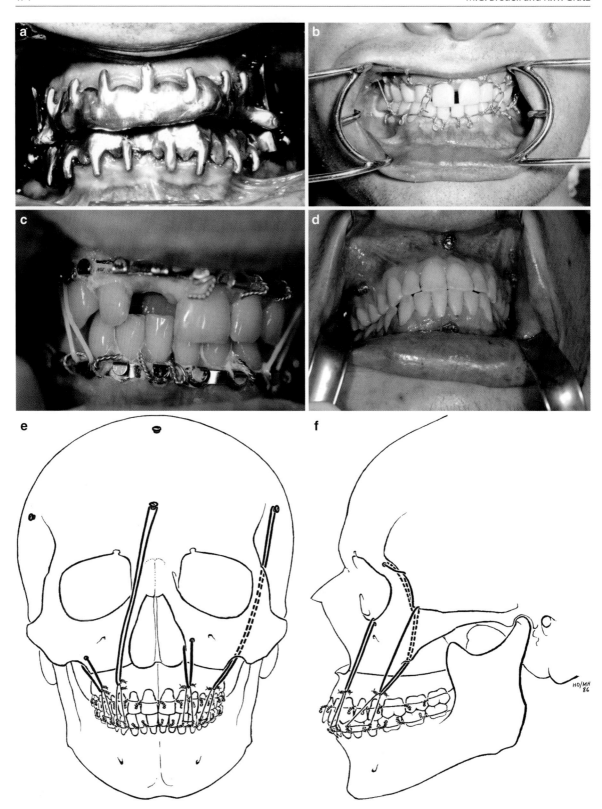

Fig. 3.24 (**a**) Silver cap splints (not commonly used anymore), (**b**) eyelets, (**c**) arch bars, (**d**) IMF screws, (**e** and **f**) wiring fixed to the piriform rim, frontal bone or zygomatic area (**g**) external fixator are all ways in which to stabilize the mandible in comminated or infected cases for instance in gunshot wounds.

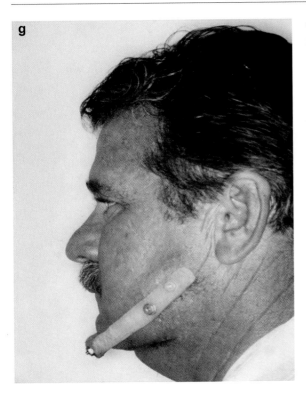

Fig. 3.24 (continued)

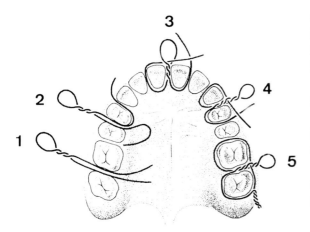

Fig. 3.25 Method of eyelet wiring demonstrated in a stepwise fashion

3.7 Midface Fractures

3.7.1 Classification

The midface may be divided into central and lateral components.

Central: Frontal sinus, nose, maxilla, medial component of the orbits.

Lateral: Zygoma as well as lateral component of the orbits.

Fractures then may classically lie within the central, lateral, or within both namely centro-lateral areas (Fig. 3.32a).

3.7.2 Maxillary Fractures

The maxilla is significantly different from the mandible as it has important fixed relations with other facial bones (zygoma, nasal bones, pterygoid plates, etc.) and contributes to facial structures like the nasal floor and maxillary sinuses.

Bone of the maxilla is much softer and thinner than that of the mandible and thus a slightly lower force is required to generate fractures, especially in older and osteoporotic patients. The maxilla is supported by facial struts or pillars (buttresses) of strengthened, thicker bone. These struts or buttresses are bilaterally located in the paranasal, zygomatico-maxillary, as well as in the more posterior pterygoid areas (Sicher and Tandler 1928).

René Le Fort described the current well-known classical facial fracture patterns after investigating the 35 cadaver skulls he subjected to various blunt forces in 1901. They represent levels of weakness in the facial bone structures.

Le Fort I: Fracture of the maxilla only, separating it from the rest of the midface.

Le Fort II: Fracture of the maxilla, running up to the infraorbital rim, then transversely to include the nasal bones.

Le Fort III: Fracture including the maxilla, zygoma, and nasal bones, the latter normally at a higher level than the Le Fort II fractures (Fig. 3.32b).

When considering these levels of weakness, it seems not to be without reason as it represents areas of energy absorption and thus has a significant role to play in the protection of the neurocranium. The honeycomb-like midface structure formed by the cortical bone buttresses and thinner bone encircling the paranasal sinuses absorbs the energy of impact and diminishes its transference to the cranium (Fig 3.32a).

In older individuals, these fracture patterns are much more common than in children due to a variety of factors. The older one gets, the more pronounced facial pneumatization becomes; second, children's bone is more elastic

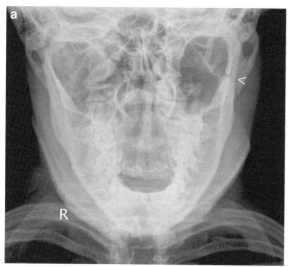

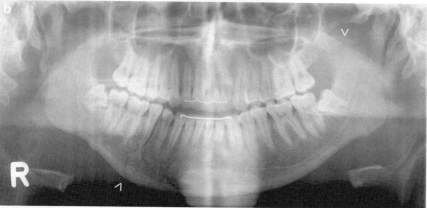

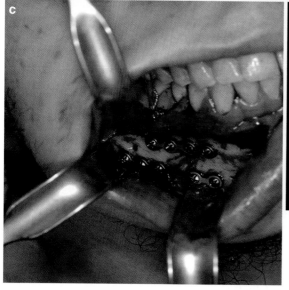

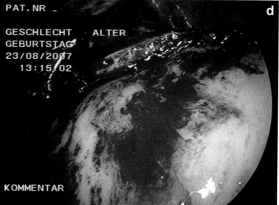

Fig. 3.26 (**a–g**) Before and after radiographs demonstrating the repositioning and fixation of facial fractures with plates and screws with a clinical picture indicating access to the mental area with preservation of the mental nerve. The left condyle was treated via an intraoral, endoscopic-assisted route

Fig. 3.26 (continued)

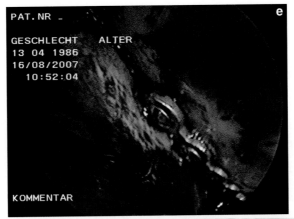

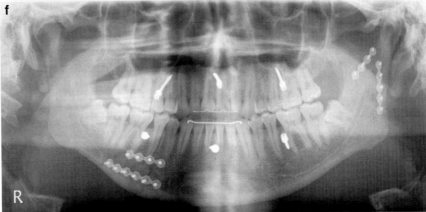

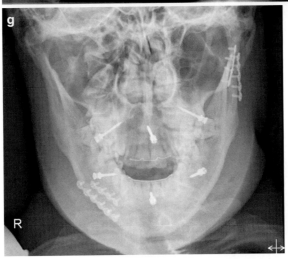

and a significant higher force is needed to cause clear fractures rather than the well-known greenstick phenomenon. A CT is the gold standard examination needed to fully grasp the extent of midfacial fractures.

In all the above cases, the maxilla may be mobile or displaced and impacted causing a disturbed occlusion with premature contact posterior, an anterior open bite. Undisplaced fractures may of course occur and usually only requires careful observation and a soft diet.

The classical Le Fort patterns of fractures do not always occur and often a combination of patterns are

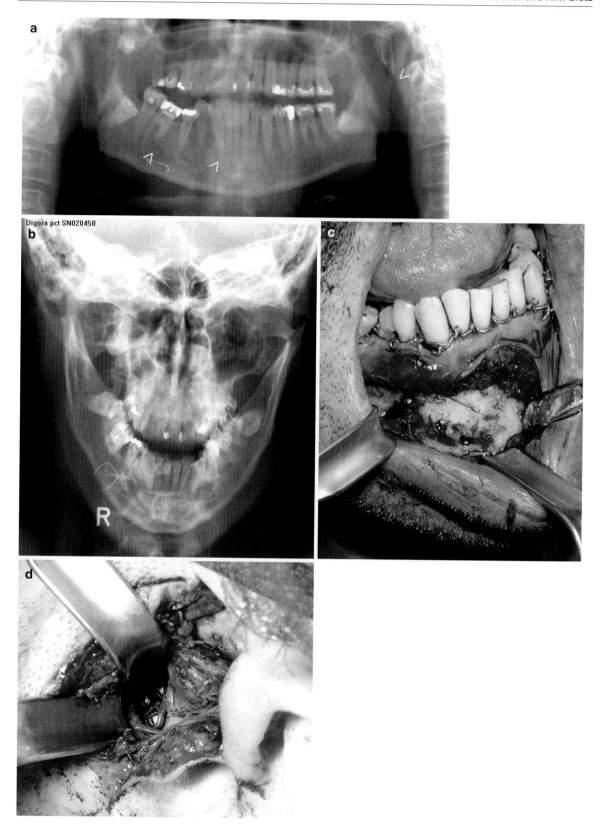

Fig. 3.27 (**a–e**) Treatment of a right mandibular sagittal fracture with lag screws. Note the simultaneous reduction and fixation of a medially dislocated condylar fracture with (**f**) showing extraoral access to the condylar area

Fig. 3.27 (continued)

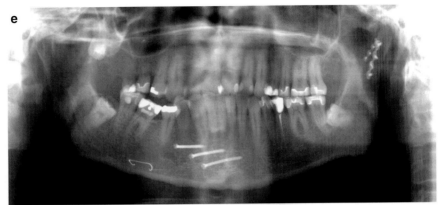

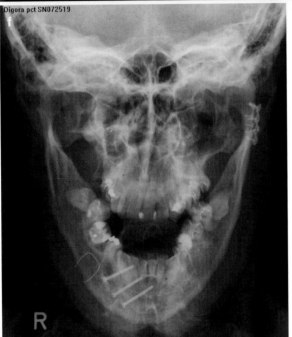

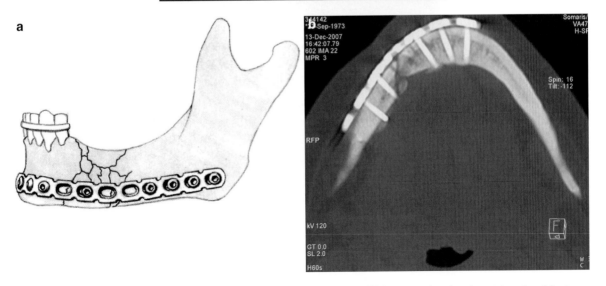

Fig. 3.28 (**a**) Bridging plate used in a comminuted fracture. (**b**) Post surgery CT demonstrating the adequately reduced fracture

Fig. 3.29 Especially challenging are treatment of the atrophied mandible fractures. (**a**) This patient was inadequately treated with small mini-plates (load sharing) instead of rigid fixation (load bearing) with a large bridging plate (**b**) with the screws placed in strong bone in the symphyseal and angle area. This is mostly done via an extraoral route, but the intraoral route is also possible in selected cases. As an alternative, an immediate rib (**c**) or iliac crest bone graft may be used. The placement of dental implants (**d**) may later be necessary as conventional dentures are seldom success after such a fracture

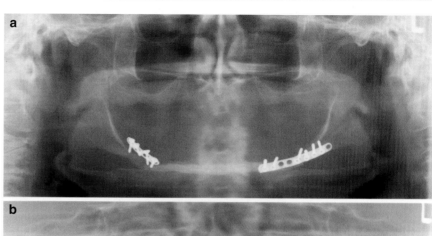

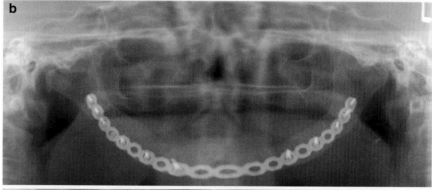

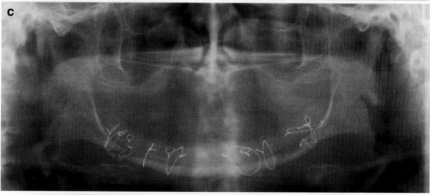

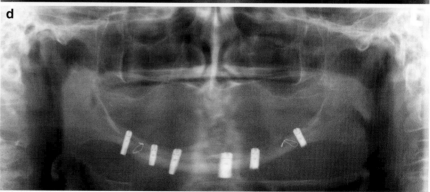

Fig. 3.30 Bilateral ankylosis in the coronoid area extending to the skull base in a patient not seeking help after a motor vehicle accident. Prolonged immobilization of coronoid and high condylar fractures may lead to ankylosis

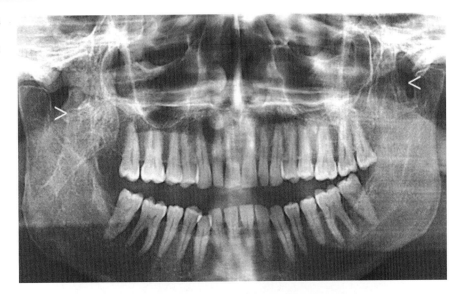

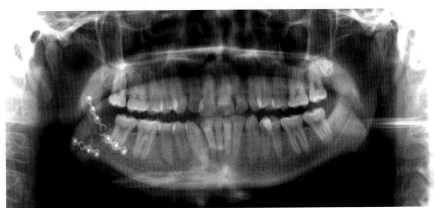

Fig. 3.31 Plate fracture due to undue chewing forces after the fixation of the fracture

present. Patients may have combined Le Fort II combined with a zygoma fracture or total comminution may be present. Sharp injuries do of course cause more localized fracture patterns with or without significant tissue loss.

3.7.2.1 Symptoms

- Patients with displaced fractures may complain that their teeth do not fit as before. (This is not always the case as much of the proprioceptive nerves have been damaged and the patient may not sense the disturbance.) Along with this, they may mention that the upper jaw teeth are loose or displaced that may in actual fact represent a mobile maxilla or segment thereof.

- They often mention a numb feeling of the cheek, nose, upper lip, gums, and teeth. (Injury of the infraorbital nerve)
- Visual disturbance is another possible complaint. This may vary from partial to total visual loss or diplopia Swelling often contributes to the complaint of visual disturbance.
- Nasal bleeding and often nasal obstruction is a common complaint.

3.7.2.2 Signs

Extraoral

- Swelling may be negligible or severe. If the patient blew his nose after the accident, he would report rapid swelling thereafter and the under the skin

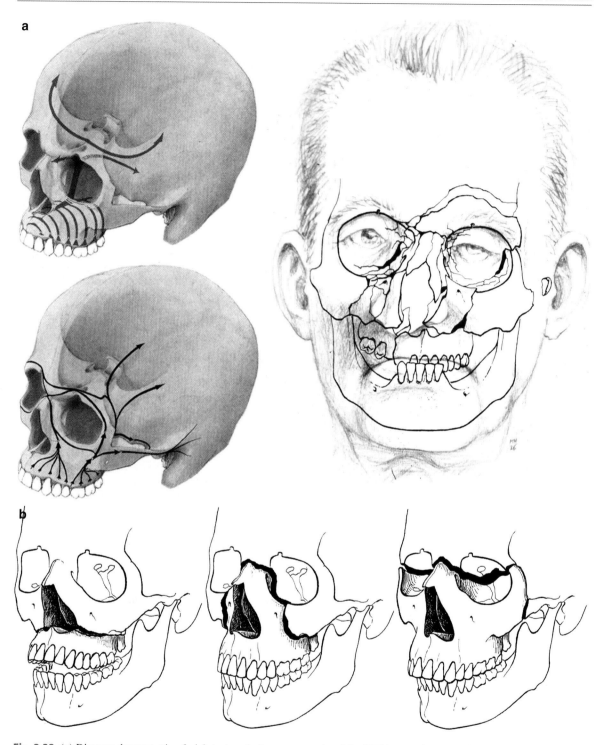

Fig. 3.32 (**a**) Diagram demonstrating facial struts or buttresses connecting the maxilla to the zygoma and skull base on the *left*. Fractures of the centro-lateral side of the left face demonstrated on the *right*. (**b**) Diagram demonstrating Le Fort I (*left*), II (*middle*), and III (*right*) fracture lines. Note the proximity of the Le Fort III fracture lines to the skull base

crepitation would be palpable due to the surgical emphysema.

- Unilocular or more often binocular periorbital hematomas, the latter more common in Le Fort II and III fractures. In all cases where involvement of the orbit is present, subconjunctival ecchymosis may be evident.
- Paresthesia or anesthesia of the infraorbital region, maxilla, nasal ala due to infraorbital nerve injury. (This would imply a fracture through the infraorbital rim or orbital floor.)
- Often, these patients present with a long face appearance due to the inferior displacement of the maxilla.
- Diplopia or disturbed eye movement. Diplopia could be uni- or bi-ocular. Uni-ocular diplopia is mostly due to lens displacement or retinal detachment. Bi-ocular displacement is mostly due to incoherent movement and different focal points. The region of diplopia should be noted. The most common diplopia is of a vertical nature due to the entrapment of the inferior rectus muscle or more commonly the perimuscular/periorbital fat.
- With impacted midface or naso-ethmoidal fractures, the nasal tip may point upward and the face will have a concave appearance laterally. Most of these patients also present with an anterior open bite. (Dish face appearance)
- Nasal deviation may be present. The nasal septum should be examined for signs of a septal hematoma.
- Steps may be palpable around the orbital rim, zygoma, and nose.
- Increased intercanthal distance may be present in isoloted naso-ethmoidal or complex midface fractures, often with accompanying epiphora. On palpation of the medial canthal area, one may be able to compress the underlying fragments and decrease the intercanthal distance. One may be able to grasp the medial or lateral canthal tissues with an instrument and displace these tissues from the underlying bony structures, confirming rupture of the ligament or fracturing of the bony attachments (Figs. 3.33–3.35).

Intraoral

- Disturbed occlusion is mostly present where the maxilla is displaced, often seen as a premature posterior occlusion presenting with an anterior open bite.

- Mobile maxilla (not necessarily in impacted cases) with bony crepitations felt during the mobilization.
- Limited mouth opening may be present. This may be relative, due to the downward displacement of the maxilla or absolute due to mechanical obstruction, mostly the medial displacement of a fractured zygoma arch.
- Steps palpable as well as hematoma visible in the vestibular area.
- The maxilla may be divided in one or more fragments. This may be associated with soft tissue tears, especially in the midpalatinal region.
- Loose teeth or fragments of teeth with bone (dentoalveolar) (Fig. 3.36) may be present and should be stabilized or removed when an imminent risk of aspiration is present.
- Bleeding into the nasopharynx and eventually into the oropharynx may be present and be visible. Significant blood loss can be hidden in this way and induce patients to vomit due to gastric irritation.

3.7.2.3 Treatment

Emergency Treatment

Aim: To ensure a safe and adequate airway and temporarily stabilize the fractures.

- Resuscitation as discussed before.
- Airway may be compromised and needs to be secured (Fig. 3.39). Care must be taken to remove or fix mobile teeth or fragments as well as dentures from the airway before potential intubation. Lost teeth may be kept in a Ringers solution and re-implanted as soon as possible, preferably within an hour.
- When intubation of a patient with Le Fort II or III or suspected anterior skull base fractures is being considered, oral intubation is the preferred route due to the risk of intracranial penetration. Orogastric tubes are also preferred to nasogastric tubes.
- If the maxilla is very mobile with associated discomfort intermaxillary fixation may be considered. A simple way of achieving the same goal is by applying a bandage around the head and under the chin, pulling the mandible against the maxilla and toward the skull base.
- Nasal bleeding may be excessive and may be controlled by manually repositioning the maxilla with a

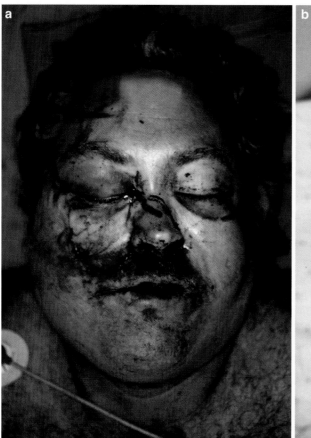 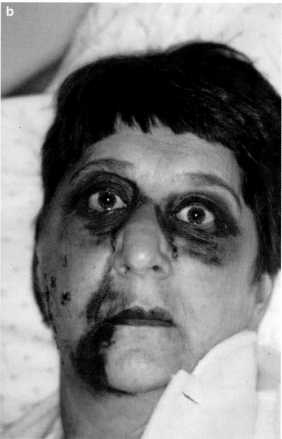

Fig. 3.33 Characteristic features of patients with midface fractures. Both patients presented with in essence the same fracture pattern, but the force required to create such fracture is much less in the older women (a) than in the young man (b) on the right who was exposed to significantly higher force and thus sustained other injuries as well. Note in both cases the periorbital hematomas indicating nasal or more probably skull base involvement

circular head bandage as described before. When no positive result is achieved, anterior packing with gauze or sponges may be impregnated with tranexamic acid. Anterior and posterior packing may be combined in more resistant cases and when nothing else helps interventional radiology may be performed with embolization (Figs. 3.37 and 3.38).

- Posterior packing is achieved by carefully placing a Foley's catheter (14 Fr) through the nose, visualizing it in the oropharynx, inflating the balloon with more or less 15 cc of saline, retracting the catheter back and thereby obstructing the posterior part of the nasopharynx. Anterior packing with hemostatic gauze is performed while lightly pull-

ing on the catheter. Maintaining the tension on the catheter is important and a plaster wound around the catheter or fixing the catheters to each other will prevent posterior dislodgement. Pressure in the cuff should be released at least partially within 24 h to prevent pressure associated necrosis of the mucosa. Once there has been no bleeding for at least 12 h after deflation, the catheters can carefully be removed.

- Instructions should be given to the patient to refrain from blowing his or her nose or to sneeze with an open mouth without obstructing the nose. Xylometazoline nasal spray or an alternative may be helpful to decongest the nose.

Definitive Treatment

Aim: To reconstruct the midface in all three dimensions and restore the patient with a functional occlusion.

- Definitive treatment of midface fractures may be delayed by up to 10 days if there is no emergency work to be done. This often allows swelling to subside and allows easier access to the fractures as well as better judgment of for instance the eye position and intraoperative changes. Where lacerations exist, which may aid in the facial reconstruction, reduction and fixation of the fractures may be performed through the lacerations and may prompt more immediate treatment.
- Approaches have changed during the past years with plates and screws enabling the surgeon to move the emphasis from the restoration of the occlusion to the complete restoration of the facial contours including the ocular position, while not forgetting the occlusion. With the previously used wire suspension techniques, this was not possible (Figs. 3.40 and 3.41).
- Addressing the central part of the face first and then working to the lateral structures like the zygoma has become popular. Starting by addressing the most stable and easily repositionable points

is a good way to start and act as a guide to the rest of the face.
- Coronal access has made the symmetrical reconstruction of the face more feasible. It also allows for the correct anterior–posterior positioning of the face by starting the reconstruction from the often more stable skull bones like the root of the zygoma and frontal bones.
- Accurate repositioning of the nasal bones is important, especially the fragments with the medial canthal ligaments attached. When this cannot be done, attachment of the ligament to the opposite side or to a well-positioned mini-plate is indicated.
- The use of navigation in more complicated cases has made a significant contribution to the more predictable outcome. This involves using the DICOM CT data set and mirroring the uninjured side of the face to the fractured side and using it as an intraoperative guide. Where both sides were fractured, the least affected side can be reconstructed first, scanning the patient thereafter and then using the reconstructed side as a template for further reconstructive efforts (Fig 3.41).
- The first attempt at reconstruction is the most important and every effort should be made to ensure the best possible outcome. All later attempts are merely a compromise to a lost opportunity.

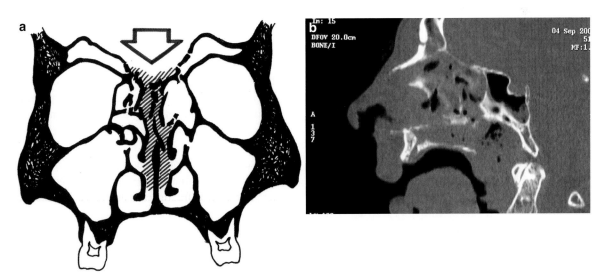

Fig. 3.34 (**a**) Area of possible cerebrospinal fluid leak through the ethmoid- and sphenoid sinus areas. In (**b**) a sagittal CT view of the anterior cranial fossa with fractures that may lead to a cerebrospinal fluid leak

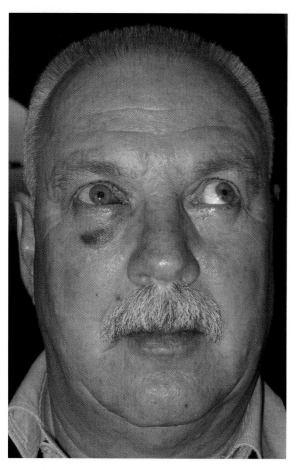

Fig. 3.35 Inhibited right eye mobility elevation due to muscular or periorbital tissue entrapment

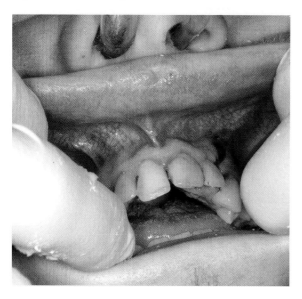

Fig. 3.36 Large dentoalveolar fracture of the left maxilla with displacement. This segment is moveable with figure pressure

3.7.2.4 Exceptions and Controversies

- Swelling may vary from patient to patient and may not be as conspicuous as expected.
- In all cases where there is comminution of the zygoma area (in Le Fort III or pure zygoma fractures) that prohibits accurate reconstruction through local incisions, a coronal access is mandatory to enable three-dimensional reconstruction of the facial skeleton.
- Removal of plates and screw fixation is not universally advocated, but should probably be performed in young patients, areas of prominence, and in colder countries where patients may complain of the temperature difference between soft tissues and the metal.
- Use of resorbable plates and screws are gaining popularity, especially in the pediatric population, but can be used in many adult midface fractures; however, there is a steep learning curve in optimal application and use of the material (Fig. 3.42a and b).

3.7.2.5 Complications

- The impacted midface may appear to be nonmobile and merely a patient with a disturbed occlusion, mostly an anterior open bite. This apparent stable situation can be overseen and later recognized. Late reconstructive attempts in this scenario remain challenging.
- Surgical emphysema may develop pre- and postoperatively in patients blowing their nose or sneezing with an occluded nose before or within 10 days after treatment.
- In cases of severe comminution and possible tissue loss, accurate reconstruction may be difficult and secondary reconstruction may be needed, although the primary reconstruction remains the most important effort.
- Immediate bone grafting should be employed where needed.
- Late reconstruction of the medial canthal position is always more challenging than at the first attempt. This highly unsightly defect is immediately noticeable (Figs. 3.42 and 3.43).

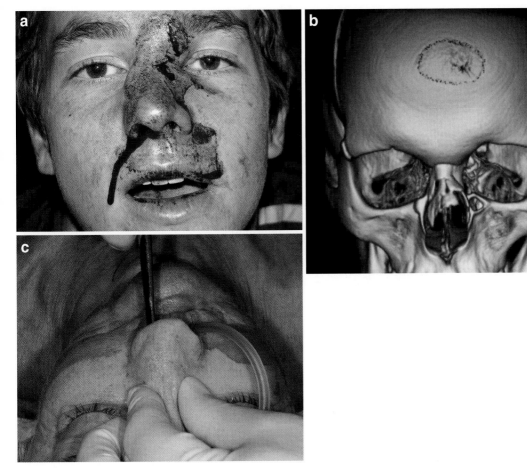

Fig. 3.37 (**a**) Isolated nasal fracture due to a hockey injury. (**b**) 3D CT reconstruction demonstrating the fractures. (**c**) After manual repositioning, a nasal splint is used for stabilization

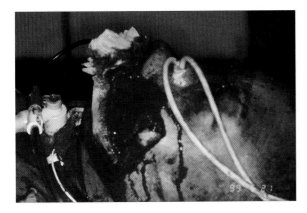

Fig. 3.38 Severe facial fractures with difficult controllable bleeding from the nasoethmoid and nasopharyngeal areas provisionally arrested with anterior and posterior packing. Embolization was required to further control the bleeding

3.7.3 *Zygoma and Orbital Wall Fractures*

Although the zygoma has been described partially in the previous section of midface fractures, it most often presents as an isolated fracture and deserves more of our attention. These fractures are often caused by more localized forces from either a lateral, anterior, and anterolateral direction.

These fractures may be subclassified as follows:

- Zygoma fracture
- Isolated zygomatic arch fracture
- Isolated wall fractures (Floor, medial wall, roof or lateral wall, or a combination thereof)

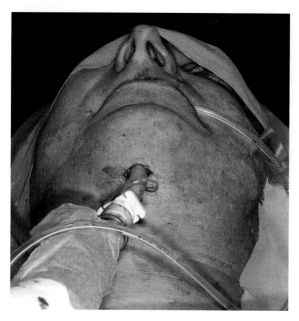

Fig. 3.39 Submental intubation where the nasal as well as the oral route is not desirable, but patient does not need tracheotomy

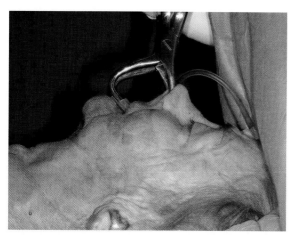

Fig. 3.40 Rowe's repositioning forceps are still used for the mobilization of the impacted midface structures

The zygoma contributes to two of the walls of the orbit and also shapes the anterolateral and lateral part of the face. If a patient sustains a zygoma fracture, there per definition has to be fractures in the frontozygomatic suture area, zygomaticotemporal suture area, as well as in the zygomaticomaxillary suture area; and this explains the commonly used term, tripod fracture.

3.7.3.1 Zygoma

Symptoms and Signs

- Paresthesia or anesthesia involving the infraorbital nerve distribution of the upper maxillary gingival tissues and teeth, cheek, upper lip, as well as lateral part of the nose.
- Nasal bleeding.
- Subconjunctival ecchymosis.
- Limited mouth opening due to the mechanical obstruction of the coronoid process (Fig. 3.47) or due to pressure of the fractured arch on the temporalis muscle.
- Swelling over the involved side with worsening if the patient blew his or her nose resulting in surgical emphysema.
- Displacement of the eye (enophthalmos, hypoglobus, or exophthalmos) and or the entrapment of eye musculature or periorbital fat in the fractured components resulting in restricted eye movement and often (Fig. 3.45 a).
- Possible flattening of the involved side that may only become evident 7–10 days after the trauma. The zygoma displacement may be significant due to inferior pull of the Masseter muscle attached to the arch and part of the body (Fig. 3.46 b).
- Palpable steps or crepitation in the infraorbital (superior portion of the zygomaticomaxillary suture), lateral orbital (frontozygomatic suture), zygomatic arch, or intraorally in the vestibulum of the affected side (zygomaticomaxillary suture).
- Pain on medial pressure on the zygoma as well as on the possible fracture lines.

Diagnosis

Of course, the diagnosis is clinical, but the gold standard today is the CT in both the coronal and axial planes.

Alternatives are the Occipitomental views (also called Waters view) angulated at 15 and 30 degrees and the Submento-vertex view or Town's view to demonstrate the zygomatic arches (Figs. 3.15 and 3.16).

Emergency Treatment

Aim: To manage the acute symptoms.

- Instruct the patient not to blow his or her nose or to sneeze with an open mouth.
- Nasal bleeding (Fig. 3.46) is normally easily controlled by local measures as previously described.
- Nasal decongestants containing phenylephrine and sprays containing oxymethazoline may be helpful in improving airflow through the congested nose.
- Antibiotics, like broad-spectrum penicillin, should be prescribed in cases where there is significant involvement of the maxillary sinus, surgical emphysema, or open fractures.
- A thorough ophthalmological consult is needed when there is any disturbed vision, diplopia, or signs of ocular injury.
- Swelling may be contained by cooling and maintaining a semi-upright position in bed.

Definitive Treatment

- Surgery may be delayed until most of the swelling has subsided, which may last up to a week.
- Undisplaced fractures do not require treatment.
- Isolated zygomatic arch fractures may be treated by elevating the fracture via a trans-temporal approach or via a trans-oral approach. Other alternatives would be elevation by placing a sharp hook transcutaneously.
- Fractures of the zygomatic body may also be treated only by elevation as described above, but may need to be stabilized with plates and screws. This is achieved either via an intraoral access, in the fronto-zygomatic area as well as the infraorbital area via small cutaneous or possibly transconjunctival access reaching the infraorbital area. Not all three areas have to be stabilized, but all three areas should be accessed to ensure accurate reduction. Where there is comminution, accurate three-dimensional

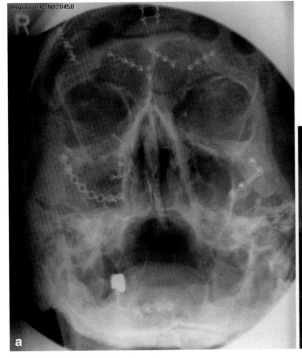
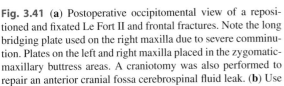
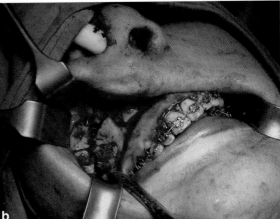

Fig. 3.41 (**a**) Postoperative occipitomental view of a repositioned and fixated Le Fort II and frontal fractures. Note the long bridging plate used on the right maxilla due to severe comminution. Plates on the left and right maxilla placed in the zygomatic-maxillary buttress areas. A craniotomy was also performed to repair an anterior cranial fossa cerebrospinal fluid leak. (**b**) Use of resorbable plates in a Le Fort I osteotomy can likewise be used in midface fractures. (**c**) Intraoperative navigation to determine if the reconstructed segments are in the correct position. Note the overcorrection at the first attempt. The green line indicates the planned postion

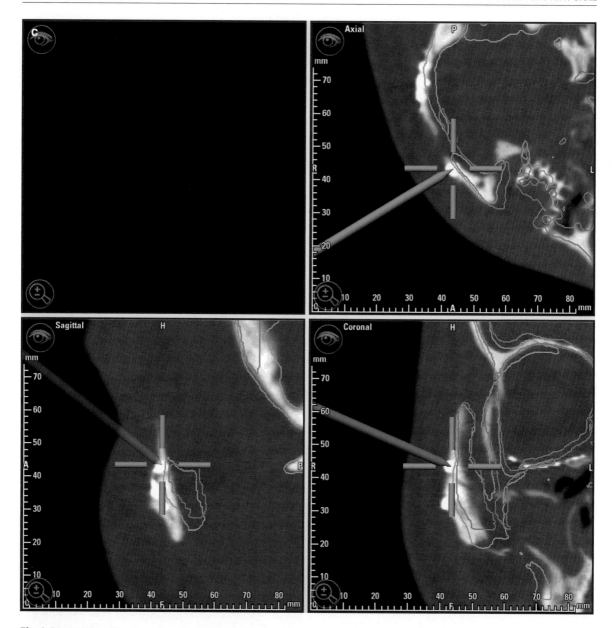

Fig. 3.41 (continued)

reposition may be difficult and reduction and fixation via a coronal access may be indicated, often in combination with navigation when available.

- It is imperative to access the orbital walls, especially the orbital floor before surgery (most common by evaluating the CT) to determine if reduction or reconstruction of the walls may have to be done simultaneously.

Exceptions and Controversies

- Accurate three-dimensional repositioning of the zygoma is imperative to get a good postoperative result. Mostly but not always, control of at least three of the fracture lines will be needed.
- Routine inspection of the orbital floor is not necessary and is only indicated in patients with ocular

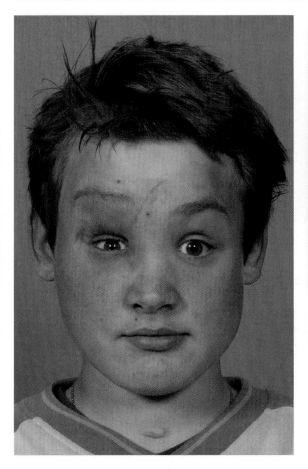

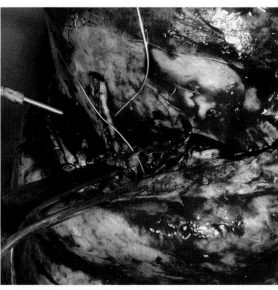

Fig. 3.43 Process of canthal reconstruction with a canthal suspension wire using the plate as stabilization and preventing migration through the bone

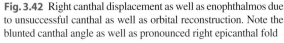

Fig. 3.42 Right canthal displacement as well as enophthalmos due to unsuccessful canthal as well as orbital reconstruction. Note the blunted canthal angle as well as pronounced right epicanthal fold

symptoms or where significant comminution or displacement is evident on the preoperative CT.

• Late orbital correction is always difficult even with the help of navigation tools. Every attempt should be made to obtain optimal restoration of the anatomy at the first intervention.

3.7.3.2 Orbital Wall

Of the four orbital walls, fractures of the floor are the most common. The medial wall is involved second most and fractures of the lateral wall and roof follows. Usually, these fractures are in combination with other facial fractures, but may be isolated when blunt trauma of the orbit occurs as for instance a ball or a fist hitting the front of the orbit and thus creating increased intraorbital pressure resulting in the thinnest wall or walls to give way (Fig. 3.48).

Symptoms and Signs

• Diplopia, possible enophthalmos, as well as limited eye movement may be present.
• Limited eye movement may be the result of entrapment of one of the extraocular muscles, mostly the inferior rectus muscle or the periorbital fat that will also restrict eye movement.

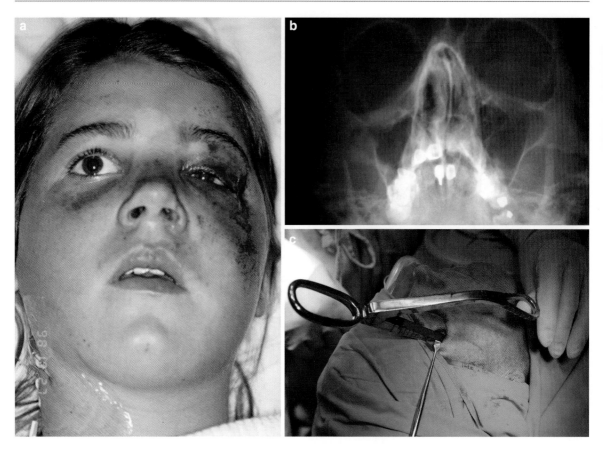

Fig. 3.44 (**a**) Clinical picture of a young girl with a left zygoma fracture. (**b**) A patient with a clear fracture of the right zygoma on the radiograph, (**c**) note the disimpaction of the fracture achieved via the right frontozygomatic (instead of the usual temporal) approach with a Rowe's elevator. After disimpaction, fixation with plates and screws was performed

- Subconjunctival ecchymosis is a common sign.
- Because of swelling or intraorbital air, the eye may be supported and enophthalmos and even diplopia may develop gradually.
- Paresthesia and anesthesia may be present in the infraorbital nerve distribution area.
- Many patients demonstrate large wall fractures without any or very minor symptoms. This may be due to the intact or partially intact periorbita as well as globe-supporting structures like Lockwood's ligament.
- Direct impact on the globe may lead to potential intraocular injuries. The most common of these is the so-called traumatic mydriasis due to paralysis of the ciliary muscle. Other common injuries are iris tears, hyphema, retinal detachment, vitreous bleeding, and damage to the optic nerve. All of these injuries would in most centers indicate the need for the involvement of an ophthalmologist.
- Ptosis may be present in a small number of patients due to direct injury to the levator palpabraae superioris muscle or ligament, injury to the third cranial nerve innervation, or directly to the superior tarsal muscle also known as Muller's muscle or its sympathetic innervation. Injury to the cervical or thoracic sympathetic trunk will lead to Horner's syndrome.
- Superior orbital fissure syndrome that develops due to pressure of fractured fragments on the superior orbital fissure may lead to ophthalmoplegia,

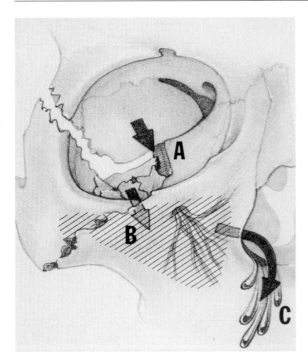

Fig. 3.45 Diagram showing the resultant bleeding in the maxillary sinus with drainage to the nasal passage. Note the potential damage to the infraorbital nerve and understandable resultant sensory disturbance

diplopia, ptosis, as well as exophthalmos (Figs. 3.49, 3.50, 3.51 and 3.53).

Diagnosis

- Clinical diagnosis is supported by a CT both in the axial and coronal planes. If not possible, an occipitomental (Water's) view should be performed where a teardrop shape protruding into the maxillary sinus is indicative of a floor fracture. There may be significant bleeding in the maxillary sinus, leaving it obliterated and making assessment difficult.
- The opinion of an ophthalmologist would usually be sought to assess the enophthalmos and calculate it with the aid of Hertel's exophthalmometry.

- Late enophthalmos may only become evident after 2–3 weeks and thus careful follow-up of patients for this period is recommended.

3.7.3.2.3 Treatment

Aim: Preventing long-standing functional problems like enophthalmos and ensuring an optimal aesthetic result.

- As with zygoma fractures, treatment is usually not urgent unless clear entrapment with strangulation is evident.
- Indications for surgery are enophthalmos of 2 mm or more and unresolving diplopia.
- Transconjunctival or transcutaneous (infraorbital or subcilliary) access is mostly used and the orbital wall is reconstructed with release of all the entrapped tissues.
- Access to the (Fig. 3.52) medial wall may be achieved via the orbital floor access or if needed via a transcaruncular incision. Coronal access as well as a medial cutaneous (Lynch) incision may also be used. The materials used may vary from titanium mesh, to outer table of the skull to resorbable materials for instance PDS foil (Fig. 3.58).
- Accurate reconstruction of the S-shaped orbital floor as seen in a sagittal plane is mandatory to achieve a good functional and aesthetic result.
- Placement of a specially shaped balloon in the maxillary sinus to elevate the floor is also used in some units.
- Endoscopic repair of the medial orbital wall is also becoming more and more popular and may indeed be a more conservative approach for some fractures (Figs. 3.54–3.56).

Complications

- The most feared early complication involving the orbits is the development of a retrobulbar hematoma. This, as the name implies, is bleeding behind the bulbus with possible dire consequences for the

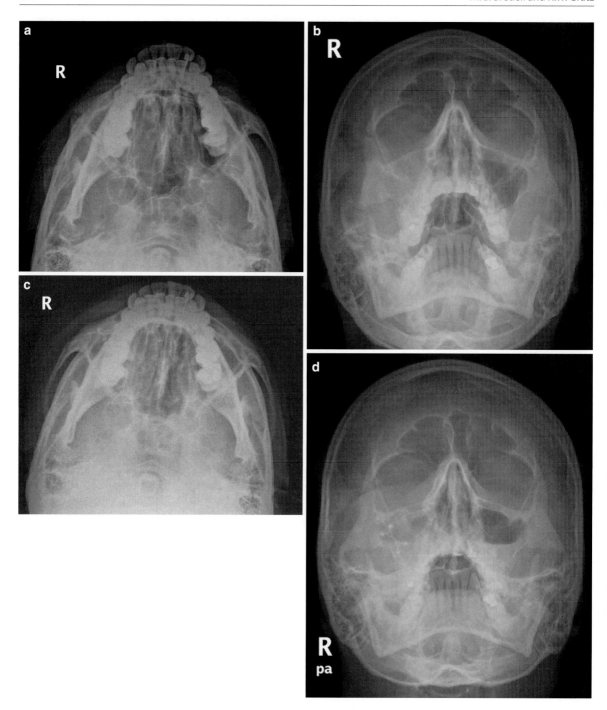

Fig. 3.46 (**a** and **b**) Preoperative X-rays of a patient with a right-sided zygoma fracture. Note the amount of displacement. This patient will have limited mouth opening due to mechanical obstruction of the coronoid process. (**c** and **d**) Postoperative view of a well-repositioned and fixed zygoma fracture with one plate on the zygoma-maxillary buttress

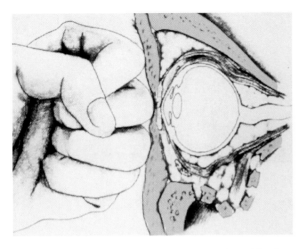

Fig. 3.47 Presssure on the orbital contents and resulting in a fracture of the orbital floor

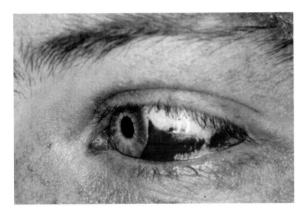

Fig. 3.48 Classic subconjunctival bleeding seen in most patients with fractures involving the orbital wall

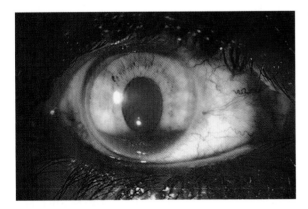

Fig. 3.49 Hyphema due to injury to the globe

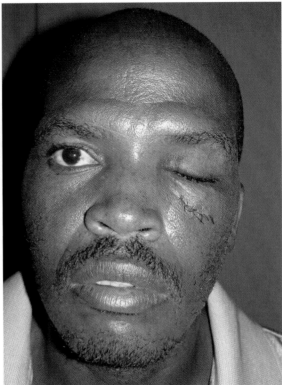

Fig. 3.50 Posttrauma ptosis due to direct injury to the levator palpebrae superior muscle

optic nerve. Patients present with progressive proptosis, ophthalmoplegia, as well as loss of vision. Immediate action is needed and in rapidly progressive cases immediate drainage and high doses of steroids (e.g., dexamethasone 8 mg) are necessary. In slower, progressive cases, an MRI may be helpful in establishing the diagnosis.

- If the orbital roof is involved, cerebrospinal fluid may leak into the orbit and periorbital tissues causing upper lid swelling and possible proptosis.
- Careless surgery may lead to muscular entrapment and damage to ocular structures.
- The infraorbital or transconjunctival access may lead to entropion or ectropion (Fig. 3.57).

Exceptions and Controversies

- There is much debate regarding the ideal material for orbital wall reconstruction; however, the most important prerequisites remain the accurate

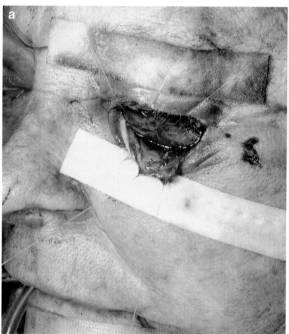
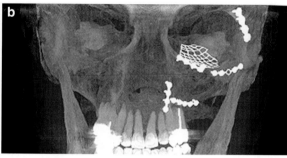

Fig. 3.51 (**a**) Inferior transconjunctival access combined with lateral canthotomy on the left to improve orbital floor, medial wall, and rim access. (**b**) The postoperative X-ray in this patient with a combined zygoma as well as orbital floor fracture

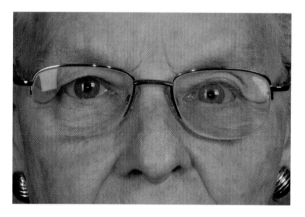

Fig. 3.52 Patient with persistent diplopia after facial fractures treated with a prism lens on the left

anatomical reconstruction with a material that will maintain dimensional stability for a long enough time. Autogenous as well as autologous bone, resorbable material, titanium mesh, or repositioning balloon catheters have all been described to be used with success.

• Timing of surgery depends on the amount of swelling and is best delayed until the eyelids can open easily and the globe position can be judged intraop-

eratively. Best results are achieved within the first 2 weeks after injury, but delayed surgery is possible in cases of late diagnosis or due to other circumstances. With very late presentation, surgery may then just as well be delayed for 6 months, allowing for the maturation of intraorbital scar tissue and less complicated surgery.

– Postoperative residual enophthalmos is usually the result of inadequate reconstruction of the orbital walls with increased orbital volume. The loss of periorbital fat is seldom the cause of such a surgical result.

3.8 Frontal and Skull Base Fractures

Above and deep to the Le Fort III level lie the frontal sinuses as well as the anterior skull base. These structures may be involved individually or in combination with other fractures. The frontal sinus acts as an airbag or crumble zone to absorb the majority of the impact, protecting the intracranial content. This is of course not the case in young children where the frontal sinus has not yet developed.

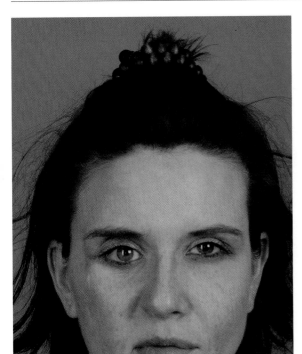

Fig. 3.53 Combination of right enophthalmos and hypoglobus of the right globe due to an untreated orbital fracture

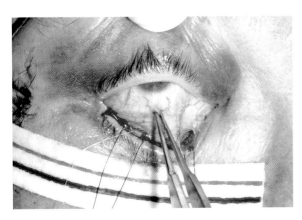

Fig. 3.54 Forced duction test ensuring that there is no muscular or periorbital fat entrapment after orbital floor reconstruction

There is a significant difference in fractures involving only the anterior wall of the frontal sinus and where the posterior wall is also involved. Most displaced posterior wall fractures need surgical exploration and cerebrospinal fluid leak repair.

In the event of blunt trauma, fractures are mostly spread over a wider area while sharper trauma of course penetrates the anterior and posterior wall as well as skull base easily and results in a more localized but not necessarily less severe injury.

3.8.1 Classification

- Anterior wall of the frontal sinus alone. (Treatment mostly just restoring the anterior wall)
- Anterior and posterior wall, but the posterior wall can be salvaged (Treatment by restoring the anterior and posterior wall where indicated as well as ensuring no persisting cerebrospinal fluid leakage)
- Anterior and posterior wall, but the posterior wall is not salvageable or the frontonasal duct's patency cannot be restored. (Treatment by either frontal sinus obliteration or cranialization)
- Fractures with commination of the naso-frontal tract should be treated with obliteration or cranialization ofter sealing off the tract.

3.8.2 Symptoms and Signs

- Depression of the frontal bone or supraorbital rim may often not be noticeable initially and is more apparent on palpation due to early swelling.
- Loss of sensation of the frontal region possible due to damage to the supraorbital and supratrochlear nerves.
- Proptosis due to impacted orbital roof and deceased orbital volume may be present.
- Cerebrospinal fluid or a bloody rhinorrhea may be apparent. When a subclinical leak is suspected, a

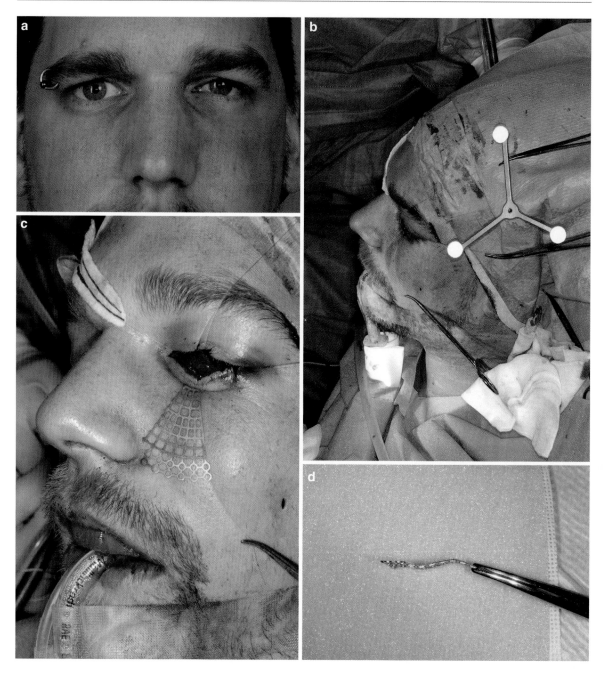

Fig. 3.55 (**a**) Patient with left-sided enophthalmos due to an orbital floor and zygoma fracture, (**b**) navigation setup, (**c**) transconjunctival access and titanium mesh ready for insertion, (**d**) S-shaped titanium mesh to reconstruct the orbital floor, (**e**) Titanium mesh reconstruction of the left orbital floor in the correct position and checked with the aid of navigation, (**f**) the 4 weeks postoperative view, and (**g**) the postoperative CT matched with the planned reconstruction indicated in green

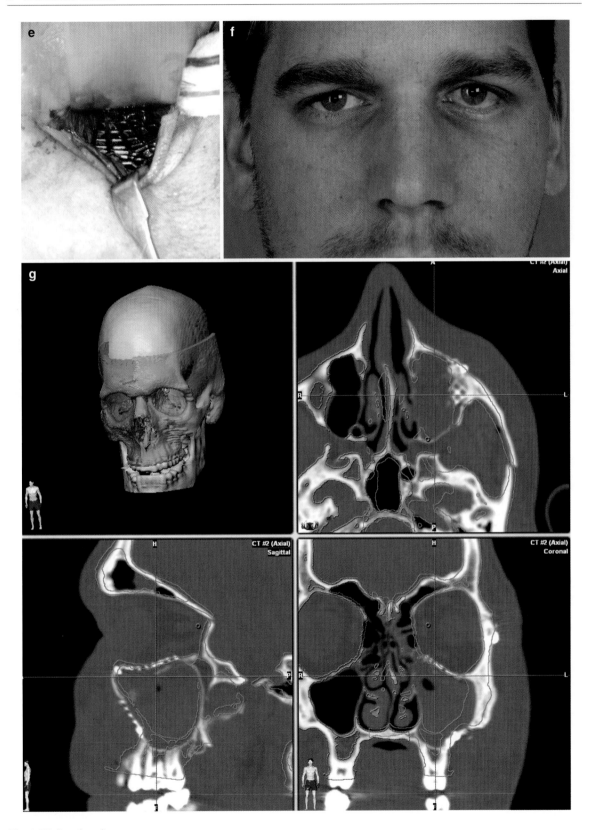

Fig. 3.55 (continued)

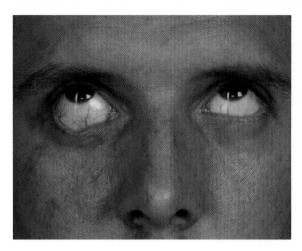

Fig. 3.56 Lower lid retraction as a complication of a transconjunctival access

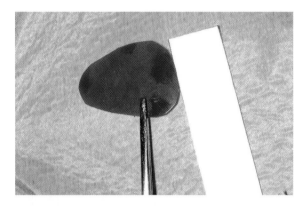

Fig. 3.57 Materials used for orbital wall reconstruction may vary widely. The PDS foil in this picture has the advantage of being resorbable, but cannot take on a three-dimensional shape

β-transferrin test may be done to confirm the presence of cerebrospinal fluid.

- Nasal bleeding or bleeding into the nasopharynx may also be present.
- Concurrent symptoms and signs of intracranial injuries should be considered.

3.8.3 Diagnosis

Verifying the clinical diagnosis with a CT in axial, coronal, as well as sagittal planes is indicated. When not available, a lateral view of the skull as well as occipitomental view (Water's) is indicated, but will not disclose the full picture.

3.8.4 Treatment

Aim: To functionally reconstruct the frontal sinus area and prevent long-term complications.

- For the most part, no urgent treatment is indicated except for the control of local bleeding.
- Antibiotics are usually described for displaced fractures due to the proximity of the frontal sinus.
- The anterior table can often be reduced via a balloon catheter, through local lacerations or when indicated by coronal approach. Fixation of the fractures is mostly done by using plates and screws and defects are closed with titanium mesh or bone grafts. As soon as the posterior table needs surgical intervention, a subcranial approach or conventional transcranial approach is indicated. Patency of the frontonasal duct should be maintained when the frontal sinus can be reconstructed. If not, obliteration or cranialization of the frontal sinus should be performed.
- When indicated, the dural repair should be performed simultaneously by using a pericranial flap (Figs. 3.59 and 3.60).

3.8.5 Complications

- Persistence of a cerebrospinal fluid leak and infection are the most common complications.
- Late development of a mucocele may be problematic and lead to significant destruction of adjoining bony structures.
- Infection of the material used for obliteration.

3.8.6 Exceptions and Controversies

- There are three potential ways to manage significant fractures of the posterior wall of the frontal sinus: Cranialization of the frontal sinus; second, obliteration with fat, muscle, bone, or bone substitutes; and third, functional reconstruction of the frontal sinus walls including the frontonasal duct in a minority of cases may be possible.
- Late reconstruction of significant defects may be performed by using computer-generated replacements

with materials like titanium, PEEK, as well as porous polyethylene. Manually shaped materials like acrylic or calcium-phosphate cements may also be used.

- Free bone grafts or, if no other alternative exists, titanium mesh may be used for frontal wall reconstruction.

3.9 Panfacial Fractures

Panfacial fractures is a term used to describe widespread fractures of the facial skeleton. This normally entails midface, mandibular fractures, as well as often the skull base.

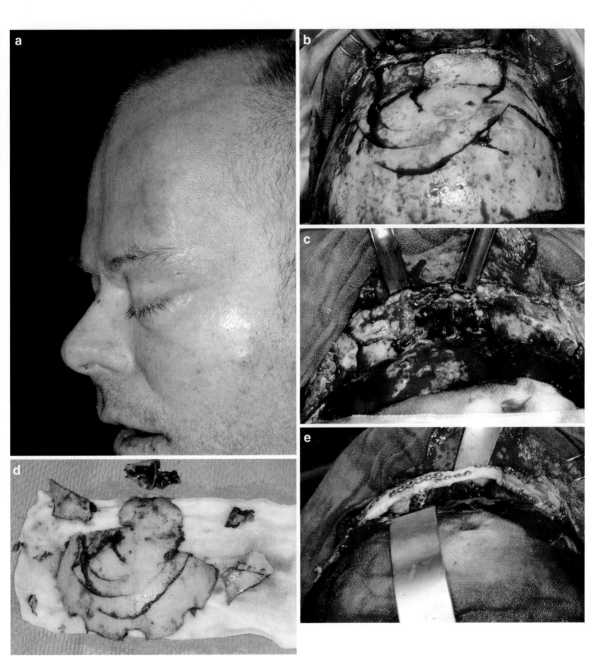

Fig. 3.58 Patient with severe frontobasal fractures. (**a**) Indented fontal area visible. (**b**) Coronal access and frontal fractures visible. (**c**) Comminuted frontonasal duct area. (**d**) Bone fragments carefully positioned to be assembled later. (**e**) Anterior frontal sinus wall and orbital roof reconstruction with cranialization of the frontal sinus. (**f**) Reconstructed frontal area with mini-plates and titanium mesh. (**g** and **h**) Early and late postoperative pictures

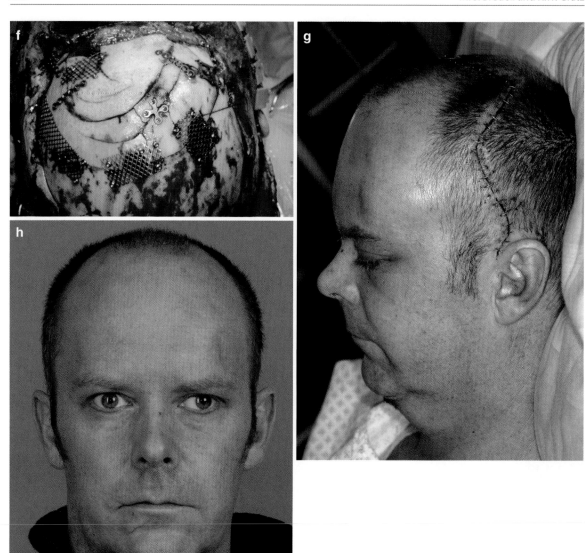

Fig. 3.58 (continued)

Clearly, higher forces are generally involved in these patients and even more care should be taken to access for possible associated injuries.

These patients' problems are compounded by the fact that the airway may be more compromised than in patients with isolated fractures. Definitive management is more complicated because both the mandible as well as the maxillary components are initially not usable as a guide or base for the reconstruction of the other.

Treatment entails first reconstruction of either the maxilla or mandible, which is then used as framework for the other. Another potential starting point is the skull base, which may be used as a reference point for reconstruction of the midface (Fig. 3.61).

3.10 High-Velocity Injuries and Gunshot Wounds

Gunshot injuries are dependent on a variety of factors, namely:

- The kinetic energy of the body proportional to mass and velocity, the projectiles deformation and fragmentation, entrance profile and path travelled through the body, as well as the biological characteristic of the tissues.
- Obviously, the characteristics of tissue damage are different with assault rifles high velocity and smaller caliber handguns low velocity. This has to be kept in mind when treating patients and their wounds.
- Smaller caliber and lower speed handgun injuries have less late sequelae than that of high-speed/high-energy injuries. This is due to the wider destructive energy distribution found in high-velocity/energy injuries. Capillary damage leads to late necrosis of tissues. Initial debridement would thus be more aggressive in the high-energy injuries. That said, it is a rule that all wounds in the face should be treated more conservatively and cautiously than for example that of the abdomen or extremities. This is due to the improved vascularity, leading to improved recovery of damaged tissues. Furthermore, the functional and aesthetic consequences due to over-zealous debridement in the facial region may be disastrous for a patient. A stepwise, careful approach is mandatory in the head and neck region.
- Immediate definitive reconstruction is only indicated in low energy (velocity) injuries where the chance of microvascular injury and late necrosis is less.

3.10.1 Treatment

3.10.1.1 Emergency treatment

Aim: To ensure an adequate airway and contain bleeding.

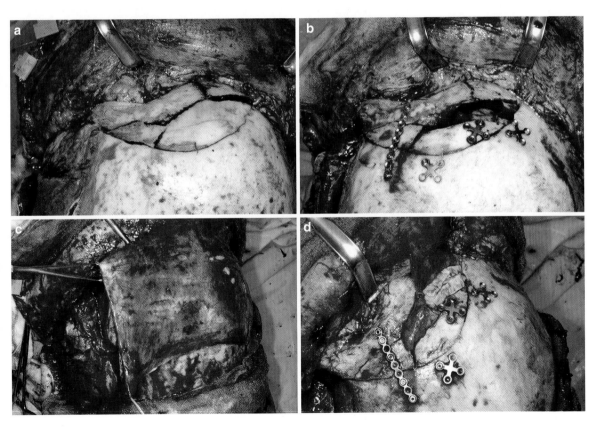

Fig. 3.59 (**a**) A patient with severe frontobasal fractures. Obturation of the frontal sinus with lyophilized cartilage was performed with reduction of the fractures and use of a pericranial flap for repair of the dural tears (**b**–**e**). The postoperative radiological control views demonstrated in (**f** and **g**)

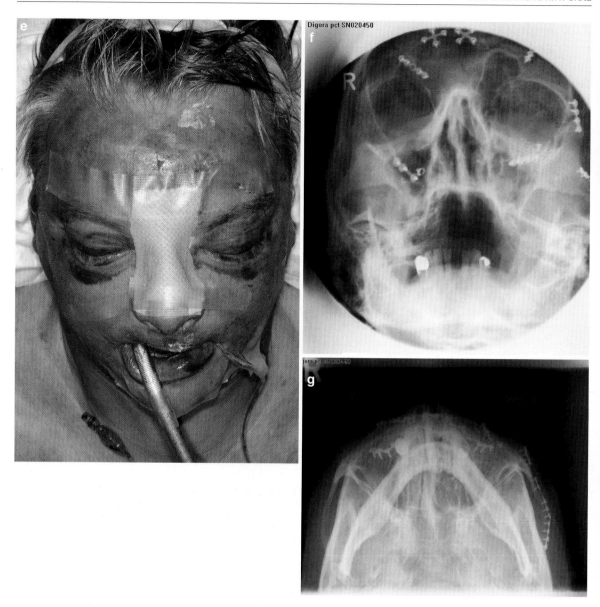

Fig. 3.59 (continued)

- Normal resuscitative principles are also indicated in this group of patients. Airway management may be a problem and securing the airway from the start is mandatory. The presence of loose fragments of teeth and bone that may be displaced in the airways should be in one's mind during the initial management. A chest X-ray is mandatory in all patients as soon as feasible.
- Bleeding should be controlled vigorously with clamps for definitive bleeders and pressure bandages for the more diffuse or hard-to-reach areas.
- Conservative debridement is indicated as discussed above and only loose, nonattached bone and tooth fragments should be removed. It often appears as if there is massive soft tissue and bone loss, but this is usually not the case, especially in lower energy gunshot wounds. Rough approximation may often contain bleeding and secure airways during the initial, emergency phase. All possible bone fragments pedicled to soft tissue should be preserved until their fate has been decided.
- Removal of the projectile is not always indicated and is mostly not a primary objective of emergency management.
- Nothing can be said against a delayed treatment protocol where at first the bleeding is managed with a very superficial debridement, repositioning sutures

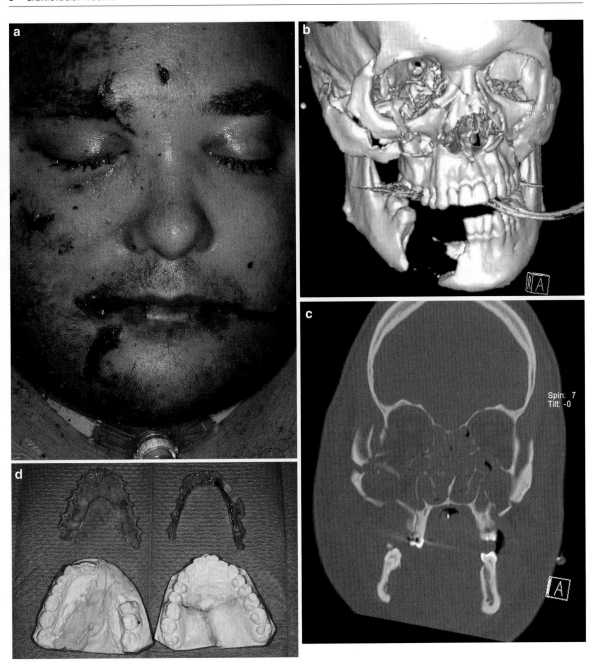

Fig. 3.60 An airplane accident victim (**a**) demonstrating severe facial fractures of a comminuted nature with segmental loss of the lower jaw (**b**, **c**). The aim in this case was to first reconstruct the lower jaw and base the midface on that. Dental casts (**d**) were made with accurate reconstruction of the occlusion and stents were prefabricated to enable accurate reconstruction of the occlusion. Adequate orbital reconstruction on the right (**e**) was not achieved during the first surgery. Accurate reconstruction (**f** and **g**) was only achieved in a stepwise method where the left orbit was first reconstructed and by using navigation tools was mirrored to the right side to achieve a symmetrical result. (**h**, **i**) demonstrates the postoperative clinical view with a satisfactory outcome with a functional occlusion shown (**j**)

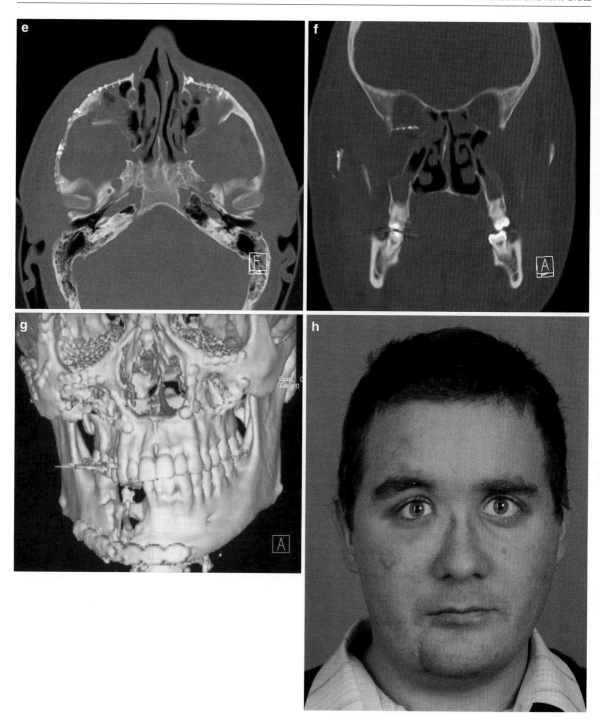

Fig. 3.60 (continued)

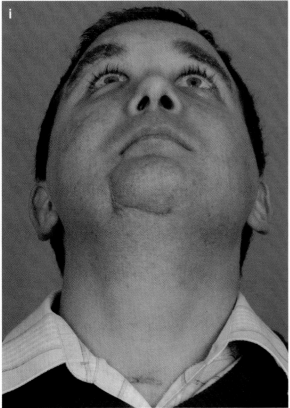

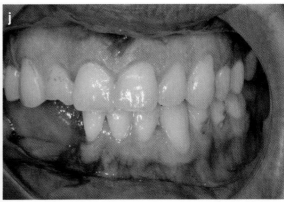

Fig. 3.60 (continued)

and compressive dressings. A more definitive reconstruction should follow within 24–48 hours.

3.10.1.2 Definitive Treatment

Aim: Full functional reconstruction in an immediate or staged approach.

- Should be deferred until the risk of infection is less. Often, there is a phase of definitive provisional treatment and final reconstruction is postponed until there is a clear indication as to which tissues will survive and which not.
- Often soft tissue coverage is the greatest challenge and local, regional as well as free flaps may have to be employed to enable bone coverage and seal the oral cavity from the cutaneous surface and nasal airways and paranasal sinuses.
- Definitive bony reconstruction can only take place if there is adequate soft tissue coverage to ensure sufficient vascularization. Depending on the situa-

tion free or free vascularized bone grafts may be employed.
- Removal of the projectile is only indicated when there is a risk of infection, migration to a high risk area for example to the carotid artery.
- In these situations, the use of large bridging load bearing plates with locking fixation is often employed acting as an internal "external" fixator. Use of external fixators as temporary or in cases of severe comminution as temporary fixation method is often of great assistance (Fig. 3.62).

3.10.2 Complications

- Aspiration, compromised airway, bleeding, and migration of the projectile or projectiles are the most common of problems.
- Infection is a major problem due to the progressive necrosis of tissues after microvascular damage.

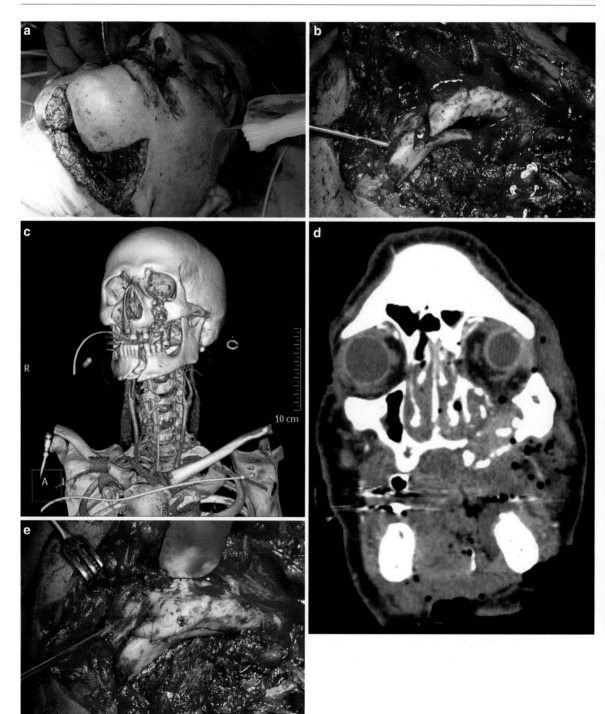

Fig. 3.61 Patient with a self-inflicted gunshot wound (**a**). Note the mandibular fracture (**b**, **c**), comminuted orbital (**d**), the reduced and fixed mandibular fracture (**e**) and (**f** and **g**) showing the early postoperative views with an iodine gauze packing in the left maxillary sinus to support some bony fragments and (**h**) showing the late postoperative results

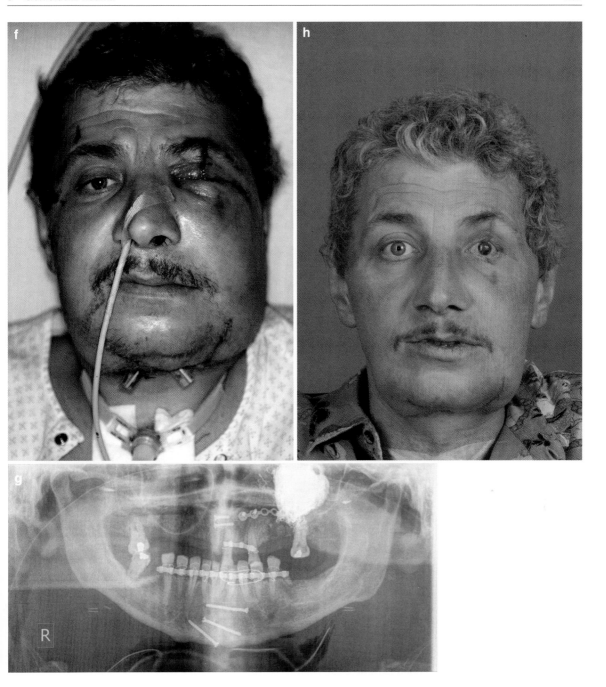

Fig. 3.61 (continued)

3.10.3 Exceptions and Controversies

- Surely, the stage at which one would commence definitive reconstruction and whether it should be free bone grafts or free vascularized grafts is the most controversial issue (Fig. 3. 63). Wounds with limited soft tissue damage usually leave the opportunity for immediate reconstruction.

- The degree of debridement performed is possibly another contentious issue (Fig. 3.63). This often depends on the degree of experience of the surgeon.

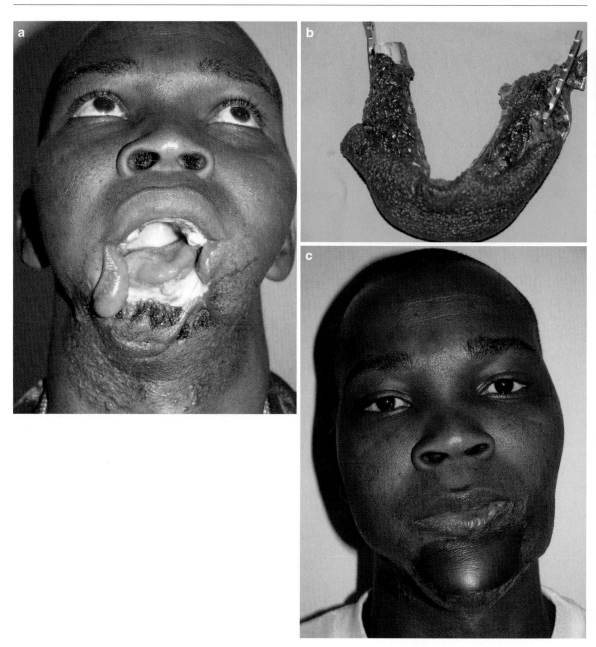

Fig. 3.62 (a) Late presentation of a patient injured during guerrilla warfare. He was fed via a PEG tube for 6 years. (b) Reconstruction with a fibula free vascularized flap. Postoperative appearance (c)

3.11 Dental and Dentoalveolar Fractures

The luxation or subluxation of teeth is fairly common, and appropriate management is imperative.

3.11.1 Dentoalveolar Fracture

Teeth displaced with the alveolar bone of the maxilla or mandible are termed dentoalveolar fractures. In these cases, the displaced fragment or fragments

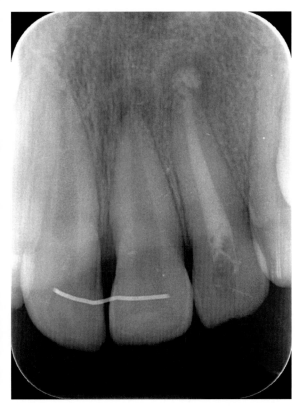

Fig. 3.63 Fractured, mobile, or luxated teeth may not regain their neurovascular innervation and then has to receive root canal treatment. The left lateral incisor in this case after receiving root canal treatment

the socket. When saline is not available, the tooth can be replaced in the socket immediately when clean, otherwise placed in the upper or lower vestibulum to keep it moist. Implantation by a dentist or maxillofacial surgeon later than 6 hours after dislodgement is seldom successful. As soon as the teeth are stable, a root canal treatment to remove the necrotic pulp is indicated. Antibiotics should be prescribed and the patient's tetanus immunization should be updated.

3.11.2.1 Subluxated Teeth

These teeth should be repositioned as soon as possible and fixed with an arch-bar or flexible wire splint joined to adjacent and the transplanted teeth with dental cement for a period of preferably shorter than 2 weeks. Fixation for too long may lead to ankylosis. If, however, a dentoalveolar fracture is present, fixation of 4–6 weeks is indicated with more rigid fixation.

Careful assessment of the relevant tooth's vitality is indicated by testing the tooth for cold sensitivity. If the tooth was severely displaced in an adult, a root canal treatment will probably be necessary; in children, the apex of the teeth may still be open and result in revascularization and innervation of the tooth.

Luxated primary teeth do not have to be re-implanted.

should be repositioned as soon as possible. This can be performed under local anesthesia or combined with sedation in compliant patients. The repositioned dentoalveolar segments can be stabilized to adjacent teeth with arch-bars, wire loops, or wire cemented to the adjacent teeth (Figs. 3.64, 3.65 and 3.66).

3.11.3 Lost Teeth

Lost teeth may in certain ideal circumstances where the wound is clean and the bone loss is minimal immediately be replaced with dental titanium implants. These in turn can also in the most ideal circumstances be fitted with a provisional crown.

Alternatively, these lost teeth can be replaced with a removable partial denture or provisional bridge as soon as most of the swelling has subsided.

3.11.2 Luxated Teeth

Teeth totally displaced out of the mouth should be found as soon as possible, rinsed off but not wiped, and placed in normal saline solution or replaced in

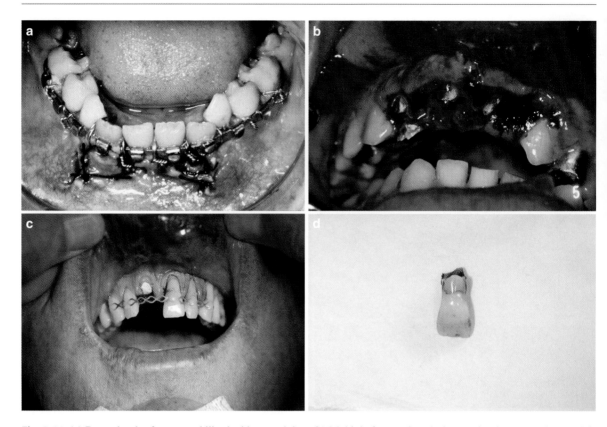

Fig. 3.64 (**a**) Dentoalveolar fracture stabilized with an arch bar. (**b**) Multiple fractured teeth that need to be removed. (**c** and **d**) Mobile teeth along with fracture of tooth 11 that can be retained and built up with a crown at a later stage

3.11.4 Complications

- Loss of teeth early or at a later stage. The latter may develop due to external or internal root resorption and/or infection.
- Incorrect repositioning may lead to an occlusal disturbance.
- Soft tissue retraction or loss leading to periodontal problems or even tooth loss.
- Decolorization, often taking on a gray/bluish color.

3.12 Soft Tissue Management

- Soft tissue injuries often accompany hard tissue injuries or may be isolated. The oral environment may be very forgiving and often superficial wounds heal without a trace of a scar. However, this is not the case where there is displacement of the tissue layers and then accurate repositioning is indicated by suturing.

Furthermore, these wounds are often soiled by fragments of teeth, plaque, or even foreign material making the deeper wounds more susceptible to infection. A thorough debridement in every case with good rinsing is thus imperative.

3.12.1 Tongue

- Deep wounds of the tongue should be sutured layer by layer. As the tongue is a constantly moving muscular structure, a sturdy vertical mattress suture for the superficial layer will prevent later opening of the wound. Sutures should be left in situ for at least 10–14 days.
- Care should be taken to adequately debride the wound surfaces ensuring the re-adaption of bleeding surfaces on another. Significant swelling may

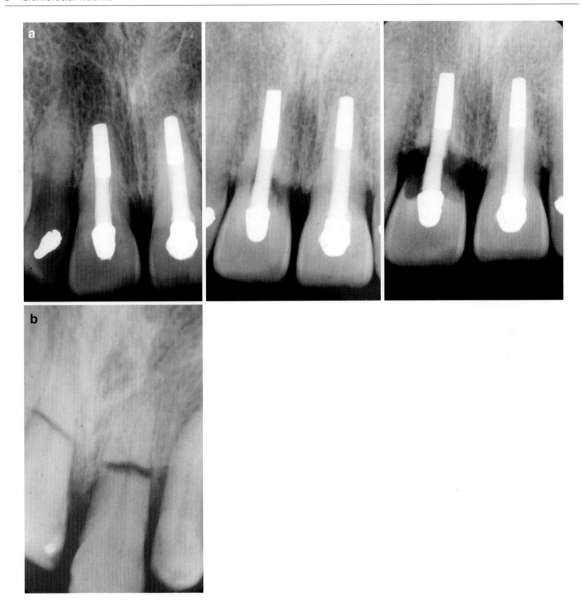

Fig. 3.65 (**a**) Progressive external root resorption after these fractured and luxated teeth were re-implanted. (**b**) Root fractures are best seen on dental films and managed by a dentist

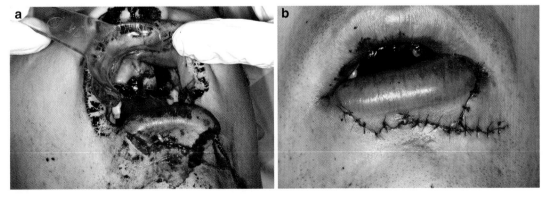

Fig. 3.66 (**a, b**) Lower lip laceration as well as upper dentoalveolar fractures with correct repositioning and suturing of the lower lip

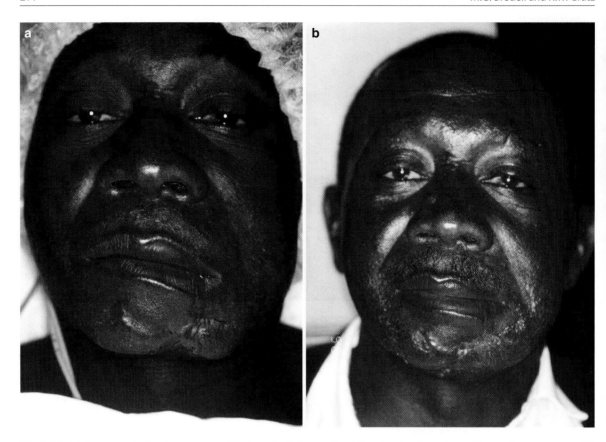

Fig. 3.67 (**a**) A poor result after incorrect repositioning of soft tissues after injury, leaving the patient with poor lip competence. (**b**) Repositioning of the soft tissues including the musculature, improving the patient's function

evolve and airway control is mandatory after suturing of larger wounds.

• Lacerations or tissue loss of especially the tongue tip should be handled with the greatest of care as this part of the tongue is important for articulation and moving the food bolus more posteriorly. Adequate tongue mobility and tip projection should always be maintained.

3.12.2 Lip

• Accurate lip reconstruction is vitally important to reestablish function and aesthetics to this very visual and functionally important part of the face.

• These injuries can be divided into those involving the skin or oral mucosa only and the group involving both the oral mucosa and outer skin or lip surface. The latter is most certainly the most challenging. Mostly, mistakes can be avoided by first performing a careful debridement, then placing an accurate, adaptive suture in the vermilion border area (skin/lip red junction). Then, the oral layer is closed with resorbable sutures, followed by rinsing from the skin surface area, suturing the periorbital musculature and lastly suturing the skin layer with fine monofilament sutures. Failure of adapting the perioral musculature will result in an unsightly whistle effect.

• In cases where there is tissue loss, these defects can be divided in those requiring just minor local excision and then closure, those requiring the utilization of local flap techniques (Bernard-Fries, Karapanski – or nasolabial flaps, etc.), and finally those requiring distant free vascularized flaps (Figs. 3.67 and 3.68).

3.12.3 Eyelid

• Meticulous reconstruction of especially the periocular musculature and more importantly the tarsal plate as well as the lacrimal system is imperative.

• When indicated, a dacryocystorhinostomy (re-cannulation of the lacrimal ductal system) should be performed to prevent epiphora. This is often easier to perform as an immediate rather than a delayed procedure.

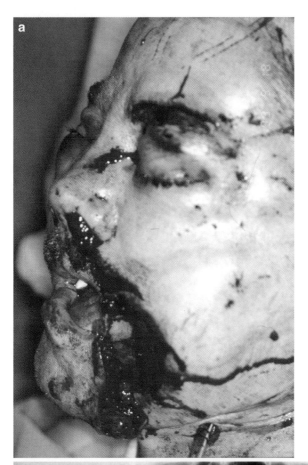

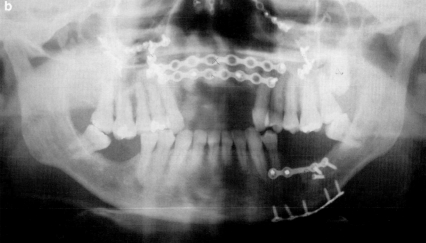

Fig. 3.68 (**a**) Severe facial trauma with loss of the total premaxilla hard and soft tissues as well as lip lacerations, Le Fort II and III fractures. (**b–d**) X-rays showing initial plate fixation as well as later reconstructive efforts with bone transplant as well as implant placement. (**e**) Showing the initial efforts of late reconstruction including a corrective rhinoplasty and (**f–h**) the final results with a satisfactory facial appearance as well as functional occlusion

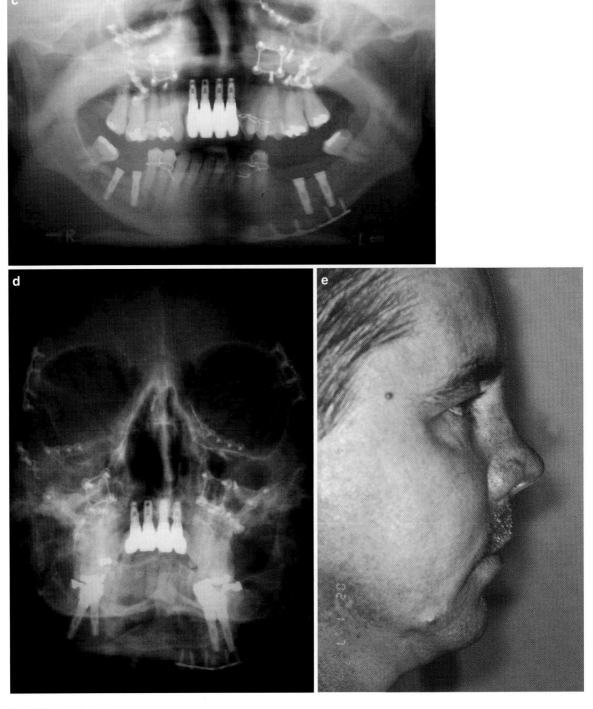

Fig. 3.68 (continued)

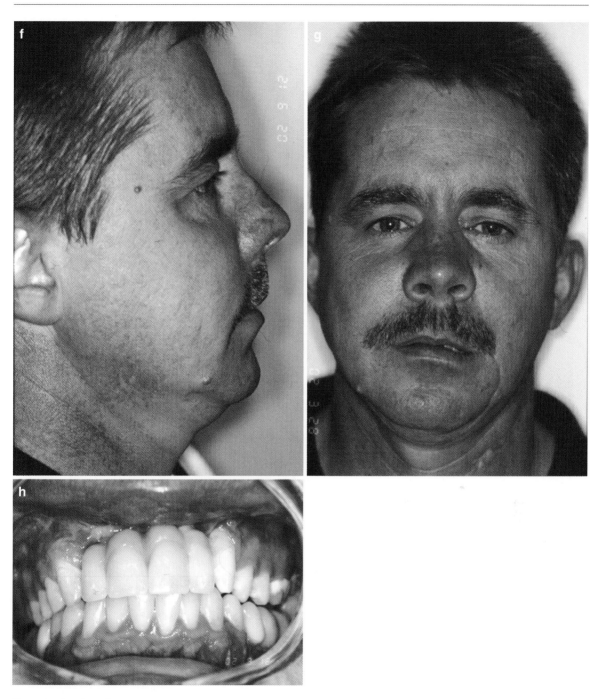

Fig. 3.68 (continued)

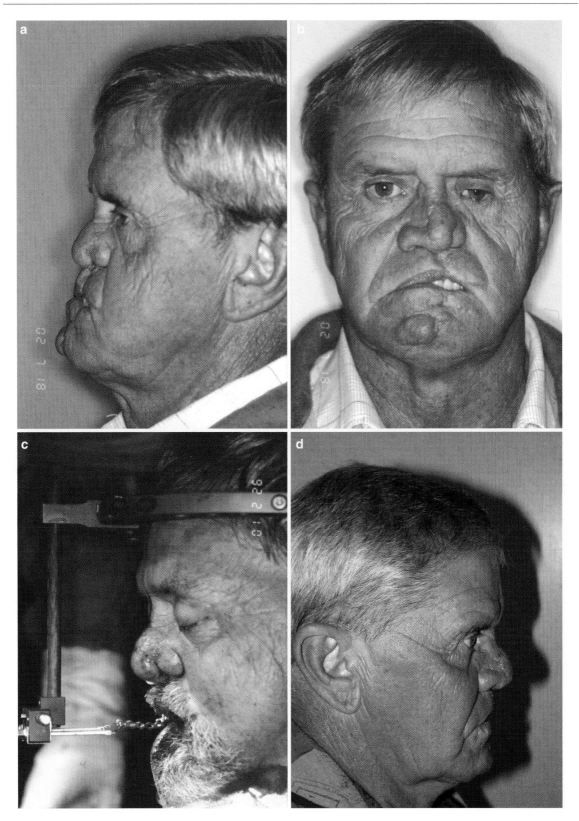

Fig. 3.69 The devestaded face (**a**, **b**) of a patient not receiving any treatment for his impacted, comminuted midface fractures as well as multiple soft tissue injuries. Treated with a RED distrac-tion device (**c**), distracting the midface after a Le Fort II osteot-omy, improving his airway as well as profile (**d** and **e**) to be utilized as a base for further reconstructive efforts

Fig. 3.69 (continued)

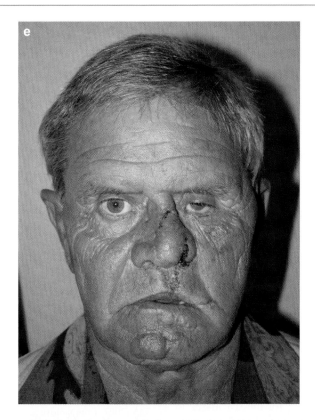

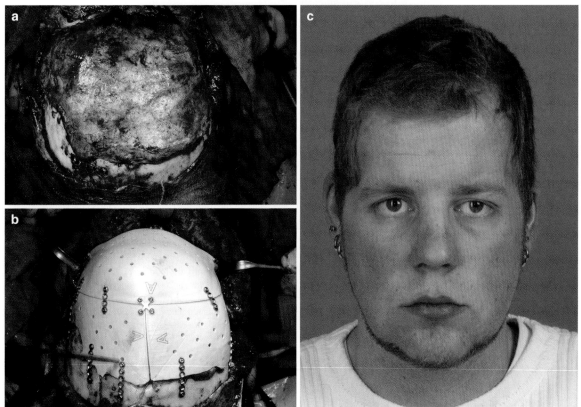

Fig. 3.70 Polyetherketone (PEEK) computer-generated reconstruction (**a** and **b**) of a large skull defect due to infection after extensive skull fractures. The postoperative stable long-term result (**c**)

3.12.4 Mouth Floor

- The mouth floor contains mainly two important structures that have to be taken into account when repair is performed. The lingual nerve has to be protected during surgery in this area as well as Whartin's duct. Probing the latter may assist in assessing potential damage as well as protecting it during the repair process.

3.13 Late Reconstruction

- Every attempt should be made to avoid the delay of reconstruction of the facial skeleton. The first opportunity is the best and scar tissue has not yet taken its toll on the wounds and structures. There are of course exceptions and this is especially the case where there is tissue loss in a contaminated field.
- Furthermore, the end result of the primary reconstruction for example enophthalmos is only apparent two or more weeks after the injury. The decision then has to be taken to either wait for the scar tissue to mature for the next 6 months or to perform an early correction when feasible. Early correction is often the way to go and should not be shied away from.
- Modern technology has made many tools available to assist us in difficult cases. Navigation tools have made mirroring possible and may assist considerably in the goal of achieving functional symmetry to the face. The major disadvantage is the lack of soft tissue predictability and up to now this still often remains a clinical judgment. In future, the role of 3D photo-imaging may assist in this, especially when individualized to the particular patient area.
- Materials like titanium, PEEK, surgical polyethylene as well as to a lesser extent, acrylic cements have made more accurate reconstruction possible, especially when assisted with 3D models and computer planning (Figs. 3.69–3.70).

The authors thank Mrs. Christa Giger and Dr Daniel Zweifel for their editing assistance.

References

Alcala-Galiano A, Arribas-Garcia IJ, Martin-Perez MA, Romance A, Montalvo-Moreno JJ, Juncos JM (2008) Pediatric facial fractures: children are not just small adults. Radiographics 28(2):441–461, quiz 618

Alvi A, Doherty T, Lewen G (2003) Facial fractures and concomitant injuries in trauma patients. Laryngoscope 113:102–106

Bakathir AA, Margasahayam MV, Al-Ismaily M (2008) Removal of bone plates in patients with maxillofacial trauma: a retrospective study. Oral Surg Oral Med Oral Pathol Oral Radiol Endod 105:e32–e37

Baumann A, Ewers R (2001) Midfacial degloving: an alternative approach for traumatic corrections in the midface. Int J Oral Maxillofac Surg 30(4):272–277

Burstein F, Cohen S, Hudgins R, Boydston W (1997) Fronto basilar trauma: classification and treatment. Plast Reconstr Surg 99(5):1314–1321

Burnstine MA (2003) Clinical recommendations for repair of orbital facial fractures. Curr Opin Ophthalmol 14(5): 236–240

Ceallaigh PO, Ekanaykaee K, Beirne CJ, Patton DW (2007) Diagnosis and management of common maxillofacial injuries in the emergency department. Part 4: orbital floor and midface fractures. Emerg Med J 24(4): 292–293

Coletti DP, Caccamese JF, Norby C, Edwards S, Von Fraunhofer JA (2007) Comparative analysis of the threaded and tapered locking reconstruction plates. J Oral Maxillofac Surg 65: 2587–2593

Donat TL, Endress C, Mathog RH (2007) Facial fracture classification according to skeletal support mechanisms. Arch Otolaryngol Head Neck Surg 124:1306–1314

Ellis E III, Miles BA (2007) Fractures of the mandible: a technical perspective. Plast Reconstr Surg 120(7 Suppl 2): 76S–89S

Hammer B, Prein J (1995) Correction of post traumatic orbital deformities: operative techniques and review of 26 patients. J Craniomaxillofac Surg 23:81–90

Huang RH, Brandt MT (2004) Traditional versus endoscope-assisted open reduction with rigid internal fixation (ORIF) of adult mandibular condyle fractures: a review of the literature regarding current thoughts of management. J Oral Maxillofac Surg 62:1272–1279

Janus SC, MacLeod SPR, Odland R (2008) Analysis of results in early versus late midface fracture repair. Otolaryngol Head Neck Surg 138:464–467

Koltai PJ, Rabkin D (1996) Management of facial trauma in children. Pediatr Clin North Am 43(6):1253–1275

Landes CA, Lipphart R (2005) Prospective evaluation of a pragmatic treatment rationale: open reduction and internal fixation of displaced and dislocated condyle or subcondylar fractures and closed reduction of non-displaced, non-dislocated fractures Part I: condyle and subcondylar fractures. Int J Oral Maxillofac Surg 34:859–870

Perry M (2008) Advanced Trauma Life Support (ATLS) and facial trauma: can one size fit all? Part 1: dilemmas in the management of multiply injured patient with coexisting facial injuries. Int J Oral Maxillofac Surg 37:209–214

Perry M, Moutray T (2008) Advanced trauma life support (ATLS) and facial trauma: can one size fit all? Part 4: 'Can the patient see?' Timely diagnosis, dilemmas and pitfalls in the multiply injured, poorly responsive/unresponsive patient. Int J Oral Maxillofac Surg 37:505–514

Pham AM, Strong EB (2006) Endoscopic management of facial fractures. Curr Opin Otolaryngol Head Neck Surg 14(4):234–241

Schaller B (2005) Subcranial approach in the surgical treatment of anterior skull base trauma. Acta Neurochir 147: 335–366

Schierle HP, Hausamen J-E (1997) Moderne Prinzipien in der Behandlung komplexer Gesichtsschädelverletzungen. Unfallchirurg 100:330–337

Stefanopoulos PK, Tarantzopoulou AD (2005) Facial bite wounds: management update. Int J Oral Maxillofac Surg 34:464–472

Manson PN, Clark N, Robertson B, Slezak S, Wheatly M, Vander Kolk C, Iliff N (1999) Subunit principles in midface fractures: the importance of sagittal buttresses, soft-tissue reductions, and sequencing treatment of segmental fractures. Plast Reconstr Surg 103(4):1287–1306

Marlow TJ, Goltra DD, Schabel SI (1997) Intracranial placement of a nasotracheal tube after facial fracture: A rare complication. J Emerg Med 15(2):187–191

Ruddermann RH, Mullen RL, Philips JH (2008) The biophysics of mandibular fractures: an evolution towards understanding. Plast Reconstr Surg 121(2):596–607

Hopper RA, Salemy S, Sze RW (2006) Diagnosis of midface fractures with CT: what the surgeon needs to know. Radiographics 26(3):783–793

Rhoner D, Tay A, Meng CS, Hutmacher D (2002) The sphenozygomatic suture as a key site for osteosynthesis of the orbitozygomatic complex in panfacial fractures. A biomechanical study in human cadavers based on clinical practice. Plast Reconstr Surg 110(6):1463–1471

Rodriques E, Stanwix M, Nam A, St Hilaire H, Simmons OP, Christy M, Grant MO, Manson PN (2008) Twenty-six-years experience treating frontal sinus fractures: A novel algorithm based on anatomical fracture pattern and failure of conventional techniques. Plast Reconstr Surg 122(6):1850–1866

Shorr N, Goldberg RA, Eshagian B, Cook T (2003) Perspective. Lateral canthoplasty. Opthalmic Plast Reconstr Surg 19(5):345–352

Suuronen R, Kallela I, Lindqvist C (2000) Bioabsorbable plates and screws: Current state of the art in facial fracture repair. J Craniomaxillofac Trauma 6(1):19–27, discussion 28–30

Tung T-C, Tseng WS, Chen CT, Lai JP, Chen YR (2000) Acute life-threatening injuries in facial fracture patients: a review of 1,025 patients. J Trauma 49(3):420–424

Ward Booth P, Schendel SA, Hausamen J-E (2007) Maxillofacial surgery, 2nd edn, vol. 1. Churchill Livingstone, Edinburgh, pp 2–256

Zimmermann CE, Troulis MJ, Kaban LB (2006) Pediatric facial fractures: recent advances in prevention, diagnosis and management. Int J Oral Maxillofac Surg 35(1):2–13

Chest Trauma

4

Demetrios Demetriades, Peep Talving, and Kenji Inaba

4.1 Thoracic Wall Injuries

4.1.1 Rib Fractures

4.1.1.1 Epidemiology and Outcomes

Fractures to the thoracic cage constitute one of the most common injuries sustained to the torso. Although the fractures themselves, in general, do not impair pulmonary mechanics in the absence of a flail segment or open chest wall defect, they are a marker of severe energy transfer. Fractures of the upper ribs are associated with an increased incidence of vascular injuries, fractures of the middle ribs are usually associated with a higher incidence of lung contusion and hemothorax, and fractures of the lower ribs are associated with an increased risk for injuries to intra-abdominal solid organ injuries.

Rib fractures can be seen at all ages. However, in the geriatric patient, the thoracic wall is much more prone to

breakage when compared to children in whom severe underlying pulmonary contusions can be seen in the absence of any fractured ribs. For the geriatric patient with rib fractures, increasing age has been consistently demonstrated as an independent risk factor for not only complications such as pneumonia but for mortality as well [6, 9, 11, 45]. For all patients, whether studied in a single center analysis [87]or as part of a large database such as the American National Trauma Database (NTDB) [41], there is a stepwise increase in mortality with each additional fracture. In the NTDB study by the Loyola group, the same held true for complications including pneumonia, ARDS, aspiration, and empyema [6].

4.1.1.2 Treatment

The mainstay of treatment for patients with rib fractures remains pain control and respiratory support ranging from incentive spirometry to mechanical ventilation. Associated complications such as pneumothorax, seen in about 40%, hemothorax in 30%, and hemo-pneumothorax in 15% [88], should be screened for and treated. Options for pain control include systemic, regional, and local delivery methods. Optimal pain control is essential for ensuring adequate pulmonary toilet. The most commonly utilized method for the majority of patients is systemic analgesia, delivered with or without patient control. In addition to the use of narcotic formulations, the addition of nonsteroidal anti-inflammatory medications may impart a synergistic effect. Epidural analgesia is also an excellent option [71]. The multitrauma patient, however, may not be a good candidate due to concurrent ongoing issues such as spine trauma, coagulopathy preventing insertion or the need to serially examine the abdomen for evolving injury. In patients without contraindications,

D. Demetriades (✉)
Director of Trauma and Surgical Intensive Care,
University of Southern California, LAC+USC Medical Center,
1200 North State Street, IPT – C5L100, Los Angeles,
CA 90033-4525, USA
e-mail: demetria@usc.edu

P. Talving
Division of Trauma and Surgical Intensive Care, LAC+USC
Medical Center, 1200 North State Street, IPT – C5L100,
Los Angeles, CA 90033-4525, USA
e-mail: peep.talving@surgery.usc.edu

K. Inaba
Division of Trauma and Surgical Intensive Care, Director
Surgical Critical Fellowship, LAC+USC Medical Center,
1200 North State Street, IPT – 5CL100, Los Angeles, CA
90033-4525, USA
e-mail: kinaba@surgery.usc.edu

H.-J. Oestern et al. (eds.), *Head, Thoracic, Abdominal, and Vascular Injuries*,
DOI: 10.1007/978-3-540-88122-3_4, © Springer-Verlag Berlin Heidelberg 2011

however, this may be an effective option. In randomized studies of patients receiving epidural analgesia, there was a significant decrease in pain, in the rate of pneumonia, and lesser mechanical ventilation requirements [12, 27]. One patient subset that requires caution, however, is the geriatric patient cohort. In a retrospective study by Kieninger, epidural analgesia was associated with an increased length of stay and complications in a patient cohort >55 years old, especially in those that were less severely injured [54]. A variety of local methods are also available for pain control ranging from regional blocks to paravertebral continuous infusion systems. The latter, utilizing bupivicaine has demonstrated efficacy in controlling pain and improving pulmonary function while minimizing systemic impact [50, 71].

Although the mainstay of treatment is analgesia, the institution of a protocolized management algorithm may be beneficial in improving outcomes. In a prospective study by Todd, a multidisciplinary clinical pathway for patients greater than 45 years of age with greater than four fractures emphasizing respiratory therapy-driven volume expansion, pain expertise, physical therapy, and nutritional support demonstrated a significant decrease in ICU and hospital length of stay by 2.4 and 3.7 days, respectively with a decrease in the incidence of pneumonia with an adjusted OR of 0.12 [98].

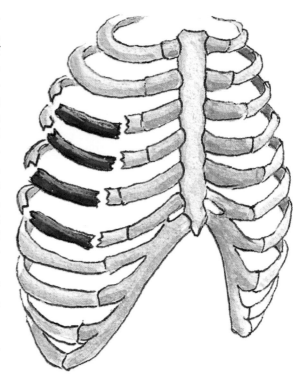

Fig. 4.1 Double fractures of at least three adjacent ribs may cause flail chest

4.1.2 Flail Chest

One distinct rib fracture pattern deserves specific mention: the flail chest. This is defined as a dysynchronous segment of the thoracic wall where three or more ribs are fractured in two or more places (Fig. 4.1). On clinical examination, the flail segment will be palpated as a dysnchronous region. In the spontaneously breathing patient, paradoxical movement of the segment (collapse with inspiration and expansion with expiration) due to the negative intrapleural pressures may be seen. On plain radiographs, multiple rib fractures in a flail pattern may be seen (Fig. 4.2). This may, however, be difficult to discern on x-ray if the fractures run through the costochondral joints. Most flail segments, however, will be clearly visible on CT. This diagnosis is a marker of severe blunt force trauma. The presence of a flail segment by itself is an independent risk factor for poor outcomes including the need for mechanical ventilation,

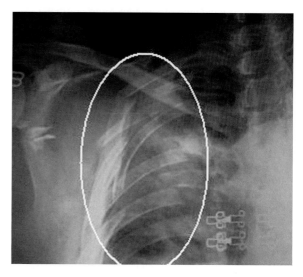

Fig. 4.2 Chest x-ray of a patient with flail chest shows multiple rib fractures and underlying lung contusion

respiratory complications, and length of stay when compared to patients with rib fractures but no flail segment [104]. As for nonflail rib fractures, the mainstay of treatment is pain control and respiratory support including noninvasive ventilatory strategies as a first-line therapy [43]. The true impact of the mechanical integrity of the chest wall is controversial. Animal studies support the contention that it is the underlying pulmonary contusion rather than the lack of chest wall integrity that is in fact responsible for the pulmonary dysfunction seen in flail chest [18]. The concept of mechanical chest wall stabilization is quite controversial as definitive outcomes data is still not available. There are a wide range of potential indications for operative fixation of the ribs, including (1) the inability to wean off of mechanical ventilation, (2) persistent pain due to malunion refractory to noninvasive pain control measures, (3) chest wall deformity impairing pulmonary mechanics, and (4) prior to closure of the chest wall after thoracotomy for other reasons [76, 79]. Small randomized trials of patients with flail chest requiring ventilatory support showed that patients with fixation required less ventilatory support, had fewer infectious complications, shorter ICU length of stay, and a higher rate of return to work [94]. Although not definitive, the data available suggests that there may be a role for mechanical stabilization in select patients. Further investigations to define patient characteristics, the optimal timing of fixation and methods are clearly warranted.

4.2 Lung Injuries

4.2.1 Pulmonary Contusion

The most common cause of lung contusion is blunt trauma to the chest. However, penetrating trauma due to gunshot wounds (GSWs), especially with high-velocity bullets, can also cause pulmonary contusion (Fig. 4.3). Blast injuries due to explosive devices are another cause of severe lung contusion. In blunt trauma, there are usually multiple associated rib fractures. However, in pediatric patients, isolated lung contusions are common because of the elasticity of the ribs.

4.2.1.1 Pathophysiology

The underlying pathology in lung contusion consists of alveolar and small blood vessel injury with flooding

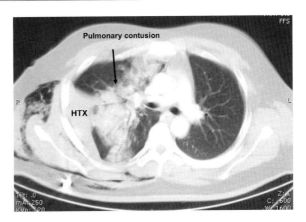

Fig. 4.3 Gunshot wound to the *right* chest with pulmonary contusion and hemothorax

of the interstitial and alveolar spaces (Fig. 4.4). This leads to perfusion without ventilation, which results in increased pulmonary shunting, reduced compliance, increased pulmonary vascular resistance, and abnormal gas exchange. Parenchymal lacerations may fill up with air and form pneumatoceles (Fig. 4.5). When these lacerations fill up with blood, there is formation of intrapulmonary hematomas. Bleeding into the bronchial tree may flood the normal parts of the lung, including the contralateral lung. In cases with extensive alveolar and vascular disruption, such as in blast injuries, the patient may suffer air embolism.

4.2.1.2 Diagnosis

The clinical presentation may vary from minor or no symptoms to severe respiratory distress, hypoxia, and hemoptysis. The initial chest x-ray (CXR) may underestimate the extent and severity of lung contusion. CT scan provides excellent information about the anatomical distribution of the pathology and the diagnosis of other associated injuries. Arterial blood gases should be performed in all significant contusions in order to assess the severity of the respiratory dysfunction and the need for mechanical ventilation.

4.2.1.3 Management

The treatment is mainly supportive and may vary from observation and oxygen administration to mechanical ventilation support. Effective pain management of associated rib fractures is critical for effective respiratory

Fig. 4.4 Lung specimen with severe lung contusion

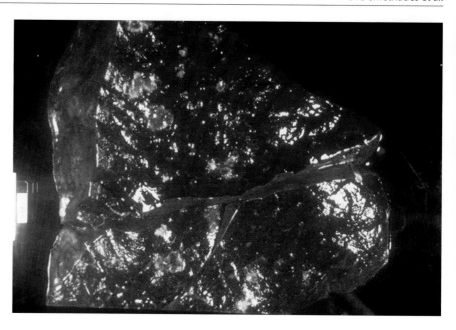

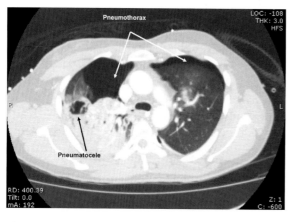

Fig. 4.5 Right pulmonary contusion with intrapulmonary laceration, pneumotocele and bilateral pneumothoraces following a gunshot wound to the chest

extracorporeal membrane oxygenation (ECMO), but we do not have any experience with this modality. In addition to the above therapeutic interventions, judicious fluid administration with moderate fluid restriction is recommended.

4.2.1.4 Prognosis

The majority of patients with lung contusions improve clinically and radiologically within the first 3–5 days. However, severe pulmonary contusions are significant factors contributing to morbidity and mortality [66]. Most common complications are ARDS and pneumonia. Failure of radiological improvement of the contusion within the first few days should alert the physician to the possibility of a superimposed pneumonia. Despite the radiological resolution of the contusion, there is evidence of long-term sequelae, which include pulmonary parenchymal fibrosis and reduced functional residual capacity [56, 57].

4.2.2 Pneumothorax

Pneumothorax is one of the most frequent pathologies following trauma and is encountered in about 20% of blunt and 30% of penetrating thoracic traumas [33, 62].

support. The threshold for mechanical ventilation should be lower in elderly patients or those with major associated injuries, because of the high incidence of rapid respiratory deterioration.

The most commonly used mechanical ventilation modality is conventional ventilation with low volumes and low pressures. Other ventilatory modalities such as noninvasive positive pressure ventilation (NPPV) [8, 92], high-frequency percussive ventilation (HFPV), and independent lung ventilation (ILV) have successfully been used in the appropriate cases [59]. In rare cases with refractory hypoxia some authors have used

The incidence of occult pneumothorax, defined as a pneumothorax not seen on plain CXRs but detected on CT scan, ranges from 4% of injured children to 64% in intubated trauma patients [42, 46].

A pneumothorax may be simple, tension, or open. A simple pneumothorax is often asymptomatic or might cause some mild to moderate dyspnea.

A tension pneumothorax is the result of air trapped in the pleural cavity under pressure resulting in compression on the heart, the major veins, and the normal lung (Fig. 4.6a and b). The clinical findings may include a restless and panicky patient in respiratory distress, tachypnea, hypotension, tachycardia, distended neck veins, deviation of the trachea, absent breath sounds, and hyperresonance on the affected hemithorax. Any patient with an undrained simple pneumothorax on mechanical ventilator is at risk of developing a tension pneumothorax (Fig. 6). Some authors reported an incidence of 20% of tension pneumothorax in patients with lung injuries on mechanical ventilation [37]. However, other authors reported that conservative management, without a chest drain, is safe in mechanically ventilated patients with occult pneumothorax [5, 10]. We believe that closely monitored patients can safely be managed without a chest drain. However, if close monitoring cannot be assured or if the patient is planned for air-evacuation or long transportation, a chest drain should be inserted. A tension pneumothorax is a life-threatening condition and requires immediate decompression by either a needle thoracostomy or a chest drain, depending on the circumstances. Prehospital needle thoracostomy is a fairly common practice by paramedics in the USA. This practice is controversial and many authors challenge its value [20, 35]. We believe that this procedure should be used with caution, only in patients with severe respiratory distress and fairly long prehospital times.

An open pneumothorax occurs in the presence of a wound in the chest wall, which allows airflow to and from the pleural cavity and results in the collapse of the lung (Fig. 4.7). The immediate management is an occlusive dressing taped only on three sides in order to create a valve permitting one way airflow from the chest cavity to the outside. A chest drain should be placed as soon as possible.

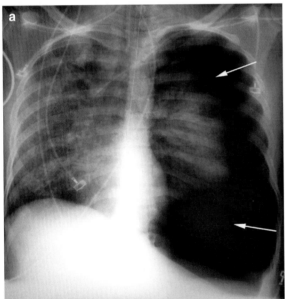

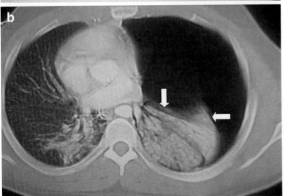

Fig. 4.6 (a) Chest x-ray with left tension pneumothorax due to a stab wound. (b)CT scan with tension pneumothorax – note the shift of the heart to the opposite side. It started as an occult hemothorax which was observed

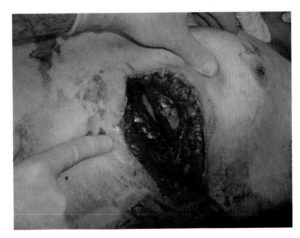

Fig. 4.7 Large open pneumothorax due to a large stab wound

4.2.3 Hemothorax

Hemothorax is defined as the collection of free blood in the pleural cavity and is diagnosed in about 50% of major trauma victims. The source of the bleeding is usually the lung parenchyma and less often the thoracic wall, heart, and great thoracic vessels or the diaphragm. The bleeding from the lung is usually self-controlled due to the low-pressure vascular system and the high concentration of tissue thromboplastin in the lung tissues.

4.2.3.1 Diagnosis of Hemo/Pneumothorax

The diagnosis of a hemothorax or pneumothorax is usually radiological, by means of plain CXRs. Ideally, the CXR should be obtained with the patient sitting up and in deep expiration, in order to diagnose small pneumothoraces or hemothoraces. However, this may not be possible in the multitrauma patient with depressed level of consciousness or hypotension and concerns about spinal injuries. The supine CXR often misses the diagnosis of significant pneumothoraces or hemothoraces (Fig. 4.8).

A chest ultrasound, as part of the trauma ultrasound, may be useful in the diagnosis of hemo/pneumothorax in the emergency room (ER) [58]. Recent prospective studies suggested that an ultrasound thoracic window is as good as or even better than a CXR in detecting pneumothoraces [34, 35, 58]. Occult hemothorax, missed by conventional CXR but diagnosed by CT scan, occurs in about 20% of severe trauma patients [90]. It is estimated that a minimum of 200–300 ml of free blood must be present in the pleural cavity in order to be detected by conventional x-rays. In the supine position, moderate-size hemothoraces may be missed. Larger hemothoraces show as increased opacification of the involved hemothorax. Massive hemothorax is defined as the presence of ≥1,000–1,500 ml of blood in the chest cavity and in this case the CXR shows a complete opacification (Fig. 4.9). Often, the distinction between a hemothorax and a lung contusion may be difficult with plain films. Chest CT scan is the best investigation, provided that the patient is fairly stable.

4.2.3.2 Management of Hemo/Pneumothorax

The role of prehospital needle thoracostomy for suspected tension pneumothorax and the safety of observational management of occult pneumothoraces have already been discussed. The definitive management of significant hemo/pneumothoraces consists of insertion of a chest drain. This allows drainage of the extravasated blood and allows re-expansion of the collapsed lung.

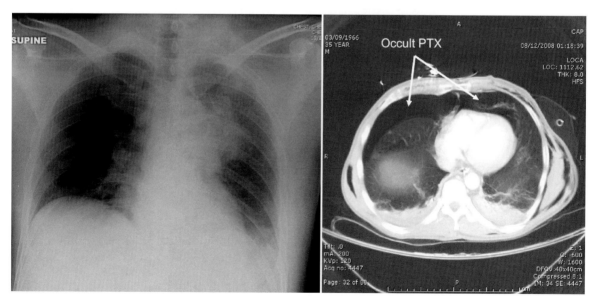

Fig. 4.8 Severe pulmonary contusion with right pneumothorax and bilateral subcutaneous emphysema. The pneumothorax was not shown on the supine chest x-ray

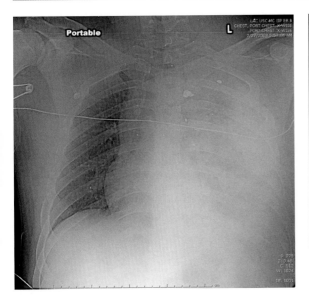

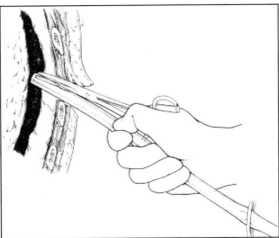

Fig. 4.11 Insertion of chest tube with the open technique is significantly invasive and painful

Fig. 4.9 Gunshot wound to the left chest with massive hemothorax

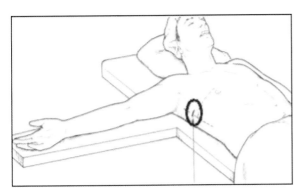

Fig. 4.10 Insertion site of the thoracostomy tube: mid-axillary line, fourth or fifth interstal space. The arm is abducted at 90°

4.2.3.3 Technique of Chest Tube Insertion

The drain should be inserted under strict antiseptic precautions. The preferred insertion site is the mid-axillary line, in the fourth or fifth intercostal space, always above the level of the nipple in a male (Fig. 4.10). At this site, the insertion is easy because of the thin thoracic wall and also it avoids injury to the diaphragm, which during expiration can easily reach the sixth intercostal space. The tube should be inserted 8–10 cm into the pleural cavity and with a direction toward the patient's head and posteriorly. The insertion can be performed with an open (Fig. 4.11) or percutaneous dilational technique (Fig. 4.12), the latter being faster and less traumatic. Immediately after insertion of the drain,

negative suction should be applied and if the patient is cooperative he should be encouraged to cough numerous times while sitting up, lying on his back, and on his sides. This encourages the re-expansion of the lung and drainage of the free blood before it clots.

Autotransfusion is an excellent and safe method of avoiding allogenic blood transfusion. The autotransfusion system is easy and cheap, and in our center, it has become part of the standard protocol for the drainage of any significant hemothorax. Citrate is added to prevent clotting of the collection blood. Any blood volume ≥ 500 ml is autotransfused.

The role of prophylactic antibiotics after this procedure is debatable. Most evidence supports the administration of one dose of antibiotic, ideally before insertion of the tube. The antibiotic should cover gram-positive cocci (staphylococcus), which is the most common cause of posttraumatic empyema. In our center, we have been using Cefazolin with successful results. Prolonged antibiotics prophylaxis (often given for the duration of the chest drain) does not offer any benefit and should be avoided [85].

Post-drain insertion, physiotherapy and ambulation are essential components of the treatment because they reduce the incidence of atelectasis and residual hemothorax. The drain should be removed as soon as possible, within 48–72 h of the initial placement. The maximum chest tube output before removal is an unresolved issue but most surgeons use 100 ml/day. The removal of the tube can take place in deep inspiration or deep expiration.

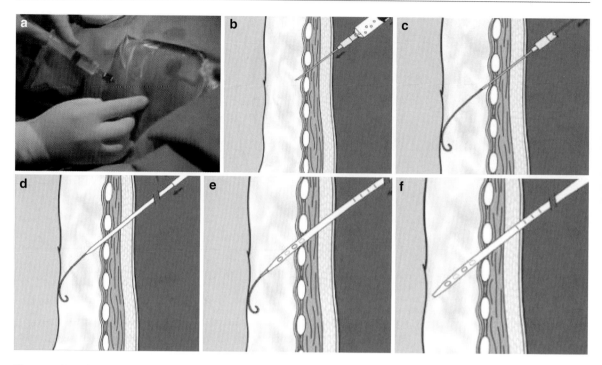

Fig. 4.12 Insertion of chest tube with the percutaneous dilational technique is less invasive and less painful than the open technique. (**a**) and (**b**) Insertion of needle attached to a syringe containing sterile water into the pleural cavity, (**c**) Insertion of the guidewire, (**d**) Sequential dilatation of the tract over the guidewire, (**e**) Insertion of the chest tube over the guidewire, (**f**) Removal of the guidewire and connection of the chest tube to the collection system

4.2.3.4 Post-Chest Tube Insertion Complications

Insertion of a thoracostomy tube is associated with significant complications. The reported overall incidence of failure or complications is about 25% [16, 31]. Some of the complications are iatrogenic and include insertion of the drain into the lung parenchyma, the heart, the diaphragm, the liver or the spleen. Sometimes, during insertion, the intercostal vessels may be injured and may bleed considerably. Other less serious iatrogenic complications include air leaks at the insertion site or kinking of the tube. Other complications or failures of the thoracostomy tube include empyema, retained hemothorax, and persistent air leak.

Empyema occurs in about 1–3% of patients with chest trauma requiring a thoracostomy tube drain. Risk factors for empyema include penetrating trauma, especially with thoracoabdominal injuries involving hollow viscus perforation, prolonged duration of the chest drain, residual hemothorax, and poor aseptic techniques [38, 51]. Most empyemas can successfully be managed with drainage and antibiotics. In loculated collections, CT-guided drainage should be considered.

Intrapleural fibrolytic therapy may be helpful in reducing the need for open surgical drainage [14]. In persistent cases, an open surgery with decortication may be necessary.

A retained significant hemothorax (Fig. 4.13a), defined as a blood collection greater than 300 ml, is by far the most common failure of thoracostomy tube drainage. An undrained residual hemothorax increases the risk of empyema and may cause fibrosis and lung entrapment. Therapeutic options for the management of this complication include intrapleural thrombolysis, video-assisted thoracoscopic surgery (VATS), and open thoracotomy. Thrombolysis should probably be the first-line intervention because of its noninvasive nature and its relative effectiveness [55, 102]. The treatment is contra-indicated in patients with recent surgery (within 48 h), stroke, or intracranial bleeding within 30 days, pregnancy, severe uncontrolled hypertension, and brain tumors. Urokinase and TPA are the most widely used agents. Our preference is Urokinase 100,000 units in 70 ml of saline injected into the pleural cavity through the thoracostomy tube, followed by an additional flush with 70 ml of normal saline. The

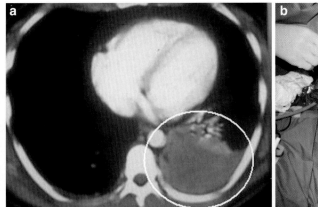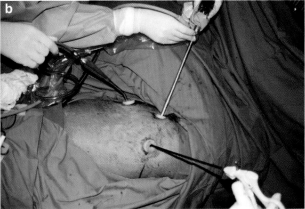

Fig. 4.13 (**a**) Persistent residual hemothorax which failed thrombolytic therapy (**b**) Thorascopic evacuation of persistent hemothorax. The thoracoscopic evacuation should be performed within the first week

tube is then clamped and the patient is encouraged to ambulate during the next 4 h. The tube is then unclamped and connected to a suction. The treatment is repeated for three consecutive days, with close radiological monitoring of the residual hemothorax, hemoglobin, and coagulation panel. If the hemothorax is successfully drained, the tube is removed. If there is a persistent significant retained hemothorax confirmed by CT scan, the next step is VATS (Fig. 4.13b).

VATS has been shown to be effective in the treatment of retained hemothorax, provided it is applied early, within the first week, before organization of the clot [100, 102]. VATS evacuation after 10 days is usually a difficult procedure and is rarely successful.

Persistent air leak is an infrequent complication. Sometimes the problem is faulty tube connections or suction system. A CXR is obtained to confirm that all holes in the chest tube are in fact in the pleural cavity. Almost all small air leaks close spontaneously and it is very rare that any surgical intervention is needed. Persistent, large air leaks should be evaluated by bronchoscopy to rule out tracheobronchial injury.

4.2.4 Indications for Emergency Thoracotomy

Less than 5% of blunt trauma patients, 10–15% of patients with stab wounds, and 15–20% of GSWs to the chest who reach the hospital alive need an emergency operation. The criteria for emergency

thoracotomy include hemodynamic instability due to blood loss or cardiac tamponade, massive initial chest tube output (>1,000–1,500 ml), persistent continuous bleeding in the chest tube of more than 250–300 ml/h for 4–5 h without any evidence of improvement, and very rarely respiratory distress due to a major tracheobronchial injury. The remaining patients should be further evaluated for occult injuries.

In patients with GSWs who are hemodynamically stable, CT scan with intravenous contrast provides excellent information about the extent of the injury and the need for further evaluation with other investigations. The direction of the bullet tract toward or away from vital structures such as the major vessels, the esophagus or the tracheobronchial tree, is very helpful in determining the need for endoscopy or esophagography (Fig. 4.14a–c). Most hemodynamically stable patients with transmediastinal GSWs can safely be managed nonoperatively on the basis of the CT scan findings.

4.2.5 Emergency Operations for Lung Injuries

4.2.5.1 Incisions

An anterolateral thoracotomy through the fourth or fifth intercostal space provides a good access to the lung and the lateral mediastinum. The incision can be extended trans-sternally into the opposite pleural cavity ("clamshell" thoracotomy), taking care to ligate

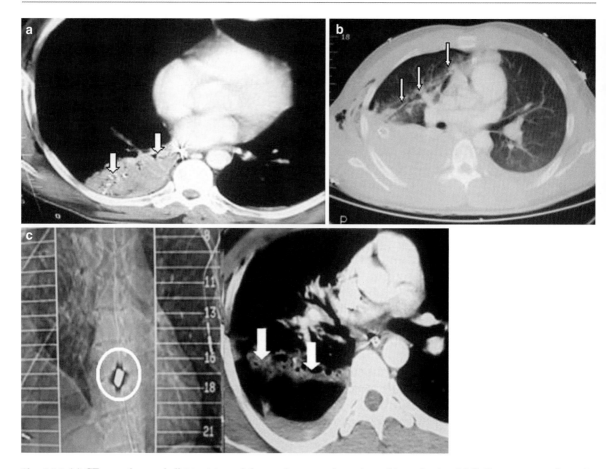

Fig. 4.14 (**a**) CT scan shows a bullet tract toward the esophagus. This patient needs further evaluation by means of esophagogram (**b**) CT bullet tract near the major vessels. This patient needs angiographic evaluation (**c**) Bullet tract away from the vital structures. There is no use for further investigation

both internal mammary arteries (Fig. 4.15). A left postero-lateral thoracotomy permits access to the aorta, the proximal left subclavian artery, the posterior heart, the entire left lung, and the distal esophagus. The right posterolateral thoracotomy provides a good exposure of the trachea, the entire right lung, and the proximal esophagus. A median sternotomy provides access to the heart and both lungs.

4.2.5.2 Operative Techniques

There are many intraoperative techniques for the management of the injured lung. The selection of method depends on the site and severity of lung injury, the shape and direction of the lung wound, the hemodynamic condition of the patient, and the experience of the surgeon. The operative techniques include application of local hemostatic agents, suturing of the bleeding lung, lung tractotomy, and resectional techniques.

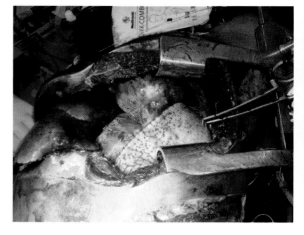

Fig. 4.15 Emergency room resuscitative thoracotomy with extension of the right thoracotomy into a clamshell incision for cardiac injury and associated bleeding in the right chest

(a) Local hemostasis may be adequate for slow, diffuse bleeding, usually found as an incidental finding during a thoracotomy for other intrathoracic injuries.

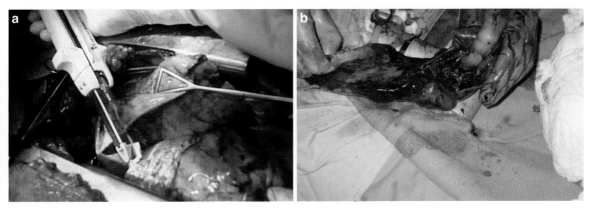

Fig. 4.16 (**a**, **b**) Lung tractotomy for bleeding from a bullet tract in the lung with GI stapling device

Electrocautery or local application of biological glue may provide good hemostasis and air leak control.

(b) Lung suturing may be effective in cases with peripheral lung lacerations. Following careful suture-ligation of major bleeders and air leaks, the laceration is repaired with figure 8 sutures, using a liver needle. Application of tissue glue before approximation of the edges of the laceration may improve hemostasis and control minor air leaks. In cases with bleeding and air leaks from deep penetrating lung injuries, suturing of the entry and exit wounds should be avoided because of the risk of air embolism, intrapulmonary hematoma, and blood flooding of the bronchial tree, including the contralateral lung. These cases should be managed with lung tractotomy or segmental resection.

(c) Lung tractotomy: This is the method of choice in cases with bleeding and/or major air leaks in deep penetrating injuries [3, 64, 101] (Fig. 4.16a and b). The wound tract is opened with a GIA stapler and any significant bleeders or air leaks are suture-ligated under direct view. Application of tissue glue might be helpful in decreasing any diffuse bleeding and minor air leaks. The tract is then closed with figure 8 absorbable sutures on a blunt liver needle. On rare occasions, tractotomy may devascularize segments of the lung, resulting in subsequent ischemic necrosis and lung abscess. The lung adjacent to the tractotomy should be always assessed for viability and any questionable areas should be resected.

(d) Lung Resections: The extent of resection can range from nonanatomic "wedge" resection to lobectomy and total pneumonectomy. These resectional techniques are rarely used. In a National Trauma

Data Bank analysis of 167,250 patients with chest trauma, only 669 patients (0.4%) required lung resection. The incidence was 1.3% in penetrating trauma, and 0.03% in blunt trauma [64]. Wedge resection was performed in 49% of cases, lobectomy in 36%, and total pneumonectomy in only 15%.

- *Wedge resection* using a stapling device, is usually the procedure of choice in fairly peripheral lung injuries. Any persisting bleeding or air leaks can be managed with sutures and/or tissue glue (Fig. 4.17).
- *Lobectomy* is the next most common resection technique. In earlier years, anatomical lobectomy was the standard technique. However, this approach has largely been replaced by nonanatomical resections, preserving as much normal lung parenchyma as possible [101]. This is best accomplished with a

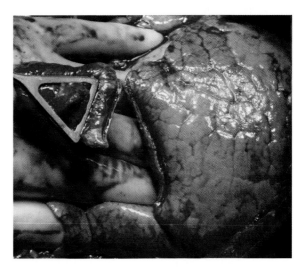

Fig. 4.17 Stapled wedge resection of bleeding lung

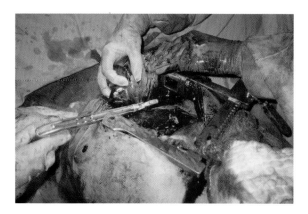

Fig. 4.18 Lung lobectomy with TA stapling device

stapling device (Fig. 4.18). During the procedure, care should be taken to avoid devascularization of the remaining normal lung parenchyma.

• *Total pneumonectomy* is rarely performed but it might be necessary in severe hilar injuries not amenable to repair. In these situations, the patient is usually hemodynamically unstable and there is severe active bleeding upon entering the pleural cavity.

The fastest way to achieve temporary bleeding control is digital compression of the hilum and subsequent application of a vascular clamp. This maneuver is critical for effective bleeding control, and prevention of air embolism and blood flooding of the normal bronchial tree. Acute occlusion often aggravates the hemodynamic condition of the patient because of acute right cardiac strain. Whenever is technically possible, repair of the hilar structures should be attempted, because total pneumonectomy is associated with a very high mortality.

The anatomical pneumonectomy involves individual isolation, ligation, and division of the hilar structures. However, this approach is time-consuming and requires significant technical skills and experience. An acceptable alternative to anatomical pneumonectomy is the en-mass stapled pneumonectomy. It has been shown clinically and experimentally that it is faster and is associated with less blood loss than the anatomical pneumonectomy [106]. The en-mass pneumonectomy can be rapidly achieved with a TA-55 staple (Fig. 4.19a–c). Additional figure of 8

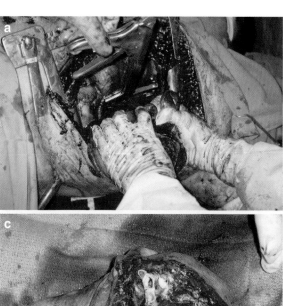
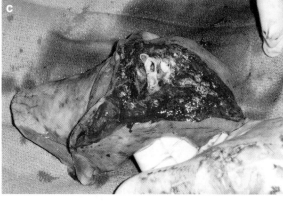
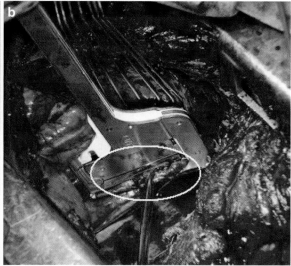

Fig. 4.19 En-mass stapled pneumonectomy: (a) Application of TA staple on the hilum (b) Removal of the lung by division above staple. Note the tissue clamp applied to the stump before release of the staple. This technique prevents retraction of the bronchial stump into the deep tissues before meticulous hemostatic (c) Lung specimen after pneumonectomy

sutures may be needed for complete hemostasis and control of air leaks from the main bronchus. Retraction of the hilar stump can make identification of any persistent bleeders difficult and may result in significant blood loss. Application of two stay sutures on the stump before removal of the stapling device can prevent this dangerous technical complication.

4.2.5.3 Outcomes

The mortality and complication rate following operative interventions on the lung increase with the complexity of the operation [48, 64, 101]. In a multivariate analysis of 669 trauma patients who underwent lung resections, there was a stepwise increase in both mortality and complications with more extensive resections that was independent of injury severity and the presence of associated injuries [64]. Analysis of 535 patients with lung resections and no major associated injuries showed a mortality of 19% for wedge resections, 27% for lobectomies, and 53% for total pneumonectomies ($p < 0.001$). Several smaller series reported a mortality of 100% for pneumonectomies. Most deaths occur in the operating room due to massive bleeding or air embolism. The remaining deaths occur in the ICU due to acute right cardiac failure, ARDS, pneumonia, and sepsis. About 70% of deaths occur within 24 h and 76% within 48 h of admission [64]. In a multivariate analysis adjusting for age, gender, mechanism of injury, hypotension on admission, base deficit, GCS, and injury severity score (ISS), the adjusted risk of death for lobectomies was 2.65 times and for pneumonectomies 5.35 times higher than wedge resections. Acute right cardiac failure is mainly due to significant increase of the pulmonary vascular resistance. The combination of pneumonectomy with shock act synergistically in increasing the pulmonary vascular resistance [19]. The most common intrathoracic complications after lung resections include pneumonia (20%), ARDS, and empyema (about 10% each). Other postoperative complications include torsion of the remaining lobe and persistent air leaks. Survivors of traumatic pneumonectomy are at risk for cor pulmonale [80].

4.3 Thoracic Aortic Injuries

4.3.1 Blunt Thoracic Aortic Injury

4.3.1.1 Epidemiology

It is estimated that 8,000–9,000 blunt trauma victims suffer injury to the thoracic aortic injury every year [40]. The majority of these injuries are due to motor vehicle crashes (about 70%) followed by motorcycle crashes (13%), falls from heights (7%), auto versus pedestrian (7%), and other mechanisms [27]. The overall incidence of thoracic aortic injuries in patients reaching the hospital alive is less than 0.5%. However, the vast majority of patients with this type of injury dies at the scene and never reaches hospital care. The incidence of aortic injuries in fatal traffic injuries is very high. In a recent analysis of 304 deaths due to blunt trauma in the county of Los Angeles, 102 patients (33%) had a rupture of the thoracic aorta. About 80% of the deaths occurred at the scene and only 20% in the hospital [95].

About 40% of patients with aortic rupture have a very severe associated injury (body area Abbreviated Injury Score ≥ 4), the most common being the head and the abdomen. The mean ISS is 40, a strong indicator of the grave condition of the victims [27]. The incidence of aortic trauma increases with age and is extremely rare to find this injury in the pediatric population. The most common anatomical site of the aortic injury is the medial aspect of the lumen, distal to the left subclavian artery (Fig. 4.20). In a prospective analysis of 185 cases of

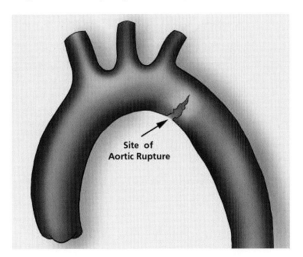

Fig. 4.20 The most common site of the aortic injury is the medial aspect of the lumen, distal to the left subclavian artery

thoracic aortic injuries, the rupture involved the isthmus in 75%, followed by the descending aorta in 22%, and the ascending aorta in 4% [27]. The most common type of injury was a false aneurysm (58%), followed by dissection (25%), and intimal tear (20%) (Fig. 4.21a and b).

4.3.1.2 Screening and Diagnosis

The supine CXR has been extensively used as the initial screening tool for the diagnosis of thoracic aortic injury. Numerous radiological findings have been described as suspicious markers for aortic trauma. They include widened upper mediastinum (>8 cm), obliteration of the aortic contour, loss of the perivertebral pleural stripe, depression of the left mainstem bronchus, deviation of a nasogastric tube to the right, an apical pleural hematoma, a massive left hemothorax, and the presence of fractures of the sternum, scapula, upper ribs or clavicle in a multitrauma patient [13, 40, 63, 68, 107] (Fig. 4.22). The widened mediastinum is the most common finding but it has a low specificity. Many conditions, such as a fracture of the thoracic spine or the sternum or supine position in an obese patient may give a widened mediastinum. The most discriminating signs are loss of the aortic knob, abnormality of the aortic arch, and deviation of the nasogastric tube [68, 99]. In earlier years, many authors suggested that a normal CXR reliably excluded a thoracic aortic injury [68, 99]. However, recent studies have shown that a significant number of aortic injuries may be missed by a plain CXR [23, 36, 39]. In summary, the current available evidence suggests that plain chest radiography is a poor screening tool. Patients with a suspicious mechanism of injury should be evaluated by CT scan, irrespective of x-ray findings [23, 36, 39].

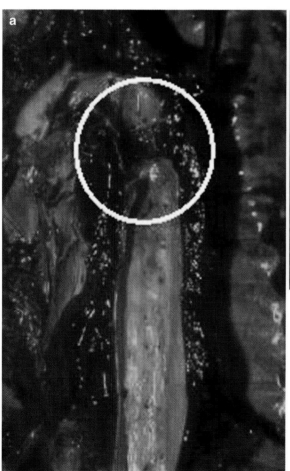
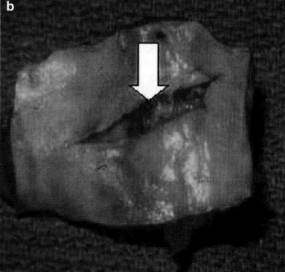

Fig. 4.21 (**a**) Free rupture of the thoracic aorta (**b**) intimal tear of the aorta

Aortography remained the gold standard for the diagnosis of thoracic aortic injury until the late 1990s. This method has significant disadvantages, including its invasiveness, the need to transport to the angio suite

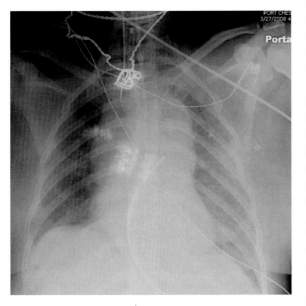

Fig. 4.22 Chest x-ray with a widened upper mediastinum due to a thoracic aortic injury

a frequently critically injured patient and the problematic immediate availability of the angiographic team after hours. The increased availability and improvement in the resolution of CT scanners has revolutionized the evaluation of suspected aortic injuries. CT scan has been shown to have almost 100% sensitivity and specificity, a 90% positive and 100% negative predictive value, and an overall diagnostic accuracy of 99.7% [69, 70] (Fig. 4.23a and b).

Transesophageal echocardiography (TEE) is another modality which was suggested as a reliable diagnostic tool [17, 89, 105]. This approach did not gain popularity because of conflicting reports and concerns regarding its accuracy and the practical problems of its availability 24 h a day [2, 67]. The dramatic shifting from angiography and TEE to CT scanning is demonstrated by a recent multicenter study sponsored by the American Association for the Surgery of Trauma [27]. The use of angiography and TEE for the diagnosis of thoracic aortic injuries decreased from 87% and 12%, respectively in 1997 to only 8% and 1% in 2007 [28].

Other diagnostic modalities such as magnetic resonance imaging (MRI) or intravascular ultrasound may be useful in rare patients where the CT scan findings are not definitive.

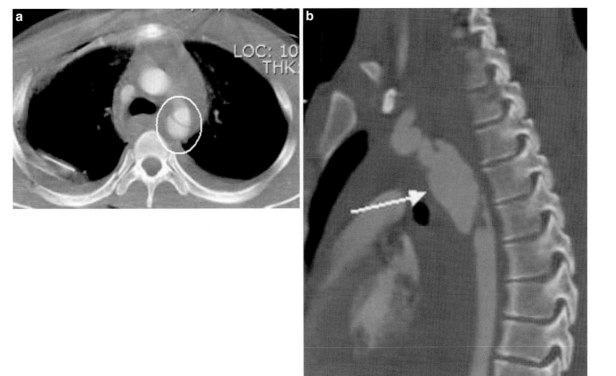

Fig. 4.23 (**a**) CT scan shows rupture of the thoracic aorta, distal to the left subclavian artery, (**b**) CT scan, sagital view, with rupture of the thoracic aorta

In summary, CT scan has become the new standard modality for the diagnosis of thoracic aortic injuries. Aortography has a diagnostic role in patients requiring angiography for other injuries such as pelvic fractures, complex liver injuries, etc. TEE might be useful in critically ill patients in the ICU who cannot be transferred safely to the radiology suite for the CT scan.

4.3.1.3 Management of Thoracic Aortic Injuries

For patients reaching the hospital alive, prompt diagnosis and early appropriate treatment remain the cornerstone for survival. The risk of free rupture is the highest in the first few hours of hospital admission and more than 90% of ruptures occur within the first 24 h [40]. The incidence of free rupture in untreated patients is about 12% [40]. Prevention of free rupture of a contained aortic injury until a definitive repair is the most urgent priority. This is best achieved pharmacologically by maintaining the systolic blood pressure as low as tolerated in most patients at about 90–110 mmHg. In elderly patients, the optimal systolic pressure may be slightly higher. Cautious restriction of intravenous fluids and administration of beta blockers, usually Esmolol drip, are the most commonly used modalities for blood pressure control. Rigorous blood pressure control reduces the risk of free rupture to 1.5% [44].

4.3.1.4 Timing of Definitive Repair

Immediate surgical repair of the injured aorta remained the standard of care for many decades. Even more recently in 2000, the Eastern Association for the Surgery of Trauma (EAST) in its Practice Management Guidelines recommended prompt repair of aortic injuries, except in patients with major associated injuries or high-risk patients [74]. There is now growing evidence that delayed semielective repair is associated with better survival than emergency repair [28, 44, 74]. In a recent multicenter prospective study of 178 eligible patients, sponsored by the AAST, delayed repair (>24 h after admission) was associated with significantly better survival than early repair (<24 h), overall, in patients with major associated injuries and in patients with no major associated injuries [29].

The concept of delayed repair has gained popularity as shown by two large prospective AAST studies in 1997 and 2007. In 1997, the mean time from injury to repair was 16.5 h and in 2007, the time increased to 54.6 h [28]. Delayed repair allows better resuscitation and performance of the repair under more optimal conditions. Rigorous blood pressure control is critical in the safe application of delayed repair. The severity of the aortic tear should also be taken into account and in large tears the repair should be performed as early as possible (Fig. 4.24).

4.3.1.5 Definitive Management of Aortic Injuries

Open surgical repair of aortic injuries remained the only therapeutic option for decades, until a few years ago. In the mid 2000s, endovascular stent-graft repair became popular and has now become the most commonly performed procedure for aortic rupture (Fig. 4.25). Another therapeutic option which has recently been used in selected patients is 'observation without any definitive repair.'

The open repair can be performed with either the clamp and sew technique or one of the various bypass techniques. The clamp and sew technique was blamed for the high incidence of paraplegia, especially if the occlusion of the aorta lasted for longer than 30 min [40]. A study sponsored by the AAST in 1997 reported an incidence of paraplegia of 16.5% with the clamp and sew technique and 4.5% with bypass techniques [40]. However, a second AAST study in 2007 showed

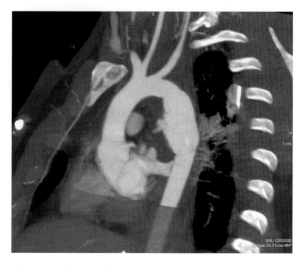

Fig. 4.24 CT scan shows a large thoracic aortic rupture with extravasation. This patient needs emergency repair because of the high risk of free rupture

Fig. 4.25 Thoracic aortic injury before and after deployment of the stent graft

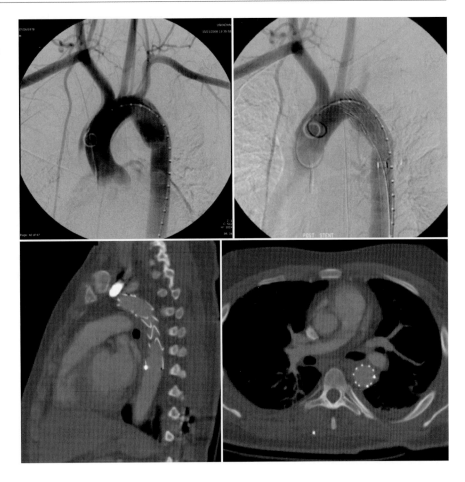

no paraplegias in the clamp and sew group but 3.5% in the bypass techniques [27]. Currently, about 85% of thoracic aortic injuries treated with open surgery are managed with bypass techniques [27].

Endovascular stent/grafts for traumatic thoracic aortic injuries were first used in 1997 [52]. This approach has become popular, especially in severe multitrauma or other high-risk patients. The procedure can be performed under sedation and local anesthesia, and is associated with lower morbidity and mortality than open repair. A systemic review of all published literature up to January 2006 showed only 284 patients from 62 centers with traumatic aortic injury treated with endovascular repair [32]. A more recent AAST study of 193 thoracic aortic injuries showed that about 65% of all patients, 60% of patients with no major extrathoracic injuries, and 57% of patients <55 years old and no major extrathoracic trauma, were managed with endovascular stent grafts [27]. Multivariate analysis adjusting for age >55, GCS ≤8,

hypotension on admission, and critical extrathoracic injuries, showed a significantly lower adjusted mortality and fewer blood transfusions in the endovascular group [27]. In the subgroup of patients with no critical extrathoracic injuries, endovascular repair was again associated with a significantly lower mortality and fewer blood transfusions than open repair.

A significant survival benefit was also identified in the subgroup of victims with associated critical extrathoracic injuries [27]. The incidence of procedure-related paraplegia was 2.9% in the open repair group and 0.8% in the endovascular group. A significant concern with the endovascular technique was the high incidence of device-related complications. Overall, 20% of patients in this group developed significant local complications, which included endoleaks, injuries to the access vessels, occlusion of the left subclavian artery or the left carotid artery, collapse of the device, and stroke (Fig. 4.26). By far, the most common complication was an endoleak and it was recorded in 14% of patients. Improvement of the devices is expected to reduce these complications significantly. There are already commercially available new devices with more appropriate shape and size, which have reduced the incidence of endoleaks and injury of the access vessels. "Branched" stent grafts will probably reduce the risk of subclavian or carotid artery occlusion. Performance of the endovascular

repair in selected high-volume centers seems to be an independent factor for better results [27].

Another major concern with endovascular stent grafts is the lack of any significant long-term follow-up. We still do not know how these devices will behave when the aorta becomes tortuous and dilated with old age or whether their mechanical properties will withstand the test of time. Despite these concerns, the very low mortality of this technique has proved very attractive to surgeons and most likely it will become the new standard of care (Table 4.1).

Nonoperative management of selected high-risk patients with small aortic injuries, such as intimal tears, has been made with very good results in a small number of patients. Follow-up studies confirmed resolution or no progression of the aortic injury [47, 53].

In summary, the diagnosis and management of traumatic thoracic aortic injuries have undergone some very major changes in the last decade. CT scan has replaced aortography and TEE in the diagnosis. Endovascularly placed stent grafts have become the most commonly used therapeutic modality, irrespective of the presence or not of any risk factors and have resulted in a major reduction of the in-hospital mortality. Rigorous initial control of the blood pressure and subsequent semielective delayed repair improved survival. Finally, the concept of nonoperative management of selected small aortic injuries has successfully been tested in a small number of patients.

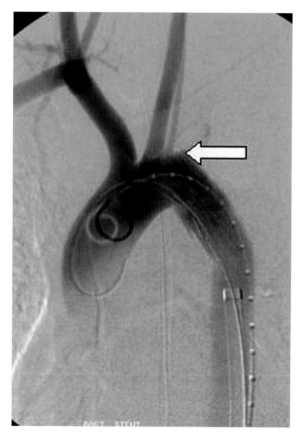

Fig. 4.26 Placement of stent-graft for traumatic aortic rupture resulted in asymptomatic occlusion of the left subclavian artery

4.3.2 Penetrating Thoracic Aortic Injuries

These are highly lethal injuries and more than 90% of the victims die at the scene or in the ER. The majority of the cases (about 80%) reaching hospital

Table 4.1 Open versus endovascular repair of thoracic aortic injuries: AAST study [27]

	All patients	Open repair	Endovascular repair	p-value
N	193	58	125	
Mean ISS	39.5	38.9	39.4	0.83
Severe associated injuries	39.2%	31.3%	43.4%	0.10
Mortality	13.0%	23.5%	7.2%	0.001
Paraplegia	1.6%	2.9%	0.8%	0.28
Systemic complication	45.1%	50.0%	42.4%	0.31

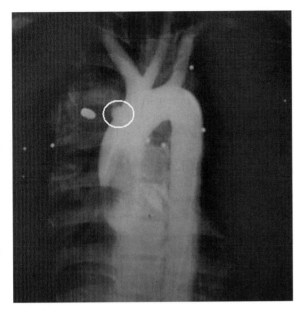

Fig. 4.27 Shotgun injury with false aneurysm of ascending aorta

care require an ER resuscitative thoracotomy because of loss of vital signs [25]. The relatively thin wall of the vessel, combined with the intraluminal high pressures and the lack of any significant tissues to contain the bleeding, result in rapid exsanguination and death. Only patients with small, contained false aneurysms survive (Fig. 4.27).

4.4 Cardiac Injuries

4.4.1 Blunt Cardiac Injury

4.4.1.1 Definition

Over the last decade, numerous publications on blunt cardiac injury (BCI) have been published [86, 93], and yet, the injury is still very poorly understood. The reported incidence varies widely from 15% to 52% [1, 7, 84]. This is due primarily to the wide spectrum of injury which ranges from a mild contusion to free wall rupture with no definitive gold standard imaging modality that can capture both structural and electrical injuries.

Practically, BCIs can be subdivided into those that are electrical and those that are structural in nature. Overall, the most commonly seen electrical abnormality

is a nonspecific ST-T wave change. The clinical significance of this finding is unknown. The most common clinically significant electrical disorders are arrhythmias, most commonly tachyarrhythmias. After sinus tachycardia, the most common arrhythmia seen is atrial fibrillation [61, 84].

The most common manifestation of a structural lesion is myocardial contusion, which is, in most cases, mild and asymptomatic. Because this condition is often asymptomatic and its clinical significance is questionable, the true incidence of clinically significant BCI remains obscure. Diagnosis and treatment should therefore be targeted at structural lesions requiring intervention and electrical dysrhythmias requiring treatment.

4.4.1.2 Screening and Diagnosis

The at-risk population is broad and includes any patient who has sustained blunt chest trauma (Fig. 4.28). In a series of studies from LAC + USC Medical Center, which included patients with major thoracic trauma (defined as multiple rib fractures, sternal fractures, pulmonary contusion > 20%, hemo-pneumothorax requiring thoracostomy tube drainage, scapular fracture, major intra-thoracic vascular injury or anterior thoracic seatbelt marks and not isolated rib or clavicle fractures), the incidence of clinically significant cardiac injuries requiring treatment was 13% [84, 103].

The diagnostic tests used for screening purposes have included serum biomarkers such as creatine

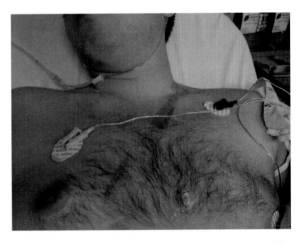

Fig. 4.28 Seatbelt mark sign on the chest is an indication for evaluation for blunt cardiac trauma by means of ECG and Troponin-I levels

phosphokinase-MB fraction and troponin-I, echocardiography, and ECG [7]. The EAST guidelines, which summarized the literature up to 1997 concluded that at that time "no single test or combination of tests has proven consistently reliable in detecting cardiac injury" [78]. Since then, however, a series of two prospective trials from LAC+USC Medical Center investigating the role of cardiac Troponin-I (Tn-I) and ECG enrolled a total of 333 consecutive patients over a 30-month period [84, 103]. All patients with the aforementioned definition of major thoracic trauma were enrolled. These patients had an admission Tn-I and ECG followed by repeat Tn-I at 4 and 8 h and a repeat ECG at 8 h. The primary outcome measure utilized in this study was a clinically significant treatment which requires BCI to be defined as cardiogenic hypotension (nonhemorrhagic, nonneurogenic), dysrhythmias, echocardiographic evidence of structural abnormality, and/or a Cardiac Index <2.5 l/min/m^2. In this cohort of patients, 13% had a diagnosis of BCI. This was a severely injured patient cohort and when compared to those patients who were screened but did not sustain a BCI, were significantly older and had a significantly higher ISS. Of the patients with BCI, 39% died, with a third of the deaths related to the cardiac injury. In these highly practical trials, the sensitivity and specificity of Tn-I alone were found to be 73% and 60%, respectively and those of ECG alone, were 89% and 67%, respectively. However, the two investigations combined had a sensitivity and specificity of 100 and 71%, respectively. From a different angle, if the Tn-I alone was positive, 7% had significant BCI and if the ECG alone was positive, 22% had significant BCI. If both were positive, the rate increased to 36%. Most importantly, however, if both the serial ECG and Tn-I measurements were normal, no clinically significant BCI were observed.

At our center, all patients with significant chest trauma are evaluated for BCI by means of ECG and Tn-I on admission and 8 h later. Patients with abnormal findings are further evaluated by transthoracic echocardiogram. Only symptomatic patients with cardiogenic shock or arrhythmias receive treatment.

4.4.1.3 Treatment

Long-term functional outcome studies, as in many trauma populations are generally lacking. However, small series of patients utilizing the New York Heart Association classification and functional testing at 1 year demonstrated excellent recovery amongst survivors [61, 91].

4.4.1.4 Blunt Cardiac Rupture

Blunt cardiac rupture is often described as a separate entity from the remainder of the BCI spectrum due to its high associated mortality. The vast majority of data accumulated on blunt ruptures is from autopsy studies including the seminal work of Parmley [77] and his study of over 200,000 autopsies. On the 50th anniversary of his work, we reviewed the current incidence of blunt cardiac ruptures in 304 victims undergoing autopsy in the Los Angeles County. Despite improvements in many systems from prehospital care to motor vehicle safety engineering, we found a strikingly similar pattern of cardiac injury. Overall, 96 (32%) victims had a cardiac injury and free rupture was identified in 61 patients (20%) [96], similar to the 65% found by Parmley. Motor vehicle collision was the most common mechanism of injury at 50%, followed by pedestrians struck by an auto at 37%. The right chambers (30% right atrium, 27% right ventricle) were most commonly injured with multiple chamber disruption in 26%. This is a catastrophic injury with a high associated mortality rate, with 78% dying at the scene and 22% en route or at the hospital.

For those patients reaching hospital care, an NTDB study [97] demonstrated that of 811,531 blunt trauma patients admitted between 2000 and 2005, 366 or 0.05% sustained a blunt cardiac rupture. With a mean age of 45 years and ISS of 58+/−19, they occurred most commonly after a motor vehicle collision (73%). The overall mortality in this selected group of patients reaching medical care was 89%. Blunt cardiac rupture is therefore a relatively rare event and although it is associated with a very high mortality rate, it is not uniformly fatal.

4.4.2 Penetrating Cardiac Injury

4.4.2.1 Epidemiology

The majority of patients sustaining cardiac injuries do not survive to present to hospital. Only 10–15% of victims reach the hospital alive [15, 26]. In a 3-year autopsy-based study from South Africa, 94% of the penetrating cardiac injuries were taken directly from the field to the morgue. In another series, also from South Africa, those victims with stab wounds had a significantly lower mortality rate of 15.6% vs 81.0% for GSWs, $p<=0.0001$ [21]. A prospective study from our center in Los Angeles demonstrated a similar figure with a stab wound survival of 65% compared to 16% for GSWs [4]. The prognostic factors determining prognosis include the mechanism of injury, the injured cardiac chamber, the presence of tamponade, prehospital time, associated injuries, and experience of the trauma team (Fig. 4.29). Right ventricular injuries have the best prognosis while intrapericardial aortic injury, the worst prognosis. Cardiac tamponade improves survival [15, 26, 30].

4.4.2.2 Clinical Presentation

High index of suspicion is the cornerstone of early diagnosis of penetrating cardiac injuries. Every penetrating injury to the chest, especially the precordium, associated with hypotension should be suspected as cardiac injury until proven otherwise. The clinical diagnosis is usually easy, although in some cases with multiple injuries it might be more complicated. The patient is often very restless and the inexperienced surgeon may mistake it for alcohol or illicit drug intoxication. Hypotension is the most common clinical finding. On rare occasions with small cardiac wounds and short prehospital times, the patient may have normal blood pressure. The Beck's triad (hypotension, distended neck veins, and distant cardiac sounds) is present in about 90% of patients with proven cardiac tamponade. Tachycardia and weak pulse are usually present. Pulses paradoxus is found in only about 10% of cases with tamponade [30]. Although the neck veins are usually distended, the surgeon should have in mind that in the presence of associated severe blood loss they might be

collapsed. In addition, besides tamponade other conditions such as tension pneumothorax or a restless patient may be the cause of distended veins.

4.4.2.3 Investigations

Trauma ultrasound (FAST) has become part of the initial clinical examination and is immediately available in every modern ER. Many series have reported excellent sensitivity and specificity in the diagnosis of cardiac tamponade [81–83]. A positive FAST in a hypotensive patient is an absolute indication for immediate operation (Fig. 4.30). However, it should be stressed that in our experience false negative trauma

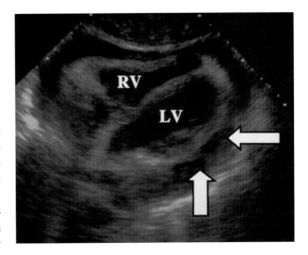

Fig. 4.30 Trauma ultrasound shows a pericardial effusion following a gunshot wound to the heart

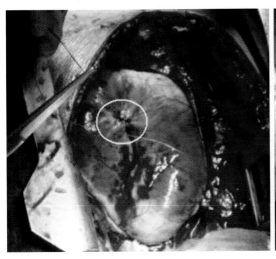 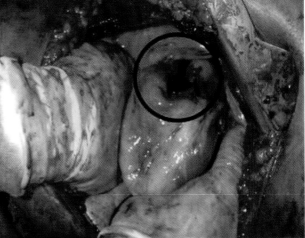

Fig. 4.29 Stab wound to the heart (*left*) and gunshot wound to the heart (*right*). Gunshot wounds have a much worse prognosis

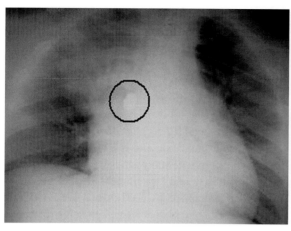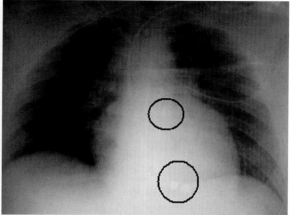

Fig. 4.31 Chest x-ray shows an enlarged cardiac shadow due to cardiac tamponade after a gunshot injury (*left*). Multiple bullets in the enlarged cardiac shadow (*right*)

ultrasounds are not infrequent and may result in delayed treatment. If time permits and the patient is hemodynamically stable, a formal echocardiogram can provide a definitive diagnosis.

Other investigations should be considered only in fairly stable patients where the diagnosis is uncertain. An erect CXR may be helpful in about 50% of patients with cardiac injury. Radiological signs suggestive of cardiac trauma include an enlarged cardiac shadow, widened upper mediastinum, and pneumopericardium [30] (Figs. 4.31 and 4.32). An electrocardiogram (ECG) is abnormal in about 50% of patients. Abnormalities may include low QRS complexes, elevated ST segments, inverted T waves, and arrhythmias [30] (Fig. 4.33).

Other investigations such as pericardiocentesis and subxiphoid window have little or no role in a hospital environment. Pericardiocentecis has an unacceptably high incidence of false negative results because of clotting in the pericardial sac (Fig. 4.34). In addition, there is a risk of iatrogenic injury to the heart, especially if there is no tamponade. It might have a place to attempt temporary relief of the cardiac tamponade in situations where there is no surgeon available.

Subxiphoid window has a very limited role in the diagnosis of cardiac tamponade and most trauma centers in the USA do not use it. It is probably the most invasive diagnostic procedure in surgery. If it is done under local anesthesia it is extremely uncomfortable and difficult and if general anesthesia is used it has the disadvantages and risks of an emergency anesthesia. On the other hand, a transdiaphragmatic window

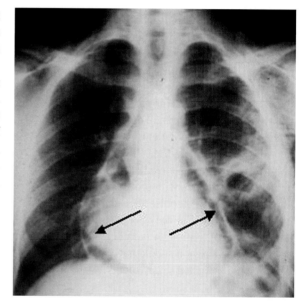

Fig. 4.32 Chest x-ray shows pneumopericardium after a stab wound to the heart

during laparotomy for associated abdominal injuries, is very useful and expeditious in ruling out a cardiac injury. The window in the pericardium is performed at the least muscular area of the diaphragm. The pericardium is grasped with two tissue forceps and is opened carefully taking meticulous hemostatic precautions in order to avoid a false positive result. If the pericardial fluid is bloody, the laparotomy incision is extended into a median sternotomy. If the pericardial fluid is clear, the window is closed with a figure of eight suture.

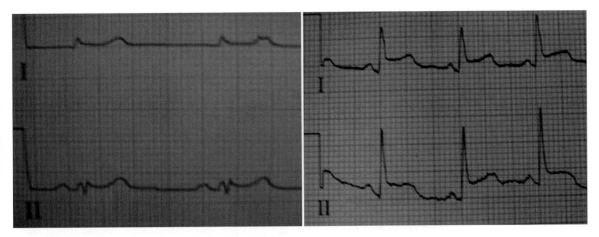

Fig. 4.33 ECG of two patients with penetrating injuries to the heart. On the left it shows low QRS complexes, on the right it shows elevated ST segments

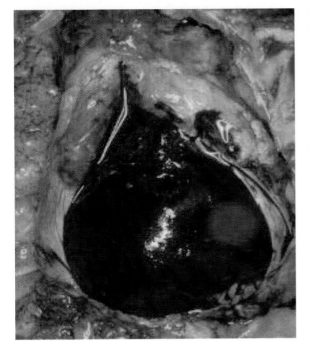

Fig. 4.34 A large clot in the pericardium in a patient with a stab wound to the heart and cardiac tamponade. The clot will give a false negative pericardiocentesis

4.4.2.4 Management

Time is the most precious commodity for the patient with penetrating cardiac injury. In the prehospital phase the "scoop and run" approach is the most appropriate approach for all victims with suspected cardiac trauma. In the ER, no attempts to stabilize the patient with intravenous fluids should be made. No time should be wasted for bladder catheterization or other procedures.

4.4.2.5 Operative Management

Emergency Room Thoracotomy

Many patients with cardiac injury arrive to the hospital in extremis or cardiac arrest and there is little or no time to transfer them to the operating room. These patients should undergo an ER thoracotomy. An ER thoracotomy tray should always be kept in every ER receiving trauma patients. The tray should be kept simple and should include only a few absolutely essential instruments (Fig. 4.35). Simultaneously with endotracheal intubation, the left arm is abducted 30° and an anterolateral thoracotomy is performed through the fourth to fifth intercostal space (below the nipple in males or the infra-mammary crease in females). The incision starts at the left parasternal border and extends to the posterior axillary line (Fig. 4.36).

The intercostal muscles are divided and the pleural cavity is entered with the use of scissors in order to avoid injury to the underlying inflated lung. A Finnochieto retractor is then applied and the ribs are spread. Any blood in the pleural cavity is evacuated and the lower lobe of the lung is grasped with tissue forceps and retracted cephalad. The left phrenic nerve is identified along the lateral surface of the pericardium (Fig. 4.37a and b). The pericardium is grasped with two hemostats in front of the nerve and a small incision

Fig. 4.35 The emergency room resuscitative thoracotomy tray should contain only the absolutely essential instruments

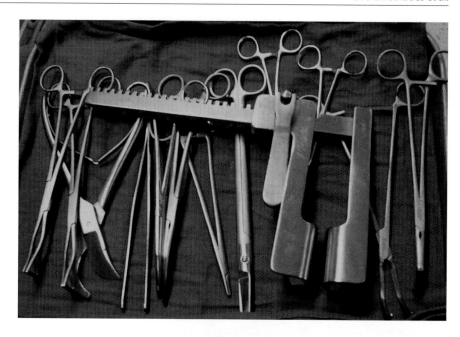

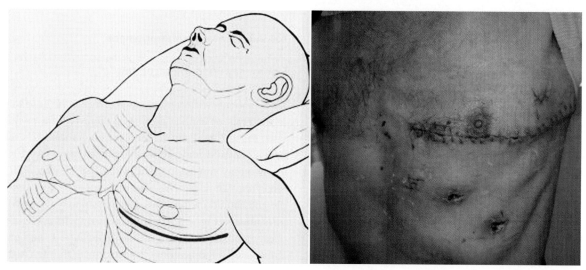

Fig. 4.36 Incision for emergency room resuscitative thoracotomy

is made. The pericardium is then opened longitudinally and parallel to the phrenic nerve (Fig. 4.37a–c) and the clot is evacuated. The cardiac bleeding is controlled by finger compression between the thumb and index or by a vascular clamp in atrial injuries. In some cases with a small wound, bleeding control may be achieved by inserting and inflating a Foley catheter (Fig. 4.38) (Caution: (a) accidental dislodgement of the balloon may enlarge the cardiac wound, (b) puncture of the balloon during suturing may result in severe bleeding.) The cardiac wound is repaired with figure of eight interrupted sutures or continuous suture, nonabsorbable 2/0 or 3/0. Injuries close to a major coronary vessel should be repaired with horizontal mattress sutures under the vessel. Skin staples may be used temporarily in knife wounds. Staples cannot be applied in most cases of GSWs associated with cardiac tissue loss. Attempts to use pledgets are ill-advised and time consuming. Injuries to the posterior wall of the heart can be exposed and repaired by grasping the apex of the heart with a Duval clamp and lifting the heart up as little as possible in order to avoid severe arrhythmias.

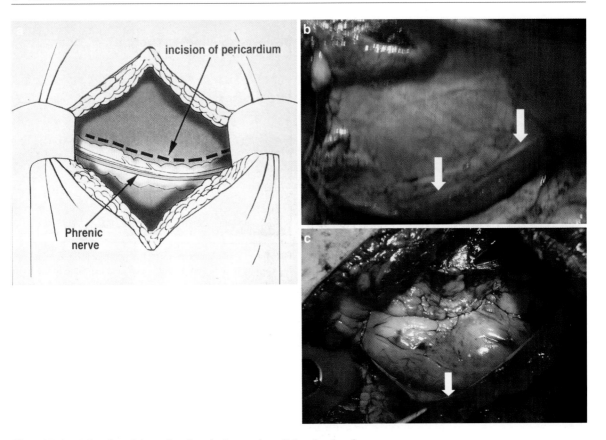

Fig. 4.37 (a–c) Opening of the pericardium in front and parallel to the phrenic nerve

Following repair, the heart is resuscitated with intravenous fluids, epinephrine, internal defibrillation (10–50 J), and aortic cross-clamping. In the presence of cardiac arrest, the thoracic aorta should be cross-clamped in order to improve the coronary and brain circulation. The most accessible site for cross-clamping is 2–4 cm above the diaphragm (Fig. 4.39). The left lower lobe of the lung is grasped and retracted upward with a Duval clamp in order to provide an adequate exposure of the aorta. The aorta is dissected with long scissors and a vascular clamp is then applied. No attempts should be made for extensive finger mobilization of the aorta because of the risk of avulsion of intercostal arteries. The aortic clamp is removed as soon as the cardiac activity returns and the carotid pulse is palpable.

In patients with cardiac arrest or severe arrhythmias who have injury to the low-pressure cardiac chambers, the lung or major veins, air embolism should be suspected. Sometimes, air can be seen in the coronary veins. In these cases, needle aspiration of the ventricles should be performed. If good cardiac activity returns, the patient is transferred to the operating room for definitive management.

Operating Room Management

Patients with suspected cardiac injuries who are not in cardiac arrest or imminent cardiac arrest should be transferred to the operating room for immediate operation. A medium sternotomy is the incision of choice for the majority of patients with suspected cardiac injuries (Fig. 4.40). The incision does not require special positioning of the patient, is fast, bloodless, provides good exposure to the heart and both lungs, and is associated with less postoperative pain and pulmonary complications than a thoracotomy. However, it is difficult to repair posterior cardiac wounds and is not possible to cross-clamp the thoracic aorta through this incision.

A left thoracotomy incision is reserved for patients requiring a resuscitative operation in the ER and in

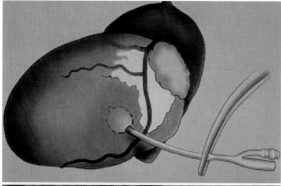

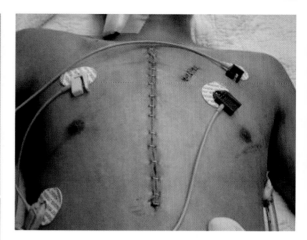

Fig. 4.40 A median sternotomy is a good incision for penetrating cardiac trauma and provides excellent exposure to the heart and the lungs

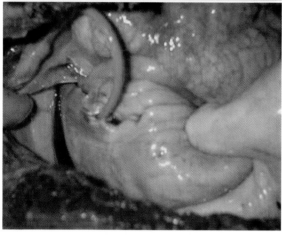

Fig. 4.38 An inflated Foley catheter through a cardiac perforation can temporarily control bleeding until definitive repair

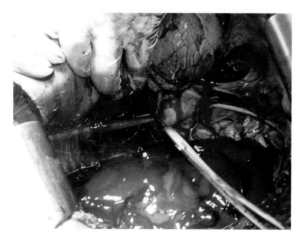

Fig. 4.39 Resuscitative thoracotomy with cross-clamping of the thoracic aorta

cases with suspected posterior cardiac injuries. The technique has been described above. Cardiac repair is performed as described in ER thoracotomy. Teflon pledgets or strips are very rarely necessary, usually in cases with fragile myocardium. Their routine use is counterproductive and delays the repair of the wounds. Partial transaction of a major coronary artery can be repaired with interrupted sutures with the help of magnifying glasses and with the heart beating. If this is not technically possible, ligation is performed and the cardiac activity is observed for a few minutes. If no arrhythmia develops the operation is completed. If arrhythmia occurs the suture is removed and gentle finger pressure is applied, while a cardiac team with cardiopulmonary bypass capabilities is mobilized.

Cardiopulmonary bypass is practically never necessary during the acute stage. The priority of the surgeon is to save the patient's life and any other intracardiac defects should be repaired electively at a later stage.

Following cardiac repair and stabilization of the patient the pericardium is closed with continuous sutures 2/0, leaving an opening near the base of the pericardium in order to avoid tamponade in case of rebleed. In some cases with acute cardiac enlargement due to cardiac failure or massive fluid resuscitation, the pericardium cannot be closed without tension, which often results in arrhythmias. In these cases, the pericardium should be left open. The sternum is closed with wire over a mediastinal drain.

4.4.2.6 Outcomes

The prognosis after penetrating cardiac trauma is grave and the overall mortality is about 80%, with many victims never reaching hospital care [15, 26]. The overall mortality for GSWs is about 90% and for stab wounds, about 65%. The overall hospital mortality is about 65% (about 85% for GSWs and 35% for stab wounds). The survival of patients who undergo a resuscitative ER thoracotomy for cardiac arrest is about 14%, although some centers report significantly lower or higher survival, depending on the indications for ER thoracotomy.

4.4.2.7 Postoperative Evaluation

All survivors should undergo routine early and late clinical, ECG, and echocardiographic evaluation to rule out significant intracardiac injuries (septal defects, valvular or papillary muscle dysfunction, myocardial dyskinesia, and late pericardial effusion). Early postoperative evaluation may miss important abnormalities and therefore it is essential for a late follow-up a few weeks after the injury. In a study of 54 patients who survived a penetrating cardiac injury, late follow-up (mean 23 months) showed ECG abnormalities in 31%, echocardiographic abnormalities in 31%, and valvular or septal defects in 19% [22].

4.5 Diaphragmatic Injuries

4.5.1 Epidemiology

About 5% of blunt trauma patients undergoing laparotomy have a diaphragmatic injury. The reported incidence of diaphragm injuries following penetrating trauma in the left thoracoabdominal area (the region bounded by the nipples superiorly and costal margin laterally and inferiorly) is particularly high. In a prospective study from our center, [72]diaphragm injury was identified in 42% of patients following penetrating trauma to the left thoracoabdominal area (59% of GSWs and 32% of stab wounds). There was no significant difference in this series between anterior, lateral, and posterior thoracoabdominal injury sites (22%, 27%, and 22%, respectively).

4.5.2 Clinical Presentation

Isolated injuries to the diaphragm may be completely asymptomatic or have only minimal abdominal tenderness or a hemothorax. About 20–25% of patients with isolated diaphragmatic injuries are completely asymptomatic on admission. [24, 60, 73]A high index of suspicion remains the cornerstone of early diagnosis, and all patients with penetrating trauma to the left thoracoabdominal area should be evaluated for diaphragmatic injury.

The natural history of unrepaired diaphragmatic injuries is not known. It is possible that some small injuries heal without adverse sequela. For right-sided diaphragmatic injuries, particularly those in posterior positions, the liver may confer some protection against the herniation of abdominal contents through the laceration, thereby permitting unimpeded healing. However, many, particularly larger injuries, fail to heal and can result in late diaphragmatic hernias. It has been suggested that the relative thinness of the diaphragm, combined with the constant motion of the muscle, may impede healing. Another possible mechanism is the early herniation of omentum through the diaphragmatic wound, which prevents healing and allows further herniation at a later stage (Fig. 4.44).

4.5.3 Diagnosis

A CXR is usually the initial study utilized in the investigation for diaphragmatic injury. The findings of plain films may range from minimal to dramatic. In a prospective study of 45 diaphragmatic injuries from our center, we reported a normal CXR in 40%, nonspecific findings in 49% and suspected diaphragmatic injury in only 11%. [72]. Radiologic signs suspicious for diaphragmatic injury include an elevated diaphragm (Fig. 4.41) or a hemopneumothorax combined with

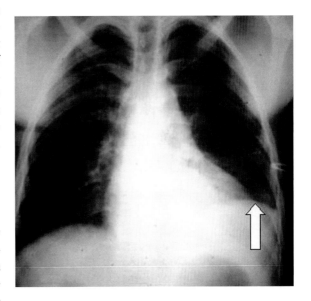

Fig. 4.41 Elevated left hemidiaphragm following a stab wound to the left thoracoabdominal area. This is a suspicious finding for a diaphragmatic injury

free air under the diaphragm. In the presence of diaphragmatic hernia, the chest film is more commonly abnormal, frequently demonstrating evidence of hollow viscus within the pleural cavity (Fig. 4.42). A small omental, gastric or bowel herniation, however, may be missed on the initial plain radiography.

Computed tomography (CT) has a definitive role in the evaluation of diaphragmatic hernias (Fig. 4.43), but has a limited role in the evaluation of uncomplicated diaphragmatic injury because of its low sensitivity. With the

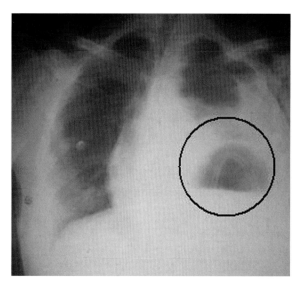

Fig. 4.42 Chest x-ray shows a nasogastric tube in the left chest in a patient with a stab wound to the left thoracoabdominal area and gastric herniation into the chest

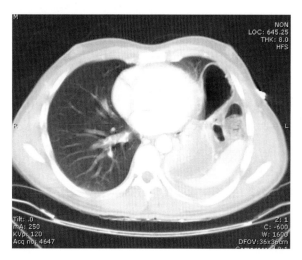

Fig. 4.43 CT scan of patient with blunt trauma and rupture of the diaphragm. The spleen, stomach and colon are in the left chest

advancing technology of helical CT and multislice scanners, however, the role of CT may be redefined. The utility of other noninvasive modalities, including ultrasound and MRI are also of little proven utility at present.

Diagnostic Peritoneal Lavage (DPL) has very limited or no role in the evaluation of diaphragmatic injuries because of the high false-negative rates. In the presence of diaphragm injury, intra-abdominal blood is preferentially diverted into the chest by the pressure gradient that occurs between the thoracic and abdominal cavities during the mechanics of respiration, decreasing the diagnostic yield of DPL.

Diagnostic laparoscopy is currently the most reliable investigation for the diagnosis of occult diaphragmatic injury and has become the standard practice in many centers, including our own (Fig. 4.44). In a prospective study from our institution, we performed routine laparoscopy in 57 asymptomatic patients with left thoracoabdominal injuries and identified occult diaphragmatic injury in 24%. [73]. Growing experience with protocolized approaches that include laparoscopy has established this method as the gold standard in the diagnosis of occult diaphragmatic injuries. Videothoracoscopy can be effectively utilized for a similar purpose, although this technique is not as commonly utilized as laparoscopy. Thoracoscopy might be the preferred approach in cases with residual hemothorax, as it permits both treatment of the diaphragmatic injury and facilitates the evacuation of the clotted blood.

As occult diaphragmatic injuries do not commonly represent an urgent threat to life on initial admission, diagnostic laparoscopy can be offered in a semielective fashion. The use of delayed laparoscopy for asymptomatic patients, hours after admission, facilitates the

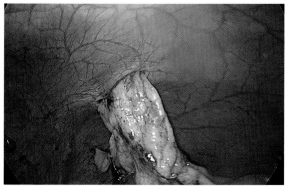

Fig. 4.44 Laparoscopy shows omentum herniating through a *left* diaphragmatic injury

reliable exclusion of hollow viscus injury through a period of serial exams and monitoring. It is our practice to offer this procedure only after appropriate evaluation and observation over a 6–8 h period for the development of peritoneal signs. Any diaphragmatic injuries can then be repaired laparoscopically without the concern of missed hollow viscus injuries.

It is important to note that when diaphragmatic hernias are suspected, tube thoracostomy placement should be avoided, if possible, until CT evaluation has been completed. In certain instances, however, a thoracostomy tube will be deemed necessary due to respiratory distress. In these situations, the thoracostomy tube should be placed above the level of the nipple by an experienced provider, and only after careful digital exploration of the chest cavity under sterile technique. Trocar techniques of thoracostomy insertion should be universally avoided.

4.5.4 Operative Management

Laparoscopic repair can easily be performed in the absence of associated intra-abdominal injuries. With open repair, after visualization of the diaphragmatic injury the suction catheter tip should be carefully inserted into the pleural cavity through the defect and any blood or gastro-intestinal contents adequately evacuated. In cases with concomitant hollow viscus injury and gross spillage of enteric contents, diligent washout of the thoracic cavity must be undertaken to prevent later empyema. The diaphragmatic laceration is repaired with "figure of eight," interrupted size 0 monofilament nonabsorbable suture material (polypropylene). A chest tube should always be inserted following repair.

4.5.5 Morbidity and Mortality

Mortality following uncomplicated diaphragmatic injury is almost universally due to associated injuries. The most common complications in this setting are atelectasis, pleural effusion, and empyema. Patients are at particular risk for the empyema if they have suffered a hollow-viscus injury in association with their diaphragmatic laceration. However, the incidence of serious complications in cases with complicated diaphragmatic hernias with hollow viscus necrosis is very high. Most of these patients develop empyema and organ failure and often die of uncontrollable sepsis.

4.6 Esophageal Injuries

4.6.1 Epidemiology

Thoracic esophageal injuries are almost always due to penetrating trauma and are very rare. Less than 0.5% of all GSWs are associated with an esophageal injury.

4.6.2 Diagnosis

The diagnosis of esophageal injuries is notoriously difficult and in many cases it is delayed resulting in complications or death [65]. There are no specific clinical signs and symptoms and the diagnosis is based on clinical suspicion and investigations. The plain CXR usually shows air in the soft tissues of the neck or the mediastinum, but may be missed if not specifically suspected. CT identifies extraluminal air with higher sensitivity. Most importantly, the CT scan may show a direction of the bullet tract toward the esophagus and prompt the physician to pursue further investigations (Fig. 4.14a). Although air in the soft tissues should always alert for further work-up, it is by no means specific for esophageal injury. Air can be present after tracheobronchial or lung injuries or just as part of the bullet trajectory without organ injury. The most common finding on chest radiograph is hemopneumothorax. Contrast esophagography localizes the site of perforation in almost all patients with an esophageal injury. Esophagoscopy is another useful investigation tool and is particularly useful in patients who cannot be evaluated by esophagography.

4.6.3 Management

All thoracic esophageal injuries should be operated on promptly because of the high risk of mediastinitis and death if left unrepaired for longer than a few hours.

4.6.4 Operative Therapy

The upper thoracic esophagus is approached through a right thoracotomy and the lower, through a left thoracotomy. In most cases, primary repair can be performed if the delay is less than 12 h. Primary repair is usually done in two layers. Pleural, intercostal muscle, diaphragmatic, or pericardial wraps have been used to reinforce the esophageal repair, but their value is uncertain [49, 65, 75]. For injuries that are diagnosed after 24 h, it is generally accepted that primary repair alone is at high risk of failure. Principles of surgical therapy under such circumstances include any combination of the following procedures: double-layer closure, buttressing with flaps, cervical esophagostomy, exclusion of lower esophagus, gastrostomy, feeding jejunostomy, and wide drainage. A second procedure may be needed following exclusion procedures, resulting in, on some occasions, the need for esophageal resection and colon interposition.

References

1. Adams JE 3rd, Davila-Roman VG, Bessey PQ et al (1996) Improved detection of cardiac contusion with cardiac troponin I. Am Heart J 131(2):308–312
2. Ahrar K, Smith DC, Bansal RC et al (1997) Angiography in blunt thoracic aortic injury. J Trauma 42(4):665–669
3. Asensio JA, Demetriades D, Berne JD et al (1997) Stapled pulmonary tractotomy: a rapid way to control hemorrhage in penetrating pulmonary injuries. J Am Coll Surg 185(5): 486–487
4. Asensio JA, Murray J, Demetriades D et al (1998) Penetrating cardiac injuries: a prospective study of variables predicting outcomes. J Am Coll Surg 186(1):24–34
5. Barrios C, Tran T, Malinoski D et al (2008) Successful management of occult pneumothorax without tube thoracostomy despite positive pressure ventilation. Am Surg 74(10):958–961
6. Bergeron E, Lavoie A, Clas D et al (2003) Elderly trauma patients with rib fractures are at greater risk of death and pneumonia. J Trauma 54(3):478–485
7. Bertinchant JP, Polge A, Mohty D et al (2000) Evaluation of incidence, clinical significance, and prognostic value of circulating cardiac troponin I and T elevation in hemodynamically stable patients with suspected myocardial contusion after blunt chest trauma. J Trauma 48(5):924–931
8. Bongard FS, Lewis FR (1984) Crystalloid resuscitation of patients with pulmonary contusion. Am J Surg 148(1):145–151
9. Brasel KJ, Guse CE, Layde P et al (2006) Rib fractures: relationship with pneumonia and mortality. Crit Care Med 34(6):1642–1646
10. Brasel KJ, Stafford RE, Weigelt JA et al (1999) Treatment of occult pneumothoraces from blunt trauma. J Trauma 46(6):987–990, discussion 990–991
11. Bulger EM, Arneson MA, Mock CN et al (2000) Rib fractures in the elderly. J Trauma 48(6):1040–1046, discussion 1046–7
12. Bulger EM, Edwards T, Klotz P et al (2004) Epidural analgesia improves outcome after multiple rib fractures. Surgery 136(2):426–430
13. Burney RE, Gundry SR, Mackenzie JR et al (1984) Chest roentgenograms in diagnosis of traumatic rupture of the aorta observer variation in interpretation. Chest 85(5): 605–609
14. Cameron R, Davies HR (2008) Intra-pleural fibrinolytic therapy versus conservative management in the treatment of adult parapneumonic effusions and empyema. Cochrane Database Syst Rev 2(2):CD002312
15. Campbell NC, Thomson SR, Muckart DJ, Meumann et al (1997) Review of 1198 cases of penetrating cardiac trauma. Br J Surg 84(12):1737–1740
16. Chan L, Reilly KM, Henderson C, Kahn F et al (1997) Complication rates of tube thoracostomy. Am J Emerg Med 15(4):368–370
17. Cohn SM, Burns GA, Jaffe C, Milner KA (1995) Exclusion of aortic tear in the unstable trauma patient: the utility of transesophageal echocardiography. J Trauma 39(6): 1087–1090
18. Craven KD, Oppenheimer L, Wood LD (1979) Effects of contusion and flail chest on pulmonary perfusion and oxygen exchange. J Appl Physiol 47(4):729–737
19. Cryer G, Mavroudis C, Yu J et al (1990) Shock, transfusion, and pneumonectomy. Death is due to right heart failure and increased pulmonary vascular resistance. Ann Surg 212:197–201
20. Cullinane DC, Morris JA Jr, Bass JG et al (2001) Needle thoracostomy may not be indicated in the trauma patient. Injury 32(10):749–752
21. Degiannis E, Loogna P, Doll D et al (2006) Penetrating cardiac injuries: recent experience in South Africa. World J Surg 30(7):1258–1264
22. Demetriades D, Charalambides D, Sareti P et al (1990) Late sequelae of penetrating cardiac injuries. Br J Surg 77:813–814
23. Demetriades D, Gomez H, Velmahos GC et al (1998) Routine helical computed tomographic evaluation of the mediastinum in high-risk blunt trauma patients. Arch Surg 133(10):1084–1088
24. Demetriades D, Kakoyiannis S, Perekh D et al (1988) Penetrating injuries of the diaphragm. Br J Surg 75:824–826
25. Demetriades D, Theodorou D, Murray J et al (1996) Mortality and prognostic factors in penetrating injuries of the aorta. J Trauma 40(5):761–763
26. Demetriades D, Van der Veen B (1983) Penetrating injuries of the heart: experience over two years in South Africa. J Trauma 23:1034–1041
27. Demetriades D, Velmahos GC, Scalea TM et al (2008) American Association for the Surgery of Trauma Thoracic Aortic Injury Study Group: operative repair or endovascular stent graft in blunt traumatic thoracic aortic injuries: results of an American Association for the Surgery of Trauma Multicenter Study. J Trauma 64(3):561–570, discussion 570–571
28. Demetriades D, Velmahos GC, Scalea TM et al (2008) Diagnosis and treatment of blunt thoracic aortic injuries: changing perspectives. J Trauma 64(6):1415–1418, discussion 1418–9

29. Demetriades D, Velmahos GC, Scalea TM, et al. (2009) Blunt traumatic aortic injuries: early or delayed repair-results of an AAST prospective study. J Trauma 66(4):967–973

30. Demetriades D (1986) Cardiac wounds. Experience with 70 patients. Ann Surg 203:315–317

31. Deneuville M (2002) Morbidity of percutaneous tube thoracostomy in trauma patients. Eur J Cardiothorac Surg 22(5):673–678

32. DePoll TL, Schurirk GW, Letham M et al (2007) Endovascular treatment of traumatic rupture of the thoracic aorta. Br J Surg 94:525–533

33. Di Bartolomeo S, Sanson G, Nardi G et al (2001) A population-based study on pneumothorax in severely traumatized patients. J Trauma 51(4):677–682

34. Dulchavsky SA, Schwarz KL, Kirkpatrick AW et al (2001) Prospective evaluation of thoracic ultrasound in the detection of pneumothorax. J Trauma 50(2):201–205

35. Eckstein M, Suyehara D (1998) Needle thoracostomy in the prehospital setting. Prehosp Emerg Care 2(2):132–135

36. Ekeh AP, Peterson W, Woods RJ et al (2008) Is chest x-ray an adequate screening tool for the diagnosis of blunt thoracic aortic injury? J Trauma 65(5):1088–1092

37. Enderson BL, Abdalla R, Frame SB et al (1993) Tube thoracostomy for occult pneumothorax: a prospective randomized study of its use. J Trauma 35(5):726–729, discussion 729–730

38. Eren S, Esme H, Sehitogullari A et al (2008) The risk factors and management of posttraumatic empyema in trauma patients. Injury 39(1):44–49

39. Exadaktylos AK, Duwe J, Eckstein F et al (2005) The role of contrast-enhanced spiral CT imaging versus chest X-rays in surgical therapeutic concepts and thoracic aortic injury: a 29-year Swiss retrospective analysis of aortic surgery. Cardiovasc J S Afr 16(3):162–165

40. Fabian TC, Richardson JD, Croce MA et al (1997) Prospective study of blunt aortic injury: multicenter trial of the American Association for the Surgery of Trauma. J Trauma 42(3):374–380, discussion 380–3

41. Flagel BT, Luchette FA, Reed RL et al (2005) Half-a-dozen ribs: the breakpoint for mortality. Surgery 138(4):717–723, discussion 723–725

42. Guerrero-Lopez F, Vazquez-Mata G, Alcazar-Romero PP et al (2000) Evaluation of the utility of computed tomography in the initial assessment of the critical care patient with chest trauma. Crit Care Med 28(5):1370–1375

43. Gunduz M, Unlugenc H, Ozalevli M et al (2005) A comparative study of continuous positive airway pressure (CPAP) and intermittent positive airway pressure (CPAP) and intermittent positive pressure ventilation (IPPV) in patients with flail chest. Emerg Med J 22(5):325–329

44. Henmila MR, Arbabi S, Row SA et al (2004) Delayed repair for blunt thoracic aortic injury: is it really equivalent to early repair? J Trauma 56:13–23

45. Holcomb JB, McMullin NR, Kozar RA et al (2003) Morbidity from rib fractures increases after age 45. J Am Coll Surg 196(4):549–555

46. Holmes JF, Brant WE, Bogren HG et al (2001) Prevalence and importance of pneumothoraces visualized on abdominal computed tomographic scan in children with blunt trauma. J Trauma 50(3):516–520

47. Holmes JH, Bloch RD, Hall RA et al (2002) Natural history of traumatic rupture of the thoracic aorta managed nonoperatively: a longitudinal analysis. Ann Thorac Surg 73:1149–1154

48. Huh J, Wall MJ Jr et al (2003) Mattox KL: surgical management of traumatic pulmonary injury. Am J Surg 186(6):620–624

49. Ivatury RR, Rohman M, Simon RF (1994) Esophageal injury. Adv Trauma Crit Care 9:245–274

50. Karmakar MK, Critchley LA, Ho AM et al (2003) Continuous thoracic paravertebral infusion of bupivacaine for pain management in patients with multiple fractured ribs. Chest 123(2):424–431

51. Karmy-Jones R, Holevar M, Sullivan RJ et al (2008) Residual hemothorax after chest tube placement correlates with increased risk of empyema following traumatic injury. Can Respir J 15(5):255–258

52. Kato N, Dake MD, Miller DC et al (1997) Traumatic thoracic aortic aneurysm: treatment with endovascular stent-grafts. Radiology 205(3):657–662

53. Kepros J, Angood P, Jaffe CC et al (2002) Aortic intimal injuries from blunt trauma: a resolution profile in nonoperative management. J Trauma 52:475–478

54. Kieninger AN, Bair HA, Bendick PJ et al (2005) Epidural versus intravenous pain control in elderly patients with rib fractures. Am J Surg 189(3):327–330

55. Kimbrell BJ, Yamzon J, Petrone P et al (2007) Intrapleural thrombolysis for the management of undrained traumatic hemothorax: a prospective observational study. J Trauma 62(5):1175–1178, discussion 1178–9

56. Kishikawa M, Minami T, Shimazu T et al (1993) Laterality of air volume in the lungs long after blunt chest trauma. J Trauma 34(6):908–912, discussion 912–913

57. Kishikawa M, Yoshioka T, Shimazu T et al (1991) Pulmonary contusion causes long-term respiratory dysfunction with decreased functional residual capacity. J Trauma 31(9):1203–1208, discussion 1208–10

58. Knudtson JL, Dort JM, Helmer SD et al (2004) Surgeon-performed ultrasound for pneumothorax in the trauma suite. J Trauma 56(3):527–530

59. Kollmorgen DR, Murray KA, Sullivan JJ et al (1994) Predictors of mortality in pulmonary contusion. Am J Surg 168(6):659–663, discussion 663–4

60. Leppaniemi A, Haapiainen R (2003) Occult diaphragmatic injuries caused by stab wounds. J Trauma 55:646–650

61. Linstaedt M, Germing A, Lawo T et al (2002) Acute and long-term clinical significance of myocardial contusion following blunt thoracic trauma: results of a prospective study. J Trauma 52(3):479–485

62. Madiba TE, Thomson SR, Mdlalose N (2001) Penetrating chest injuries in the firearm era. Injury 32(1):13–16

63. Marnocha KE, Maglinte DD (1985) Plain-film criteria for excluding aortic rupture in blunt chest trauma. AJR Am J Roentgenol 144(1):19–21

64. Martin MJ, McDonald JM, Mullenix PS et al (2006) Operative management and outcomes of traumatic lung resection. J Am Coll Surg 203(3):336–344

65. Michel L, Grillo HC, Malt RA (1982) Esophageal perforation. Ann Thorac Surg 33:203–210

66. Miller PR, Croce MA, Bee TK et al (2001) TC: ARDS after pulmonary contusion: accurate measurement of contusion

volume identifies high-risk patients. J Trauma 51(2):223–228, discussion 229–30

67. Minard G, Schurr MJ, Croce MA et al (1996) A prospective analysis of transesophageal echocardiography in the diagnosis of traumatic disruption of the aorta. J Trauma 40(2):225–230

68. Mirvis SE, Bidwell JK, Buddemeyer EU et al (1987) Value of chest radiography in excluding traumatic aortic rupture. Radiology 163(2):487–493

69. Mirvis SE, Shanmuganathan K, Buell J et al (1998) Use of spiral computed tomography for the assessment of blunt trauma patients with potential aortic injury. J Trauma 45(5):922–930

70. Mirvis SE, Shanmuganathan K (2007) Diagnosis of blunt traumatic aortic injury 2007: still a nemesis. Eur J Radiol 64(1):27–40

71. Moon MR, Luchette FA, Gibson SW et al (1999) Prospective, randomized comparison of epidural versus parenteral opioid analgesia in thoracic trauma. Ann Surg 229(5):684–691, discussion 691–2

72. Murray JA, Demetriades D, Cornwell EE 3rd et al (1997) Penetrating left thoracoabdominal trauma: the incidence and clinical presentation of diaphragm injuries. J Trauma 43:624–626

73. Murray JA, Demetriades D, Ascensio JA et al (1998) Occult injuries to the diaphragm: prospective evaluation of laparoscopy in penetrating injuries to the left lower chest. Am Coll Surg 187:626–630

74. Nagy K, Fabian T, Rodman G et al (2000) Guidelines for the diagnosis and management of blunt aortic injury: an EAST Practice Management Guidelines Work Group. J Trauma 48(6):1128–1143

75. Nesbitt JC, Sawyers JL (1987) Surgical management of the esophageal perforation. Am Surg 53:183–191

76. Nirula R, Diaz JJ Jr, Trunkey DD et al (2009) Rib fracture repair: indications, technical issues, and future directions. World J Surg 33(1):14–22

77. Parmley LF, Mattingly TW, Manion WC et al (1958) Nonpenetrating traumatic injury of the aorta. Circulation 17(6):1086–1101

78. Pasquale M, Fabian TC (1998) Practice management guidelines for trauma from the eastern association for the surgery of trauma. J Trauma 44(6):941–956, discussion 956–957

79. Pettiford BL, Luketich JD, Landreneau RJ (2007) The management of flail chest. Thorac Surg Clin 17(1):25–33

80. Richardson JD (2004) Outcome of tracheobronchial injuries: a long-term perspective. J Trauma 56:30–36

81. Rozycki GS, Ballard RB, Feliciano DV et al (1998) Surgeon-performed ultrasound for the assessment of truncal injuries: lessons learned from 1540 patients. Ann Surg 228(4):557–567

82. Rozycki GS, Feliciano DV, Ochsner MG et al (1999) The role of ultrasound in patients with possible penetrating cardiac wounds: a prospective multicenter study. J Trauma 46(4):543–551, discussion 551–552

83. Rozycki GS, Feliciano DV, Schmidt JA et al (1996) The role of surgeon-performed ultrasound in patients with possible cardiac wounds. Ann Surg 223(6)):737–744, discussion 744–746

84. Salim A, Velmahos GC, Jindal A et al (2001) Clinically significant blunt cardiac trauma: role of serum troponin levels combined with electrocardiographic findings. J Trauma 50(2):237–243

85. Sanabria A, Valdivieso E, Gomez G et al (2006) Prophylactic antibiotics in chest trauma: a meta-analysis of high-quality studies. World J Surg 30(10):1843–1847

86. Schultz JM, Trunkey DD (2004) Blunt cardiac injury. Crit Care Clin 20(1):57–70

87. Sharma OP, Oswanski MF, Jolly S et al (2008) Perils of rib fractures. Am Surg 74(4):310–314

88. Sirmali M, Turut H, Topcu S et al (2003) A comprehensive analysis of traumatic rib fractures: morbidity, mortality and management. Eur J Cardiothorac Surg 24(1):133–138

89. Smith MD, Cassidy JM, Souther S, Morris EJ, Sapin PM, Johnson SB, Kearney PA (1995) Transesophageal echocardiography in the diagnosis of traumatic rupture of the aorta. N Engl J Med 332(6):356–362

90. Stafford RE, Linn J, Washington L (2006) Incidence and management of occult hemothoraces. Am J Surg 192(6):722–726

91. Sturaitis M, McCallum D, Sutherland G, Cheung H, Driedger AA, Sibbald WJ (1986) Lack of significant long-term sequelae following traumatic myocardial contusion. Arch Intern Med 146(9):1765–1769

92. Sutyak JP, Wohltmann CD, Larson J (2007) Pulmonary contusions and critical care management in thoracic trauma. Thorac Surg Clin 17(1):11–23

93. Sybrandy KC, Sybrandy KC, Cramer MJ, Burgersdijk C (2003) Diagnosing cardiac contusion: old wisdom and new insights. Heart 89(5):485–489

94. Tanaka H, Yukioka T, Yamaguti Y et al (2002) Surgical stabilization of internal pneumatic stabilization? A prospective randomized study of management of severe flail chest patients. J Trauma 52(4):727–732, discussion 732

95. Teixeira P, Inaba K, Georgiou C, Barmparas G, Talving P, Green D, Plurad D, Demetriades D (2009) Blunt thoracic aortic injuries: lesson learned from the coroner Southern California Chapter of the American College of Surgeons Annual Meeting, Santa Barbara, California, USA

96. Teixeira PG, Inaba K, Oncel D et al Blunt cardiac trauma: Lessons learned from the coroner. Southern California Chapter of the American College of Surgeons Annual Meeting, Santa Barbara, California, USA

97. Teixeira PG, Inaba K, Oncel D et al (2009) Blunt cardiac rupture: a 5-year NTDB analysis. J Trauma 67(4):788–791

98. Todd SR, McNally MM, Holcomb JB et al (2006) A multidisciplinary clinical pathway decreases rib fracture-associated infectious morbidity and mortality in high-risk trauma patients. Am J Surg 192(6):806–811

99. Ungar TC, Wolf SJ, Haukoos JS, Dyer DS, Moore EE (2006) Derivation of a clinical decision rule to exclude thoracic aortic imaging in patients with blunt chest trauma after motor vehicle collisions. J Trauma 61(5):1150–1155

100. Vassiliu P, Velmahos GC, Toutouzas KG (2001) Timing, safety, and efficacy of thoracoscopic evacuation of undrained post-traumatic hemothorax. Am Surg 67(12):1165–1169

101. Velmahos GC, Baker C, Demetriades D, Goodman J, Murray JA, Asensio JA (1999) Lung-sparing surgery after penetrating trauma using tractotomy, partial lobectomy, and pneumonorrhaphy. Arch Surg 134(2):186–189

102. Velmahos GC, Demetriades D, Chan L, Tatevossian R, Cornwell EE 3rd, Yassa N, Murray JA, Asensio JA, Berne TV (1999) Predicting the need for thoracoscopic evacua-

tion of residual traumatic hemothorax: chest radiograph is insufficient. J Trauma 46(1):65–70

103. Velmahos GC, Karaiskakis M, Salim A et al (2003) Normal electrocardiography and serum troponin I levels preclude the presence of clinically significant blunt cardiac injury. J Trauma 54(1):45–50, discussion 50–1

104. Velmahos GC, Vassiliu P, Chan LS, Murray JA, Berne TV, Demetriades D (2002) Influence of flail chest on outcome among patients with severe thoracic cage trauma. Int Surg 87(4):240–244

105. Vignon P, Lang RM (1999) Use of transesophageal echocardiography for the assessment of traumatic aortic injuries. Echocardiography 16(2):207–219

106. Wagner RB, Crawford WO Jr, Schimpf PP (1988) Classification of parenchymal injuries of the lung. Radiology 167(1):77–82

107. Woodring JH (1990) The normal mediastinum in blunt traumatic rupture of the thoracic aorta and brachiocephalic arteries. J Emerg Med 8(4):467–476

Diaphragm

5

Luke P. H. Leenen

5.1 Introduction

The diaphragm forms the dome-shaped, partly muscular and partly fibrous separation between the thorax and the abdomen. Because of this particular shape it raises higher than generally expected, up to the fifth inter-costal space. It attaches to the front side of the thorax and ribs, approximately at nipple level and dorsally also to the ribs, however at a lower level, whereas the crurae attach to the corpora of the first to third lumbar vertebral body. The muscular crurae form the portals of inferior vena cava (level Th8), aortic (level Th12), and esophageal (level Th10) structures. It is innervated on both sides individually by the phrenic nerves originating from C3 to C5.

The diaphragm can be compromised both, thoracic, but also after abdominal trauma. Pelvic trauma is also associated with diaphragmatic injury [1, 2].

5.2 Trauma Mechanism and Epidemiology

Diaphragmatic rupture is present in 1–3% of admitted patients with thoracoabdominal trauma to trauma centers [1, 3, 4]. Motorvehicle accidents are the most common cause of blunt traumatic rupture and account for 90% of these injuries [5]. Left-sided ruptures are most common and are found in 75% of the patients; bilateral injuries, though very uncommon, can occur [4, 6–9]. A special feature is the diaphragmatic lesion accompanied by luxation of the heart through the diaphragm [10].

As a result of the rupture, abdominal organs may strangulate into the thoracic cavity causing functional problems or even incarceration and necrosis of the herniated organ, which is associated with an increased morbidity and mortality [6, 7]. Surgical repair in the acute phase is therefore necessary to restore anatomical boundaries.

Penetrating trauma of the diaphragm is seen in 6% of cases with mid torso injuries [11].

Associated injuries are present in up to 75% of cases [5, 12]. In blunt trauma chest, abdominal, pelvic, and long bone trauma are seen often. In penetrating injuries, commonly accompanying gastric and hepatic injury are found.

Blunt diaphragmatic injury can go with a high mortality of up to 15–25% [9, 13].

5.3 Diagnostic Procedures

Early diagnosis of diaphragmatic injury remains a challenge as both clinical and radiographic signs may be absent or missed. It can be graded by the American Association for the Surgery of Trauma from simple contusion, up to severe laceration with severe tissue loss (Table 5.1). The difference between penetrating and blunt trauma should be determined.

5.3.1 Penetrating Injury

In penetrating trauma, diagnosis is not very complicated as, from the point of entry, a diaphragmatic lesion

L.P.H. Leenen
Department of Surgery, University Medical Center, Utrecht,
Heidelberglaan 100, 3584 CX Utrecht, The Netherlands
e-mail: lleenen@umcutrecht.nl.

H.-J. Oestern et al. (eds.), *Head, Thoracic, Abdominal, and Vascular Injuries*,
DOI: 10.1007/978-3-540-88122-3_5, © Springer-Verlag Berlin Heidelberg 2011

Table 5.1 The American Association for the Surgery of Trauma organ injury scale for the diaphragm [31]

Grade	Injury	Description
I	Contusion	Contusion without disruption of normal anatomy
II	Laceration	Laceration smaller than 2 cm of length
III	Laceration	Laceration between 2 and 10 cm length
IV	Laceration	Laceration longer than 20 cm or tissue loss of up to 25 cm^2
V	Laceration	Los of diaphragmatic tissue more than 25 cm^2

can be suspected. Diagnosis can be confirmed with either thoracoscopy or laparoscopy. Leppäniemi et al. [14] evaluated 97 patients with anterior thoracoabdominal stab wounds and found that a high percentage of asymptomatic patients have hollow viscus herniation and therefore recommended evaluation with invasive diagnostic methods like thoracoscopy or laparoscopy.

The advantage of laparoscopy is that concomitant injury to other abdominal organs also can be evaluated. Thoracoscopy, however, is easier to perform and gives a nice overview of the entire diaphragm. Suturing can be performed during the same procedure.

5.3.2 Early Diagnosis in Blunt Injury

Early diagnosis of traumatic diaphragmatic injury in blunt trauma is a challenge. A high percentage of patients present with dyspnea, chest, or abdominal pain; however, these are mostly indiscriminate findings [9, 15].

In a clear-cut case with substantial displacement of abdominal organs into the thorax, at physical exam, diminished breath sounds with a dull percussion can be found. A differential diagnosis between hemothorax and diaphragmatic injuries is not easy. If a thorax drain is placed and only a small amount of blood is evacuated, suspicion is raised; however, massive hemorrhage can also ensue with a diaphragmatic rupture, as for instance, a ruptured spleen can be dislodged into the thorax.

Immediately after the initial assessment a chest X-ray should be taken. It allows diagnosis in 23–60% on left-sided diaphragmatic injuries and 17% of the right-sided injuries [16–20]. Repeated chest radiography increases the detection rate of traumatic diaphragmatic rupture [13, 21]. The conventional chest X-ray, however, can miss up

to 40% of traumatic diaphragmatic injury [5, 15]. The smallest signs of disturbance of the diaphragmatic contour should raise suspicion. These are, for instance, elevated diaphragm and obliteration of diaphragmatic contours. Protrusion of organs (Figs. 5.1–5.4) and an air bubble sign can signify the injury on the chest X-ray.

After passing a naso- or orogastric tube, a renewed chest X-ray should be taken to see whether the position of this tube is above contour of the diaphragm, signifying a diaphragmatic lesion. Another technique is the use of swallow studies, locating the stomach or other hollow viscus above the diaphragm.

Nowadays, more and more trauma patients are subjected to CT scanning in an early phase after the initial

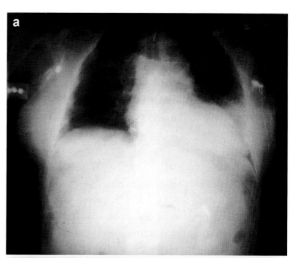

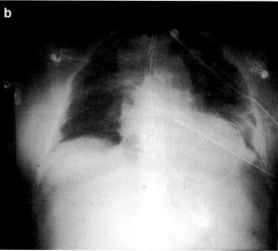

Fig. 5.1 (**a**) Chest X-ray of a motor vehicle accident victim. Note the blurred *left* diaphragm. (**b**) Same patient as in Fig. 5.1a. Chest X-ray after passing an oral-gastric tube. Note the clear visualization of the tube in the stomach above the diaphragm

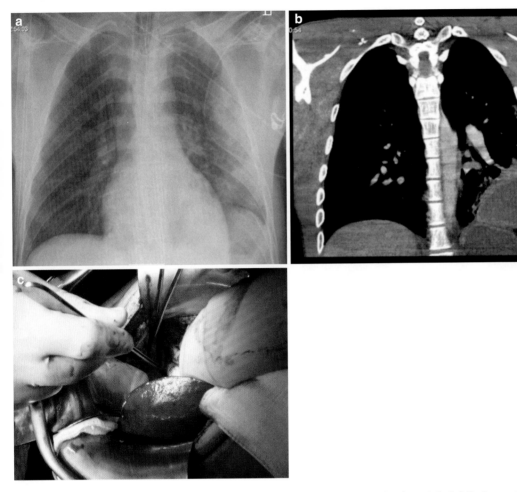

Fig. 5.2 (**a**) Chest X-ray of a patient after falling down from a roof. Blurred *left* diaphragm. (**b**) Multiplanar reconstruction after CT scanning of patient in Fig. 5.2a. Clear visualization of stomach penetrating through the *left* diaphragm. (**c**) Intraoperative view of same patient as in Fig. 5.2a and b

assessment, provided they are hemodynamically stable. The diaphragm should be evaluated thoroughly after every substantial thoracic, abdominal, or pelvic injury because these injuries are easily missed even with these diagnostic modalities. Subtle signs should not be neglected as they can be the early signs of a diaphragmatic rupture developing a hernia at a later stage. Patients who are on positive pressure ventilation in an early stage can especially hide a diaphragmatic injury because of the positive pressure on the thoracic side, which tends to push the organs into the abdominal cavity. Moreover, special attention should be given to those patients with pelvic fractures, as this devastating injury is related to the development of a diaphragmatic tear [1, 2]. Signs signifying diaphragmatic injury on CT are a segmental unrecognized diaphragm, constriction of herniated organs at the level of the diaphragm, the so-called collar sign, elevated abdominal organs, visualization of the herniated viscera against the posterior chest wall (dependent viscera sign), and a thickened diaphragm [22–26].

During trauma laparotomy for any reason, both diaphragmatic sides should be explored and examined for smaller or larger tears. Nevertheless, even during laparotomy right-sided lesions can be missed [8].

5.3.3 Late Diagnosis

The diagnosis of traumatic diaphragmatic rupture can be delayed for even several years. In these late cases, a full workup with CT scanning preferably with intraluminal and intravenous contrast should be done in order to evaluate the full extent of the hernia and to define

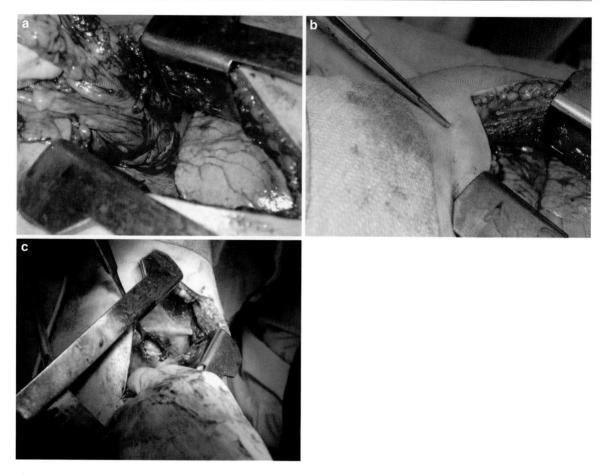

Fig. 5.3 (**a**) Patient with a late presentation after a small stab wound in the left thoracoabdominal transition. (**b**) Note the small scar in the *left upper* quadrant of the abdomen, signifying the old original stab wound. (**c**) Intra-operative view after reposition of the hernia contents

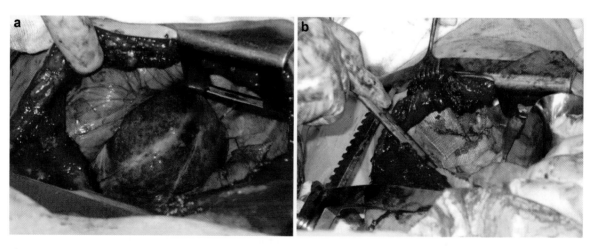

Fig. 5.4 (**a**) Intra-operative view of a patient with a delayed representation of a *right* sided diaphragmatic rupture with necessity of thoraco-phrenico-laparotomy. (**b**) Intrathoracic view after reposition and repair of the diaphragm from above

the rim of the diaphragmatic lesion. At operation, it can be difficult to define the rim of the diaphragm, as most times the herniated organs are blossoming over the diaphragmatic remnant.

Nevertheless, a substantial portion of patients is diagnosed during surgery for other injuries or even present with chronic complaints caused by herniated organs.

5.4 Therapy

Once the diagnosis of a diaphragmatic rupture is established it should be repaired, because even small lesions tend to give herniation of hollow viscus and solid organs through the defect. In blunt trauma, most times, larger defects are present. In a right-sided rupture small lesions can be observed; however, it has been the authors' experience that most times these evolve in larger defects with herniation of the liver and even colon, resulting in a more complicated repair at a later stage. Therapy of the diaphragmatic lesions is straightforward. In acute lesions, a laparotomy is preferred as most times abdominal organs are injured and/or are a bleeding source, making a trauma laparotomy mandatory.

Every trauma laparotomy should have a thorough exploration of the diaphragm on both sides. In case of a rupture of the diaphragm, the herniated organs should be gently withdrawn from the tear. The defect should be defined, grasped with, for example, Allis clamps, and sutured with interrupted or running nonabsorbable sutures in an airtight fashion. Long-lasting resorbable sutures will also do in most cases. It should not be forgotten to place a drain in the thoracic cavity as a pneumothorax, by definition, remains, and most times there is a concomitant lung injury. If there is a laceration of a hollow viscus before closing the thoracic cavity, it should be rinsed thoroughly with warmed saline. In case of larger defects, a nonabsorbable mesh , for example, Gore Tex ® or silastic patches may be used. When the diaphragm is totally detached from the thoracic wall special attention should be given to suturing the remnants to the ribs. This can be done with tags or sutures around the ribs.

In case of a late presentation (months or years) of a diaphragmatic rupture, the approach should be from the thoracic side, because the herniated organs, most times, have thoroughly adhered to the intrathoracic organs, mostly the lungs. A tedious dissection, avoiding

damage to the lung, avoiding an air leak, is carried out to free the herniated organs. Thereafter, the organs are relocated in the abdomen and the defect is closed as mentioned above. In case of a late presentation of a right-side herniation, many times the liver has "blossomed" above the diaphragm causing trouble to get it relocated into the abdomen. Enlarging the defect is often the only feasible option, in which the liver can be relocated in the abdomen. Care should be taken of the liver caval vein which are riding over the edges of the diaphragmatic rupture before entering the caval vein.

5.5 Prognosis

Complications of diaphragmatic lesions can be related to the lesion itself, but also to the, most times, accompanying injuries. Complication rates between 40% and 60% have been reported [26, 27,28].

The diaphragmatic injury and repair itself can be complicated by suture line dehiscence or phrenic paralysis. Secondary to surgery and trauma in this area can be pulmonary atelectases [9], subdiaphragmatic abscesses, empyema, and lung or liver abscesses. In case of herniated organs, perforation can lead to substantial morbidity and even mortality. This can be preceded with episodes of recurrent abdominal bowel obstruction.

Moreover, sequelae like wound infection, pneumonia, sepsis, multiple organ failure, and ARDS are associated with diaphragmatic rupture as part of the associated high energy injuries.

Diaphragmatic injuries have been associated with mortality rates of up to 40% [29]. Ruptures due to blunt trauma are reportedly associated with a higher mortality than penetrating trauma [30].

References

1. Rodriguez-Morales G, Rodriguez A, Shatney CH (1986) Acute rupture of the diaphragm in blunt trauma, analysis of 60 patients. J Trauma 26:438
2. Grage TB, MacLean LD, Cambell GS (1959) Traumatic rupture of the diaphragm. Surgery 46:669
3. Waldschmidt ML, Laws HL (1980) Injuries of the diaphragm. J Trauma 20:587–592
4. Simpson J, Lobo DN, Shah AB, Rowlands BJ (2000) Traumatic diaphragmatic rupture: associated injuries and outcome. Ann R Coll Surg Engl 82:97–100

5. Moore EE, Feliciane DD, Mattox KL (2003) Trauma. McGraw-Hill Professional, New York
6. Payne JH Jr, Yellin AE (1982) Traumatic diaphragmatic hernia. Arch Surg 117:18–24
7. de OF, Oliveira FJ, Queiros A (1982) Traumatic diaphragmatic hernias: a report of 19 cases. Can J Surg 25:658–659, 662
8. Sirbu H, Busch T, Spillner J, Schachtrupp A, Autschbach R (2005) Late bilateral diaphragmatic rupture: challenging diagnostic and surgical repair. Hernia 9:90–92
9. Leppäniemi A, Pohjankyro A, Haapiainen R (1994) Acute diaphragmatic injury after blunt trauma. Ann Chir Gynaecol 83:17–21
10. van Brussel JP, Vles WJ, Leenen LP (2000) Luxatio cordis in blunt-trauma thoraco-abdominal injuries. Ned Tijdschr Geneeskd 144:1073–1075
11. Boffard KD (2003) Manual of definitive surgical trauma care. Arnold, London
12. Mihos P, Potaris K, Gakidis J et al (2003) Traumatic rupture of the diaphragm: experience with 65 patients. Injury 34:169–172
13. Matsevych OY (2008) Blunt diaphragmatic rupture: four year's experience. Hernia 12:73–78
14. Leppäniemi A, Haapiainen R (2003) Occult diaphragmatic injuries caused by stab wounds. J Trauma 55:646–650
15. Sangster G, Ventura VP, Carbo A, Gates T, Garayburu J, D'Agostino H (2007) Diaphragmatic rupture: a frequently missed injury in blunt thoracoabdominal trauma patients. Emerg Radiol 13:225–230
16. Hanna WC, Ferri LE, Fata P, Razek T, Mulder DS (2008) The current status of traumatic diaphragmatic injury: lessons learned from 105 patients over 13 years. Ann Thorac Surg 85:1044–1048
17. Athanassiadi K, Kalavrouziotis G, Athanassiou M et al (1999) Blunt diaphragmatic rupture. Eur J Cardiothorac Surg 15:469–474
18. Shanmuganathan K, Mirvis SE (1999) Imaging diagnosis of nonaortic thoracic injury. Radiol Clin North Am 37:533–551, vi
19. Gelman R, Mirvis SE, Gens D (1991) Diaphragmatic rupture due to blunt trauma: sensitivity of plain chest radiographs. Am J Roentgenol 156:51–57
20. Koroglu M, Ernst RD, Oto A, Mileski WJ (2004) Traumatic diaphragmatic rupture: can oral contrast increase CT detectability? Emerg Radiol 10:334–336
21. Eren S, Kantarci M, Okur A (2006) Imaging of diaphragmatic rupture after trauma. Clin Radiol 61:467–477
22. Killeen KL, Mirvis SE, Shanmuganathan K (1999) Helical CT of diaphragmatic rupture caused by blunt trauma. AJR Am J Roentgenol 173:1611–1616
23. Nchimi A, Szapiro D, Ghaye B et al (2005) Helical CT of blunt diaphragmatic rupture. AJR Am J Roentgenol 184:24–30
24. Iochum S, Ludig T, Walter F, Sebbag H, Grosdidier G, Blum AG (2002) Imaging of diaphragmatic injury: a diagnostic challenge? Radiographics 22:S103–S116
25. Murray JG, Caoili E, Gruden JF, Evans SJ, Halvorsen RA Jr, Mackersie RC (1996) Acute rupture of the diaphragm due to blunt trauma: diagnostic sensitivity and specificity of CT. AJR Am J Roentgenol 166:1035–1039
26. Bergin D, Ennis R, Keogh C, Fenlon HM, Murray JG (2001) The "dependent viscera" sign in CT diagnosis of blunt traumatic diaphragmatic rupture. AJR Am J Roentgenol 177:1137–1140
27. Chen JC, Wilson SE (1991) Diaphragmatic injuries: recognition and management in sixty two patrients. Am Surg 57:810
28. Meyers BF, McCabe CJ (1993) Traumatic diaphragmatic hernia. Ann Surg 218:783
29. Mansour KA, Clements JL, Hatcher CR et al (1973) Diaphragmatic hernia caused by trauma: experience with 35 cases. Am Surg 41:97
30. Asensio JA, Demetriades D, Rodriguez A (1996) Injury to the diaphragm. In: Feliciano DV, Moore EE, Mattox KL (eds) Trauma, 3rd edn. Appleton and Lange, Stamford Connecticut
31. Moore EE, Malangoni MA, Coggbill T et al (1994) Organ injury scaling IV: thoracic, lung, cardiac and diaphragm. J Trauma 36:299

Esophageal and Gastric Injuries

6

Paul M. Schneider, Georg Lurje, Peter Bauerfeind, and Marc Schiesser

6.1 Esophageal Injuries

6.1.1 Classification

Traumatic lesions of the esophagus can be classified into:

Primary lesions

- Perforations
- Ruptures

Secondary lesions

- Fistulas
- Strictures

Perforations: Perforations are due to internal or external forces. The vast majority of esophageal perforations occur iatrogenic (e.g., endoscopy, dilatation, transesophageal echocardiography (TEE), Sengstaken–Blakemore tubes, endotracheal tubes). Penetrating injuries due to external forces (e.g., stab wounds, gunshots) are less frequent. For the therapeutic concept it should always be kept in mind whether a normal or already diseased organ (e.g., peptic stenosis, achalasia, carcinoma) is perforated.

A complete or true perforation affects all layers of the esophageal wall and can be contained (cervical fascia or mediastinum) or uncontained by connecting the esophageal lumen with the pleural or peritoneal cavity. An incomplete perforation is characterized by an isolated injury of individual layers of the esophageal wall.

Ruptures: Esophageal ruptures occur most frequently in the distal esophagus (*locus minoris resistentiae*) and are commonly induced by gas or fluid (e.g., compressed air) barotrauma. A particular form of rupture is the so-called Boerhaave's syndrome. It occurs as a consequence of an episode of forced vomiting. Rare cases of spontaneous rupture may also occur in achalasia.

Fistulas: Fistulas can result as a consequence of a traumatic injury and connect the esophageal lumen to other organs (internal fistula, e.g., esophago-bronchial fistula) or to the body surface (external fistula). Fistulas can be complete or incomplete (blind end). Posttraumatic fistulas have to be separated from postoperative fistulas, which are mainly due to anastomotic leakage.

Strictures: Strictures can develop as a result of esophageal trauma in the recovery period. They are a particular problem in caustic injuries with alkalines when injuries involve deeper layers than the mucosa. Cumbersome repeated dilatations and ultimately esophageal resection may be necessary treatment options.

P.M. Schneider (✉)
Department of Surgery, University Hospital Zurich,
Raemistrasse 100, 8091 Zurich, Switzerland
e-mail: paul.schneider@usz.ch

G. Lurje and M. Schiesser
Department of Surgery, University Hospital Zurich,
Zurich, Switzerland
e-mail: georg.lurje@usz.ch
e-mail: marc.schiesser@usz.ch

P. Bauerfeind
Department of Gastroenterology, University of Zurich,
Zurich, Switzerland
e-mail: peter.bauerfeind@usz.ch

H.-J. Oestern et al. (eds.), *Head, Thoracic, Abdominal, and Vascular Injuries*,
DOI: 10.1007/978-3-540-88122-3_6, © Springer-Verlag Berlin Heidelberg 2011

6.1.2 Pathophysiology, Diagnosis, and Treatment of Esophageal Injuries

6.1.2.1 External Trauma and Iatrogenic Lesions

Perforation of the esophagus from an external trauma is mainly due to a penetrating injury. In a retrospective multicenter study of the American Association for the Surgery of Trauma involving 405 patients with known penetrating esophageal injuries, it was shown that the predominant mechanism of injury was gunshot trauma in 78.8% and stabbing in 18.5% of patients [5]. Injuries were located in the cervical esophagus in 57%, thoracic esophagus in 30%, and abdominal esophagus in 17%, with combined injuries occurring in 4% of patients. The overall mortality rate was 19%. Penetrating esophageal trauma in the cervical esophagus is commonly associated with vascular, tracheal or spinal cord injuries with injuries of the trachea being the most often co-injured structures [34]. Esophageal perforation from blunt trauma is a very rare event. It is usually related to a high-speed motor vehicle crash. Beal and co-workers [6] reported 96 patients with blunt esophageal trauma and in 80%, a perforation occurred in the cervical and upper thoracic esophagus. Early signs and symptoms of esophageal perforation due to blunt trauma especially in patients presenting with multiple blunt injuries are easily overseen. It is therefore mandatory to pay particular attention while assessing this injury in patients with high-energy neck and chest trauma.

Meanwhile, iatrogenic esophageal perforation is the most common cause of esophageal perforation and is found in more than 80% of patients. The leading causes are diagnostic and interventional endoscopic procedures and TEE. Esophageal perforation during upper GI endoscopy occurs at a frequency of 0.03% using flexible endoscopes and is higher (0.11%) during a rigid endoscopy [18, 35]. Perforations due to diagnostic endoscopy are most frequently located in the hypopharynx or cervical esophagus. The risk of esophageal injury, however, increases with therapeutic manipulations (e.g., dilatation for strictures or achalasia) in a diseased organ. They occur at frequencies between 2% and 6% [39]. TEE has been recognized to be a common risk factor for iatrogenic esophageal perforation with an incidence of 0.18% [11, 29]. Rarely, perforation of the esophagus occurs with a Sengstaken–Blakemore tube, nasogastric tube, endotracheal tube, during endoscopic retrograde cholangiopancreatography (ERCP)

or endoscopic ultrasound-guided interventions. The same is true of esophageal injuries during surgical procedures in the vicinity of the organ.

Serious consequences of traumatic esophageal perforations are, in principle, independent of the nature of the trauma. Infectious material can enter the mediastinum or pleural cavity and lead to mediastinitis and pleural empyema. Even perforations in the cervical part of the esophagus can lead to descending mediastinitis. Especially in instrumental perforation in the fasting patient (e.g., prior to endoscopy), there is less contamination and symptoms can be less severe and occur with a delay. Thoracic lesions are initially characterized by a more severe cause due to mediastinitis and abdominal perforations manifest themselves as an acute abdomen.

The diagnostic work-up is based on four examinations:

- Chest X-ray/plain abdominal X-ray
- Upper flexible endoscopy (esophagus and stomach) ± flexible bronchoscopy
- Computed tomography (CT) of the neck, chest, and abdomen
- Pharyngo-esophagography with water-soluble contrast medium

X-rays can detect a cervical lesion with the appearance of paraesophageal air in the neck (Minnegerode's sign). In thoracic lesions, pneumo- or seropneumothorax, mediastinal widening or emphysema can be discovered. In abdominal perforation, free air below the diaphragm is commonly seen. Endoscopy can give important and reliable information about the localization and size of the defect. CT with water-soluble contrast material (oral route or by an esophagogastric tube) can discriminate between a free perforation and a contained perforation. It identifies pleural effusions, mediastinal emphysema or empyema. Pharyngo-esophagography with water-soluble contrast material can directly demonstrate a perforation.

At our institution, the routine diagnostic work-up for suspected esophageal perforation comprises the usage of flexible upper endoscopy in combination with CT with water-soluble contrast medium given orally or preferentially through a nasogastric tube. In some cases, flexible bronchoscopy is necessary to rule out involvement of the tracheobronchial tree.

The choice of the therapeutic procedure depends mainly on the cause of the perforation, the presence of a diseased organ (achalasia, carcinoma, benign steno-sis), localization and extent of the defect, interval between injury and the diagnosis, age, and general condition of the patient.

Fresh accidental surgical lesions should always be immediately repaired.

There is a trend toward conservative therapy especially in instrumental esophageal perforation. The advantage is that contamination during the early phase is diminished since patients are usually fasting before the examination.

Circumscribed lesions of the cervical esophagus and contained perforations of the thoracic esophagus can be treated by nasogastric suction-tubes, antibiotic treatment, and total parenteral or enteral nutrition [2, 10]. Otherwise, cervical lesions are surgically treated through a left cervical access along the anterior border of the sternocleidomastoid muscle (Fig. 6.1) and are directly sutured or receive external drainage.

In early detected (≤24 h) thoracic instrumental per-forations or abdominal perforations in a diseased esophagus, we prefer the combination of placement of a covered self-expandable stent and if necessary addi-tional drainage (e.g., chest tube, laparoscopically placed drain). In patients with early instrumental per-forations (≤24 h), there are encouraging results sug-gesting favorable outcome with the usage of covered self-expandable stents [26, 30, 41]. Thoracic perfora-tions with delayed detection (>24 h) draining into the chest can be approached through a right thoracotomy and repaired by direct suturing and reinforcement (e.g., pleural flap, diaphragmatic flap, muscle flap, or omental flap). In severe cases or when the clinical con-dition deteriorates, resection of the esophagus with closure at the level of the cardia and creation of a left cervical esophagostomy is necessary. Reconstruction after esophagectomy is always delayed for several weeks to months and is performed via the anterior mediastinal (substernal) route. A rarely necessary alternative for an unstable patient (septic shock) is the exclusion by a cervical esophagostomy and distal clo-sure (band, stapling line ± balloon catheter) at the level of the cardia plus wide drainage (Fig. 6.2).

In distal perforations, the surgical approach involves a laparotomy with a wide longitudinal opening of the hiatus. This access provides a good exposure for per-forations up to 10 cm proximal the cardia. Surgical repair is established by direct suturing of the lesion and coverage with a fundoplasty according to Thal [38] (Fig. 6.3a–e).

At our institution, we routinely perform double-layer sutures of the mucosa/submucosa and muscle/adventitia typically as running sutures over a large bougie (42–54 Ch) as depicted in Fig. 6.3d.

It is important to clearly identify the proximal and distal ends of the mucosal tear before suturing.

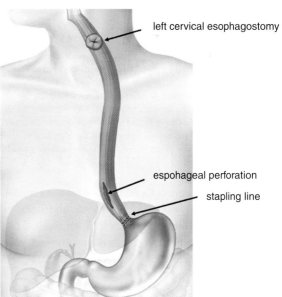

Fig. 6.2 Exclusion of an esophageal perforation with a cervical esophagostomy and distal closure (reflux prevention). We prefer a stapling line across the cardia without transsection. In addi-tion, a ballon catheter can be placed into the esophageal lumen proximal the stapling line

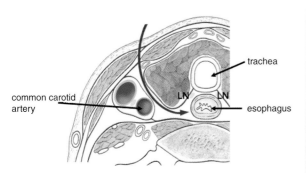

Fig. 6.1 Surgical access to the cervical esophagus and hypo-pharyx by an incision along the anterior border of the left sterno-cleidomastoideus muscle and dissection medial to the common carotid artery and lateral to the thyroid gland (*red line*). The omohyoideus muscle and inferior thyroid artery have to be divided (not shown). The recurrent laryngeal nerve (NL) is located in the tracheo-esophageal groove and has to be identified to prevent injury

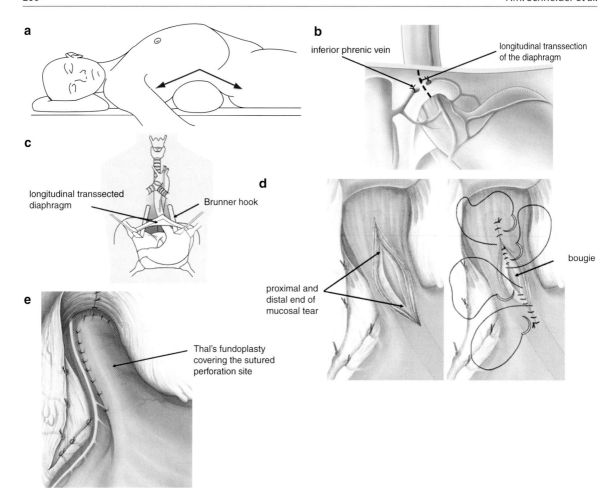

Fig. 6.3 (**a**) Positioning of the patient. (**b**) Longitudinal opening (marked by *black dotted incision line*) of the diaphragm to expose the distal esophagus. The inferior V. phrenica has to be divided and we use this landmark to start division of the diaphragm. Directly underneath is the pericardium. (**c**) Positioning of the patient and insertion of long Brunner hooks to expose the lower mediastinum after longitudinal opening of the diaphragm. The *red* area is the space of direct vision. Both chest cavities can be easily opened, extensively rinsed and drained. (**d**) Double layer suturing of the mucosa/submucosa and muscle layer/adventitia of the esophagus. We prefer running sutures coming out of both edges. Sometimes the muscle layer at the proximal and distal end has to be further divided to clearly identify the end of the mucosal/submucosal tear. A large bougie (45–54 Ch) is always in place to prevent stenosis while suturing. (**e**) Reinforcement of the suture repair by a fundoplasty according to [38]

Our current treatment algorithm is shown in Fig. 6.4.

With the advent of improved diagnostic and therapeutic strategies, the overall mortality from esophageal perforation has dramatically decreased over the last years and may now be below 5% in experienced centers [37].

6.1.2.2 Boerhaave's Syndrome

Boerhaave's syndrome is characterized by a transmural rupture of the esophageal wall and is induced by an episode of forced vomiting. This syndrome was described by Herman Boerhaave [1], Professor at the University of Leiden, the Netherlands in 1724 following the autopsy of his friend, Baron von Wassenaer, Grand Admiral of the Dutch fleet. After indulging himself to an opulent dinner and wine, he developed an excruciating chest pain following self-induced vomiting. The term spontaneous esophageal rupture does not reflect the pathophysiology and is therefore misleading.

The pathophysiology of Boerhaave's syndrome is related to an intraluminal barotrauma. It is speculated that the velocity of pressure-increase is more

Algorithm Esophageal Perforation

1. Endoscopy
2. CT Chest / Abdomen

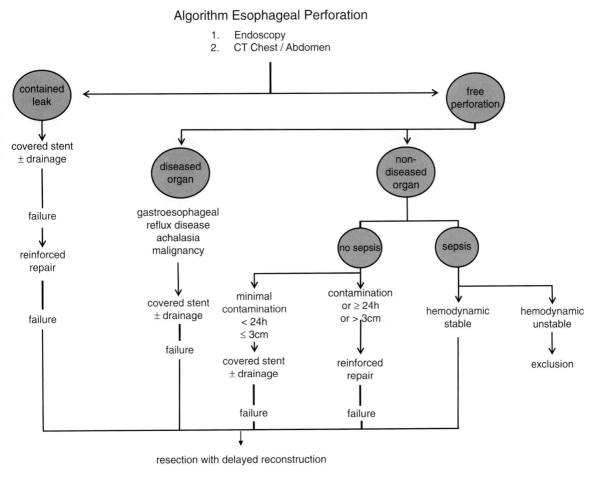

Fig. 6.4 Current treatment algorithm for thoracic or abdominal esophageal perforations in our institution. It has to be noted however, that individual decisions are frequently necessary

important than the absolute pressure achieved in the esophageal wall. Most common, there is a distal supracardial left lateral longitudinal complete defect of the esophageal wall. Higher localized ruptures are extremely rare. Occasionally, ruptures can be incomplete and can develop secondarily to a complete lesion of the wall.

The classical triad (Mackler's Triad) of Boerhaave's syndrome consists of:

- Episode of forced vomiting
- Acute chest or epigastric pain
- Mediastinal or cutaneous emphysema

Pathognomonic is the development of a pneumo- or sero-pneumothorax. A typical sign is the development of mediastinal emphysema, progressing rapidly to a cutaneous emphysema of the neck and upper chest. In one-third of the cases, there are clinical signs of an acute abdomen due to irritation of the basal pleura or free perforation into the abdominal cavity. Symptoms and medical findings are variable and the clinical diagnosis can be difficult. Within the context of chest pain work-up it is therefore mandatory to ask for an episode of forced vomiting and to rule out Boerhaave's syndrome.

Keep in mind: chest pain – always ask for vomiting!

In the presence of the classical triad, the clinical diagnosis of Boerhaave's syndrome is almost certain. Despite this, a complete diagnostic work-up has to be performed. In the majority of cases, a mediastinal emphysema can be seen in chest X-rays. Esophagography with water-soluble contrast medium is accurate in approximately 70% of cases. The two main diagnostic procedures at our center are endoscopy and CT with the

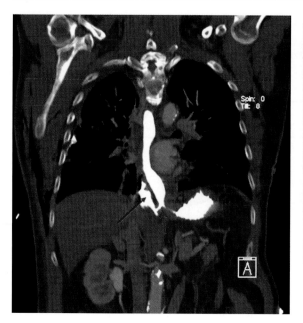

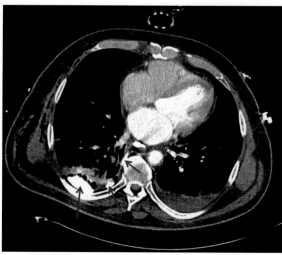

Fig. 6.6 CT scan demonstrating an uncontained perforation of the esophagus draining into the right chest cavity (*arrows*)

Fig. 6.5 CT scan demonstrating a contained perforation of the distal esophagus (Boerhaave's syndrome) on the right side (*pink arrow*) that does not drain into the right chest cavity. The perforation site is marked with a *red arrow*

use of water-soluble contrast medium given by mouth or through a nasogastric tube. Upper endoscopy shows the length and the exact location of the lesion. CT scans show even a minimum amount of free air in the mediastinum or upper abdomen which can be easily overseen in X-rays. In addition, application of water-soluble contrast material can clarify, if the perforation is contained (Fig. 6.5) or uncontained (Fig. 6.6). In case of an injured mediastinal pleura, contrast medium enters into the chest cavity, preferentially on the left side.

The two most important criteria next to the general condition of the patient is the presence of a contained or free rupture and the time elapsed between perforation and diagnosis (more or less than 24 h).

Even though conservative therapy with nasogastric-suction tubes, total parenteral nutrition, and antibiotic treatment is possible in cases of contained esophageal rupture, we prefer the placement of a covered, self-expandable stent, which is removed between 2 and 3 weeks after initial placement as shown in Fig. 6.7a and b [25, 26]. Additional drainage (chest tube, laparoscopic placement of a mediastinal drain) might be necessary.

In free ruptures with exit of contrast material into the chest (Fig. 6.6), we usually perform a laparotomy with wide longitudinal opening of the hiatus that easily

exposes the esophagus up to 10 cm above the cardia. As such, direct repair of the defect can be performed with a double-layer running suture of the mucosa/submucosa and of the muscle layer over a large bougie (42–54 Ch). This primary repair is reinforced with a fundoplasty according to Thal [38] as shown in Fig. 6.3a–e.

More recently, small free perforations (<3 cm) with no or minimal contamination of the mediastinum, a short delay (<24 h) and no signs of sepsis, were successfully treated in our institution by placement of a covered, self-expandable stent that also overlaid the cardia. Additionally, broad spectrum antibiotic treatment is given and a nasogastric tube over the stent is installed.

Repair in rarely higher locations is performed through a right thoracotomy with a diaphragmatic flap, pleural flap, muscle flap or a simple T-tube [9, 21].

In patients with rapid clinical deterioration (sepsis) following primary surgical repair, or in cases of late clinical diagnosis, a transmediastinal esophagectomy with closure of the stomach at the level of the cardia and left cervical esophagostomy should be performed. In addition, the mediastinum and the pleural cavities have to be extensively lavaged and drained. Convincing data from [33] justify to proceed with esophagectomy, since mortality was 13% in patients with esophagectomy compared to 68% with late repair and drainage in patients with delayed diagnosis (>24 h). There should not be any attempt for a primary reconstruction in this situation; instead, reconstruction should be delayed for a variable

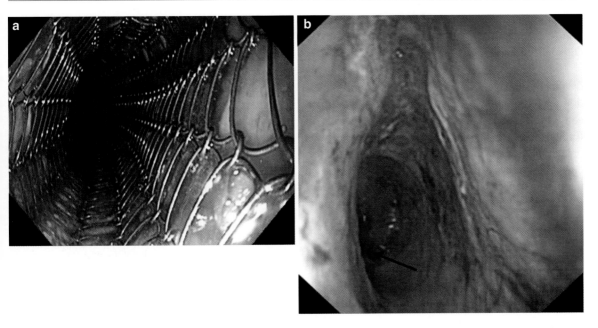

Fig. 6.7 (**a**) Self-expandable covered stent in a patient with Boerhaave's syndrome.(**b**) Complete healing after endoscopic stent removal (cardia is marked with an *arrow*)

interval of several weeks to months. In the meantime, enteral nutrition is performed through a percutaneous gastric feeding tube or placement of a jejunal feeding tube especially when the stomach will be used for reconstruction. Of course, antibiotic treatment is mandatory.

Our current treatment algorithm is shown in Fig. 6.4.

Prognosis of Boerhaave's syndrome is largely dependent on the type of perforation, the general condition of the patient, and the presence of sepsis. A timely diagnosis and immediate treatment are critical. Compromised clinical outcome is a frequently encountered problem if the diagnostic work up and treatment is delayed for more than 24 h. Until several years ago, mortality was more than 50% in many retrospective series. However, it can be lower than 10% in some experienced centers [12] and was lower than 5% in the series of Stein et al. [37].

6.1.2.3 Ingestion of Foreign Bodies

Foreign body ingestions typically occur in children and patients with psychiatric disorders. Between 80% and 90% of ingested foreign bodies pass the gastrointestinal tract without any problems [14]. Open surgery is rarely necessary (<1%) and the majority of objects can be removed using flexible endoscopy. In the largest series by [24] that included 5,848 patients with documented foreign body ingestion, only eight patients suffered from esophageal perforation (0.001%). All perforations were located in the cervical esophagus.

Symptoms of accidental ingestion of foreign bodies are odynophagia, dysphagia, or asphyxia. Aphagia and hypersalivation are indicative of complete obstruction of the esophagus. Cutaneous or mediastinal emphysema, hematemesis, and peritonitis are clinical signs of the rare event of esophageal perforation. In rare cases, foreign bodies in the esophagus and stomach are detected after a longer uneventful interval through the occurrence of local complications [40]. It is important to emphasize that in cases of foreign body ingestion, the patient needs to be immediately sent to a hospital for diagnostic work-up and if necessary, therapeutic intervention.

The first diagnostic procedure is the thorough inspection of the oral cavity.

The indication for foreign body extraction located in the esophagus or stomach has to take into account the risks and benefits. Type of the material, size, shape, location, as well as the presence of a diseased organ and the interval between ingestion and diagnosis are important [28]. It is very helpful if the patient brings an example of the swallowed object to the emergency room.

If the foreign body is localized in the hypopharynx or upper esophageal sphincter, there is a vital indication for foreign body extraction because of a dramatically increased risk of asphyxia. The presence of foreign bodies in the stomach is not necessarily an indication for extraction if the type and size of the foreign body allow a passage through the pylorus and there is no expected harm from ingested substances.

More than 85% of foreign bodies that pass through the esophagus will leave the body spontaneously (via naturalis).

In case of asphyxia, the oral cavity has to be digitally explored and the Esmarch maneuver needs to be performed. Small infants can be held on the legs upside down and clapped on the back to spontaneously remove the foreign body. The Heimlich maneuver is a life-saving measure for aspirated foreign bodies; however, the dangers of severe complications like splenic rupture or esophageal rupture have to be kept in mind when performing this maneuver. In rare cases of supra- or infraglottic ingestion, a coniotomy needs to be performed.

Foreign bodies in the hypopharynx are generally removed by laryngoscopy. In contrast to rigid esophagoscopy, using a flexible instrument significantly reduces the complication rate. Therefore, flexible endoscopy is the preferred intervention worldwide for extraction of foreign bodies in the esophagus [7, 15]. Dormia baskets, retrieval forceps, polypectomy snares, Roth nets, tripods, and other devices have been successfully used. It has to be kept in mind that every attempt to remove a foreign body from the upper gastrointestinal tract has to be done under the precaution that intubation can be immediately performed to protect the airways. Dangerous sharp foreign bodies have to be removed under general anesthesia [28].

Although complications from endoscopic foreign body extractions are rare, they can be severe and ultimately even lead to death. Lacerations and perforations during extraction generally occur in the cervical region and hypopharynx and can be treated conservatively [8]. The indication for surgical removal of a foreign body is rare. Sharp objects, batteries, and magnets constitute a serious problem [4]. Batteries contain corrosive substances and may cause necrosis in case of leakage. Complications related to the ingestion of

magnetic foreign bodies by children represent an affirmed health hazard in the USA. Responsible for complications is the ingestion of at least two magnets, or one magnet and a metallic foreign body, with a time interval between ingestions. In these cases, the endoscopic extraction of the foreign body is strongly recommended if it has not yet passed the pylorus. For those that have already passed the pylorus, continuous observation is warranted and surgical extraction is indicated on apparition of the first clinical symptoms.

In case a foreign body cannot be localized by endoscopy but the patient still has persistent symptoms from foreign body ingestion, a CT-scan should be performed. The negative predictive value and diagnostic accuracy were reported to be 97% and 94%, respectively [27].

In a retrospective analysis by [23], 1,338 cases of suspected foreign body ingestion, presenting from 1996 to 2000 in Hong Kong were reported. Fish bone (62.7%) was the most common type of foreign body ingestion. In general, only a salt-water fish has bones that are rigid enough to penetrate the intestinal wall. It is therefore important to ask the patient which kind of fish he has eaten. Most of the objects were impacted at/ or above the cricopharyngeal muscle, with the valleculae (31.4%) being the most frequent site of impactation. Multivariate analysis showed that a delayed presentation for more than 2 days ($p<0.001$), positive cervical radiographic findings ($p < 0.001$), and foreign body impaction at the cricopharyngeal muscle ($p=0.009$) or upper esophagus ($p = 0.005$) were significant independent risk factors associated with the development of complications after foreign body ingestion. Awareness should be raised when these risk factors are present. The algorithm suggested by Lai and co-workers for the diagnosis and treatment of foreign body ingestions is shown in Fig. 6.8.

6.1.2.4 Caustic Injuries

Accidental ingestion represents the vast majority of caustic injuries that occur in children under 5 years of age. Less frequent, ingestion of caustic agents is observed in adults in an attempt to commit suicide. The severity and extent of esophago-gastric injuries depend on the nature, amount, and concentration of the caustic substance, and on the duration of mucosal contact [32].

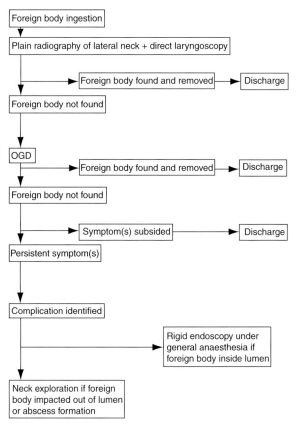

Fig. 6.8 Treatment algorithm for foreign body ingestion according to [23]

Injuries with acid or alkaline solutions can reduce the pressure in the lower esophageal sphincter that may lead to continuous reflux of ingested substances, accounting for generally more extensive injuries of the lower esophageal region. The most common chemicals are alkalines or acids. Alkaline solutions cause a deep burn with a colliquation necrosis compared to a coagulative necrosis that limits the depth of tissue penetration with acid burns. Alkaline ingestion is further complicated by a pylorospasm with regurgitation that aggravates both gastric and esophageal injuries [36]. Although acid passes more quickly through the esophagus it can also induce pylorospasms with acid accumulation in the gastric antrum inducing severe gastritis and full thickness necrosis ultimately leading to gastric perforation within 24–48 h.

Caustic injuries of the esophagus and stomach can be classified according to histopathological criteria as described by Kikendall and co-workers [22]:

- First degree: superficial mucosal injury with isolated small defects and edema; no specific therapy is necessary and healing is uneventful.
- Second degree: mucosa is destroyed and submucosa or muscle layer are partially damaged. Healing is by scarring.
- Third degree: complete necrosis of all organ layers. Consequences can be early perforation with mediastinitis, peritonitis, and erosion of intrathoracic and intra-abdominal organs.

The following phases of inflammation and regeneration can be defined [22]:

- Acute initial stage (up to 4 days):
Acute tissue necrosis is present as a consequence of coagulation (acid) or colliquation (alkaline). It is delineated by infiltrating leucocytes following bacterial and hemorrhagic infiltration.
- Granulation phase (up to 4 weeks):
Further demarcation of necrotic material with spontaneous bleeding from eroded small vessels. Formation of a granulation tissue and collagen fibers. In this period, the esophageal wall is at risk.
- Scarring phase (up to 4 months):
80% of strictures will present within the first 8 weeks and over 90% during the first year.

Common symptoms of caustic injuries are pain in the mouth and throat, odynophagia, dysphagia, thirst, and hypersalivation. A toxic edema of the glottis may also be present.

In an emergency situation, a principal differentiation in weak or strong acid or alkaline solutions is important. In any case, a toxicologist has to be consulted since various substances can induce complex injuries in the body. The most important task is an immediate diagnostic work-up, which includes endoscopic evaluation of the localization, extent, and depth of the organ damage [32].

For clinical reasons, an endoscopic classification of the extent of damage is performed since histopathologic differentiation is not readily available.

Caustic injuries are classified into three endoscopic categories:

- First degree: mild caustic injury defined by edema and erosions.
- Second degree: severe caustic injury defined by thrombosed vessels, bleeding, ulcers, necrotic areas

of the mucosa next to islands of intact mucosa, bleeding following biopsies.

- Third degree: very severe caustic injury characterized by complete necrosis of the mucosa with no bleeding when multiple deep biopsies are taken.

Further examination by CT with water-soluble contrast material is helpful to exclude and/or demonstrate a perforation (Fig. 6.9).

Initial therapy aims at stabilization of the patient and early intubation, aggressive fluid resuscitation, treatment of metabolic acidosis and coagulation disorders. A nasogastric tube is inserted during endoscopy. Lavage of the stomach, induced vomiting by emetic agents or chemical antagonizing are absolutely contraindicated.

The presence of a perforation or a third-degree injury is an indication for a surgical intervention (Fig. 6.9a and b). In second-degree injuries, surgical intervention is indicated if the clinical course shows a rapid deterioration of vital functions despite maximal intensive care therapy.

The first step in the operative strategy is a laparotomy. In case of an esophageal perforation, a transhiatal esophagectomy is performed [20, 43] using the same approach as described above. If a total gastrectomy is performed and the esophagus does not to have to be removed, a cervical esophagostomy and a distal closure of the esophageal stump are carried out Fig. 6.2). A jejunal feeding tube should be inserted in every patient to ensure enteral nutrition. Reconstruction should be performed at a stage when all the possible late consequences of the initial injury are established. In any instance, the extent of possible stricture formation in the cervical esophageal remnant has to be awaited. We therefore perform definitive reconstruction 1 year after the incident. Either a gastric tube reconstruction, if the stomach was not injured or a colon interposition is performed.

In endoscopic grade I and II injuries, when surgical resection is not necessary, conservative therapy is undertaken. This therapy comprises the placement of a nasogastric tube, parenteral nutrition, blockage of the acid production of the stomach by proton pump inhibitors, and regular endoscopic follow-up.

Broad spectrum antibiotic treatment is mandatory. As prospective clinical trials have not demonstrated a significant benefit of early systemic corticosteroid therapy, its use in the prevention of posttraumatic esophageal strictures remains questionable [3, 17].

Early bouginage is the most effective measure to prevent stricture formation in the esophagus after a second- and third-degree injury and should be started toward the end of the second week following the injury. [37] advocate to start even earlier between day 6 and 12. It should be performed in intervals of 2–4 days over a guide wire. Nevertheless, it has to be kept in mind that despite all efforts, an esophagectomy may be necessary following conservative treatment due to extensive scarring and stricture formation that cannot be

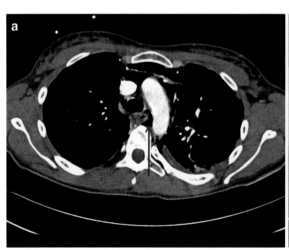
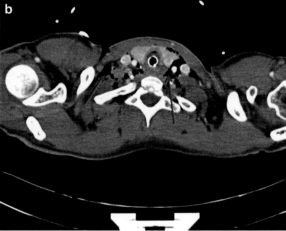
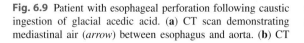

Fig. 6.9 Patient with esophageal perforation following caustic ingestion of glacial acedic acid. (**a**) CT scan demonstrating mediastinal air (*arrow*) between esophagus and aorta. (**b**) CT scan demonstrating air in the neck (*arrows*) that can also be felt as subcutaneous emphysema

successfully treated by long-term bouginage [16]. The incidence of malignant degeneration is increased [19] particularly after alkaline ingestion. Its potential risk of malignant degeneration however, does not justify prophylactic esophagectomy. Therefore, endoscopic follow-up starting 10 years after caustic ingestion with stricture formation appears reasonable.

6.2 Gastric Injuries

Traumatic perforation or ruptures of the stomach by internal or external forces are rare events [42]. In contrast to esophageal perforation, spontaneous healing by sealing with omentum or neighboring organs can occur. Large ruptures however, lead to peritonitis and the development of an acute abdomen [31]. If a stomach perforation is clinically suspected, free subdiaphragmatic air can be seen in chest X-rays and plain abdominal films. CT with water-soluble contrast material can show a small amount of free air and extravasation of contrast material. It is important to keep in mind that endoscopy is not at all contraindicated in case of suspected stomach perforation and may enable the correct diagnosis in unclear cases. Symptomatic contained perforations without peritoneal irritation can be treated conservatively by placement of a nasogastric tube [13]. In general, perforations are treated by local excision and direct suturing using either a laparoscopic (e.g., in instrumental perforation) or more frequently open approach. Large defects can necessitate partial gastric resections and rarely, gastrectomy.

References

1. Adams BD, Sebastian BM, Carter J (2006) Honoring the admiral: Boerhaave-van Wassenaer's syndrome. Dis Esophagus 19(3):146–151
2. Altorjay A, Kiss J, Vörös A, Bohák A (1997) Nonoperative management of esophageal perforations. Is it justified? Ann Surg 225(4):415–421
3. Anderson KD, Rouse TM, Randolph JG (1990) A controlled trial of corticosteroids in children with corrosive injury of the esophagus. N Engl J Med 323(10):637–640
4. Arana A, Hauser B, Hachimi-Idrissi S, Vandenplas Y (2001) Management of ingested foreign bodies in childhood and review of the literature. Eur J Pediatr 160(8):468–472
5. Asensio JA, Chahwan S, Forno W, MacKersie R, Wall M, Lake J, Minard G, Kirton O, Nagy K, Karmy-Jones R, Brundage S, Hoyt D, Winchell R, Kralovich K, Shapiro M,
Falcone R, McGuire E, Ivatury R, Stoner M, Yelon J, Ledgerwood A, Luchette F, Schwab CW, Frankel H, Chang B, Coscia R, Maull K, Wang D, Hirsch E, Cue J, Schmacht D, Dunn E, Miller F, Powell M, Sherck J, Enderson B, Rue L 3rd, Warrenc R, Rodriquez J, West M, Weireter L, Britt LD, Dries D, Dunham CM, Malangoni M, cFallon W, Simon R, Bell R, Hanpeter D, Gambaro E, Ceballos J, Torcal J, Alo K, Ramicone E, Chan L (2001) American Association for the Surgery of Trauma. Penetratingesophageal injuries: multicenter study of the American Association for the Surgery of Trauma. J Trauma 50(2):289–296
6. Beal SL, Pottmeyer EW, Spisso JM (1988) Esophageal perforation following external blunt trauma. J Trauma 28(10): 1425–1432
7. Berggreen PJ, Harrison E, Sanowski RA, Ingebo K, Noland B, Zierer S (1993) Techniques and complications of esophageal foreign body extraction in children and adults. Gastrointest Endosc 39(5):626–630
8. Brady PG (1991) Esophageal foreign bodies. Gastroenterol Clin North Am 20(4):691–701
9. Brinster CJ, Singhal S, Lee L, Marshall MB, Kaiser LR, Kucharczuk JC (2004) Evolving options in the management of esophageal perforation. Ann Thorac Surg 77(4):1475–83
10. Cameron JL, Kieffer RF, Hendrix TR, Mehigan DG, Baker RR (1979) Selective nonoperative management of contained intrathoracic esophageal disruptions. Ann Thorac Surg 27(5):404–408
11. Daniel WG, Erbel R, Kasper W, Visser CA, Engberding R, Sutherland GR, Grube E, Hanrath P, Maisch B, Dennig K et al (1991) Safety of transesophageal echocardiography. A multicenter survey of 10,419 examinations. Circulation 83(3):817–821
12. De Schipper JP, ter Gunne AF Pull, Oostvogel HJ, van Laarhoven CJ (2009) Spontaneous rupture of the oesophagus: Boerhaave's syndrome in 2008. Literature review and treatment algorithm. Dig Surg 26(1):1–6
13. Durham R (1990) Management of gastric injuries. Surg Clin North Am 70(3):517–527
14. Eisen GM, Baron TH, Dominitz JA, Faigel DO, Goldstein JL, Johanson JF, Mallery JS, Raddawi HM, Vargo JJ 2nd, Waring JP, Fanelli RD, Wheeler-Harbough J (2002) American Society for Gastrointestinal Endoscopy Guideline for the management of ingested foreign bodies. Gastrointest Endosc 55(7):802–806
15. Fischer A, Thomusch O, Benz S, von Dobschuetz E, Baier P, Hopt UT (2006) Nonoperative treatment of 15 benign esophageal perforations with self-expandable covered metal stents. Ann Thorac Surg 81(2):467–472
16. Han Y, Cheng QS, Li XF, Wang XP (2004) Surgical management of esophageal strictures after caustic burns: a 30 years of experience. World J Gastroenterol 10(19):2846–2849
17. Howell JM, Dalsey WC, Hartsell FW, Butzin CA (1992) Steroids for the treatment of corrosive esophageal injury: a statistical analysis of past studies. Am J Emerg Med 10(5): 421–425
18. Kavic SM, Basson MD (2001) Complications of endoscopy. Am J Surg 181(4):319–332
19. Kochhar R, Sethy PK, Kochhar S, Nagi B, Gupta NM (2006) Corrosive induced carcinoma of esophagus: report of three patients and review of literature. J Gastroenterol Hepatol 21(4):777–780

20. Horváth OP, Oláh T, Zentai G (1991) Emergency esophago-gastrectomy for treatment of hydrochloric acid injury. Ann Thorac Surg 52(1):98–101

21. Kiernan PD, Sheridan MJ, Hettrick V, Vaughan B, Graling P (2006) Thoracic esophageal perforation: one surgeon's experience. Dis Esophagus 19(1):24–30

22. Kikendall JW (1991) Caustic ingestion injuries. Gastroenterol Clin North Am 20(4):847–857

23. Lai AT, Chow TL, Lee DT, Kwok SP (2003) Risk factors predicting the development of complications after foreign body ingestion. Br J Surg 90(12):1531–1535

24. Lam HC, Woo JK, van Hasselt CA (2003) Esophageal perforation and neck abscess from ingested foreign bodies: treatment and outcomes. Ear Nose Throat J 82(10):786, 789–94

25. Lam HC, Woo JK, van Hasselt CA (2001) Management of ingested foreign bodies: a retrospective review of 5240 patients. J Laryngol Otol 115(12):954–957

26. Leers JM, Vivaldi C, Schäfer H, Bludau M, Brabender J, Lurje G, Herbold T, Hölscher AH, Metzger R (2009) Endoscopic therapy for esophageal perforation or anastomotic leak with a self-expandable metallic stent. Surg Endosc 23(10):2258–62

27. Luk WH, Fan WC, Chan RY, Chan SW, Tse KH, Chan JC (2009) Foreign body ingestion: comparison of diagnostic accuracy of computed tomography versus endoscopy. J Laryngol Otol 123(5):535–540

28. Mannegold BC (1992) Fremdkörper im Bereich von Ösophagus und Magen. In: Siewert JR et al. (ed) Chirurgische Gastroenterologie, Band 2, 2. Auflage, Springer, Berlin Heidelberg Tokyo New York

29. Min JK, Spencer KT, Furlong KT, DeCara JM, Sugeng L, Ward RP, Lang RM (2005) Clinical features of complications from transesophageal echocardiography: a single-center case series of 10, 000 consecutive examinations. J Am Soc Echocardiogr 18(9):925–929

30. Mumtaz H, Barone GW, Ketel BL, Ozdemir A (2002) Successful management of a nonmalignant esophageal perforation with a coated stent. Ann Thorac Surg 74(4): 1233–1235

31. Pikoulis E, Delis S, Tsatsoulis P, Leppäniemi A, Derlopas K, Koukoulides G, Mantonakis S (1999) Blunt injuries of the stomach. Eur J Surg 165(10):937–939

32. Poley JW, Steyerberg EW, Kuipers EJ, Dees J, Hartmans R, Tilanus HW, Siersema PD (2004) Ingestion of acid and alkaline agents: outcome and prognostic value of early upper endoscopy. Gastrointest Endosc 60(3):372–377

33. Salo JA, Isolauri JO, Heikkilä LJ, Markkula HT, Heikkinen LO, Kivilaakso EO, Mattila SP (1993) Management of delayed esophageal perforation with mediastinal sepsis. Esophagectomy or primary repair? J Thorac Cardiovasc Surg 106(6):1088–1091

34. Sheely CH 2nd, Mattox KL, Beall AC Jr, DeBakey ME (1975) Penetrating wounds of the cervical esophagus. Am J Surg 130(6):707–711

35. Silvis SE, Nebel O, Rogers G, Sugawa C, Mandelstam P (1976) Endoscopic complications. Results of the 1974 American Society for Gastrointestinal Endoscopy Survey. JAMA 235(9):928–930

36. Spitz L, Lakhoo K (1993) Caustic ingestion. Arch Dis Child 68(2):157–158

37. Stein HJ, von Rahden BHA, Bartels H, Siewert JR (2006) Verletzungen von Oesophagus und Magen. In: Siewert, Rothmund, Schumpelik (eds) Praxis der Viszeralchirurgie. Springer, Heidelberg

38. Thal AP (1968) A unified approach to surgical problems of the esophagogastric junction. Ann Surg 168(3):542–550

39. Vaezi MF, Richter JE (1998) Current therapies for achalasia: comparison and efficacy. J Clin Gastroenterol 27(1):21–35

40. von Rahden BH, Feith M, Dittler HJ, Stein HJ (2002) Cervical esophageal perforation with severe mediastinitis due to an impacted dental prosthesis. Dis Esophagus 15(4):340–344

41. White RE, Mungatana C, Topazian M (2003) Expandable stents for iatrogenic perforation of esophageal malignancies. J Gastrointest Surg 7(6):715–719, discussion 719–20

42. Wilkinson AE (1989) Injuries of the stomach. An analysis of 95 cases. S Afr J Surg 27(2):59–60, discussion 60–1

43. Wu MH, Lai WW (1993) Surgical management of extensive corrosive injuries of the alimentary tract. Surg Gynecol Obstet 177(1):12–16

Liver

Luke P. H. Leenen

7.1 Introduction

The liver as the major and largest solid organ in the abdomen is identified as the most injured organ in abdominal trauma. Its position in the upper abdomen just under the lower ribcage and extending from the right to left side makes it vulnerable for any injury in the thoraco-abdominal transition.

The treatment of liver injuries has changed dramatically over the years. From operative therapy of virtually every laceration of the liver, the paradigm has changed to a nonoperative management (NOM) of these injuries as long as it is hemodynamically feasible.

Concomitant injuries can play an important role for the ultimate prognosis [1]; however, hemodynamic stability dictates the indication for urgent laparotomy.

Because of the huge developments in radiological techniques, more sophisticated treatment options have been developed over the years making the treatment of liver injuries a very versatile task, which should be tailored to the particular situation of the patient.

7.2 Trauma Mechanism and Epidemiology

Because of its anatomical position the liver is vulnerable to all injuries in the thoraco-abdominal transition. Both direct blunt and penetrating injuries can threaten

the liver. Deceleration injuries cause laceration of the liver along the ligamentous structures, hepatobiliary tract, and in rare cases venous structures can be lacerated because of the massive deceleration forces put upon the organ. There is a 15–45% chance for the liver being injured [2, 3]. The most common mechanism is a motor vehicle injury. The rapid deceleration causes laceration of the liver by seatbelts or by the steering wheel [4]. Nevertheless, the wearing of seatbelts is of utmost importance as older data show that more than half of the patients with hepatic injuries were unrestrained [5].

Because of its ligamentous anatomy, the liver is vulnerable to deceleration injuries along these ligaments [6].

Mortality developed over the years from 30% to 40% before the second world war to around 20% in the postwar era [7]. This was attributed to the changing injury pattern from penetrating to mostly blunt injury nowadays. Blunt trauma goes with the highest mortality of up to 45%, whereas penetrating injury comes with a lower mortality rate. Gunshot wounds go with 26.0% mortality rate, whereas stab wounds have a mortality of 3.4%. In a National Trauma Data Bank (NTDB) analysis by Hurtuk [8], average annual rate for mortality of entries with hepatic injury was 16.8%. In a recent analysis by Tinkhof and coworkers [4] also through the NTDB, mortality rate for all hepatic injuries was shown to be 16.7%.

Demetriades showed that major risk factors for associated liver injury were motor vehicle crash and pelvis AIS 4 or greater [9].

The American Association for the Surgery of Trauma published a grading system for liver injuries (Table 7.1), addressing hematoma and lacerations in various grades and stipulated vascular (venous) lesions in the higher grades of injury. The system was validated by Tinkhof and coworkers using the NTDB [10]. They showed that when isolated liver injury is analyzed, increasing organ

L.P.H. Leenen
Department of Surgery, University Medical Center,
Heidelberglaan 100, 3584 CX Utrecht, The Netherlands
e-mail: lleenen@umcutrecht.nl

H.-J. Oestern et al. (eds.), *Head, Thoracic, Abdominal, and Vascular Injuries*,
DOI: 10.1007/978-3-540-88122-3_7, © Springer-Verlag Berlin Heidelberg 2011

Table 7.1 The American Association for the Surgery of Trauma organ injury scale for the liver

Grade*	Injury	Description
I	Hematoma	Subcapsular, <10% surface area
II	Hematoma	Subcapsular, 10–50% surface area: intraparenchymal <10 cm in diameter
	Laceration	Capsular tear 1–3 cm parenchymal depth, <10 cm in length
III	Hematoma	Subcapsular, >50% surface area of ruptured subcapsular or parenchymal hematoma; intra parenchymal hematoma >10 cm or expanding 3 cm parenchymal depth
	Laceration	Parenchymal disruption involving 25–75% hepatic lobe or 1–3 Couinaud's segments
IV	Laceration	Parenchymal disruption involving >75% of hepatic lobe or >3 Couinaud's segments within a single lobe
V	Vascular	Juxtahepatic venous injuries, i.e., retrohepatic vena cava/central major hepatic veins
VI	Vascular	Hepatic avulsion

*Advance one grade for multiple injuries up to grade III

injury grade is associated with increasing mortality, and this association continues to be present for high-grade injuries, even when injuries with severe traumatic brain injury are excluded. However, also in patients with combined injuries, the organ injury grading was associated with mortality, suggesting that organ injury grading may be a surrogate for general severity and complexity of patient injury. Major vein disruption, sometimes associated with retrohepatic caval injuries, comes with substantial higher mortality rates, whereas arterial disruption is currently with the use of arterial transcathether embolization and a scala of operative tricks associated with lower mortality rates.

Operative risk is also related to grading of the hepatic injury. Up to 85% of hepatic injuries can be managed nonoperatively, with risk of failure related to the grade of organ injury [10].

Bile duct injury is found in 6% of liver trauma and can result in persistent fistula. The incidence is rising with the severity of the liver injury [11]; however, the fistula volume is not related to proximal or more distal biliary injury [12].

7.3 Diagnostic Procedures

Diagnostic evaluation should be appropriate to the condition of the patient. In an hemodynamically unstable patient only the minimum of diagnostic effort should be given. After establishing a patent airway and adequate ventilation, the hemodynamically unstable patient should undergo a focused sonography to rule out intraabdominal bleeding. In the case of such a bleeding focus in the abdomen, immediate transfer to the operating room (OR) should ensue for exploratory laparotomy, without further delay and diagnostic evaluation.

7.3.1 Clinical Evaluation

During clinical evaluation, signs of impact should be evaluated; bruises, seatbelt sign, tenderness over the lower thorax should be warning signs for underlying hepatic injury. In case of a hemoperitoneum, only 60% of cases show rigidity of the abdomen [13]; therefore, additional evaluation should follow.

7.3.2 Diagnostic Peritoneal Lavage

Although currently of limited value, the diagnostic peritoneal lavage (DPL) still has to be mentioned as a diagnostic tool in the evaluation of abdominal solid organ trauma. A major drawback is that DPL is so sensitive that minor injuries that have already ceased bleeding at the time of operation are also diagnosed.

7.3.3 Radiological Evaluation

If the patient is hemodynamically unstable, a focused sonography of the abdomen (focused assessment sonography in trauma) (FAST)) should be performed. The sole goal of FAST is determination of free fluid in the abdomen. It should be performed immediately after the evaluation and treatment of the airway and breathing, according to the ATLS® protocol [14]. FAST is used as a quick, first assessment tool in the evaluation of the circulation. Appropriate IV lines should be instituted and warm O negative blood should be held ready.

FAST has definite advantages, because it is portable, easy and very efficacious in detecting free fluid in the peritoneal cavity. The lack of specificity of where the blood comes from, and the lack of grading of the organ injury are drawbacks. In a series of over 1,000 ultrasound evaluations [15], a negative predictive value of 94.0% was found, with only 1.7% delayed diagnoses, without clinical consequences. False negative FAST is reported [16] in case of concomitant pelvic injury. In these cases, a computed tomography (CT) for evaluation of the abdominal cavity is recommended as a higher number of occult lesions are detected.

Recently, in an animal study, dye-enhanced sonography showed better grading possibilities [17]; however, until now, no clinical experience has been reported.

If there is no ultrasound available a DPL should be considered.

In the unstable patient, further delay for diagnostic purposes should be precluded and the patient should go immediately to the OR for resuscitative laparotomy.

Other sources of bleeding such as thoracic cavity or pelvic bleeding should be evaluated.

CT has become the gold standard and the most important diagnostic tool for hepatic trauma. It gives the possibility of adequate grading of hepatic injuries. If nonoperative treatment is contemplated, CT scanning is mandatory. CT also gives possibilities of evaluating missile tracts through the liver after penetrating trauma [18–21]. In Fig. 7.1, an example is shown of a grade IV injury. In case of an arterial blush (Fig. 7.2), transcatheter arterial embolization should be considered.

Angiography is becoming increasingly popular in the diagnostic armamentarium for liver injury. Most times preceded by CT scanning, an obvious blush (Fig. 7.3a) can be treated with transcathether embolization (Fig. 7.3b) obviating operative therapy. Problems with this approach can be necrosis of substantial parts of the liver, needing secondary operation for necrotectomy.

In persistent or suspected bile leakage, choices in diagnostic modalities can be endoscopic retrograde cholangiopancreatography (ERCP) or magnetic resonance

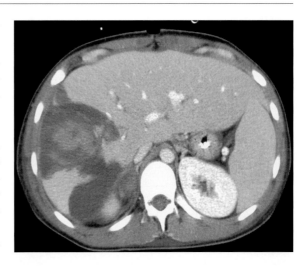

Fig. 7.1 CT scan of a Grade 4 injury

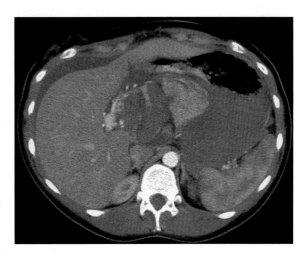

Fig. 7.2 Blush on CT scan after liver injury

cholangiopancreatography (MRCP). The advantage of ERCP is that it can be performed without specific measures for metallic objects and anesthesia teams. However, the manipulation of the bile duct and the instrumentation of the bile system can result in additional damage and/or infection. Nevertheless, an advantage of the method is that the sphincter of Oddi can be manipulated and/or cut, and when a significant lesion is found, a stent can be positioned through the sphincter in order to alleviate the pressure in the bile system. MRCP (Fig. 7.4) is also a very useful method for detecting bile duct injury and can detect even small-size duct lesions [22].

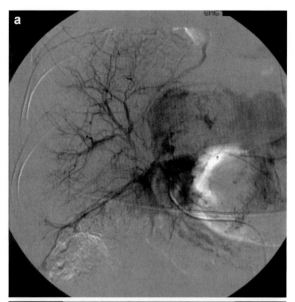

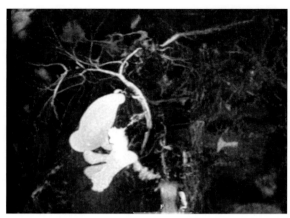

Fig. 7.4 MRCP of the same patient as in Fig. 4a with biliary leakage

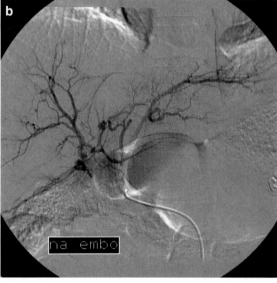

Fig. 7.3 (**a**) Diagnostic angiography diagnosing liver bleeding, (**b**) same patient as in Fig. 3a after transcatheter embolization

7.4 Therapy

Because of today's more sophisticated diagnostic possibilities a more differentiated therapeutic approach is possible. Therapy is guided by the physiological situation of the patient. NOM is indicated in the physiologically normal patient or a patient who can be managed with only limited hemodynamic support. In the unstable patient, immediate laparotomy is indicated and a whole spectrum of therapeutic interventions to damage-control techniques are used in the patient in extremis.

7.4.1 Non Operative Therapy

Currently, NOM is the most used treatment modality in liver injury. This can be augmented with arterial embolization in selected cases. Nonoperative therapy had a bad reputation in the early twentieth century. Invariably all patients with liver injury, in whom nonoperative therapy was tried, died [7]. Currently, those patients who are hemodynamically stable can be considered for NOM. A good insight of the grading of the injury is mandatory. Grading can be obtained with preferably, volume CT scanning. The success rate for NOM is dependent on grade and concomitant injuries and host of factors like Coumadin ® use, but is between 85% and 95% [23–25]. Other reports mention the success rate for NOM as 80% [10].

NOM can be allowed with patients with up to four units of packed red blood cell transfusion [7].

Late problems like hemobilia are likely to occur and should be treated with angio-embolization. Bile leaks can occur and need every now and then ERCP with stenting to lower the pressure in the biliary tree. Major bile collections should be drained [26]. Some authors advise laparoscopic drainage of the abdomen in case of major abdominal collections after NOM of liver injuries.

Major questions remain unanswered: admission time, mobilization schemes, return to full activity, sports activity, and repeat CT scanning are unanswered for still.

7.4.2 Operative Therapy

In case of suspected laparotomy, the personnel of the operation theater should be warned well in advance and should prepare for an emergent laparotomy and possibilities of an autotransfusion. The anesthesia team should continue the resuscitative efforts, however, keeping blood pressure around 100 mmHg until an initial control of the bleeding has taken place. Measures for the prevention of hypothermia should be taken.

7.4.2.1 Draping

The patient with a significant liver injury, who is quite hemodynamically unstable, should have a generous trauma draping from the clavicle to the thigh. In case of a major problem, the thorax should be accessible be it through a sternotomy, or an anterolateral thoracophrenico-laparotomy (Fig. 7.5). Such an approach makes the retrohepatic vena cava, as well as the hepatic veins, accessible. Also, a hepatic exclusion maneuver is possible through such an exposure.

7.4.2.2 Initial Actions

After opening the abdomen all four quadrants should be packed and blood removed from the abdominal cavity. Pressure should be placed on the bleeding liver. By manual compression most bleeding of the liver can be stopped.

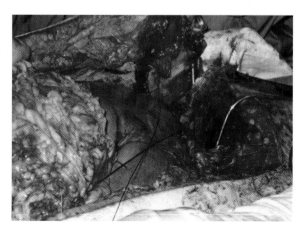

Fig. 7.5 Thoracophrenicolaparotomy for cephalad approach to the vena cava

Let the anesthetist catch up before embarking on further exploration. The lesion should then be evaluated and a plan made for the treatment of the injury. In case of ongoing bleeding from the liver, consider a Pringle maneuver, plugging of lesions, and packing again. Many injuries stop bleeding after initial packing. Allow the anesthetist to regain normal blood pressure. Do not probe deeper lesions in order to prevent renewed bleeding. If bleeding has ceased, the liver can be left alone; however, packing should be considered in case of coagulopathy, hypothermia or extensive damage (see below).

7.4.2.3 Access to the Liver

Operating upon a patient with a liver injury should be done through an incision from the xiphoid to the symphysis. In general, to provide adequate access to the liver in case of severe damage, the coronary ligaments should be taken down. Starting at the right-side, the liver can be exposed and turned left to get access to the right-side of the liver and the veins on that side. The left lobe is easily mobilized by taking down the cranial ligaments attached to the diaphragm. If sufficient access cannot be obtained on the cranial side and the inferior cava and liver veins, a sternotomy can be performed to gain access to the pericardium and the outflow trajectory of the liver. This is also the way to go if a hepatic exclusion is contemplated, e.g., with a cava-atrial shunt.

7.4.2.4 Pringle Maneuver

After the initial description of the inflow control by Pringle [27], it was long forgotten; however, it was re-popularized again in the 1960s of the last century. Brisk arterial bleeding diffusely from the hepatic parenchyma can be diminished by inflow control by cross- clamping of the hepatic ligament. The easiest way is to digitally probe the foramen of Winslow, behind the hepaticduodenal ligament and clamp the ligament from left to right.

Even hepatic artery ligation is possible, however necrosis should be expected. Nowadays, provided good and quick access to the angiosuite transcathether angio-embolization is possible. In the currently developing operating suites with angiographic facilities, transport could be omitted in the first place and this procedure can be performed in the OR after the initial operation.

7.4.2.5 Packing

Feliciano revived the use of perihepatic packing [28], where it rapidly was associated with damage-control procedures. This category of patients with a need for definitive packing goes with a high mortality rate, however was shown in number of reports very successful [29–31]. Indications for definitive packing are coagulopathy, hypothermia, extensive damage, extensive uncontrollable bleeding, expanding subcapsular hematoma, transfer of a borderline stable patient, and retrohepatic venous injury. The technique is to mobilize the liver (see above) when necessary. Put packs subdiaphragmatic, subhepatic, under the ribs, and behind the injured lobe (Fig. 7.6). Try to restore the contours of the liver as much as possible. There is no plastic lining necessary if the packs are removed timely.

No attempt of closure of the fascia should be made. Most times, with an adequate technique, the intrinsic pressure of the packs is enough to overcome the venous pressure. If not, additional measures should be taken,

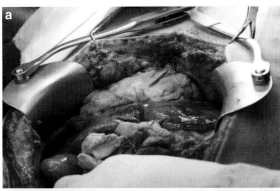
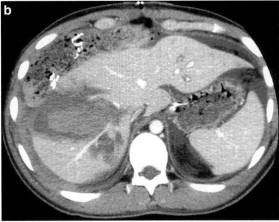

Fig. 7.6 Packing of the liver: (**a**) Intraoperative view, (**b**) postoperative CT (different patient as in Fig. 6a)

as described elsewhere in this chapter. Moreover, as these patients mostly need huge amounts of fluid for resuscitation, the chance of an ensuing abdominal compartment syndrome is very large [32]. Drains are generally not used unless bile leakage is suspected. In those cases, drainage of the common bile duct with a T-drain should be considered.

Removal of the packs should be as early as the correction of coagulopathy, typically 1–2 days after the initial operation.

7.4.2.6 Selective Resection

Generally, resectional therapy of the liver is not advocated [13]. Recently, however, Polanco and co-workers [33] evaluated a series of 56 patients from a series of 216 patients with complex liver injuries who underwent some form of resectional liver surgery. The main mechanism was blunt trauma from which 16 patients had venous injuries. Apart from anatomic resections, nonanatomic, lobectomies and one hepatectomy with immediate liver transplantation was performed with an overall mortality of 17.8%, however with a morbidity of over 60%. They conclude that in selected cases, with the adequate expertise at hand, resectional surgery for complex liver trauma is an option. However, if this expertise is not available, packing and transfer is an adequate option in these devastating cases.

Generally speaking, resectional therapy is indicated for injuries to the left lobe because only limited compression by packing is achieved and in free segments. When returning for pack removal necrotic tissue should be resected. The technique used is most times finger fraction technique and vessel ligation, assisted by other tools like electrocautery, CUSA, argon beam coagulation, and recently good experience has been gained with various glues and local hemostatic agents.

7.4.2.7 Tubes and Catheters

In case of penetrating wounds or deep lacerations with brisk bleeding, preferably venous origin application of Foley catheters can be considered (Fig. 7.7). An alternative is to mount a (finger) part of a surgical glove or a penrose drain over a chest tube, which then is filled with saline or water, which can be used as a tamponade in deep liver lacerations. These can be left in the liver after closure of the abdomen. Most times, if the patient

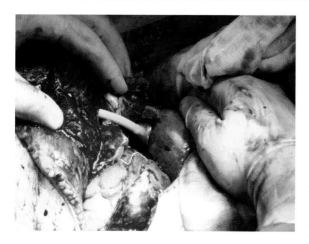

Fig. 7.7 Balloon catheter in penetrating liver injury

returns to the OR after normalizing his physiologic condition, these devices can be removed without any problem. In case of arterial bleeding, this temporary tamponade can be used as a bridge to angiography if deep unreachable injuries have to be managed.

7.4.2.8 Miscellaneous Techniques

Several other tricks during operation of a severe hepatic lesion can be used. A tourniquet can be used to compress the injured lobe for instance with a Penrose drain wrapped around the liver. Also, deep sutures have been used with or without felt pledges; however, this should be used with caution as further damage can be done by rupturing the friable liver tissue further.

7.4.2.9 Arterial Injuries

If after packing there is continued blood loss, most times an arterial injury is probable. The bleeder can be deep in the laceration and sometimes, the lesion has to be extended to expose the bleeding artery to tie or clip it. In case of massive bleeding, the Pringle maneuver can be used in which the liver ligament is clamped, providing inflow occlusion from both the porta hepatis as well as the common hepatic artery.

7.4.2.10 Venous Injuries

Perihepatic venous injuries are very problematic to manage and highly lethal, too. The mention of the atrio-caval shunt is found many times in the literature;

however, the actual use is rather scarce. The results are also disappointing with only a very few survivors [34, 35]. Direct repair without shunt was reported with a somewhat more favorable results [36, 37]. Principles are compression of the liver during resuscitation, early appreciation of venous injuries, portal triad occlusion, and the use of finger fraction techniques. An alternative technique was described by Carrillo et al. [38] in which they temporarily clamped the venous structures with small clamps, packing and temporary closure for return after 24 h and removing the clamps, mostly without major bleeding after removal of the clamps. Alternatively, when brisk venous bleeding emerges from underneath the liver indicating a venous lesion, compressing the liver most times ceases bleeding, giving the opportunity to leave the lesion, pack, and wait 24 h for removing the packs from the abdomen.

7.4.3 Interventional Radiology

As discussed above, when an arterial blush is diagnosed as selective as possible catheterization should be tried for diagnosis, followed by transcathether embolization (Fig. 7.3a and b) [40, 41].

Complications are inherent to the technique as necrosis is the result of obstruction of major arterial vessels. In some instances, necrosectomy has to follow the initial procedure. Some reports mention gall bladder infarction [41, 42].

Indications for an angiography, generally speaking, are blushes on CT. The indication for embolization is enforced when multiple blood transfusions are needed. Some authors advise to have angiography in every considerable damage of the liver and not just for blushes on the CT alone.

7.5 Prognosis

7.5.1 Mortality Rate

Mortality has declined dramatically over the years [7]. Over the last years, it has stabilized to 10–15% in polytraumatized patients [8, 43]. In these patients, late deaths are most times attributed to head injury, sepsis, and multiple organ failure. Early death is, most times, related to persistent hemorrhage at or shortly after surgery [1]. Mortality related to liver injury solely is estimated at approximately 5% and is related to the grade of liver injury [1]. The collateral damage from concomitant injuries is responsible for significantly more deaths than the liver injury itself [1].

Complications with NOM are dependent on the grade of liver injury and range from 0% to 7% [39, 44]. High-grade lesions, however, have a complication rate of up to 13% [45]. Grade of liver injury and transfusion requirements are related to the complication rates.

7.5.2 Infections and Abscesses

Hepatic or intra-abdominal abscesses can be treated with percutaneous, preferably CT-guided approach; however, in selected cases, a surgical approach is needed.

7.5.3 Necrosis

Necrosis of torn hepatic tissue is one of the complications that can lead to secondary surgery and partial resection of necrotic tissue.

7.5.4 Bile Leakage

Biliary leakage occurs in 6% of cases. Richardson [7] advises laparoscopic evacuation of bile in the abdomen. Persistent leakage can be treated with ERCP and stenting of the sphincter of Oddi in order to lower the pressure in the system and achieve preferable flow of the bile in the duodenum instead of the free abdominal cavity (26).

7.5.5 Prognosis Depends on Concomitant Injuries

Prognosis has been improved as mentioned earlier, mostly by the increased use of NOM. Schnüriger and coworkers [1] evaluated 183 patients with high-grade (grade III–V) injuries of the liver, for which in 35 patients, an immediate laparotomy was required for extrahepatic abdominal injuries. Thirty one of these patients died eventually; of which 22 died because of the concomitant injuries. Sixty three patients were managed without surgery and liver-related complications were seen in 11% of cases. Extra hepatic complications were seen in 17% of cases and related to grade IV and V hepatic injuries.

7.5.6 Non-Liver Related Complications

Many of the nonliver-related complications are attributed to concomitant injuries. SIRS, respiratory failure, pulmonary embolism, pneumonia, multiple organ failure, and sepsis are to be expected in patients with extensive injuries; major transfusion requirements and multiple surgeries, however, are related to the severity of the hepatic injury [1].

References

1. Schnüriger B, Inderbitzin D, Schäfer M, Kickuth R, Exadactylos A, Candinas D (2009) Concomitant injuries are an important determinant of outcome of high grade blunt hepatic trauma. British J Surgery 96:104–110
2. Cox EF, Flancbaum L, Dauterive AH et al (1988) Blunt trauma to the liver. Analysis of management and mortality of 323 consecutive patients. Ann Surg 207:126
3. Fisher RP, Miller-Crotchett P, Reed RL II et al (1988) Gastrointestinal disruption: the hazard of non-operative management in adults with blubt abdominal injury. J Trauma 28:1445
4. Lau IV, Horsch JD, Viano DC, Andrzejak DV (1987) Biomechanics of liver injury by steering wheel loading. J Trauma 27(3):225–235
5. McGarvey N, Indeck M (1991) Epidemiology of liver trauma. Trauma Q 7:22
6. Rulli F, Galata G, Maura A, Cadeddu F, Olivi G, Farinon AM (2008) Dynamics of liver trauma: tearing of segments III and IV at the level of the hepatic ligament. Chir Ital 60:659–669
7. Richardson JD (2005) Changes in the management of injuries to the liver and spleen. J Am Coll Surg 200:648–669
8. Hurtuk M, Reed RL, Esposito TJ et al (2006) Trauma surgeons practice what they preach: the NTDB story on solid organ injury management. J Trauma 61:243–254
9. Demetriades D, Karaiskakis M, Toutouzas K, Alo K, Velmahos G, Chan L (2002) Pelvic fractures: epidemiology and predictors of associated abdominal injuries and outcomes. J Am Coll Surg 195:1–10
10. Tinkoff G, Esposito TJ, Reed J, Kilgo P, Fildes J, Pasquale M, Meredith JW (2008) American association for the surgery of

trauma organ injury scale I: Spleen, liver, and kidney, validation based on the national trauma data bank. J Am Coll Surg 207:646–655

11. Vassiliu P, Toutouzas KG, Velmahos GC (2004) A prospective study of post-traumatic biliary and pancreatic fistuli. The role of expectant management. Injury 35:223–227

12. Hollands MJ, Little JM (1991) Post-traumatic bile fistulae. J Trauma 31:117–120

13. Boffard KD (ed) (2003) Manual of definitive surgical care. Arnold, London

14. ATLS manual (2008) 8th edn. ACS Committee on Trauma, Chicago

15. Bakker J, Genders R, Mali W, Leenen L (2005) Sonography as the primary screening method in evaluating blunt abdominal trauma. J Clin Ultrasound 33:155–163

16. Ballard RB, Rozycki GS, Newman PG, Cubillos JE, Salomone JP, Ingram WL, Feliciano DV (1999) An algorithm to reduce the incidence of false-negative FAST* examinations in patients at high risk for occult injury. J Am Coll Surg 189:145–151

17. Tang J, Wang Y, Mei X, An L, Li J, Lin Q (2007) The value of contrast-enhanced gray-scale ultrasound in the diagnosis of hepatic trauma: an animal experiment. J Trauma 62:1468–1472

18. Meredith JW, Trunkey DD (1988) CT scanning in acute abdominal injuries. Surg Clin North Am 68:255–268

19. Federle MP, Jeffrey RB Jr (1983) Hemoperitoneum studied by computed tomography. Radiology 148:187–192

20. Federle MP, Goldberg HI, Kaiser JA et al (1981) Evaluation of abdominal trauma by computed tomography. Radiology 138:637–644

21. Toombs BD, Lester RC, Ben-Menachem Y et al (1981) Computed tomography in blunt trauma. Rad Clin North Am 19:17–35

22. Kelly MD, Armstrong CP, Longstaff A (2008) Characterization of biliary injury from blunt liver trauma by MRCP: case report. J Trauma 64:1363–1365

23. Kemmeter PR, Hoedema RE, Foote JA et al (2001) Concomitant blunt enteric injuries with injuries of the liver and spleen: a dilemma for trauma surgeons. Am Surg 267:221–226

24. Buckman RF, Piano G, Dunham CM et al (1988) Major bowel and diaphragmatic injuries associated with blunt spleen or liver rupture. J Trauma 28:1317–1321

25. Fischer RP, Miller-Crotchet P, Reed RL (1988) The hazards of nonoperative management of adults with blunt abdominal injury. J Trauma 28:1445–1449

26. Ackerman NB, Sillin LF, Suresh K (1985) Consequences of intraperitoneal bile: bile ascites versus bile peritonitis. Am J Surg 149:244–248

27. Pringle JH (1908) Notes on the arrest of hemorrhage due to trauma. Ann Surg 48:546–566

28. Feliciano DV, Mattox KL, Jordan GL Jr (1981) Intra-abdominal packing for control of hepatic hemorrhage: a reappraisal. J Trauma 21:285–290

29. Cue JI, Cryer HG, Miller FB et al (1990) Packing and planned reexploration for hepatic and retroperitoneal hemorrhage critical refinements of a useful technique. J Trauma 30:1007–1014

30. Caruso DM, Battistella FD, Owings JT et al (1999) Perihepatic packing of major liver injuries. Arch Surg 134:958–963

31. Estourgie SH, Werken Chr, Leenen LPH (2002) The efficacy of gauze packing in liver trauma: an evaluation of the management and treatment of liver trauma. Eur J Trauma 28:190–195

32. Morris JA, Eddy VA, Blinman TA et al (1993) The staged celiotomy for trauma: issues in unpacking and reconstruction. Ann Surg 217:576–586

33. Polanco P, Leon S, Pineda J, Puyana JC, Ochoa JB, Alarcon L, Harbrecht BG, Geller D, Peitzman AB (2008) Hepatic resection in the management of complex injury to the liver. J Trauma 65:1264–1270

34. Cogbill TH, Moore EE, Jurkovich GJ et al (1988) Severe hepatic trauma: a multi-institutional experience with liver injuries. J Trauma 28:1433–1438

35. Ciresi KF, Lim RC Jr (1990) Hepatic vein and retrohepatic vena cava injury World. J Surg 14:472–477

36. Evans S, Jackson RJ, Smith SD (1993) Successful repair of major retrohepatic vascular injuries without the use of shunt or sternotomy. J Pediatr Surg 28:317–320

37. Bethea MC (1977) A simplified approach to hepatic vein injuries. Surg Gynecol Obstet 145:78–80

38. Carrillo EH, Spain DA, Miller F et al (1997) Intrahepatic vascular clamping in complex hepatic vein injuries. J Trauma 43:131–133

39. Pachter HL, Spencer FC, Hoffstetter SR (1986) The management of juxtahepatic venous injuries without an atrio-caval shunt: preliminary clinical observations. Surgery 99:569–575

40. Scalfani SJA, Shaftan GW, McAuley J et al (1984) Interventional radiology in the management of hepatic trauma. J Trauma 24:256–262

41. Mohr AM, Lavery RF, Barone A et al (2003) Angiographic embolization for liver injuries: low mortality, high morbidity. J Trauma 55:1077–1082

42. Takayasu K, Moriyama N, Nuramajsu Y et al (1985) Gallbladder infarction after hepatic artery embolization. AJR 144:135–138

43. Asensio JA, Demetriades D, Chahwan S, Gomez H, Hanpeter D, Velmahos G et al (2000) Approach to the management of complex hepatic injuries. J Trauma 48:66–69

44. Velmahos GC, Toutouzas K, Radin R, Chan L, Rhee P, Tillou A et al (2003) High success with nonoperative management of blunt hepatic trauma: the liver is a sturdy organ. Arch Surg 138:475–480

45. Kozar RA, Moore FA, Cothren CC, Moore EE, Sena M, Bulger EM et al (2006) Risk factors for hepatic morbidity following nonoperative management: multicenter study. Arch Surg 141:451–458

Splenic Injuries

Selman Uranues and Abe Fingerhut

8

8.1 Introduction

The spleen is the most commonly injured intra-abdominal organ in blunt trauma, involved in more than 60% of cases. Historically, splenectomy has been the most widely used treatment of splenic injury, since Reigner reported the first splenectomy for blunt trauma in 1892 [10]. The first splenic salvage in trauma using partial splenectomy goes back to 1581. It was Viard, who performed partial resections in two patients for spleens purportedly prolapsed through abdominal wounds [10]. Although splenic preservation had been conceived of so early and even successfully performed, Kocher stated in 1911, "Injuries of the spleen demand excision of the gland; no evil effects follow its removal while the danger of hemorrhage is effectively stopped." This dogma remained unchanged until the first description of overwhelming sepsis in splenectomized children in 1952. The real revolution in surgical handling followed upon the pioneering work of the Brazilian surgeon Marcel Campos Christo and Leon Morgenstern in the early 1960s and 1970s [17]. Christo first reported experimental segmental splenectomy in animals. He then applied these techniques to eight patients with splenic injuries. In 1966, Morgenstern reported subtotal splenectomy in myelofibrosis [8]. These publications on partial splenic conservation in trauma and massive splenomegaly

attracted the attention of not only pediatric but also general surgeons. Mishalany (1974) reported successful splenic salvage utilizing catgut sutures after incorporating a pedicle of omentum over the injury site [7]. It was also the development of new hemostatic techniques and equipment that led to the desired breakthroughs in the 1970s and 1980s. In 1979, Morgenstern outlined the techniques of modern splenic surgery, emphasizing the important points in management [9].

The armamentarium for the management of splenic injuries embraces three major alternatives: nonoperative management (NOM), surgical preservation of the spleen, and splenectomy. The treatment of splenic injury has changed over the past decade from prompt splenectomy in all cases to splenic salvage when possible. Each of these management strategies has a role in the treatment of splenic injury; it is important to know when each of these therapies should be used, and perhaps more importantly, when it should not, with the aim of ensuring the best outcome for the patient. The most important factor influencing this change is the recognition of the risk of infection after splenectomy.

8.2 Reasons for Splenic Preservation

With a high perfusion rate of 10 l/min, the spleen has an important role of filtering erythrocytes, white blood cells, and bacteria. The main immunological task of the spleen is filtering out pathogens and antigens. Clearance is markedly impaired after splenectomy, increasing the infection rate. The incidence of severe infection in the asplenic state ranges from 0.4% to 30% (Table 8.1).

In contrast to the lymph nodes and mucosal-associated lymphoid tissue, there are no afferent lymphatic

S. Uranues (✉)
Department of Surgery, Medical University of Graz,
Graz, Austria
e-mail: selman.uranues@medunigraz.at

A. Fingerhut
Digestive and General Surgery Unit, Centre Hospitalier
Intercommunal, Poissy, France
e-mail: abefinger@aol.com

H.-J. Oestern et al. (eds.), *Head, Thoracic, Abdominal, and Vascular Injuries*,
DOI: 10.1007/978-3-540-88122-3_8, © Springer-Verlag Berlin Heidelberg 2011

Table 8.1 Physiology of the spleen

Physiological functions of the spleen
• 10 l blood flow per hour
• Connected to major vessels
• Has only efferent but no afferent lymphatic vessels
• Plays key role by hematogenic infections

Table 8.2 Important immunologic functions of the spleen

Immunologic functions of the spleen
• Trapping and processing of antigen
• "Homing" of lymphocytes
• Lymphocyte transformation and proliferation
• Antibody and lymphokine production
• Macrophage activation

vessels in the spleen, and it mainly reacts to disseminated blood-borne antigens such as circulating bacteria in septicemia. This is accomplished in two ways, based on the histological structure of the organ: on the one hand, by the white pulp, which, as the central lymphoreticular organ, is the single largest lymphoid organ of the body; and on the other, by the red pulp, which contains numerous cells of macrophage/monocyte lineage, and also a great number of natural killer cells (Table 8.2).

Altered humoral and cellular parameters of the specific and nonspecific immune response characterize asplenic patients, who are prone to frequent infections. There is a significant decrease in IgM and IgG, and an increase in the platelet count. A clear connection has been found between diminished IgG2 and increased lung and bronchial infections. IgG1 and IgG3 impairment seems to be responsible for abdominal infections, frequently associated with increased permeability and translocation of bacteria from the colon. In the postoperative phase, translocated bacteria can be responsible for impaired wound healing and abscesses as well as for lung and urinary tract infections. Fibronectin is decreased in asplenic patients, impairing the phagocytosis of monocytes. The migration rate as well as the phagocytosis of mononuclear cells is reduced to 50% in asplenic patients. Other effects of splenectomy include depressed T-cell functions and decreased opsonization of bacteria.

The deficiency in the clearance of intravascular antigen in asplenic patients is the basis for infectious complications, including overwhelming postsplenectomy infection (OPSI), increased early and late septic morbidity, and increased septic mortality. The most common causative organism is Streptococcus pneumoniae, accounting for at least 50% of OPSI. Other possible agents include Escherichia coli, Haemophilus influenzae, Neisseria meningitidis, and Staphylococcus aureus. OPSI is a life-threatening event that usually develops suddenly in a previously healthy person. Symptoms begin with a sore throat, fever, or malaise and progress quickly to headache, vomiting, and hyperexia; hypotension and septic shock; death can follow within 24–48 h. Disseminated intravascular coagulation has also been associated with OPSI. The risk of developing OPSI is greatest in the first year after splenectomy. Case reports have noted OPSI up to 42 years after splenectomy. The reported lifetime incidence in the adult population varies from 0.34% to 2.6%, with an overall mortality of 0–2.5%.

The best and most effective measure for preventing OPSI is orthotopic conservation of the spleen itself. An orthotopically preserved spleen with its natural vascular supply and an adequate residual parenchymal mass of at least 25% are prerequisites for normal hematologic and immunologic function.

8.3 Accessory Spleen, Splenosis, and Autotransplantation

Accessory spleen is a common splenic anomaly. The accessory spleens, supplied by capillaries, are usually near the splenic hilus, embedded in fatty tissue or the omentum. Splenosis occurs when small particles of the spleen regenerate focally in the abdomen following injury or splenectomy. This regenerative capacity of spleen particles is utilized in autotransplantation of splenic pulpa, whereby the regenerating spleen particles can be demonstrated scintigraphically after autotransplantation. The initial euphoria surrounding autotransplantation as an effective means of preventing immune deficiency after splenectomy, however, soon died down, as neither accessory spleens nor accidentally or incidentally regenerated spleen tissue can provide the immune competence of an orthtopic spleen with its main vessels preserved. There have been reports of OPSI in patients with documented splenosis or accessory spleens as well as in patients with functional, autotransplanted splenic tissue. Hematologically functioning spleen does not equate to retention of immunologic function.

8.4 Diagnostic Procedures

A number of procedures, both invasive and noninvasive, have been proposed as being helpful in making a diagnostic decision. As the course and mechanism of the injury can indicate what kind of damage can be expected, a careful history should precede the diagnostic work-up of every trauma patient.

Physical examination and *laboratory findings* are not reliable diagnostic criteria for splenic injury but they can be indicative of abdominal injury in general.

In Europe, *ultrasonography* (US) is the method of choice for the detection of splenic injury. It is noninvasive, nonstressful, can readily be performed in the emergency room and can be repeated as necessary. With portable equipment, US can be performed simultaneously with ongoing resuscitation without sedation, and it can also be done at the bedside without moving the patient. Experienced operators can achieve a sensitivity of 89%, specificity of 97%, and accuracy of 96% with ultrasound [3].

CT scan is noninvasive and can provide valuable supplemental information about the injured organs. CT examinations of the traumatized patient are usually performed during rapid i.v. infusion of contrast medium. Computed tomography(CT) is independent of the examiner; it permits evaluation of the extent of hemoperitoneum, and the degree of splenic injury and other abdominal injuries (Fig. 8.1). Its overall specifity

is nearly 100%, with sensitivity of 93% and accuracy of 97% [14, 16]. CT has poorer sensitivity and specificity for mesenterial tears and intestinal injuries, and this should be taken into consideration in the nonoperative management of splenic injuries [2]. In some hospitals, CT has the disadvantage of being physically remote from the areas equipped for emergency resuscitation.

Angiography is rarely used to evaluate splenic injury, but it may be of limited value if splenic artery embolization is contemplated [15].

8.5 Grading of Splenic Injuries

In 1989, the internationally recognized classification (Table 8.3) of the Organ Injury Scale (OIS) Committee of the American Association for the Surgery of Trauma (AAST) was published. The classification used by the authors at that time (Table 8.4) is simpler and more

Table 8.3 Organ Injury Scale of the AAST

Splenic injury scale		
Grade		Injury Description
I	Hematoma:	Subcapsular, nonexpanding <10% surface area
	Laceration:	Capsular tear, nonbleeding, <1 cm parenchymal depth
II	Hematoma:	Subcapsular, nonexpanding, 10–50% surface area; intraparenchymal, nonexpanding, <2 cm in diameter
	Laceration:	Capsular tear, active bleeding; 1–3 cm parenchymal depth which does not involve a trabecular vessel
III	Hematoma:	Subcapsular, >50% surface area or expanding; ruptures subcapsular hematoma with active bleeding; intraparenchymal hematoma >2 cm or expanding
	Laceration:	>3 cm parenchymal depth or involving trabecular vessels
IV	Hematoma:	Ruptured intraparenchymal hematoma with active bleeding
	Laceration:	Laceration involving segmental or hilar vessels producing major devascurarization (>25% of spleen)
V	Laceration: Vascular:	Completely shattered spleen Hilar vascular injury which devascularizes spleen

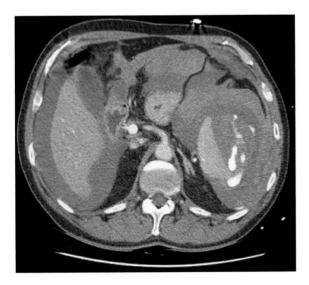

Fig. 8.1 CT-scan showing severe splenic injury with contrast blush

Table 8.4 Splenic injury grading, Medical University of Graz

Classification of splenic rupture		Organ-preserving treatment
Grade O	Subcapsular hematoma	Nonoperative
Grade I	Capsular injury	Tissue sealing, coagulation
Grade II	Superficial injury without involvement of the hilus	Tissue sealing, coagulation, suture
Grade III	Deep parenchymal laceration, partly extending to the hilus with involvement of the segmental arteries and/ or massive fragmentation of a pole	Splenorrhaphy with absorbable mesh, partial stapler resection
Grade IV	Massive fragmentation of the entire organ and/ or total detachment of the hilus	Splenectomy

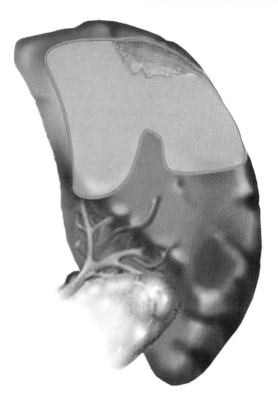

Fig. 8.2 Degree 0 splenic rupture

practical, but in general agreement with the OIS classification. In both systems, splenic injuries are classified on a five-point scale.

Degree 0 (Graz classification)/Grade I injuries (OIS classification) (Fig. 8.2).

These patients usually have stable cardiovascular signs and can be treated nonoperatively. If laparotomy is indicated because of other associated injuries, the spleen can be secured with fibrin glue and/or collagen fleece to prevent secondary bleeding from a ruptured hematoma.

First-degree (Graz classification)/Grade II injuries (OIS classification) (Fig. 8.3).

This degree of injury is characterized by superficial capsular tears, usually with only minimal bleeding; such patients are also good candidates for nonoperative treatment. If laparotomy is indicated because of ongoing bleeding or other associated injuries, the splenic lesions can be treated using adhesives and coagulation.

Second-degree (Graz classification)/Grade III injuries (OIS classification) (Fig. 8.4).

These injuries are usually at right angles to the axis of the spleen and run along the segmental boundaries; the large vessels near the hilus are intact. These transverse injuries bleed only moderately. Lengthwise lacerations that cross the segmental borders may produce more severe bleeding. Frequently there are multiple

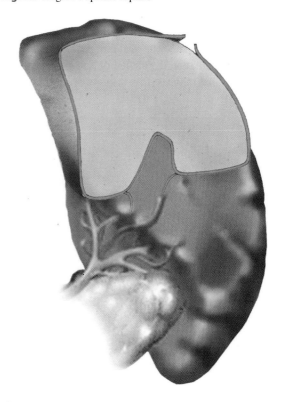

Fig. 8.3 Degree 1 splenic rupture

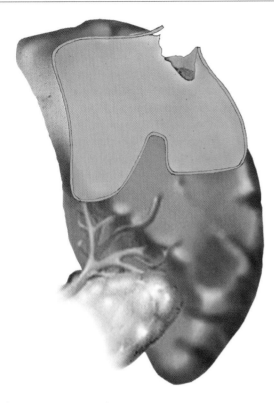

Fig. 8.4 Degree 2 splenic rupture

lacerations. These injuries can be treated very adequately with coagulation and adhesives. Stapler resection of one segment can also be useful if the injuries are limited to one pole.

Third-degree (Graz classification)/Grade IV lesions (OIS classification) (Fig. 8.5).

Injuries of this grade are the most difficult to manage with splenic salvage. They are deep, extending to the hilus on both surfaces and causing severe bleeding. The best course with these injuries is splenorrhaphy to produce compression with an absorbable mesh, which quickly and effectively stops the bleeding. Injuries involving only one pole or one half of the spleen can be treated with partial resection.

Fourth-degree (Graz classification)/Grade V injuries (OIS classification) (Fig. 8.6).

These injuries should be treated by splenectomy. In the rare cases when the upper pole is intact and the upper polar artery branches off early, subtotal resection with preservation of the upper pole would be a possibility for preserving part of the organ. But as these patients usually show severe blood loss, a fast and safe splenectomy is usually the appropriate treatment.

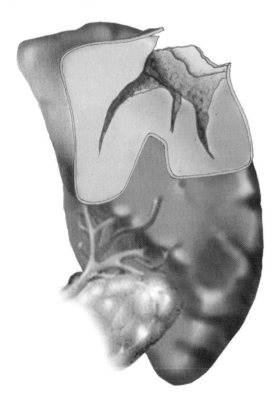

Fig. 8.5 Degree 3 splenic rupture

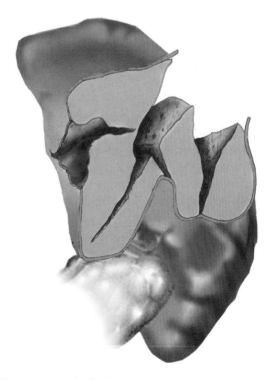

Fig. 8.6 Degree 4 splenic rupture

8.6 Strategies in Splenic Injuries

8.6.1 Nonoperative Management

Nonoperative management has been widely accepted in selected cases of splenic injuries; excellent results have been reported with children. The rate of successful nonoperative treatment of splenic injuries in children is about 95% [1]. Surgeons have been more reluctant to use this technique in adults although nonoperative management of splenic injuries with proper selection of patients is as safe and practicable in adults as in children [5]. With proper selection, non-operative management has a variety of advantages. Patients require fewer units of blood, hospitalization is shorter and the mortality rate is reduced [6]. Organ salvage without surgery is feasible for grades 0 and 1 and in some grade-2 and -3 splenic injuries. In any case, the patient selected for nonoperative treatment must be hemodynamically stable (Table 8.5). Initially unstable patients can also be managed with NOM if they can be quickly stabilized in course of the resuscitation and remain stable. After initial resuscitation, patients with signs of progressive hypovolemia and worsening abdominal symptoms should be treated operatively; the same applies to patients in whom concomitant injury to hollow viscus organs cannot definitely be ruled out. One of the most important selection criteria after hemodynamic stability should the absence of extravasation of contrast medium ("contrast blush") upon CT; this latter counts as a sure sign of active bleeding (Fig. 8.1). Stable patients with contrast blush can profit from a highly selective angioembolisation followed by safe NOM. An altered state of consciousness due to injury, medication, alcohol, or drugs are not absolute contraindications for NOM but these patients are particularly poor candidates and need special attention. The current recommendation is that an immediate operation is indicated when a splenic injury requires more than four units of blood.

The prerequisite for successful nonoperative management is careful clinical and laboratory observation, preferably in the surgical intensive care unit, including strict bed rest for 24–72 h depending on the severity of injury. The patient should be evaluated at least twice a day by the same surgeon, preferably with experience in visceral trauma surgery [11]. Bedside ultrasonography or CT scan should be performed for close monitoring in the first days after the splenic injury. After discharge, follow-up sonography or CT-scan should be scheduled depending on the injury pattern and patient-related conditions [18].

Another factor that influences treatment success is the degree of thrombosis prophylaxis and/or the need of heparin. Even with lower injury grades, high-dose thrombosis prophylaxis, continuous administration of heparin or hemodialysis can compromise the success of NOM.

There is evidence in the literature that careful choice of indication for the administration of heparin is an important factor in successful conservative management [4].

The enthusiasm for the nonsurgical approach can lead to a dangerous mind-set in which most patients, even those who are not particularly good candidates for nonoperative management, are subjected to protracted imaging studies, while a necessary operation is delayed. Delayed bleeding is reported to occur in 0.3–1% of all splenic injuries.

Unsuccessful NOM may more frequently result in splenectomy than does splenorrhaphy. Laparoscopy is perhaps another means for selection of the patients and for exclusion of intestinal damage.

Possible complications and long-term effects that may be produced by NOM are delayed bleeding, probably so-called posttraumatic cysts, and splenosis.

Table 8.5 Criteria for non operative treatment

Criteria for nonoperative management
• Local tenderness – no diffuse abdominal rigidity
• No progressive hypovolemia
• Hemodynamic stability after two to four units of blood
• Rapid correction of hypotension and tachycardia
• Exclusion of associated hollow viscus injuries
• Experienced surgical judgment

8.6.2 Laparoscopy in Splenic Trauma

Minimally invasive surgery has both diagnostic and therapeutic applications in the surgical treatment of injuries to visceral organs. The basic requirement for laparoscopic surgery is that the patient be hemodynamically stable; an unstable patient is not a good candidate for laparoscopic exploration.

Stable patients with splenic injury are worked up in the shock room with ultrasound and a CT scan, then treated conservatively. If there is uncertainty with regard to intestinal injury, laparoscopic exploration is a good supplementary diagnostic measure with treatment potential. During this exploration, splenic injuries that have ceased to bleed can be protected from renewed bleeding with fibrin adhesive and collagen fleece, but the spleen must be handled with eggshell delicacy to prevent further injury and re-bleeding.

Partial resection of one of the two poles of the spleen may be done laparoscopically only in exceptional cases. In these cases, the patient should be placed in a contralateral semilateral position so that there is good view of the spleen in its fossa.

Mesh splenorrhaphy requires complete mobilization of the spleen and in trauma cases it should only be done where there is active bleeding. These patients are usually hemodynamically unstable and should be operated with open rather than laparoscopic technique.

8.6.3 Methods of Splenic Repair

The primary prerequisite for fast, uncomplicated surgery on the spleen is a good view with generous exposure of the surgical field. A midline incision is the standard, since it makes it easier to explore for other organic injuries and attend to them. Another basic prerequisite is complete mobilization. Only a completely mobilized spleen can be rotated onto the abdominal wall, allowing satisfactory exposure and quick and safe salvage of the spleen. To avoid any additional tears, capsular avulsions and stripping, the spleen should be handled with "egg shell" delicacy. Here, it is helpful to insert a gastric tube before or during the operation to decompress the stomach and provide a better view. Blood-saving devices, such as the Cell Saver®, can be used in cases without injury to hollow viscus organs. Using the Cell Saver® should not consume valuable time and so increase blood loss. Patients who require surgery for a splenic injury are generally unstable, or borderline unstable, and need to have their bleeding controlled. Blood and clots so should be evacuated from the abdominal cavity with all due speed; this is best accomplished by hand and with sponges. After a quick survey, the spleen is raised ventromedially with the nondominant hand, so pulling the

peritoneal fold in the dorsal direction. The peritoneum can then be cut with scissors from caudal to cranial to mobilize the spleen. The splenic fossa is then packed with warm towels and the spleen lifted onto the abdominal wall. In this position, the splenic hilus can be compressed with an atraumatic clamp or, better yet, digitally, and the bleeding reduced. Care must be taken that the tail of the pancreas is not injured when the hilar vessels are clamped off. The next step is to sever the short gastric vessels between ligatures or with a modern coagulation device (ultrasound activated or ligature-sealing device). Only then can all injuries and their extent be properly assessed and a decision for the further procedure, splenic preservation or splenectomy, made. In any case, splenic preservation should not take significantly longer than splenectomy. For this reason, the choice of the technique that is most advantageous for the particular degree of injury is of immense importance. The most important methods and those that are most suitable for trauma are described below. When splenic salvage or splenectomy has been completed, drainage of the splenic fossa is useful.

8.6.3.1 Parenchymal Suture (Fig. 8.7)

Because the splenic parenchyma is fragile and the capsule is thin and without tensile strength, care must be taken when suturing not to tear the capsule, extending the laceration. Slowly absorbable monofilic atraumatic sutures are the most suitable for suturing by hand. Of the many hand sutures described to date, mattress sutures, U-sutures, and pledget-armed sutures are most

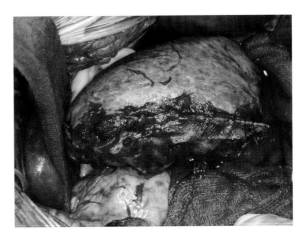

Fig. 8.7 Partial splenectomy in trauma with collagen fleece and hand suture closure of the resection line

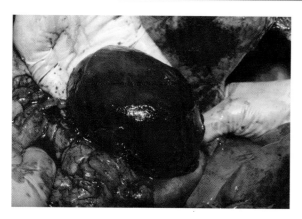

Fig. 8.8 Use of collagen fleece and fibrin sealing in superficial lacerations

commonly used. On the whole, however, hand sutures are complicated and time consuming, and unsuitable for extensive ruptures. The new adhesive and coagulation techniques have increasingly encroached upon the position of the hand suture.

8.6.3.2 Use of Adhesives (Fig. 8.8)

Of the adhesives currently available, fibrin glue is the most suitable for treating splenic lesions. Fibrin sealing is based on the conversion of fibrinogen to fibrin as in the final phase of blood clotting; fibrin promotes clotting, tissue adhesion, and wound healing through interaction with the fibroblasts. Fibrin glue can be applied with a sprayer.

Collagen fleece is also suitable for covering bleeding surfaces. It is composed of heterologous collagen fibrils obtained from devitalized connective tissue and is fully resorbable.

Fibrin sealant (Tisseel[R], Baxter) or a hemostatic matrix (FloSeal[R], Baxter) in combination with a collagen fleece (Lyostypt[R], B.Braun, TissuFleece[R]; Baxter) is used preferentially in the treatment of first- and second-degree splenic ruptures. The bleeding parenchymal surface is covered briefly with a warm laparotomy pad; then, fibrin is applied and the collagen fleece is pressed upon it for about 1 min. Sprayers have proved to be advantageous for the application of the fibrin glue. First, air alone is sprayed before the fibrin is applied. This creates a surface that is free of blood and nearly dry.

A major advantage of these hemostatic agents is that they can be combined with the other techniques described below.

8.6.3.3 Coagulation Techniques

Argon beam coagulation has proved to be most useful in spleen trauma. Coagulation is valuable for controlling the bleeding in first- and second-degree lacerations. In contrast to adhesive procedures, during coagulation the parenchymal surface need not be completely free of blood. It is not suitable for extensive deep injuries with intensive bleeding, because too much valuable time is lost before adequate hemostasis is achieved. The ratio of coagulation necroses to healthy residual parenchyma is also unfavorable in these cases.

The argon beam coagulator is a noncontact monopolar electrocoagulator. It emits argon gas, which blows away blood and clears the injured field of pooled coagula. The device transfers radiofrequency electrical energy through the stream to the tissue, causing coagulation.

8.6.3.4 Partial Resection

A partial resection may be necessary with second-, third-, and fourth-degree ruptures limited to one pole or half of the spleen. The most suitable strategy for both quick and effective hemostasis and parenchymal preservation is resection with a TA-stapler. Prior to stapler application, vessels supplying the segment to be resected should be selectively severed by ligation or coagulation. This creates an immediate demarcation (Fig. 8.9). Then the splenic parenchyma should be compressed digitally adjacent to the injured area (Fig. 8.10). The compression presses the splenic parenchyma in the direction of the injury so that a thin layer of parenchyma and vessels with an intact capsule

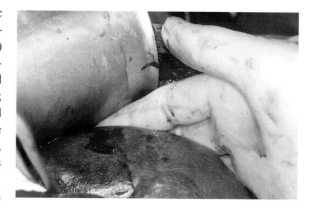

Fig. 8.9 Bluish demarcation line after ligature of the respective vessels

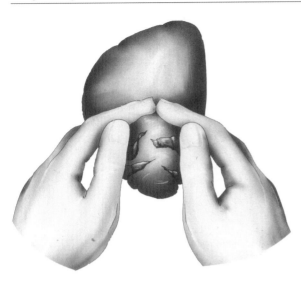

Fig. 8.10 Digital fracture of the splenic tissue at the resection line

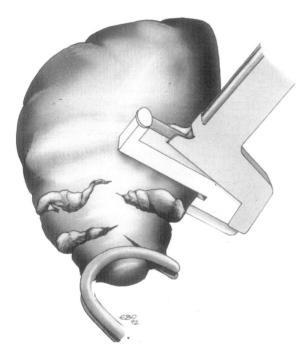

Fig. 8.11 Technique of stapling hemisplenectomy

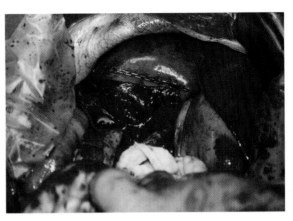

Fig. 8.12 Stapler line after partial resection

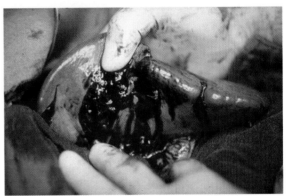

Fig. 8.13 Spleen with deep laceration on both surfaces

8.6.3.5 Mesh Splenorrhaphy

When deep, extensive tears involve both hilar and diaphragmatic surfaces, it is too time-consuming and mostly impossible to attempt to achieve hemostasis with sutures, coagulation, and/or fibrin sealing (Fig. 8.13). The best approach in these cases is splenorrhaphy with an absorbable mesh. The meshes available on the market (Vicryl[R], Ethicon, Johnson & Johnson) are shaped to fit the spleen and come with three purse-string sutures in place, so that the suture that best suits the respective spleen can be used quickly. If no such ready-to-use mesh is available, one may use an appropriately sized piece of absorbable mesh with an absorbable thread that, depending on the size of the spleen, is threaded through the mesh like a purse string (Fig. 8.14). When the mesh is wrapped around the spleen, and the thread is pulled together on the hilar face to produce hemostasis without compromising intraparenchymal circulation. It is extremely important that the

remains between the surgeon's fingers. The stapler can be applied and the resection performed without tearing the capsule (Fig. 8.11). The cut edge can be sealed with fibrin glue and collagen fleece. The advantages of this technique are its simplicity, and the reduction in time and blood loss. The equipment needed is available in most operating theaters (Fig. 8.12).

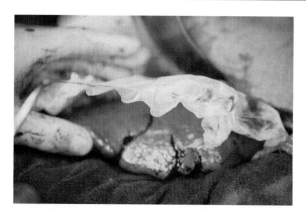

Fig. 8.14 Wrapping of the mesh in third degree injury

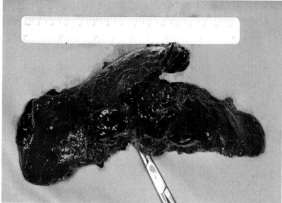

Fig. 8.16 Totally shattered spleen

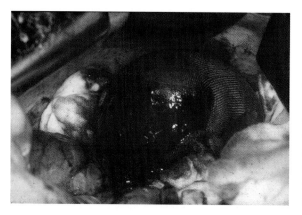

Fig. 8.15 Conization of the spleen after mesh splenorrhaphy with slight oozing of blood through the holes

pouch be slightly smaller than the spleen itself, so that the thread lies on the margin when it has been pulled taut. Because of the tension of the mesh on the hilar aspect, the splenic tissue forms a cone over the hilus. The mesh does not cover the tissue on the visceral surface and so there is a sufficiently large space around the hilus for vessels to enter and emerge. The conization itself compresses the splenic parenchyma on the concave surface, facilitating the desired hemostasis even in deep ruptures of this surface. On the convex diaphragmatic surface, the mesh lies taut over the surface and compresses the ruptured parenchyma. Any slight oozing of blood through the holes in the mesh can be arrested with fibrin glue and collagen fleece (Fig. 8.15).

8.6.4 Splenectomy

Massive fragmentation of the entire spleen and/or separation of the splenic hilus are definite indications for

splenectomy (Fig. 8.16). Severe, concomitant intra- and/or extraabdominal injuries, lack of experience in spleen-preserving surgery, and lack of the necessary equipment are contraindications for organ-conserving surgery with splenic trauma. In these cases, a fast and safe splenectomy should be performed. This is best done via a median laparotomy. The spleen is mobilized and rotated medioventrally onto the abdominal wall. In this position, the hilar vessels can be ligated without injuring the pancreas and other neighboring organs. The short gastric vessels should be carefully ligated and severed. Their stumps should be attached to the serosa on the gastric fundus with a few single button stitches so that overextension of the stomach due to upper abdominal atonia will not cause them to slip, resulting in afterbleeding. It is usually advantageous to drain the splenic fossa for a few days, and administration of antibiotics is helpful. Splenectomized patients should be immunized with pneumococcus vaccine as soon as possible after the operation as long as they are free of infection.

8.7 Sequelae to Splenectomy

Loss of the spleen can have long-term, or even lifelong aftereffects. Patients undergoing splenectomy for any reason are more susceptible to infections. The most dangerous sequel to splenectomy is still OPSI, which can develop many years after surgery as a complete surprise in an apparently healthy individual. Mortality is up to 80%. After splenectomy certain prophylactic measures aimed especially at preventing OPSI should be taken. Most important here is active immunization against pneumococci (Imovax Pneumo R, Institut Merieux, Lyon, France; PneumovaxR-23, Merck Sharp

& Dohme, West Point, PA 19486, USA). These vaccines contain capsular polysaccharides of 23 pneumococcal serotypes responsible for 90% of the most frequently reported organisms (about 90 different serotypes have been identified to date). Active immunization should be administered as soon as possible after splenectomy when the patient is afebrile and in good general condition. Prophylactic antibiotics should be administered for this period if required. Later, boosters with pneumococcal vaccine should be given only when the titer has been determined. Active immunization against meningococcus is not currently advised as a satisfactory type-B vaccine is not available. The meningococcus vaccine currently available (Mencevax[R]) contains groups A, C, W 135, and Y capsule polysaccharides from Neisseria meningitidis. A single subcutaneous injection provides 95% protection for 3–5 years. This vaccination is recommended for asplenic travelers to tropic areas.

A yearly influenza immunization is also recommended. Patients should also be advised that they may be especially susceptible to infections. They should use antibiotics generously and should always have a broad-spectrum antibiotic with them when traveling. At the first sign of an upperespiratory infection, they should take a prophylactic antibiotic.

Children can also be immunized against pneumococcus. In July 2000, the American Academy of Pediatrics (AAP) recommended childhood pneumococcal immunization. The safety of the pneumococcus vaccine for pregnant women has not yet been studied. There is no evidence that the vaccine is harmful to either the mother or the fetus.

Another potential aftereffect of splenectomy may be thrombocytosis, which usually disappears in a short time, but it can become chronic in up to 30%. The thrombocytes probably also undergo changes that predispose to thrombosis and embolism in conjunction with other factors, such as the appearance of atypical erythrocytes, as a result of diminished cellular clearance, loss of equilibrium in the leukocytic system, relative increase of electrophoretically slow proteins, and increase in blood viscosity [12]. This provides an objective basis for Robinette's finding that ischemic heart disease was 5.5% more common in splenectomized World War II veterans than in controls [13].

References

1. Bond SJ, Eichelberger MR, Gotschall CS et al (1996) Nonoperative management of blunt hepatic and splenic injury in children. Ann Surg 3:286–289
2. Elton C, Riaz AA, Young N et al (2005) Accuracy of computed tomography in the detection of blunt bowel and mesenteric injuries. Br J Surg 92:1024–1028
3. Hoffmann R, Nerlich M, Muggia-Sullarn M et al (1992) Blunt abdominal trauma in cases of multiple trauma evaluated by ultrasonography: a prospective analysis of 291 patients. J Trauma 32:452–460
4. Kornprat P, Uranues S, Salehi S et al (2007) Preliminary results of a prospective study of nonoperative treatment of splenic injuries caused by blunt abdominal trauma. European Surg (ACA) 39(1):33–38
5. Mc Connell DB, Trunkey DD (1990) Nonoperative management of abdominal trauma. Surg Clin North Am 70: 677–684
6. Meguid AA, Bair HA, MR HGA et al (2003) Prospective evaluation of criteria for the nonoperative management of blunt splenic trauma. Am Surg 69:238–242
7. Mishalany H (1974) Repair of the ruptured spleen. J Pediatr Surg 9:175–178
8. Morgenstern L (1966) Subtotal splenectomy in myelofibrosis. Surgery 60:336
9. Morgenstern L (1979) Techniques of splenic conservation. Arch Surg 114:449
10. Morgenstern L (1997) A history of splenectomy. In: Hiatt JR, Phillips EH, Morgenstern L (eds) Surgical diseases of the spleen. Springer, Berlin/Heidelberg
11. Myers JG, Dent DL, Stewart RM et al (2000) Blunt splenic injuries: Dedicated trauma surgeons can achieve a high rate of nonoperative success in patients of all ages. J Trauma 48:801–805
12. Pimpl W, Dapunt O, Kaindl H et al (1989) Incidence of septic and thromboembolic-related deaths after splenectomy in adults. Br J Surg 76:517–521
13. Robinette CD, Fraumeni JF (1977) Splenectomy and subsequent mortality in veterans of the 1939–1945 war. Lancet 2:127–129
14. Rodriguez C, Barone JE, Wilbanks TO et al (2002) Isolated free fluid on computed tomographic scan in blunt abdominal trauma: a systematic review of incidence and management. J Trauma 53:79–85
15. Sclafani FJA, Weisberg A, Scalea TM (1991) Blunt splenic injuries: nonsurgical treatment with CT, arteriography and transcatheter arterial embolization of the splenic artery. Radiology 181:189–196
16. Shanmuganathan K, Mirvis SE, Sover ER (1993) Value of contrast-enhanced CT in detecting active hemorrhage in patients with blunt abdominal or pelvic trauma. AJR Am J Roentgenol 16:65–69
17. Uranües S (1995) Introduction and historical survey. In: Uranüs S (ed) Current spleen surgery. Zuckschwerdt München Bern Wien New York
18. Uranues S, Pfeifer J (2001) Nonoperative treatment of blunt splenic injury. World J Surg 25:1405–1407

Pancreas, Duodenum, Small Bowel

9

Ari K. Leppäniemi

9.1 Introduction

Pancreatic and duodenal injuries are not common and their detection can be challenging both preoperatively and during explorative laparotomy. Their protected location in the retroperitoneum can give subtle symptoms and signs in isolated injuries leading to delayed diagnosis and management. Penetrating injuries of the pancreas and duodenum are often associated with major abdominal vascular injuries that require urgent operative intervention. After achieving hemostatic control the detection or exclusion of pancreatic and duodenal injuries require adequate exposure and mobilization of the adjacent organs. The rest of the small bowel, the jejunum, and the ileum, occupy a considerable part of the abdominal cavity and multiple perforations are common after penetrating abdominal trauma. Intraperitoneal perforation of the small bowel is associated with rapid chemical irritation of the peritoneal surface followed by a significant local and systemic inflammatory and septic challenge to the natural defense systems of the body. Although the contamination of the peritoneal cavity by enteric content can occasionally be limited by sealing the perforation with greater omentum or surrounding organs followed by an abscess or fistula, the most common consequence is generalized peritonitis and the associated systemic sepsis.

9.2 Trauma Mechanism and Epidemiology

9.2.1 Small Bowel and Mesentery

The majority of small bowel injuries (the jejunum and ileum) are caused by penetrating injuries (Fig. 9.1) and the frequency of small bowel injury is about 29% after operatively treated penetrating trauma and 7% following blunt trauma, respectively [8]. Blunt injuries of the small bowel are rare but sudden compression of the abdomen caused by vehicle restraints, for example, can create sudden increase of intraluminal pressure in a closed bowel loop resulting in a blow-out perforation of the bowel wall.

Mesenteric injuries are seldom recorded separately. In a study of 72 patients with abdominal gunshot wounds, the mesentery or mesocolon were injured in

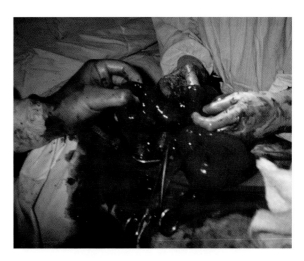

Fig. 9.1 Small bowel perforation caused by an abdominal gunshot wound

A.K. Leppäniemi
Department of Surgery, Meilahti hospital, University of
Helsinki, Haartmaninkatu 4, P.O. Box 340, FIN-00029 HUS
Helsinki, Finland
e-mail: ari.leppaniemi@hus.fi

H.-J. Oestern et al. (eds.), *Head, Thoracic, Abdominal, and Vascular Injuries*,
DOI: 10.1007/978-3-540-88122-3_9, © Springer-Verlag Berlin Heidelberg 2011

12 cases (17%) [17]. In another study of 111 blunt small bowel and mesenteric injuries in 70 patients, there were 22 mesenteric tears, 11 resulting in devascularized bowel [10].

9.2.2 Duodenum and Pancreas

Whereas the mechanism of injury in penetrating duodenal trauma is a direct violation of the duodenal wall by the wounding agent, blunt injury causes duodenal disruption by complex mechanisms. The duodenum, which is retroperitoneal and not very mobile, is fixed at two sites by the common bile duct and the ligament of Treitz, lying against the bony vertebral column. Because of such a configuration and position, disruption of the duodenum by blunt forces can occur by crushing followed by a direct blow to the abdomen, shearing associated with sudden deceleration, or bursting energy associated with sudden abdominal compression [13]. Intramural duodenal hematoma is a rare injury usually following blunt abdominal trauma most commonly presenting with signs of progressive high intestinal obstruction (Fig. 9.2).

The mechanism of injury in penetrating pancreatic trauma is direct violation of the pancreatic gland by the wounding agent. Pancreas is a fixed organ in the retroperitoneum that lies against a rigid vertebral column and is therefore prone to crush injuries following blunt trauma.

In the USA, about 70–80% of duodenal and pancreatic injuries are caused by penetrating trauma, whereas in Europe, blunt trauma is a more common cause of

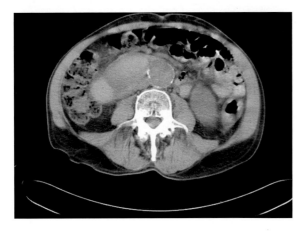

Fig. 9.2 Intramural duodenal hematoma on CT

pancreatic injury [2, 16]. The reported incidences of duodenal and pancreatic trauma in the literature are 3.7–5.0% and 1–2%, respectively [14, 26].

9.3 Diagnostic Procedures

9.3.1 Clinical Evaluation

Hemodynamically unstable patients with the likely source of the bleeding in the abdomen and patients with generalized abdominal tenderness should undergo immediate laparotomy without further diagnostic studies [18]. In stable patients with penetrating anterior abdominal trauma, the aim of the clinical evaluation is to determine whether the peritoneum has been penetrated. Peritoneal penetration is associated with a 60% risk of organ injury requiring surgical repair, whereas establishing an intact peritoneum rules out an intraperitoneal injury in stab wounds and low energy gunshot wounds [18]. There are isolated reports of small bowel injuries caused by penetrating extraperitoneal gunshot wounds thought to be caused either by the immediate extreme blast overpressure with immediate intestinal laceration, or secondarily manifesting in a few days as multiple perforations caused by the intramural hemorrhage, inflammatory cell infiltration, and patchy necrosis [23, 28]. Inspection of the penetrating wounds with assessment of the knife or bullet tract and surgical exploration of the wound under local anesthesia may reveal peritoneal penetration. Diagnostic laparoscopy is useful in assessing peritoneal penetration in equivocal findings after local wound exploration and in detecting occult diaphragmatic injuries, especially on the left side, but its value in evaluating small bowel or pancreatic injuries is limited [19, 20].

Bowel injuries from blunt trauma pose a diagnostic challenge. Whereas intraperitoneal small bowel perforation can lead to a generalized peritonitis within a few hours, blunt duodenal injuries in the retroperitoneal part of the organ may only produce minimal and vague symptoms such as abdominal, back or flank pain. Isolated pancreatic injuries can remain silent at the early stage and manifest later as pancreatic pseudocysts, abscesses or fistulas.

In blunt trauma, the history of abdominal bruising indicative of the use of seatbelt should alert to the possibility of small bowel injury. Diagnostic peritoneal lavage (DPL) with visual and laboratory assessment of the lavage fluid may reveal components of intraperitoneal blood, bile, pancreatic juice or intestinal contents, but its use has greatly diminished in recent years. Serum or urine amylase levels are not reliable in detecting or excluding a pancreatic injury. However, an abnormal serum amylase level warrants further investigations to exclude an injury to the main pancreatic duct.

Findings strongly suggesting gastrointestinal perforation, such as generalized peritonitis on physical examination, bowel content seen in the wound, upper gastrointestinal hemorrhage, or DPL positive for bile or gross intestinal content warrant early explorative laparotomy.

9.3.2 Radiological Investigations

Plain abdominal x-rays can identify extraluminal air in the intra- or retroperitoneal areas indicative of gastrointestinal perforation, as well as assess the level of mechanical intestinal obstruction and follow-up of the resolution (enhanced with oral contrast medium) in patients with suspected intramural duodenal hematomas. Contrast studies with water-soluble contrast medium to reveal upper gastrointestinal perforations are useful when positive, but are not reliable in excluding a perforation. Ultrasound examination is useful in detecting intraperitoneal fluid especially, if performed rapidly in unstable patients with multiple injury sites identifying a major hemoperitoneum requiring early surgical intervention.

Computed tomography (CT) of the abdomen with intraluminal and intravenous contrast has become the mainstay for the evaluation of blunt abdominal trauma. It is sensitive in detecting small amount of intra- or retroperitoneal air, and the presence of free fluid in the abdomen in the absence of solid organ injury may be a sign of blunt small bowel injury [7]. It should be noted that about 13% of patients with perforated small bowel injury after blunt trauma found at surgery have a normal preoperative abdominal CT scan [9]. However, abdominal CT remains the most reliable method to detect subtle retroperitoneal perforations of the duodenum and it can be enhanced with oral contrast medium.

In blunt pancreatic trauma, CT is the primary diagnostic tool even if it sometimes misses a pancreatic injury at the initial stage. Findings suggesting the presence of a pancreatic injury include a peripancreatic hematoma, fluid in the lesser sac or thickening of the left anterior renal fascia, and parenchymal lacerations or transections of the main pancreatic duct may be visible on the CT [26]. Endoscopic retrograde cholangiopancreatography (ERCP) is very useful in identifying injuries to the main pancreatic duct, but it is seldom available in the acute setting. Magnetic resonance cholangiopancreatography (MRCP) can detect pancreatic injuries but its reliability has not yet been established. To characterize delayed manifestations of main pancreatic duct injuries, such as fistulas and pseudocysts, both ERCP and MRCP are very useful.

9.3.3 Grading of Organ Injuries

The American Association for the Surgery of Trauma has published the most commonly used scales for grading individual organ injuries. The injuries are graded from I to V with increasing severity. Although useful in determining the management strategy for pancreatic injuries (Table 9.1), its role in managing small bowel injuries is less important.

Table 9.1 The American Association for the Surgery of Trauma organ injury scale for pancreas

Grade	Injury	Description
I	Hematoma	Minor contusion without duct injury
	Laceration	Superficial laceration without duct injury
II	Hematoma	Major contusion without duct injury or tissue loss
	Laceration	Major laceration without duct injury or tissue loss
III	Laceration	Distal transection or parenchymal injury with duct injury
IV	Laceration	Proximal transection or parenchymal injury involving ampulla
V	Laceration	Massive disruption of pancreatic head

9.4 Therapy

9.4.1 Nonoperative Management

Pancreatic contusions and minor lacerations can be treated nonoperatively provided that no other injuries requiring surgical repair are present, and that an injury to the major pancreatic duct has been excluded [6]. A minor leak or a side-fistula of the pancreatic duct can usually be managed with an endoscopically placed stent.

In the absence of associated injuries requiring surgery, the treatment of an intramural duodenal hematoma is nonoperative consisting of nasogastric suction and parenteral fluid administration. Prolonged obstruction may require parenteral nutrition and even operative treatment if the obstruction persists for more than 2 weeks.

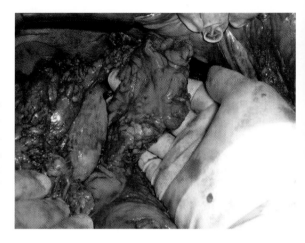

Fig. 9.3 Mobilization of the distal pancreas and spleen

9.4.2 Operative Management

9.4.2.1 Pancreas and Duodenum

Visualization of the entire pancreas requires several maneuvers including transection of the gastrocolic ligament to allow inspection of the anterior surface and inferior border of the gland, and the Kocher maneuver to allow for the exposure of the head and uncinate process of the pancreas. Additional exposure of the superior border of the head and body of the pancreas can be achieved by transection of the gastrohepatic ligament. Finally, lateral mobilization of the spleen and splenic flexure of the colon and the dissection of the retroperitoneal attachments of the inferior border of the pancreas allows the visualization and bimanual palpation of the posterior surface of the tail and body of the gland [1] (Fig. 9.3).

After adequate exposure of the pancreas, the next step is to determine whether the main pancreatic duct is intact. Complete transection of the pancreas that sometimes can be sealed with a hematoma under the pancreatic capsule, central perforation, large vertical laceration, and severe contusion especially in the distal part of the gland are indicative of disruption of the main pancreatic duct. Attempts at verifying the ductal injury with radiological means or injecting dye are often cumbersome and unreliable.

Injuries with intact main pancreatic duct (Grades I and II) found at operative exploration can be managed with simple hemostatic sutures and peripancreatic drainage. Grade III injuries with ductal disruption at or to the left of the superior mesenteric vein are best treated with distal pancreatectomy. Splenic preserving distal pancreatectomy can be performed under favorable conditions. To avoid endocrine insufficiency, distal resections involving more than 80% of the gland should be avoided, except in unstable patients with major associated injuries.

Injuries involving the main pancreatic duct at the head of the gland are challenging injuries, and in most cases, the best option in multiple injured patients is just to ensure adequate peripancreatic drainage with one or more well-placed drains. A recent study indicated that even in damage-control situations packing combined with adequate pancreatic drainage effectively controls both hemorrhage and abdominal contamination in patients with either life-threatening physiological parameters or proximal pancreatic injuries [24].

Under favorable conditions, proximal (Grade IV) injuries can be treated with duodenum-preserving resection of the pancreatic head (avoiding the intrapancreatic portion of the common bile duct), closure of the proximal stump, and draining the distal pancreas into a Roux-en-Y limb of jejunum with a distal pancreaticojejunostomy. The other alternative is to perform a distal pancreatectomy accepting the risk of the development of diabetes.

Any suspicion of a duodenal injury should prompt a thorough exploration and visualization of all four

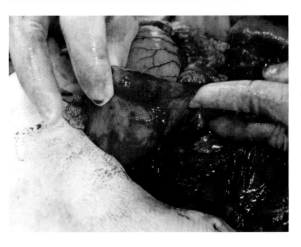

Fig. 9.4 Kocher maneuver to mobilize the duodenum

portions of the organ. A Kocher maneuver is performed by incising the lateral peritoneal attachments of the duodenum, and sweeping both the second and third portions medially using a sharp and blunt dissection (Fig. 9.4). The fourth portion of the duodenum can be visualized by transecting the ligament of Treitz while identifying and preserving the inferior mesenteric vein and rotating the duodenum laterally from left to right. Thereafter, the third portion or transverse portion of the duodenum can most often be adequately visualized anteriorly and digitally palpated posteriorly. In severe injuries of the right side of the transverse duodenum, the exposure can be dramatically improved by mobilizing the right hemicolon and hepatic flexure medially and incising the retroperitoneal attachments of the small bowel from the right lower quadrant upwards enabling the complete reflection of the small bowel out of the abdominal cavity (Cattell and Braasch maneuver) [1].

Small duodenal perforations encountered early after injury heal well after debridement and tension-free transverse closure in two layers. A through- and-through perforation with a narrow duodenal strip in between can be formed in to one defect and closed as a simple laceration. Injuries facing the head of the pancreas can be sutured from inside through the anterolateral defect. In injuries close to the ampulla of Vater, careful placement of the sutures is important to avoid accidental closure of the distal common bile duct. The intact bile duct system can be confirmed by placement of a soft, small-caliber feeding tube through a separate choledochotomy incision in the hepatoduodenal ligament down through the ampulla before duodenal closure.

More extensive lacerations in the first, third, and fourth parts of the duodenum can be treated with segmental duodenal resection and end-to-end anastomosis. In distal duodenal injuries, a Roux-en-Y duodenojejunostomy with or without resection is often the easiest way to restore gastrointestinal continuity.

In patients with large or multiple duodenal perforations associated with extensive loss of duodenal tissue, and in patients seen after more than a few hours after injury with generalized peritonitis, duodenal wall edema and maceration of surrounding tissues, duodenal repair is associated with a high risk of duodenal leak and subsequent mortality and morbidity. A variety of duodenal exclusion procedures have been introduced to protect the duodenal repair. Exclusion of the duodenal repair from gastric secretions allows time for adequate healing. Following duodenal repair, the pyloric exclusion procedure consists of closure of the pyloric ring from inside through a gastrotomy incision at the greater curvature of the antrum with a running polypropylene suture and a gastrojejunostomy placed at the gastrotomy site. In spite of the initial successes following the pyloric exclusion procedure, however, recent evidence based on an analysis of 147 patients with severe duodenal injuries suggested that pyloric exclusion is not superior to simple duodenal repair and might even contribute to longer hospital stays [5].

In devastating duodenal injuries, a more complete exclusion is achieved with a duodenal diverticulization procedure that consists of suture repair of the duodenal injury, antrectomy and gastrojejunostomy, tube duodenostomy, and periduodenal drainage. Truncal vagotomy and biliary drainage are useful additions.

Minor co-existing injuries of duodenum and pancreas can be treated separately with duodenal repair and peripancreatic drainage, respectively. More extensive duodenal injuries combined with minor pancreatic head injuries are best treated with duodenal repair combined with pyloric exclusion and drainage.

Major lacerations in the head of the pancreas with ductal involvement, devascularizing lesions of the duodenum, or duodenal lacerations with destruction of the ampulla and distal common duct may require pancreaticoduodenectomy as a debridement procedure during damage-control surgery [4, 13].

Even a simple duodenal repair should be accompanied with a nasogastroduodenal tube equipped with extra side holes and placed so that it decompresses both the stomach and the duodenum. A more extensive decompression can be achieved with a lateral tube duodenostomy or retrograde tube jejunostomy. Biliary decompression with a T-tube placed in the common bile duct is useful in delayed presentation of duodenal injuries. External drainage of the periduodenal space is useful in all duodenal injuries and can sometimes be used to treat a small duodenal leak. All complex or delayed duodenal injuries are associated with a high risk of duodenal leak warranting the placement of a feeding tube jejunostomy at the primary operation. All pancreatic injuries, even peripheral ones, require adequate placement of peripancreatic drains.

9.4.2.2 Small Bowel and the Mesentery

Lacerations and hematomas in the mesentery should be carefully assessed and large hematomas at the base of the mesentery should be explored to exclude major superior mesenteric vessel injury. The small bowel must be examined loop by loop and the removal of debris from the surface of the bowel with a swab is important in order to detect minor perforations.

Small bleeding vessels in the mesentery can be ligated and the mesenteric defect closed with sutures placed carefully through the peritoneal covering of the mesentery to avoid further injury to mesenteric blood vessels. After completion of the mesenteric closure, the viability of the nearby segment of bowel should be reassessed.

Small isolated bowel perforations can be managed with excision of the wound edges and closure in one or two layers without causing narrowing of the bowel lumen. Wide laceration, multiple closely located perforations or extensive mesenteric injuries with vascular compromise require resection and reconstruction with an end-to-end anastomosis. To avoid a short bowel syndrome after injuries requiring extensive resections, a minimum of 100 cm of small bowel should be preserved including the distal ileum.

9.5 Prognosis

9.5.1 Pancreas and Duodenum

The mortality rate after blunt pancreatic injury is less than 10%, but the morbidity remains high. In a series of 48 patients with blunt major (Grade III-V) pancreatic injuries, the complication rate was significant (62%), especially when treatment was delayed for more than 24 h [21]. The mortality rate following penetrating pancreatic injuries is about 15–20% and most often due to hemorrhage from associated vascular injuries or devastating injuries from close range gunshot wounds [15, 22, 25]. The pancreatic fistula rate following penetrating pancreatic injury is about 10% and seldom contribute to death, whereas postoperative hemorrhagic pancreatitis is associated with a mortality rate as high as 80% [15, 22]. Postoperative pancreatitis, pseudocyst formation, and pancreatic fistulas can in most cases be managed nonoperatively. Advanced endoscopic procedures can be used to stent the pancreatic duct and internally drain a pseudocyst. Dehiscence of a pancreaticojejunal anastomosis after a Roux-en-Y pancreaticojejunostomy is a severe complication requiring early reoperation. In most cases, total removal of the distal pancreas is the only viable option.

The mortality rate after penetrating duodenal trauma is about 15–20%, and in the majority of cases caused by early uncontrollable hemorrhage from associated vascular and hepatic injuries. The duodenum-related mortality rate is 1–2% and associated with duodenal repair dehiscence. The duodenal fistula rate in patients surviving the first 24 h is about 5%, and associated with both duodenorrhaphy and pyloric exclusion or duodenal diverticulization procedures although pyloric exclusion seems to be more often related to spontaneous resolution of the fistula [3, 27].

Worsening general condition, fever and tachycardia, increasing abdominal pain, decreasing urinary output, and increasing respiratory distress a few days after initially good recovery from duodenal repair may point towards suture line or anastomotic dehiscence. Bile-stained secretions from the drains or wound confirm the diagnosis. Positive finding in methylen blue test through the nasogastric tube or an upper gastrointestinal contrast study confirms the diagnosis but the absence of contrast leak or extraluminal air in the abdomen does not exclude anastomotic dehiscence.

A controlled duodenal leak into a drain with good general condition of the patient can be managed expectantly, whereas progressive sepsis and uncontrolled leakage of the duodenal content outside the confined area of drainage require a reoperation, diversion of the duodenal content, luminal decompression and insertion of a feeding jejunostomy, if not placed at the primary operation. The peritoneal cavity should be irrigated with large amounts of warm normal saline to dilute the toxic effects of the intestinal content and prevent formation of retention abscesses.

9.5.2 Small Bowel

The mortality rate associated with small bowel injuries is about 5–7% and in most cases related to associated head, thoracic and vascular injuries [11,12]. Postoperative intra-abdominal abscess and bowel obstruction are encountered in about 6% and 6–10%, respectively, whereas leakage from a small bowel suture line or anastomosis is rare [11, 12].

References

1. Asensio JA, Demetriades D, Berne JD et al (1997) A unified approach to the surgical exposure of pancreatic and duodenal injuries. Am J Surg 174:54–60
2. Asensio JA, Petrone P, Roldan G et al (2002) Pancreatic and duodenal injuries complex and lethal. Scand J Surg 91:81–86
3. Cogbill TH, Moore EE, Feliciano DV et al (1990) Conservative management of duodenal trauma: a multicenter perspective. J Trauma 30:1469–1475
4. Degiannis E, Glapa M, Loukogeorgakis SP et al (2008) management of pancreatic trauma. Injury 39:21–29
5. DuBose JJ, Inaba K, Teizeira PG et al (2008) Pyloric exclusion in the treatment of severe duodenal injuries: results from the National Trauma Data Bank. Am Surg 74:925–929
6. Duchesne JC, Schmieg R, Islam S et al (2008) Selective nonoperative management of low-grade blunt pancreatic injury: are we there yet? J Trauma 65:49–53
7. Ap E, Saxe J, Walusimbi M et al (2008) Diagnosis of blunt intestinal and mesenteric injury in the era of multidetector CT technology – are results better? J Trauma 65:354–359
8. Fabian TC, Croce MA (1996) Abdominal trauma, including indications for celiotomy. In: Feliciano DV, Moore EE, Mattox KL (eds) trauma. Appleton and Lange, Stamford
9. Fakhry S (2007) Blunt small bowel injuries – just as difficult, just as dangerous. Panam J Trauma 14:17–19
10. Frick EJ Jr, Pasquale MD, Cipolle MD (1999) Small-bowel and mesentery injuries in blunt trauma. J Trauma 46: 920–926
11. Guarino J, Hassett JM Jr, Luchette FA (1995) Small bowel injuries: mechanism, patterns and outcome. J Trauma 39:1076–1080
12. Hackam DJ, Ali J, Jastaniah SS (2000) Effects of other intra-abdominal injuries on the diagnosis, management, and outcome of small bowel trauma. J Trauma 49:606–610
13. Ivatury RR, Nassoura ZE, Simon RJ et al (1996) Complex duodenal injuries. Surg Clin North Am 76:797–812
14. Ivatury RR, Malhotra AK, Aboutanos MB et al (2007) Duodenal injuries: a review. Eur J Trauma Emerg Surg 33:231–237
15. Jones RC (1985) Management of pancreatic trauma. Am J Surg 150:698–704
16. Leppäniemi A, Haapiainen R, Kiviluoto T et al (1988) Pancreatic trauma: acute and late manifestations. Br J Surg 75:165–167
17. Leppäniemi A, Cederberg A, Tikka S (1996) Truncal gunshot wounds in Finland, 1985 to 1989. J Trauma 40(suppl 3): 217–222
18. Leppäniemi A, Voutilainen P, Haapiainen R (1999) Indications for early mandatory laparotomy for abdominal stab wounds. Br J Surg 86:76–80
19. Leppäniemi A, Haapiainen R (2003) Diagnostic laparoscopy in abdominal stab wounds – a prospective randomized study. J Trauma 55:636–645
20. Leppäniemi A, Haapiainen R (2003) Occult diaphragmatic injuries caused by stab wounds. J Trauma 55:646–650
21. Lin B-C, Chen R-J, Fang J-F et al (2004) Management of blunt major pancreatic injury. J Trauma 56:774–778
22. Madiba TE, Mokoena TR (1995) Favourable prognosis after surgical drainage of gunshot, stab or blunt trauma of the pancreas. Br J Surg 82:1236–1239
23. Sasaki LS, Mittal VK (1995) Small bowel laceration from a penetrating extraperitoneal gunshot wound: a case report. J Trauma 39:602–604
24. Seamon MJ, Kim PK, Stawicki SP et al (2008) Pancreatic injury in damage control laparotomies: is pancreatic resection safe during the initial laparotomy? Injury. doi:10.1016/j.injury.2008.08.010
25. Sorensen VJ, Obeid FN, Horst HM et al (1986) Penetrating pancreatic injuries, 1978–1983. Am Surg 52:354–358
26. Subramanian A, Feliciano DV (2008) Pancreatic trauma revisited. Eur J Trauma Emerg Surg 34:3–10
27. Timaran CH, Martinez O, Ospina JA (1999) Prognostic factors and management of civilian penetrating duodenal trauma. J Trauma 47:330–335
28. Velitchkov NG, Losanoff JE, Kjossev KT et al (2000) Delayed small bowel injury as a result of penetrating extraperitoneal high-velocity ballistic trauma to the abdomen. J Trauma 48:169–170

Colorectal Injuries

10

Alexander Woltmann and Christian Hierholzer

10.1 Introductory Statements

Colorectal injuries have the highest priority in trauma surgery. If these injuries are missed or treated with delay, consequences may be deleterious. Specifically, patients are endangered by septic complications.

For the therapeutic strategy, the medical infrastructure in which the injury is treated is critical. If the injury is occurring in a war scenario, different levels of qualities are applied than in civil circumstances of injury. With this background the circular letter from the office of the Surgeon´ general No. 178 in world war II must be read that military surgeons once faced court martial if patient did not undergo stoma creation after colon injuries [10].

Improved medical infrastructure has contributed to amelioration of prognosis of these injuries. Mortality of colorectal injuries was calculated as 60% in world war I, was reduced to 37% in world war II, and has currently dropped to 3–22% in civilian life [7].

It is important to distinguish if colorectal injury occurs as monotrauma or in the setting of polytrauma. In monotrauma, treatment is generally possible using a single and definitive procedure. In polytraumatized patients, surgical treatment is performed using a staged approach. For complex injuries, the concept of damage-control surgery has been established. The term damage-control originates from the navy and describes the captain's reaction on a sinking ship. In this situation, the captain pursues a strategy that saves as many lives as possible.

10.2 Anatomy

In principle, the structure of the intestinal wall is identical in every section of the intestine and is composed of: serosa, muscularis propria, submucosa, and mucosa. The intestinal wall of the colon however, is significantly thinner than the wall of the small intestine. Therefore, and due to the fecal intestinal content, primary sutures of the colon are prone to failure and result more often in insufficiencies of anastomosis compared to the small intestine.

Because the colon ascendens and descendens are located retroperitoneally, they usually do not have mesentery. In contrast, the caecum, the colon transversum, and sigma are located intraperitoneally and are covered completely by visceral peritoneum and have mesentery. The rectum is located extraperitoneally. Therefore, injuries occurring to the secondary retro- and extraperitoneal areas may not necessarily cause peritonitis. Injuries of colon segments located intraperitoneally with perforation of the intestinal lumen result in extravasation of feces into the abdominal cavity and will always cause peritonitis.

The secondarily retroperitoneal areas are more protected from injuries due to their localization. Due to its central mesentery and its length, the small intestine is more mobile compared to the large intestine and, therefore, is injured more frequently. Blunt and penetrating trauma affect, in order of frequency, primarily the small intestine followed by the intraperitoneal and lastly the secondary retro- and extraperitoneal areas of colon and rectum [3, 5, 16, 19].

Every surgical procedure must respect arterial perfusion of superior and inferior mesenteric artery and the Riolan's anastomosis. Extended rupture of the mesentery without rupture of the large intestine may

A. Woltmann (✉) and C.Hierholzer
Department of Surgery, Trauma Center Murnau
Prof.-Küntscsher-Str.8, 82418 Murnau, Germany
e-mail: woltmann@bgu-murnau.de

H.-J. Oestern et al. (eds.), *Head, Thoracic, Abdominal, and Vascular Injuries*,
DOI: 10.1007/978-3-540-88122-3_10, © Springer-Verlag Berlin Heidelberg 2011

require segmental resection. If the injury affects an area of end-perfusion, and if ischemia has occurred colon segments have to be resected according to the segmental blood supply. Injuries of the rectum have additional perfusion provided by the internal iliac artery and therefore, are less endangered by ischemia.

10.3 Ethiology

Ethiologically, distinction is made between war and civil victims [3, 18]. In war, incidence of colorectal injuries is higher and therefore, significant experience in surgical treatment of these injuries has accumulated. In civil life, penetrating injuries, which prevail in the US and Africa, result more often in colorectal injuries than blunt trauma.

In penetrating trauma, injuries are caused by bomb explosions, high caliber rounds, improvised explosive devices and other missiles, gunshot, and stab wounds, and impalement (Figs. 10.1 and 10.3). The latter predominately affects the rectum. In Europe, colorectal injuries are predominately caused by blunt trauma including seat belt injuries (Fig. 10.2) or collision with an obstacle.

In contrast to penetrating trauma that often results in open wounds, blunt trauma is predominately associated with contusion or safety belt marks. In addition, rectal injury typically occurs following pelvic trauma (Fig. 10.3). Colorectal injuries are most often associated with head injuries followed by pelvic trauma [15].

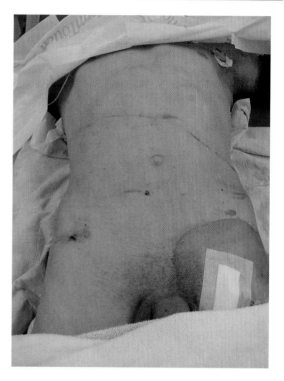

Fig. 10.2 Seat belt mark with perforation of the sigma and small bowel

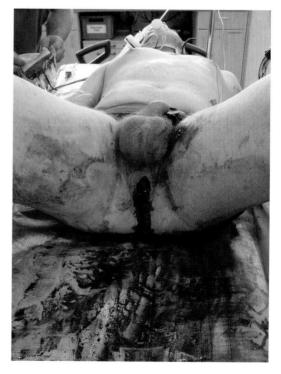

Fig. 10.3 Open rectal injury after motorcycle accident with additional sacrum fracture

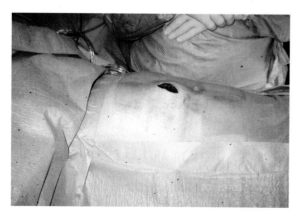

Fig. 10.1 Stab wound with perforation of the right colon

10.4 Diagnostic Work-up

Urgency, extent, and direction of the diagnostic work-up are dependent on the cardio-vascular circulation, respiratory function, and pain symptoms of the patient. In the conscious and awake patient, a thorough physical exam may reveal essential findings that point to colorectal injury. If the patient is unconscious, therapeutic procedure is dependent on findings of an extended diagnostic work-up. This time-consuming approach is feasible only when open wounds that require invasive exploration are not present.

10.5 Past Medical History

Type and intensity of the impaction force may direct attention of the treating physician towards colorectal injury. Blunt anterior hit to the abdomen caused for example by a hoof kick or steering bars, fall from a height, and deceleration injury in motor vehicle accidents with primary onset of back pain (combined spinal and abdominal trauma) are typical mechanisms of injury for colorectal injury. In penetrating injury, the mechanism for colorectal injury is obvious.

All symptoms listed in Table 10.1 require specific attention. In the digital rectal palpation, a prostate dislocation or blood on gloved examination finger may be important findings. Palpation of the spine and the pelvic ring may point to associated injuries, which in turn may be indicative of colorectal injury. Clinical findings have to be correlated with findings from the diagnostic work-up and additional diagnostic studies or acute therapeutic procedures have to be determined.

Table 10.1 Clinical symptoms of colorectal injury

Open wounds
Abrasions
Seat belt marks and contusion
Hematoma of abdominal wall/ecchymosis
Expansion of intraabdominal fluid
Pain symptoms and peritonitis
Rectal bleeding

10.6 Extended Diagnostic Work-up

10.6.1 Ultrasound

Ultrasound studies of the abdomen are basic surgical tools. Vital therapeutic decisions may depend on ultrasound findings. Focus of ultrasound studies is detection of free intra-abdominal fluid with relative volume quantification and not to perform differentiated imaging of organ pathology. Three categories are distinguished: no free fluid present, little quantity, or major quantity present [16].

These diagnostic studies have to be concluded within 2 min. If free abdominal fluid has been excluded, exsanguination into the abdominal cavity is unlikely. However, organ injury is not excluded. Little free fluid is indicative of intra-abdominal injury and additional diagnostic work-up is required to rule out injury to intra-abdominal hollow organs.

If major quantities of free fluid are detected and the patient is hemodynamically unstable immediate laparotomy has to be performed. If little quantity of fluid is detected, sequential evaluation of quantity of free abdominal fluid using ultrasound is indicated. Additional imaging studies such as computed tomography (CT) scan are required to explain the origin of free fluid if conservative therapeutic approach is chosen (e.g., rupture of liver capsule without hemodynamic instability).

10.6.2 Laboratory Work-up

The laboratory testing listed in Table 10.2 is beneficial for diagnosis of colorectal injury. A reduced hematocrit is indicative of bleeding and not hemodilution until the contrary is proved. Laboratory findings revealing increased lactate and negative base excess indicate condition of imminent or manifested shock. If parameters are deteriorating during the phase of diagnostic work-up and treatment, this may be a warning sign to re-evaluate and alter the therapeutic strategy.

10.6.3 Conventional X-Ray

If intra-abdominal bleeding has been ruled out by the diagnostic work-up mentioned above, additional x-ray studies are indicated: plain chest view, plain anterior–posterior

Table 10.2 Laboratory testing with colorectal injuries

Blood group
Blood testing (testing and preparation of six blood units)
Hemoglobin
Hematocrit
Thrombocyte count
Prothrombin time (PT)
Blood gas analysis
Lactate
Base excess
Amylase, Lipase
Urine test

(ap) view, and left lateral radiography of the abdomen. In the ap abdominal view, foreign bodies such as projectiles may be visible and in the left lateral view, free intra-abdominal air may be detected. Other x-ray studies are beneficial in diagnosing associated injuries, which are indicative of colorectal injury.

10.6.4 CT Scan

A conventional CT scan with contrast media is complementing the previous diagnostic work-up, a spiral CT scan of the core body may replace conventional x-ray studies. CT scan is utilized to assess organ lesions in detail, to detect free intra-abdominal air (Fig. 10.4), and

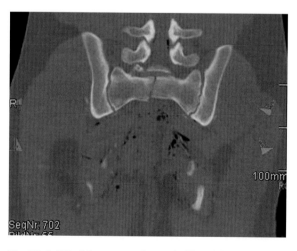

Fig. 10.4 CT of the same patient as in Fig. 10.3. Mention the free air in the retroperitoneal space

to assess the extent of hematoma formation retroperitoneally and in the rectus sheat. In contrast to ultrasound studies, assessment of CT scan images is not impaired by superposition of air caused by skin emphysema. Measurement of density using Haunsfield units enables to differentiate various types of free fluids (e.g., blood, ascites). In addition, perfusion of various organ systems can be assessed. CT studies are performed using plain images and contrast media (enteral and intravenous). Currently, CT scanning can be performed within 5–15 min. Leakage of contrast media out of the intestinal lumen connotes presence of perforation.

10.6.5 Invasive Diagnostics

10.6.5.1 Procto-Rectoscopy

In impalement injuries and in posttraumatic peranal hemorrhage, a procto-rectoscopy is indicated to assess rectal injury and to perform local treatment if necessary.

10.6.5.2 Peritoneal Lavage

Establishment of peritoneal lavage in 1965 [13] was a major improvement in the diagnostic work-up of abdominal trauma. Abdominal injuries that required a laparotomy were detected at an earlier time point. The rate of missed injuries declined. In contrast, the rate of nontherapeutic laparotomy increased. In peritoneal lavage, only the quality of the free fluid can be assessed. Small amounts of blood stain the collected peritoneal fluid red and therefore, the results do not support conclusions relevant for valid decisions for consecutive treatment. Iatrogenic lesions during this procedure are possible. Adhesions impair placement of the catheter. Therefore, this method is not in current practice.

10.6.5.3 Laparoscopy

Spectrum of indication for laparoscopy is similar to peritoneal lavage. This method facilitates differentiation of both type and source of free intra-abdominal fluid. However, organ systems with secondary retroperitoneal localization can only be assessed in part. Precise evaluation of the entire intestine "hand by

Table 10.3 Indication for explorative laparotomy

Major amount of abdominal fluid and hemodynamic instability
Typical associated injuries and cardinal symptoms of abdominal trauma
(example : thoraco-lumbar slice fracture and ecchymosis of abdominal wall)
Posttraumatic peritonitis
Posttraumatic free intraabdominal air
Penetrating injuries

Table 10.4 Classification of the colorectal injury

Serosal tear
Simple perforation
≤25% of wall
>25% of wall
Perforation and bleeding of mesentery

hand" requires time and expertise. Therefore, indication to perform laparoscopy in these cases is rare. [12]. In patients with impaired ventilation or increased intracranial pressure laparoscopy in contraindicated. Good indication for laparoscopy is exploration of abdominal stab wound to assess if the peritoneum has been perforated and if organ injury has occurred. Depending on findings the treatment concept is determined. Basic prerequisite for laparoscopy is hemodynamic stability of the injured patient. In our practice, the optical trocar is inserted paraumbilically using a mini-laparotomy. Exploration is performed with optic assessment, atraumatic grasping forceps, and combined suction-irrigation probe.

In unclear findings, laparotomy is performed. In some cases, stab wounds perforating the colon may be treated by laparoscopic primary suturing.

10.6.5.4 Explorative Laparotomy

Suspected perforating colorectal injury is the major indication for explorative laparotomy specifically if conditions listed in Table 10.3 are present. The surgical technique of laparotomy in trauma patients is described in detail in chapter 12. In our practice, we prefer median laparotomy.

10.7 Classification

Abdominal trauma is classified according to the "Penetrating Abdominal Trauma Index" by Moore et al. 1981 [9] or the "Abdominal Trauma Index" by Borlase et al. 1990 [1]. Individual organ systems are scored based on risk factors for complications such as abscess formation, intestinal fistula, wound infection, pneumonia, or multi-organ failure as well as injury severity and required therapy. Scoring points range from 1 = minimal, 2 = minor, 3 = moderate, 4 = severe, to 5 = maximal.

Calculation of the risk factor of the colon for complications listed above is 4 and therefore, is four times higher than the risk factor of the small intestine. The pancreas with a score of 5 points is the only organ system that is considered more dangerous. Injury severity of the colon is classified as described in Table 10.4.

10.8 Therapy

10.8.1 Conservative

Limited colorectal injury without rupture such as small serosal tears or intramural hematoma may be treated conservatively. Treatment goal is spontaneous healing without complications. Organ entity and function should be preserved. Complications caused by surgery including burst abdomen and incisional hernia are prevented.

Decision for conservative treatment is dependent on surgical experience and may be supported by physical examination, direct inspection, and findings of laparoscopy or laparotomy. However, during conservative treatment, direct local control of the site of injury is impossible and the risk of underestimation of these injuries and late detection of the development of peritonitis is increased.

Additionally, for the treating physician it is more difficult to change the treatment strategy from a conservative to an operative approach compared to primary decision for operative treatment.

10.9 Operative Therapy

10.9.1 Patient Consent

The alert and awake patient is informed that treatment goal of laparoscopy/laparotomy is a detailed assessment of organ injuries. If organ injuries are diagnosed that require surgery, surgical treatment is continued as a single-step procedure. It is important to mention that second-look procedures and application of colostomy may be required. The standard complications of abdominal surgery are explained including insufficiency of anastomosis, incisional hernia, etc. In an unalert or unconscious patient, medical decision is based on the assumed will of the patient.

10.9.2 Patient Preparation for Surgery

It is not necessary to respect the fasting period. In patients with penetrating injuries the status of tetanus vaccination has to be evaluated or refreshed, accordingly. Bacterial cultures and photo documentation are recommended. Antibiotic medication using third-generation cephalosporin and Metronidazol or combination of Ampicillin/Sulbactam is recommended for 5 days if the laparotomy is therapeutic. A gastric tube is inserted and 6 units of erythrocyte concentrates are prepared. In case of emergency, transfusion of group 0 Rh-negative blood can be done if there is no time for specific blood testing. A urinary catheter is administered preoperatively or a suprapubic urinary catheter intraoperatively under direct visual and digital control. Coverage of the patient using warm blankets or warm touch air flow blankets prevents hypothermia.

Procedures to treat colorectal injury require instruments such as the abdominal tray, vascular tray, and abdominal wall retractors. General anesthesia and relaxation of the patient are required. The patient is positioned into the lithotomy position with the left arm adjacent to the body. The operating surgeon is standing on the right, two assistants on the left side of the patient. If necessary, one assistant can be positioned between the legs of the patient.

10.9.3 Priorities

In explorative laparotomy, control of hemorrhage is the highest priority. In hemodynamically unstable patients, control of hemorrhage is critical to establish hemodynamic stability. Consecutively, assessment of injuries can be performed. Bacterial decontamination is the second priority. Injuries of abdominal cavity organs are temporarily occluded for preparation of segmental resection or definitively using excision of wound margins and direct suturing.

The general rule for the treatment of injured intestinal segments is to resect as much as needed and as little as possible. Typically, mobilization of the injured intestinal section is recommended for good overview, detailed assessment, and tension-free anastomosis.

10.9.4 Principles

The strategy of damage-control surgery is applied to all conditions listed in Table 10.5. The goal of surgical treatment includes control of hemorrhage, decontamination, and temporary closure of the abdomen. In summary, secure control of active bleeding as rapidly as possible is the highest priority. Injuries of cavernous organs are resected. The intestinal ends are closed without reconstruction of intestinal continuity and without application of colostomy. The abdominal wall is closed temporarily and provisorily. The goal of treatment is to stabilize general condition of the patient prior to performing definitive surgery for the injury, such as reconstructing the intestinal passage in a second look or with additional staged operations [14].

Serosal tears and small stab wounds are occluded by primary suture (Fig. 10.5a and b). In traumatic perforation

Table 10.5 Indication for damage control surgery in colorectal injuries

Polytraumatization with injuries of multiple body areas that require primary
treatment
Imminent or manifested hemorrhagic or septic shock
Hypothermia
Impairment of coagulation

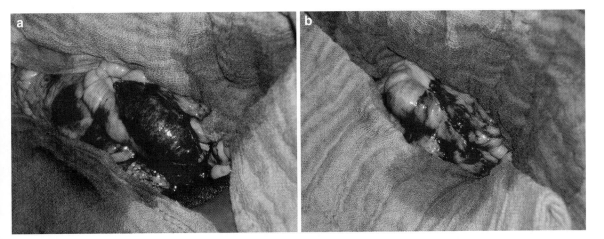

Fig. 10.5 (**a**) Major serosal tear of the right colon after blunt trauma (**b**) Primary suture of the serosa lesion

of the colon, adjacent areas of the intestinal wall are also affected due to the thinness of the colon wall. Therefore, simple excision and direct suturing of the defect is too risky and jeopardizes wound healing. It is safer to resect the injured colon segment with a safety margin in the healthy tissue (Fig. 10.6). This technique requires adequate mobilization. Mobilization of the right flexura for the right hemicolon and mobilization of the left flexura for the left hemicolon are necessary (Fig. 10.6).

Prior to performing anastomosis, orthograde intestinal wash-out is performed intraoperatively. Wash-out requires appendectomy following insertion of a large volume catheter into the appendix basis. The entire colon is mobilized and the afferent limb is completely cleansed using warm Ringer solution at the site of resection. Wash-out solution is collected via a large volume catheter, which is securely attached and sealed to the oral resection stump (Fig. 10.7a–c). The efferent limb is also cleansed either by orthograde wash-out toward or by retrograde wash-out from the anus. Following cleansing of the intestinal section, tension-free and well-perfused anastomosis of the large intestine is performed. Adequate suturing technique includes running single layer stitches and a monophil 4–0 suture, or alternatively, a circulary stapler that is inserted rectally (Fig. 10.8).

If cardio-circulatory condition deteriorates or becomes critical intraoperatively, it is advisable to blindly occlude the intestinal ends following resection and to reconstruct intestinal continuity in a second-look operation. If this concept imposes too much risk on the patient the colon should be diverted by administration of a colostomy (Fig. 10.9).

This Hartmann procedure is indicated only for injuries of the left hemicolon. Otherwise, the blindly occluded anal limb is too long. This Hartmann condition can be resolved after 6 months and reconstruction of intestinal continuity is achieved.

As a general rule, ano-rectal injuries do not require resection. The injuries are sutured or drained from either the abdominal or transanal route. In these situations, administration of a protective loop ileostoma or transverse loop colostomy is recommended (Fig. 10.10). The colostomy for diversion of the intestinal passage is preferentially administered at the terminal ileum or sigma. It is important that the protective stoma completely blocks the intestinal passage into the efferent limb.

The ileostoma has the advantage that relocation is associated with fewer complications compared to relocation of a colostomy. The complication rate varies from 5% to 30% [11]. As a general rule, relocation of a protective stoma is performed with an interval of at least 6 weeks because inflammatory adhesion of the operation site may render the procedure more difficult and may cause complications.

If surgical treatment was delayed and peritonitis has already developed, eradication of infection is performed in a single surgery. In diffuse peritonitis (Fig. 10.11) and septic shock, open treatment of the abdomen and temporary closure of the abdominal wall is indicated following decontamination and closure of the perforation. Preferentially, vacuum sealing is utilized for temporary closure (Fig. 10.12) and consists of abdominal pads with attached perforated foil placed with the foil side onto the greater omentum and covered with

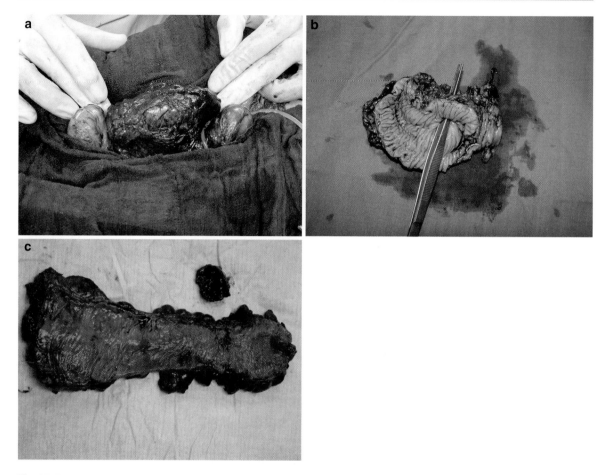

Fig. 10.6 (**a**) Rupture of the colon sigmoideum after blunt trauma (**b**) Iatrogenic left colon injury after splenectomy (**c**) Iatrogenic double perforation of the rectum after puncture of the urinary bladder in order to insert a cystofix catheter

vacuum-sealing foil. The negative vacuum suction should not exceed 20 cm H$_2$O [17]. Staged irrigation procedures of the abdominal cavity are necessary every 24–48 h until definitive closure of the abdomen. If direct closure of the abdomen following successful termination of staged irrigation is impossible, abdominal closure may be achieved secondarily by mesh graft that is transplanted onto the greater omentum or a vicryl net, which is placed between the fascia (Fig. 10.13).

10.9.5 Complications and Results from Literature

Mortality following colorectal injury is dependent on injury severity, associated injuries, time point of surgical therapy, and medical infrastructure available for the patient. Similar criteria apply for the morbidity of infection that currently is calculated at 25–35%. Additional complications listed in Table 10.6 may occur. The concept of open treatment of the abdomen, successful control of hemorrhage, staged eradication of infection, and stabilization of circulation followed by secondary abdominal closure offers a good basis for the successful healing of colorectal injuries.

The surgical strategy for the treatment of colorectal injuries remains controversial [6]. American trauma surgeons did not favor primary reconstructive treatment of blunt colon injuries and primary suturing was suggested only for small stab wounds in 1998 [4]. In perforating injuries, the complication rate for insufficiency of anastomosis is calculated at approximately 2% following direct suturing and approximately 6% following

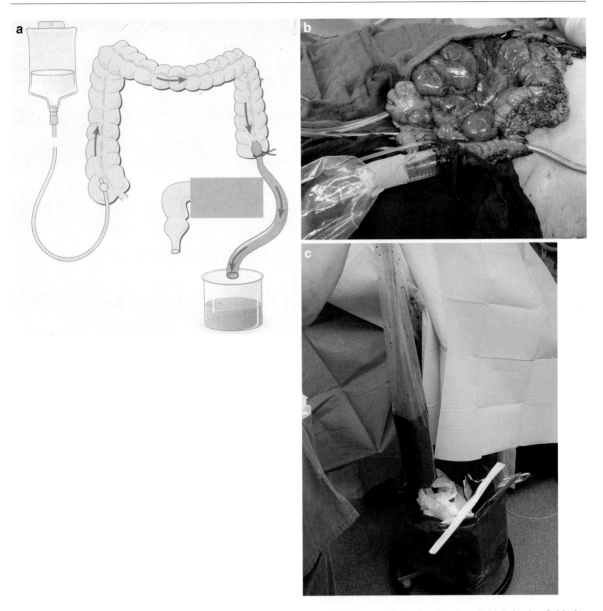

Fig. 10.7 (**a**) Cartoon of the intraoperative colon "wash-out" principle (**b**) Intraoperative colon "wash-out" (**c**) Irrigation fluid after colon "wash-out"

resection and anastomosis [15]. Preferentially, direct suturing should be performed using a transverse and not a longitudinal suturing technique. Alternatively to the therapeutic concept of diversion colostomy, primary resection and anastomosis is possible for the treatment of blunt colon injuries. In addition to primary reconstruction of the intestinal passage, we favor administration of a protective stoma to support and ensure healing of intestinal anastomosis.

The necessity and benefit of diversion colostomy remains unclear. Woo et al. [19] reported that rate of intra-abdominal abscess formation was 12% following administration of colostomy compared to 5% following resection and anastomosis. Significant differences between the groups were found for posttraumatic respiratory complications with 28% in the colostomy group compared to 7% in the anastomosis group. However, these results reflect the severity of injury

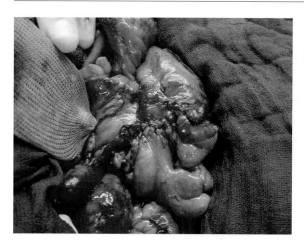

Fig. 10.8 Primary anastomosis after segmental resection of the sigma

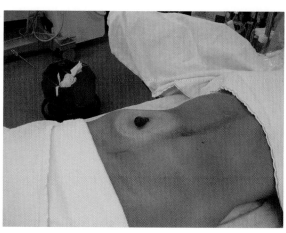

Fig. 10.10 Protective ileostoma after resection and anastomosis of the sigma

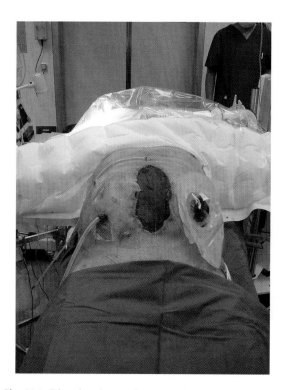

Fig. 10.9 Diversion sigma colostomy and temporary closure of the abdomen by vacuum dressing because of diffuse peritonitis after perforation of the colon

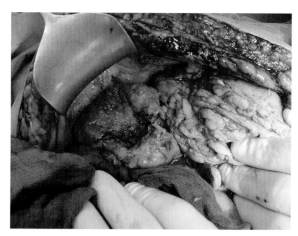

Fig. 10.11 Perforation of the right colon, delayed laparotomy and diffuse peritonitis

more than the quality of surgical treatment. Patients treated with colostomy demonstrated an increased ISS score, rate of shock, and transfusion of blood units compared to patients of the anastomosis group.

In conclusion, it is not possible to provide evidence-based recommendations for treatment modalities in these patients. Definitive treatment with primary resection and

reconstruction of the intestinal passage may be performed if the general condition of the patient and medical infrastructure allow this single-step approach. According to Schumpelick [15], favorable conditions for primary definitive treatment of colon injuries without administration of a colostomy are summarized in Table 10.7.

In 2001, Demetriades [2] demonstrated in a prospective study that the surgical method of colon management after resection for penetrating trauma does not affect the incidence of abdominal complications. In contrast, severe fecal contamination, transfusion of ≥4 units of blood within the first 24 h, and single-agent antibiotic prophylaxis are independent risk factors for abdominal complications [2]. In these cases, damage-control surgery is recommended followed by delayed anastomosis administered in a subsequent

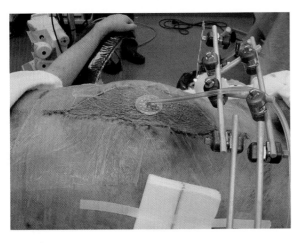

Fig. 10.12 Temporary abdominal closure with vacuum dressing

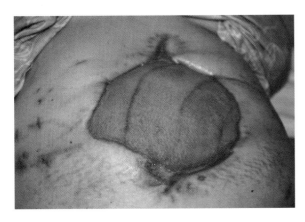

Fig. 10.13 Laparostoma closed with mesh graft

Table 10.6 Complications following colorectal injuries

Abdominal compartment syndrome
Peritonitis
Insufficiency of anastomosis
Abscess formation
Rupture of abdominal wall
Retraction of muscle fascia
Hernia
Ileus caused by adhesions

operation [8]. This concept demonstrated similar results compared to the group undergoing immediate anastomosis after destructive colon injury with respect to anastomotic leakage.

Table 10.7 Favorable conditions for primary definitive repair of colorectal injuries without colostomy

Limited extension of perforation with clean edges
Absence of contusion/hematoma
Vitality of injured intestinal segment
Hemodynamic stability
Blood loss under 20%
Associated injuries of less than two organ systems
Operation within 6 h following trauma
Age less than 60 years
ASA < 3

References

1. Borlase BC, Moore EE, Moore FA (1990) The abdominal trauma index – a critical reassessment and validation. J Trauma 30:1340–1344
2. Demetriades D, Murray JA, Chan L et al (2001) Penetrating colon injuries requiring resection: Diversion or primary anastomosis? An AAST prospective multicenter study. J Trauma 50:765–775
3. Duncan JE, Corwin CH, Sweeney WB (2008) Management of colorectal injuries during operation Iraqi freedom: patterns of stoma usage. J Trauma 64:1043–1047
4. Eshraghi N, Mullins RJ, Mayberry JC et al (1998) Surveyed opinion of American trauma surgeons in management of colon injuries. J Trauma 44:93–98
5. Exadaktylos A, Stettbacher A, Edu S et al (2003) Erfolgreiches selektives Management abdomineller Stichverletzungen durch klinische Evaluation. Unfallchirurg 3:215–219
6. Gonzalez RP, Merlotti GJ, Holevar MR (1996) Colostomy in penetrating colon injury: is it necessary? J Trauma 41:271–275
7. Jurkovich GJ, Carrico CJ (1991) Trauma: management of acute injuries: colon and rectum. In: Sabsiton DC (ed) Textbook of surgery, 14th edn. W.B. Saunders, Philadelphia/London/Toronto, pp 271–272
8. Miller PR, Chang MC, Hoth JJ et al (2007) Colonic resection in the setting of damage control laparotomy: is delayed anastomosis safe. Am Surg 76:605–610
9. Moore EE, Dunn EL, Moore JB, Thompson JS (1981) Penetrating abdominal trauma index. J Trauma 21:439–445
10. Office of the Surgeon General (1943) Circular Letter No.178, October 23
11. Riesener KP, Lehnen W, Hofer M (1997) Morbidity of ileostomy and colostomy closure: impact of surgical technique and perioperative treatment. World J Surg 21:103–106
12. Röthlin M, Trentz O (1997) Stellenwert der diagnostischen Laparoskopie beim Abdominaltrauma. Unfallchirurg 100:595–600
13. Root HD, Hauser CW, McKinley CR (1965) Diagnostic peritoneal lavage. Surgery 57:633

14. Rotondo MF, Zonies DH (1997) The damage control sequence and underlying logic. Surg Clin North Am 77:761–777
15. Schumpelick V, Ambacher T, Riesener KP (1999) Aktuelle Therapie der Verletzungen von Colon und Retroperitoneum. Chirurg 70:1269–1277
16. Vidmar D, Pleskovic A, Tonin M (2003) Diagnosis of bowel injuries from blunt abdominal trauma. Eur J Trauma 29:220–227
17. Woltmann A, Trentz O (2004) Abdominalverletzungen. Trauma Berfuskrankh 6:73–83
18. Welling DR, Hutton JE, Place RJ et al (2008) Diversion defended – military colon trauma. J Trauma 64:1119–1122
19. Woo K, Wilson MT, Killeen K et al (2007) Adapting to the changing paradigm of management of colon injuries. Am J Surg 194:746–750

Abdominal Compartment Syndrome, Abdominal Decompression, and Temporary Abdominal Closure

Christoph Meier

11.1 Intra-Abdominal Hypertension and Abdominal Compartment Syndrome

11.1.1 Introduction

Normal intra-abdominal pressure (IAP) varies with the respiratory cycle. In a healthy individual, mean IAP is 6.5 mmHg with a range from slightly sub-atmospheric to 16 mmHg. It is slightly increased in mechanically ventilated patients due to pressure transmission of pleural pressures across the diaphragm into the abdominal cavity.

Some of the deleterious effects of intra-abdominal hypertension (IAH) on human physiology were described in the second-half of the nineteenth century, but it has lasted a very long time for IAH and the abdominal compartment syndrome (ACS) to be recognized to their full extent. With the widespread applied concept of damage-control surgery and supranormal fluid resuscitation for severely injured patients, IAH and ACS have been encountered in increasing numbers. Today, ACS may be seen as a consequence of successful treatment of patients who formerly died due to profound hemorrhagic or septic shock.

In 2004, the World Society on Abdominal Compartment Syndrome (WSACS) was founded and 2 years later, consensus definitions and recommendations were published. These definitions provide substantial clarification in the diagnostic criteria of IAH

and ACS and should uniformly be used in clinical practice and research as well.

11.1.2 Definitions

In 2004, an international ACS Consensus Definitions Conference was organized by the WSACS. The herein-explained definitions are based on the results of this conference [9, 16]. All definitions, algorithms, and recommendations can be found on the society's webpage (www.wsacs.org).

The abdomen is considered a closed box with rigid and flexible walls. IAP increases with inspiration and decreases with expiration. It is affected by the state of its contents and the compliance of the abdominal wall. The normal IAP is approximately 5–7 mmHg in critically ill adult patients.

Analogous to the well-accepted concept of cerebral perfusion pressure, abdominal perfusion pressure (APP) is calculated as mean arterial pressure minus IAP (APP = MAP–IAP). As APP considers both arterial inflow (MAP) and restriction to venous outflow (IAP), it has evolved as a superior resuscitation endpoint compared to other endpoints such as urinary output, arterial lactate, arterial pH or base deficit. A target APP of ≥60 mmHg has been demonstrated to correlate with improved survival from IAH and ACS [9].

IAH is defined by a sustained or repeated pathological elevation in IAP ≥12 mmHg (Table 11.1). *Acute IAH* develops over a period of hours and is primarily seen in surgical patients after trauma or intra-abdominal hemorrhage. *Subacute IAH* is more often encountered in medical patients. It results from a combination of predisposing conditions (risk factors) and causal factors. Usually, it develops over a period of days. *Chronic IAH*

C. Meier
Division of Trauma Surgery, Department of Surgery
Zürich General Hospital Waid, Tièchestrasse 99, 8037 Zürich, Switzerland
e-mail: christoph.meier@waid.zuerich.ch

H.-J. Oestern et al. (eds.), *Head, Thoracic, Abdominal, and Vascular Injuries*,
DOI: 10.1007/978-3-540-88122-3_11, © Springer-Verlag Berlin Heidelberg 2011

Table 11.1 IAH Grading (from [16])

Grade I	IAP 12–15 mmHg
Grade II	IAP 16–20 mmHg
Grade III	IAP 21–25 mmHg
Grade IV	IAP>25 mmHg

Table 11.2 Classification of ACS (from [16])

Primary ACS	Primary ACS is characterized by acute or subacute IAH of relatively brief duration associated with injury or disease in the abdomino-pelvic region that frequently requires early surgical or interventional radiological intervention (e.g., abdominal trauma, ruptured abdominal aortic aneurysm, peritonitis, pelvic trauma).
Secondary ACS	Secondary ACS refers to conditions that do not originate from the abdominopelvic region. It is characterized by the presence of subacute or chronic IAH that develops as a result of conditions requiring massive fluid resuscitation (e.g., sepsis, capillary leak, major burns).
Recurrent ACS	Recurrent ACS refers to the condition in which ACS redevelops following previous surgical or medical treatment of primary of secondary ACS.

is encountered in morbid obesity, pregnancy, intra-abdominal tumors, ascites, and other conditions. Developing over a longer time period, the abdominal wall progressively distends in response to increasing IAP allowing time for the body to adapt physiologically. Chronic IAH may place the patient at risk for developing either acute or subacute IAH when critically ill.

The ACS is defined as a sustained IAP>20 mmHg (with or without an abdominal perfusion pressure (APP)<60 mmHg) which is associated with a new organ dysfunction or failure. In contrast to IAH, ACS is not graded, but rather considered as an "all or nothing" phenomenon. ACS can be classified as either primary, secondary, or recurrent, according to the duration and cause of the patient's IAH (Table 11.2).

11.1.3 Pathophysiological Effects of IAH and ACS

The effects of IAH include not only the abdomen and its contents but also the patient's hemodynamics, the central nervous system, pulmonary function, and other organ systems. In this respect, the ACS should be considered a systemic disease or complication rather than just a local problem of the abdomen. In the following, the effects of IAH on different organ systems are discussed in more detail.

11.1.3.1 Cardiovascular System

Cardiovascular dysfunction and failure are commonly seen in patients with critical IAH. Preload, cardiac contractility, and afterload are affected. Blood flow through the inferior caval vein back to the heart is compromised in IAH due to elevated intra-thoracic pressure. Furthermore, the inferior caval vein may be mechanically narrowed as it passes through the diaphragmatic crura by a cephalad deviation of the diaphragm. Reduced preload immediately results in a reduced cardiac stroke volume and subsequently in a reduced output. Elevated IAP also causes venous blood pooling in the pelvis and lower extremities. Increased hydrostatic venous pressure promotes edema in this regions and the formation of deep venous thrombosis.

Compression of the lung parenchyma increases pulmonary artery pressure, resulting in a reduction of left ventricular preload and increased right ventricular afterload. In response to worsening right ventricular afterload, the right ventricle may dilate with a decrease of the ejection fraction and an increased myocardial oxygen demand. This may lead to myocardial ischemia and further reduction of right heart contractility and function.

Elevated intra-thoracic pressure and IAP also increase systemic vascular resistance. More commonly, an increase of systemic vascular resistance is observed as compensation for reduced venous blood return and decreased cardiac output in the situation of intravascular volume depletion. Thus, mean arterial pressure remains stable in the early stages of IAH.

11.1.3.2 Respiratory System

Increased IAP displaces the diaphragm in a cephalad direction causing a reduction of intrathoracic volume. As a consequence, loss of lung volume with atelectasis formation, decrease of functional residual capacity, ventilation perfusion mismatch, and a rise of the intrathoracic pressure are observed. A decrease of lung and chest wall compliance results in hypoxia, hypercapnia, and the need for mechanical ventilation. High-peak inspiratory pressures are needed during mechanical ventilation to maintain adequate lung function. Worsening hypercapnia, deteriorating respiratory system compliance, and excessively increased airway pressures have been recognized as critical indicators of pulmonary failure in the situation of critical IAH which may warrant surgical decompression of the abdomen. Although surgical decompression results in immediate reversal of respiratory failure, the lung may also be damaged by systemic release of proinflammatory cytokines with neutrophil accumulation in the lung due to intestinal and hepatic tissue hypoxia. Lung damage in association with ACS may be seen as either caused by direct effects of IAH or as organ dysfunction due to a second hit at a later stage in full blown ACS.

11.1.3.3 Renal Implications

IAH and ACS have been recognized as a predisposing cause of renal failure. Decreased renal function has been observed to be one of the earliest signs of impending ACS. A impaired cardiac output causes a decrease of renal blood flow. Furthermore, this leads to a drop in renal perfusion pressure and subsequently also a decreased glomerular filtration rate and urinary output. In milder cases, glomerular filtration rate is preserved by compensatory responses such as increased renin release and increased angiotensin I/II levels. Angiotension II induces preferential constriction of efferent arterioles which maintains intraglomerular pressure and therefore, glomerular filtration rate as well. However, in critical IAH, these compensatory mechanisms are overwhelmed resulting in acute renal failure. Normalizing cardiac output by restoration of the intravascular volume has shown to improve urinary output but fails to fully correct the renal derangements in the presence of IAH. Besides cardiac output, direct compression of the renal parenchyma and the renal veins by elevated IAH is considered a possible contributing factor of renal pathophysiology.

11.1.3.4 Gastrointestinal Effects

From experimental research we know that mesenteric and gastro-intestinal mucosal blood flow decrease with increasing IAP. Noteworthy, a similar effect has been shown for hepatic arterial blood flow despite maintained

cardiac output. In line with these observations, measurements of gastric tissue pH demonstrated acidotic levels in patients with elevated IAP indicating mucosal ischemia. Microvascular oxygen saturation in the gastric mucosa may be decreased despite unchanged system oxygenation. Data from laparoscopy studies show a decrease of hepatic microcirculation even when IAP is only moderately elevated. Recently, the effects of IAH on the splanchnic circulation have been identified as a potential trigger (second hit) for the development of multiple organ failure MOF). In the experimental setting, oxygen-free radical production and bacterial translocation from the gut lumen into the mesenteric lymph nodes, liver, and spleen is associated with increased IAP indicating ischemia-reperfusion injury. In animal models, IAH causes liver necrosis and mucosal damage in the bowel and it may also have an adverse effect on colonic anastomosis healing.

11.1.3.5 Central Nervous System

The rise of intra-cranial pressure (ICP) in patients with IAH is thought to be caused by an obstruction to the cerebral venous drainage. Patients with head trauma are more susceptible to high IAP levels than patients without head trauma. It has been speculated that in the presence of elevated ICP, the effect of IAH may induce a more profound and hazardous increase in the ICP due to a different starting ICP with a reduced compensatory capacity. Thus, careful and repeated assessment of IAP is essential in patients with head trauma and elevated ICP.

11.1.3.6 ACS and Multiple Organ Failure

Recent experimental and clinical studies have convincingly demonstrated an association of the ACS with MOF. With the introduction of damage-control surgery, more severely injured patients have been salvaged by abbreviating life-saving surgery including hemorrhage and infection control together with decompression of compartment syndromes and temporary fracture fixation. However, despite the undisputable advantage and success of this concept, a new set of morbid complications have been recognized in this patient group with ACS being one of the most devastating. To date, it is still unclear whether ACS is a cause of MOF or merely an end result.

Clinical studies have shown that patients with subsequent ACS after damage-control surgery develop MOF more frequently than patients without ACS but otherwise show identical indices such as demographics, injury severity score, initial vital signs on admission or 24 h fluid resuscitation [20]. Incidence of MOF was significantly higher in the presence of ACS than in patients who did not develop ACS (32% vs. 8%). Overall mortality of the patients with ACS was 43% compared to 12% in patients without ACS. Even more impressive is the fact that mortality of patients with ACS and subsequent MOF reached 85%.

Despite immediate improvement or even normalization of organ function upon surgical decompression is seen in patients with ACS, a considerable part of these patients develop MOF in the later course and die. This clinical observation is supported by several animal studies which showed that critical IAH provoked the release of pro-inflammatory cytokines which may trigger the induction of MOF (two-hit model) [22]. There is evidence from these experiments that ACS may serve as a second hit promoting the path to fatal MOF.

Thus, the avoidance of critical IAH seems to be the much more promising approach to lower mortality of ACS than therapeutic decompression of apparent ACS. In this respect, early identification of high-risk patients for the development of IAH, not only pressure- but also functional monitoring of this patient group, and a new fluid resuscitation regimen that avoids massive gut edema are in the focus of current ACS research.

11.1.4 Intra-Abdominal Pressure Measurement Techniques

In critically ill patients at risk for IAH, accurate IAP measurement is needed to evaluate its role in the development of organ dysfunction. It has been clearly demonstrated that clinical examination of the abdomen is unreliable to assess IAP. Direct IAP measurement techniques have been evaluated in both animal and human studies but are not commonly used in the daily routine. Indirect IAP measurement via the bladder (intra-vesical pressure [IVP]) is the most popular technique in clinical practice. Intermittent IVP measurement is the current gold standard for indirect IAP measurement as proposed by the WSACS. The manometer technique (Fig. 11.1) is a good and cheap alternative without the need for any

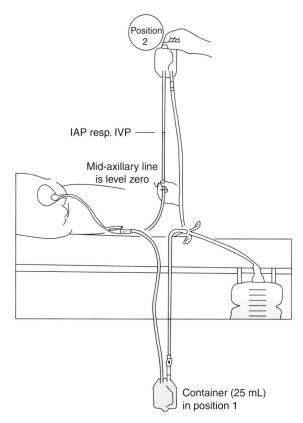

Fig. 11.1 Manometer technique: The container fills with urine during drainage (position 1). When lifted to position 2 urine flows back into the bladder. The scaled manometer tube is zeroed by using the mid-axillary line and IAP resp. IVP can be read from the level of the meniscus

additional electronic equipment. Another technique which allows free urinary drainage and continuous IVP measurement by using a standard 18-Fr three-way urinary catheter in which continuous normal saline perfusion (4 mL/h) is maintained via the irrigation port represents an interesting alternative [3]. An important advantage of all continuous IAP measurement techniques is the possibility of simultaneous monitoring of abdominal perfusion pressure. However, this method has not yet been sufficiently evaluated and thus, its widespread use cannot be recommended at this time.

Transgastric IAP measurement is another option. Evaluation of different variations of this technique has demonstrated good agreement with IAP. However, it is not frequently used in clinical practice, but remains an alternative when IVP measurement is not feasible. The use of a balloon-tipped catheter allows measurement in a continuous or semicontinuous fashion which is an advantage over current IVP measurement techniques.

One of the problems associated with this technique is a possible interference with gastric contents and nutrition and the influence of intestinal peristalsis.

Other techniques such as uterine or rectal pressure measurement have no clinical relevance. Inferior vena cava pressure measurement shows a very good agreement with IAP. Continuous pressure monitoring is possible but this technique is not commonly used in the clinical setting due to possible catheter-related complications (e.g., infections, septic shock, thrombosis).

11.1.4.1 Indirect Intra-Vesical Pressure Measurement Via the Bladder

For reliable and reproducible IVP measurement readings the following points are essential. To avoid any confusion, IAP should always be expressed in mmHg. The measurement should be performed in correct supine position at end expiration. The mid-axillary line serves as the zero level. Before IVP measurement, the bladder must be completely emptied and then instilled with 25 mL of saline (bladder priming). The measurement should be performed 30–60 s after the volume instillation to allow bladder detrusor muscle relaxation. IVP measurement may produce erroneous elevation of intrabladder pressure in the presence of pelvic fractures with hematomas or pelvic packing. Furthermore, IVP readings may not be reliable in patients with bladder trauma or neurological bladder disorders.

Figure 11.2 shows "the revised closed system repeated measurement technique" as proposed by Malbrain [14]. A ramp with three stopcocks is inserted in the drainage tubing connected to an ordinary Foley catheter. A sterile 1,000 mL bag with normal saline is attached to the first stopcock. A syringe is connected to the second stopcock allowing precise fluid instillation (25 mL) from the infusion bag into the bladder for priming prior to IVP measurement after the system has been flushed and the bladder has completely been drained. Once the bladder is primed, the third stopcock which connects the bladder with the pressure transducer is opened for pressure reading after proper zeroing. Unlike other techniques, this closed system minimizes the risk of urinary tract infections. It is easy to use and requires less nursing time than other techniques. This technique is recommended to be used for up to 3 weeks for screening and monitoring. Its main disadvantage is that it interferes with urine output without the possibility of obtaining a continuous trend.

11.1.4.2 Indirect IAP Measurement Via the Stomach

The IAP can also be measured with a nasogastric tube. This route is preferred when IVP measurement is considered inappropriate. It has the advantage that it does not interfere with urinary output and there is no risk of infection. Different modifications of gastric pressure

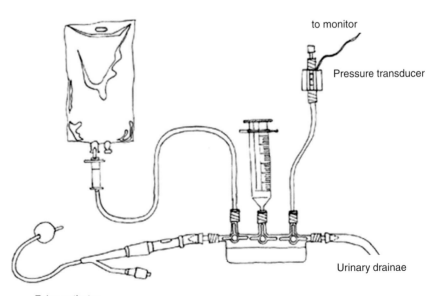

Fig. 11.2 The revised closed system repeated measurement technique allows repeated indirect IAP measurements for a time period up to 3 weeks

measuring have been described in the literature [14]. The revised semicontinuous technique uses an esophageal balloon catheter which is inserted into the stomach. The catheter is connected to a pressure transducer and a glass syringe which is used to fill 1–2 mL air into the balloon for calibration. Unlike other methods, this is a dry system which is not flushed with normal saline in order to avoid air-fluid interactions. The disadvantage of this method is air resorption in the balloon after a couple of hours. Thus, frequent recalibration of the system is necessary.

The continuous fully-automated technique [14] uses a special IAP-catheter with an air pouch at its tip. This device comes with a pressure transducer, electronic hardware, and a device for automatic filling of the air-pouch which are all integrated in the IAP-monitor. The system recalibrates itself automatically and it provides continuous monitoring of IAP together with abdominal perfusion pressure. Like other fluid-free systems, it does not need a conductive fluid column for pressure transmission. Thus, it is free from interference caused by wrong transducer positions.

11.1.5 Identification of Risk Patients and Prevalence of IAH and ACS

One of the most important factors for successful management of IAH and ACS is the identification of patients at risk to develop critical IAH. In most cases, IAH is a complication of ICU patients either surgical or medical. Table 11.3 displays a list with 34 risk factors associated with IAH and ACS as issued by the WSACS. The most common risk factor is a history of massive fluid resuscitation, mainly with crystalloids. This risk factor alone encompasses a large number of ICU patients and highlights the importance of always considering the possibility of IAH development in critically ill patients with a subsequent proactive approach to IAP measurement. In this respect, baseline measurement of IAP is advised when two or more risk factors are present.

In a recent prospective multicenter study, prevalence of IAH in a mixed ICU population accounted for over 50% and ACS was diagnosed in 8% [15]. Burns, major elective or emergency abdominal surgery, and major trauma are frequently associated with critical IAH. In a group of major torso trauma patients,

Table 11.3 Risk factors for IAH/ACS (Adapted from [16])

Related to diminished abdominal wall compliance

- Mechanical ventilation, especially fighting with the ventilator and the use of accessory muscles
- Use of positive end expiratory pressure (PEEP) or the presence of auto-PEEP
- Basal pleuropneumonia
- High body mass index (> 30)
- Pneumoperitoneum
- Abdominal surgery, especially with tight abdominal closure
- Pneumatic anti-shock garments
- Prone and other body positioning
- Abdominal wall bleeding or rectus sheath hematoma
- Correction of large hernias, gastroschisis or omphalocele
- Burns with abdominal eschars

Related to increased intra-abdominal contents

- Gastroparesis/Gastric distension/Ileus
- Volvulus
- Colonic pseudo-obstruction (Ogilvie's syndrome)
- Retroperitoneal or abdominal wall hematoma
- Enteral feeding
- Intra- or retroperitoneal tumor
- Damage control laparotomy

Related to abdominal collections of fluid, air or blood

- Liver dysfunction with ascites
- Abdominal infection (e.g., pancreatitis, peritonitis, abscess)
- Haemoperitoneum
- Pneumoperitoneum
- Laparoscopy with excessive inflation pressure
- Major trauma
- Peritoneal dialysis

Related to capillary leak and fluid resuscitation

- Acidosis (pH < 7.2)
- Hypothermia (core temperature < 33°C)
- Coagulopathy (platelets < 55,000/mm³ or activated partial thromboplastin time (APTT) more than two times normal or higher or prothrombin time (PTT) < 50% or international standardized ratio (INR) > 1.5)
- Polytransfusion (>10U of packed red cells/24 h)
- Sepsis (as defined by the American-European Consensus Conference definitions)
- Bacteremia
- Septic shock
- Massive fluid resuscitation (>5 L of colloid or A > 10 L of crystalloid/24 h with capillary leak and positive fluid balance)
- Major burns

IAP > 25 mmHg in combination with organ dysfunction was found in 14% [2]. In another case series, ACS, defined according to the ACS definition, developed in 36% of the patients who had to undergo postinjury damage-control laparotomy [20].

11.1.6 Prevention of ACS

The prevention of ACS may be much more successful than its treatment to lower ACS-related MOF and ACS. Despite adequate surgical decompression and rapid improvement of hemodynamic, pulmonary, and renal indices, development of fatal MOF may have already been triggered. One of the major challenges is the reduction of the incidence of MOF. Critical IAH should be detected and treated before it provides a second insult to the patient's inflammatory response culminating in an MOF with fatal outcome. However, this second insult may happen before ACS is clinically evident. Thus, new functional monitoring strategies such as microdialysis of the abdominal rectus muscle or near-infrared spectroscopy of the abdominal wall are under evaluation [17, 25]. The common goal of this research is the identification of those patients at high-risk to develop critical IAH and treat them early enough to prevent the development of MOF before ACS is clinically evident.

Shock, no matter of the origin, and subsequent reperfusion of ischemic tissue due to successful resuscitation causes increased endothelic permeability (capillary leak). In addition, the dilution of solute and protein in the intravascular space promotes the shift of water into the interstitium causing edema. In this respect, the more severe the shock state and the more aggressive the fluid resuscitation are, the more likely is the appearance of critical IAH . In the opinion of most experts in the field, many cases of ACS are complications of overaggressive supranormal crystalloid fluid resuscitation to achieve elevated oxygen delivery indices [1]. Supranormal crystalloid resuscitation improves not only cardiac preload and output, it also decreases oncotic pressure and increases hydrostatic pressure in the capillary vascular bed. When administered in patients with hemorrhagic shock and postischemic reperfusion injury with capillary leak, this resuscitation regimen may result in a massive bowel edema with subsequent IAP increase and further organ dysfunction. Massive fluid resuscitation saves patients' lives but causes problematic edema in the brain, lungs, and the intestine. Thus, definition of better resuscitation endpoints and the development of new fluid resuscitation regimen may help to lower the incidence of ACS. In this respect, hypertonic saline has evolved as an interesting resuscitative adjunct. It requires much less volume than isotonic crystalloids while mesenteric blood flow is increased and acute lung injury is decreased compared to lactated Ringer's. Furthermore, recent research has demonstrated that hypertonic saline may prevent gut injury by inducing local protective anti-inflammation [1].

In addition to optimizing fluid resuscitation, rapid hemorrhage control, correction of coagulopathy, and prevention of hypothermia are crucial cornerstones in the prevention of ACS by reducing the severity and duration of the hemorrhagic shock state. As a consequence, volume requirement is also decreased.

Besides better patient surveillance, evolving new monitoring techniques, and changing resuscitation strategies, prophylactic abdominal decompression and TAC are established measures to prevent the development of ACS in high-risk patients. Indication and technique are described in detail in 11.2 (blue).

11.1.7 IAP Monitoring

Prevalence and incidence of IAH in an intensive care unit (ICU) population is considerably high, although routine IAP monitoring is neither reasonable nor justified for all patients admitted to an ICU. The WSACS recommends a baseline IAP measurement if the patient has at least two risk factors for IAH (Table 11.3) in combination with one of the following criteria: (1) new ICU admission or (2) new organ dysfunction. In patients with elevated IAP and in patients with evolving organ dysfunction, intermittent IAP measurement should be performed at least every 4–6 h. If IAP is within normal range at baseline measurement, repeated IAP measurements are not necessary, but IAP should be rechecked in the situation of clinical deterioration. For patients with IAH, appropriate therapeutic measures should be initialized. IAP monitoring may be stopped when the risk factors for IAH have resolved or the patient does not show any signs of organ dysfunction with IAP levels within normal limits (<12 mmHg) for 24–48 h. However, in the situation of sequential closure of a left-open abdomen after decompressive laparotomy, regular IAP measurements are recommended until the abdomen is completely closed without relevant IAP elevation.

11.1.8 Management of IAH and ACS

The WSACS has developed a very useful algorithm for the clinical management of IAH and ACS (Fig. 11.3).

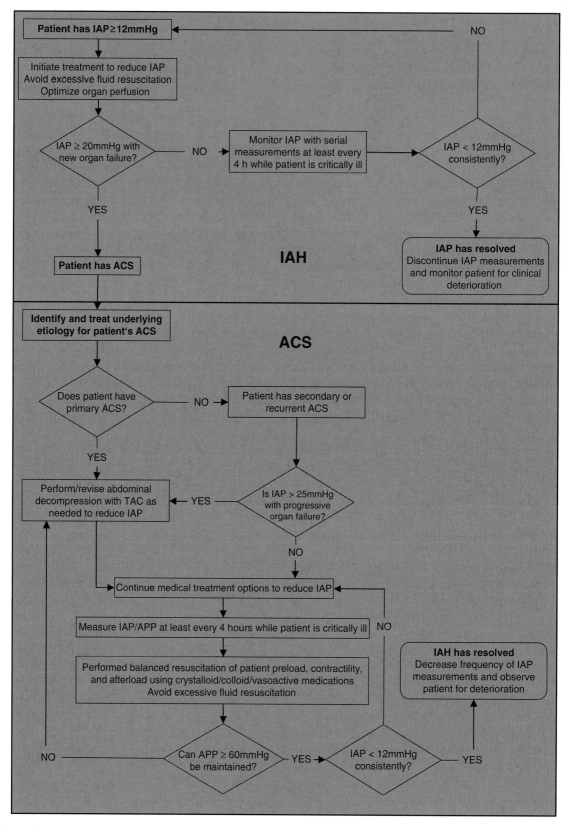

Fig. 11.3 Algorithm for the clinical management of IAH and ACS adapted from WSACS

In the following, different treatment modalities are discussed in more detail.

11.1.8.1 Medical Treatment

Maintaining adequate tissue perfusion and oxygenation are the cornerstones of any successful treatment strategy in the ICU, regardless of the specific situation. As IAH represents a specific situation, the resuscitation target values may have to be adjusted in this patient group. In the situation of IAH, conventional hemodynamic parameters such as central venous pressure and pulmonary artery occlusion pressure do often overestimate the hemodynamic status. Reliance on such pressure-based measurements may mislead therapeutic management due to falsely high estimation of the patient's preload status. Pulse contour analysis and volumetric assessment via transpulmonary thermodilation is a more appropriate monitoring technique to assess the cardiovascular status in these patients.

There is a clear association between the administration of large amounts of fluids and the development of IAH. However, aggressive fluid administration may be inevitable in the early phase after major trauma or in various other life-threatening conditions. There are promising reports from alternative fluid resuscitation regimen with hypertonic saline which supposedly lowers capillary leak-associated edema and – as a consequence – the development of IAH as well [1]. Maintaining abdominal perfusion pressure >60 mmHg may represent a more appropriate resuscitation target than mean arterial pressure [8]. This is particularly true of renal function, which is exceptionally vulnerable to the adverse effects of IAH.

There is still no reliable data on noninvasive techniques to decrease IAP. Most of these concepts aim at either decreasing intra-abdominal volume or increasing abdominal wall compliance. Evacuation of intraluminal contents by gastric or rectal tubes or endoscopic decompression may represent successful options in some situations. Prokinetics such as metoclopramid or prostigmine may be used as well. All these measures may help to lower IAP in patients with massive dilatation of the bowel but may be inadequate in most situations in which IAH is caused by intra- or retroperitoneal hematoma, packing or generalized edema.

CT- or US-guided evacuation of ascites or intra- and retroperitoneal hematoma represents another option. Abdominal wall compliance may be improved by sedation, neuromuscular blockade, body positioning or a negative fluid balance [9].

As capillary leak is one of the main factors in the development of IAH, correction of capillary leak and a well-balanced fluid resuscitation management may be very effective in decreasing IAP. Euvolemia and adequate intravascular fluid status are essential since hypovolemia leads to splanchnic hypoerfusion and organ dysfunction whereas overresuscitation aggravates edema formation and IAH. In this respect, mobilization of edema by application of diuretics can be attempted if hemodynamically tolerated by the patient. Fluid removal by ultrafiltration has also been shown to have a beneficial effect on IAP.

11.1.8.2 Surgical Management of IAH and ACS

Surgical decompression of the abdomen is the only available definite method and the current gold standard in the treatment of a full-blown ACS [10]. Decompressive laparotomy reliably decreases IAP. However, in a considerable number of patients, IAP may not reach physiological levels despite adequate decompression [10]. There is still no consensus at which IAP threshold level decompressive laparotomy should be performed. However, with increasing recognition of the bad outcome of ACS, many experts in the field suggest that an IAP of 20 mmHg in combination with a new organ dysfunction should be treated by immediate surgical decompression leaving other measures for lower IAP levels and without IAP-related organ dysfunction. Others suggest an even more aggressive approach with an IAP threshold at 15 mmHg in selected patients. To date, the literature is not sufficient to provide a reliable recommendation.

Recently, less invasive alternatives to decompressive laparotomy have been described. Subcutaneous linea alba fasciotomy performed in patients with pancreatitis-associated ACS can result in an adequate decrease of IAP [13]. This technique may be suitable for patients with secondary ACS or patients who do not need a laparotomy for any intra-abdominal injury or pathology. In contrast to temporary abdominal closure (TAC) techniques, no special wound care or dressings are necessary and the risk of infection may be smaller. However, subcutaneous linea alba fasciotomy may be less invasive than decompressive laparotomy, but expansion of the abdominal cavity is also limited and intraoperative inspection of the intra- and retroperitoneal content is not possible. The effect of the fasciotomy may immediately be monitored by intraoperative IAP measurement. If IAP decrease is considered insufficient, surgery may be converted to a formal decompressive laparotomy. By incising the linea alba, a large incisional hernia is created leaving the peritoneum intact. Thus, secondary abdominal wall repair is also necessary despite an initial limited surgical approach. More research is necessary to identify patients benefiting from subcutaneous linea alba fasciotomy.

Abdominal wall components separation as described by Ramirez et al. is an established technique for secondary abdominal closure due to incisional hernias [21]. This technique including some modifications performed either by open surgery or endoscopically has also been evaluated as potential therapeutic measure to decrease IAP [6]. With these techniques, IAP may be lowered by an improved compliance of the abdominal wall allowing an increased volume of the abdominal cavity. In contrast to subcutaneous linea alba fasciotomy, the risk for hernias is reduced avoiding later hernia repair. While these arguments undoubtedly appear appealing, one must consider that surgical dissection, even by endoscopic means, is extensive and time-consuming making this approach in the emergency situation probably not feasible. As the current literature does not provide sufficient data, no reliable recommendation can be provided in this respect.

11.2 Abdominal Decompression and Temporary Abdominal Closure

11.2.1 Introduction

The open abdomen is an established concept in the management of critically ill patients after a laparotomy. By definition, it is a nonclosure of the fascia and skin in order to increase the abdominal volume capacity. By providing an extension of the abdominal volume, IAP is considerably decreased. An open abdomen also facilitates repeated access to the peritoneal cavity either for monitoring (e.g., bowel ischemia) or therapeutic measures (e.g., repeated debridements, hemorrhage control, delayed bowel anastomoses). On the other hand, it is associated with serious disadvantages

such as fistula formation, septic complications, and abdominal wall retraction resulting in large defects.

11.2.2 Pathophysiological Considerations and Complications Related to Open Abdomen

An open abdomen performed after injury or sepsis is generally associated with massive capillary leak (e.g., bowel edema), significant fluid loss, and amplified inflammatory response caused by ischemia-reperfusion injury following abdominal decompression. These edemas and fluid losses can cause significant nursing problems. Furthermore, protein loss is increased in patients with an open abdomen.

Entero-atmospheric fistulas are a serious complication of the open abdomen. The formation of fistulas is provoked by several factors, such as a dry-up of bowel serosa when exposed to air, frequent handling of edematous bowel during repeated re-explorations, breakdown of anastomoses or direct contact of prosthetic material with the bowel.

Repeated dressing changes may damage the fascia, the rectus abdominis muscle, and the skin. The longer the abdomen is left open, the more likely is the retraction of the abdominal wall . Incautious handling of the fascia may result in necrosis of the fascial edges and wound infection making subsequent successful fascial closure unlikely.

11.2.3 Avoidance and Management of Complications Related to the Open Abdomen

Avoidance of complications is better than their treatment. In this respect, several details have to be respected. Direct contact of the bowel with adherent dressings must be avoided, only nonadherent dressings should be used. Whenever possible, the omentum should be positioned between bowel and the dressing. In the situation of intestinal anastomoses, contact of the dressing with the anastomosis must be avoided. It is important to protect the anastomosis by placing it deep in the peritoneal cavity. All re-explorations and dressing changes should be performed with great care to diminish serosa lesions.

Early closure of the fascia minimizes the risk of complications. However, fascial closure must not be forced, otherwise recurrent IAH may occur.

Cytokine production is increased in the open abdomen. This is of particular concern since a relationship between cytokine stimulation and the triggering of MOF has been shown. In this respect, drainage of third-space fluid may play a role in reducing systemic complications associated with an open abdomen.

Special considerations are warranted regarding tubes or stomas traversing the abdominal wall. If possible, stomas and surgically placed feeding tubes should be avoided in the initial phase of capillary leakage and progressive edema whenever possible. Edema of the abdominal wall and bowel can result in retraction of the bowel, tubes or drains. Later, as the edema resolves, the relative position of the viscera again changes. Drains and stomas should be brought out through the oblique muscles to avoid damage to the rectus muscle. These flank stomas are well away from the open abdomen and its dressings, avoiding soilage of the laparotomy wound and the abdominal contents. Furthermore, intact rectus components improve later abdominal wall reconstruction.

Once a fistula formation has occurred, its closure while the abdomen is still open is not recommended. The goal of treatment should be contamination control [12]. This should include appropriate drainage, repeated peritoneal lavage, and dressing changes. Exterioration of the fistula, proximal diversion of the bowel, or removal of a distal bowel obstruction are other valuable measures. Furthermore, it is important to correct fluid loss and electrolyte abnormalities and to provide adequate nutrition. The effect of somatostatin to enhance closure of enteric fistula remains questionable.

In the situation of chronic fistulas, the abdominal wound is allowed to close around the fistula. Resection of the fistula combined with reanastomosis of the bowel is performed usually a few months after the open abdomen has been established when the patient has recovered and intra-abdominal infection has healed.

11.2.4 Methods of Temporary Abdominal Closure Techniques

In the situation of an open abdomen, the abdomen must be temporarily closed to provide a barrier to

Table 11.4 Requirements for the ideal temporary abdominal closure technique

Universal availability
Low cost
Simple and quick application/removal
Good drainage capacity
Protection from evisceration and contamination (barrier function)
Tissue friendliness (no skin or fascia destruction with multiple applications)
Prevention of entero-atmospheric fistula formation (non-adhesive)
Expansion of abdominal volume (Prevention of IAH)

prevent bowel evisceration and to allow easy access for repeated surgery. Furthermore, a reliable decrease of IAP must be achieved. Raeburn investigated the development of ACS following damage-control laparotomy [20]. Abdominal closure following damage-control surgery was performed by skin closure only, by bag silo closure (bogota bag) or by primary fascial closure according to the surgeon's preference and judgment. Overall, development of ACS was observed in 36% of their patients. Intriguing, the type of abdominal closure did not influence the development of ACS.

Table 11.4 lists different qualities required for the ideal TAC technique [4]. However, the ideal TAC has not been invented yet. In the following, different TAC techniques currently in use are described in more detail. During the last years, the vacuum-assisted wound closure (VAWC) technique in different modifications has gained increasing popularity among surgeons. Thus, the pros and cons of this particular technique are more extensively discussed.

11.2.4.1 Towel Clip Closure/Skin Closure Only

This is a simple and cheap technique which allows quick abdominal re-exploration. The towel clips are placed through the skin edges at 2–3 cm intervals to approximate the wound [4]. Alternatively, the skin may be closed with a running suture. There are considerable disadvantages associated with this technique. Among others, these include skin damage and poor drainage of intra-abdominal fluids. Furthermore, this technique does not provide volume expansion of the abdomen resulting in a high risk of IAH development. During damage- control laparotomy, towel clip closure may be used for a short period after abdominal packing for hemorrhage control in order to gain time to catch up with fluid resuscitation, patient rewarming, and correction of coagulation abnormalities before better hemorrhage control can be achieved.

11.2.4.2 Bag Silo Closure (Bogota Bag)

For this technique, a sterile 3 L plastic cystoscopy fluid irrigation bag is cut into shape to cover the abdominal wall defect in a silo-like manner [11]. The bag is either sutured to the skin or the fascia. Since its first description, many modifications have been developed. The bag silo is a low-cost technique and its surface is nonadherent. It is simple and quick to apply and evisceration is reliably prevented. Due to the transparency of the bag, continuous visual assessment of bowel viability is possible. It is very important to avoid damage to the fascia and the underlying abdominal rectus muscle in order to facilitate delayed primary fascial closure at a later stage.

Disadvantages of this technique are the limited drainage capacity, the risk of hypothermia, and considerable nursing problems due to leakage and skin maceration. However, expansion of the abdominal volume with a bag silo closure exceeds the capacity provided by other techniques currently in use. Thus, the risk of IAH and ACS may be lower compared to other techniques. For many experts, bag silo closure is the preferred TAC technique for the initial phase after abdominal decompression, either prophylactically after damage-control surgery or by therapeutic means in the presence of critical IAH. With decreasing organ swelling and edema, the bag silo may be replaced by a VAWC technique, which facilitates fascial approximation and sequential fascial closure. In some patients, fascial closure may already be possible at that stage without recurrent increase of IAP.

11.2.4.3 Zipper Technique

Zipper systems allow repetitive and easy access to the abdominal cavity once mounted. The polyester-based fabric can be cut into shape and be sutured to the fascia. If formed in a bag silo-like manner, this technique may provide additional volume for intra-abdominal expansion. Disadvantages are similar to the bag silo technique (Fig. 11.4).

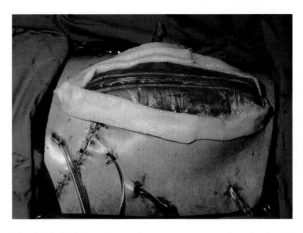

Fig. 11.4 TAC by using a zipper system sutured to the fascial edges

11.2.4.4 Synthetic Mesh Closure

Another popular TAC technique is synthetic mesh closure. Typically, the mesh is sewn to the fascia in a rather loose manner. Absorbable mesh can safely be used in an infected environment. It is easy to place, facilitates re-exploration with the ability to open and reclose the abdomen. Moist dressings are placed on top of the mesh. These dressings must not dry up. The pores of the mesh allow egress of abdominal fluids which can also cause nursing problems and skin maceration. The fistula rate associated with absorbable mesh closure is low (about 5%). Whenever possible, omentum should be interposed between mesh and bowel. The mesh promotes granulation tissue and once granulation tissue has incorporated the mesh, a split skin graft can be applied to close the wound. However, this technique results in large ventral hernias requiring abdominal wall reconstruction at a later stage.

The application of a nonresorbable polypropylene mesh is associated with a high fistula rate up to 50%; it cannot be used in an infected field, and if infected it will require removal. Some synthetic material allow staged abdominal closure by application of controlled tension to pull the fascial edges closer until a formal tension-free fascial closure is possible in the majority of patients [23].

11.2.4.5 Vac Pac Closure

This technique allows a cheap and rapid closure of the abdominal wall [5]. A nonadherent and fenestrated polyethylene sheet is placed over the viscera. This layer is covered by moist surgical towels and silicone drains are placed. The dressing and wound edges are sealed with an adhesive dressing and wall suction is applied to the drains to control abdominal secretions. The fistula rate is low but the technique fails to approximate the abdominal wall resulting in a relatively low fascial closure rate of about 50% compared to newer modifications such as VAWC [5].

11.2.4.6 Abdominal Vacuum-Assisted Closure (VAS)

A commercially available perforated nonadherent plastic sheet with an encapsulated polyurethane sponge is placed directly over the viscera. This sheet is extended laterally to separate the abdominal wall from the viscera. This layer is covered with a large polyurethane sponge which can be loosely fixed to the fascia with a few sutures. The dressing is sealed with an adherent sheet and an aspiration system is placed with suction between 75 and 150 mmHg [19].

The VAC technique provides good fluid drainage and prevents leakage which avoids nursing problems. Subatmospheric pressure promotes wound healing, the formation of granulation tissue, reduction of edema, and potential removal of inflammatory substances. Overall, all these effects may contribute to an improved condition of the laparotomy wound increasing the chances for successful delayed fascial closure superiorly to other TAC techniques reported in the literature [23].

However, there is no consensus about the ideal magnitude of negative pressure applied to the system for TAC. Experimental studies have clearly demonstrated that a negative pressure of 125 mmHg is superior to both higher and lower pressure values to achieve the best results concerning promotion of wound healing [18]. However, the influence and the magnitude of negative pressure on containment of the abdominal volume in the situation of IAH and the risk of fistula formation remains unclear. In this respect, it has also been reported, that when the VAC was connected to suction, there was an immediate increase in IAP due to a decrease of the sponge volume reversing some of the effects provided by surgical decompression (Fig. 11.5a and b). This is in line with a very recent experimental comparative study, which has demonstrated that alternative TAC techniques such as bag silo closure and zipper systems provide significantly more abdominal volume expansion than the VAC [7]. Thus, the VAC may not be recommended immediately after decompressive laparotomy because it provides insufficient volume expansion and therefore holds an increased risk for

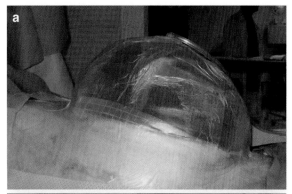

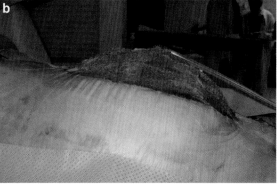

Fig. 11.5 (**a**) The mounted system before installation of negative pressure. (**b**) After application of negative pressure the volume of the decompressed abdomen is markedly reduced

recurrence of IAH. In our experience, the VAC may safely be applied at a later stage after regression of the abdominal volume when application of the VAC does not have an adverse effect on IAH anymore. Usually, the change to the VAC is feasible after 2–4 days following decompression in most cases. Once the VAC is applied, the dressing needs to be changed in intervals of 2–5 days. Longer intervals are not recommended because it gets difficult to separate the sponge from ingrowing granulation tissue. These dressing changes are combined with sequential narrowing of the laparotomy at both ends with interrupted tension-free sutures of the fascia until the fascia is completely closed. In some patients, delayed fascial closure may be achieved only a few days after decompressive laparotomy, others take considerably longer. When delayed fascial closure is not possible mesh closure and split skin grafting may be necessary.

11.2.4.7 Bogota-VAC

An interesting modification of the established bag silo closure is the combination of the Bogota bag with a

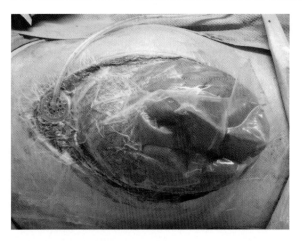

Fig. 11.6 In contrast to the VAC system (Fig. 11.5), the sponge does not reduce the effect of abdominal decompression. The ring-shaped sponge is used for a proper wound sealing and conditioning of the wound edges while the combination with the bag silo provides a better volume expansion of the decompressed abdomen

commercially available vacuum-assisted wound dressing system (Fig. 11.6) [24]. Instead of a cystoscopy bag, a thin nonadherent polyurethane drape is loosely sutured to the fascia forming a bag silo. A ring-shaped polyurethane sponge is positioned into the wound between the wound edges and the bag silo. The wound is sealed with adhesive dressing tapes, the sponge is connected to a vacuum pump and topic negative pressure is applied.

The technique can be applied in short time without technical difficulties. The vacuum part of the system has got all the characteristics of the VAC technique. Overall, all these effects may contribute to an improved condition of the laparotomy wound increasing the chances for successful delayed fascial closure while the bag silo allows additional volume for intra-abdominal expansion effectively reducing the risk of recurrent critical IAH.

11.2.5 Fascial Closure and Abdominal Wall Reconstruction after an Open Abdomen

One of the major goals of modern TAC techniques is to achieve a later tension-free fascial closure without provoking recurrent IAH. Thus, frequent monitoring of IAP is essential during sequential fascial closure. The current literature demonstrates that secondary fascial closure is possible in the majority of patients without the need for abdominal wall granulation and skin grafting leaving an often disabling hernia for subsequent extensive abdominal wall reconstruction [23]. However, when secondary fascial closure is not feasible, abdominal wall reconstruction is necessary to close the defect.

Abdominal wall defects, which are not suitable for immediate complete or sequential closure, may be closed by an absorbable polyglactin mesh accepting the inevitable incisional hernia. This closure prevents bowel evisceration and allows the formation of granulation tissue. As soon as possible, usually after 2–3 weeks, the now conditioned abdominal defect is covered with a split skin graft. As the abdomen is closed, the fascial defect has to be addressed a few months later.

Definitive reconstruction may be done by either abdominal wall components separation or repair with a synthetic nonabsorbable mesh (e.g., polypropylene). Local and distant flaps are other options [4]. Unlike synthetic nonabsorbable mesh, flaps can also be used in contaminated wounds. Mesh closure has also the disadvantage of adherence to the bowel with the risk of fistula formation. Interposition of peritoneum or omentum may be ideal to overcome this problem but not always possible. Free tissue transfer (free flaps) is the last resort for abdominal wall reconstruction. Regarding potential later abdominal wall reconstruction, initial abdominal decompression is preferably performed by a midline laparotomy. In contrast to other incisions, these defects may be more difficult to close, but the innervation and blood supply of the abdominal wall are well preserved, making later reconstruction easier.

References

1. Zsolt B, McKinley BA, Cox CS et al (2003) Abdominal compartment syndrome: the cause or effect of postinjury multiple organ failure. Shock 20:483–492
2. Balogh Z, McKinley BA, Holcomb JB et al (2003) Both primary and secondary abdominal compartment syndrome can be predicted early and are harbingers of multiple organ failure. J Trauma 54:848–859
3. Balogh Z, Jones F, D'Amours S et al (2004) Continuous intra-abdominal pressure measurement technique. Am J Surg 188:679–684
4. Balogh Z, Moore FA, Goettler CE et al (2006) Management of abdominal compartment syndrome. In: Ivatury RR, Cheatham ML, Malbrain MLNG, Sugrue M (eds) Abdominal compartment syndrome. Landes Bioscience, Georgetown, pp 264–294

5. Barker DE, Kaufman HJ, Smith LA et al (2000) Vacuum pack technique of temporary abdominal closure: a 7-year experience with 112 patients. J Trauma 48:201–207

6. Barnes GS, Papasavas PK, O'Mara MS et al (2004) Modified extraperitoneal endoscopic separation of parts for abdominal compartment syndrome. Surg Endosc 18:1636–1639

7. Benninger E, Laschke MW, Cardell M et al (2009) Intra-abdominal pressure development after different temporary abdominal closure techniques in a porcine model. J Trauma 66(4):1118–1124

8. Cheatham ML, White MW, Sagraves SG et al (2000) Abdominal perfusion pressure: a superior parameter in the assessment of intra-abdominal hypertension. J Trauma 49:621–626

9. Cheatham ML, Malbrain MLNG, Kirkpatrick A et al (2007) Results from the conference of experts on intra-abdominal hypertension and abdominal compartment syndrome. Part II: recommendations. Intensive Care Med 33:951–962

10. De Waele JJ, Hoste EA, Malbrain ML (2006) Decompressive laparotomy for abdominal compartment syndrome – a critical analysis. Crit Care 10:R51

11. Fernandez L, Norwood S, Roettger R et al (1996) Temporary intravenous bag silo closure in severe abdominal trauma. J Trauma 40:258–260

12. Goettler CE, Rotondo MF, Schwab WC (2006) Surgical management of the open abdomen after damage control or abdominal compartment syndrome. In: Ivatury RR, Cheatham ML, Malbrain MLNG, Sugrue M (eds) Abdominal compartment syndrome. Landes Bioscience, Georgetown, pp 271–282

13. Leppaniemi AK, Hienonen PA, Siren JE et al (2006) Treatment of abdominal compartment syndrome with subcutaneous anterior abdominal fasciotomy in severe pancreatitis. World J Surg 30:1922–1924

14. Malbrain MLNG (2004) Different techniques to measure intra-abdominal pressure (IAP): time for a critical re-appraisal. Intensive Care Med 30:357–371

15. Malbrain MLNG, Chiumello D, Pelosi P et al (2004) Prevalence of intra-abdominal hypertension in critically ill patients: a multicentre epidemiological study. Intensive Care Med 30:822–829

16. Malbrain MLNG, Cheatham ML, Kirkpatrick A et al (2006) Results from the conference of experts on intra-abdominal hypertension and abdominal compartment syndrome. Part I: definitions. Intensive Care Med 32:1722–1732

17. Meier C, Contaldo C, Schramm R et al (2007) Microdialysis of the rectus abdominis muscle for early detection of impending abdominal compartment syndrome. Intensive Care Med 33:1434–1443

18. Morykwas MJ, Faler BJ, Pearce DJ et al (2001) Effects of varying levels of subathmospheric pressure on the rate of granulation tissue formation in experimental wounds in swine. Ann Plast Surg 47:547–551

19. Perez D, Wildi S, Demartines N et al (2007) Prospective evaluation of vacuum-assisted closure in abdominal compartment syndrome and severe abdominal sepsis. J Coll Am Surg 205:586–592

20. Raeburn CD, Moore EE, Biffl WL et al (2001) The abdominal compartment syndrome is a morbid complication of postinjury damage control surgery. Am J Surg 182:542–546

21. Ramirez OM, Ruas E, Dellon AL (1990) "Components separation" method for closure of abdominal wall defects: an anatomic and clinical study. Plast Reconstr Surg 86:519–526

22. Rezende-Neto JB, Moore EE, Masuno T et al (2003) The abdominal compartment syndrome as a second insult during systemic neutrophil priming provokes multiple organ injury. Shock 20:303–308

23. Van Hensbroek PB, Wind J, Dijkgraaf MGW et al (2009) Temporary Closure of the open abdomen: a systematic review on delayed primary fascial closure in patients with an open abdomen. World J Surg 33:199–207

24. Von Rueden C, Benninger E, Mayer D et al (2008) Bogota-VAC- a newly modified temporary abdominal closure technique. Eur J Trauma Emerg Surg: 34:582–586

25. Widder S, Ranson MK, Zygun D et al (2008) Use of near-infrared spectroscopy as a physiologic monitor for intra-abdominal hypertension. J Trauma 64:1165–1168

Trauma Laparotomy: Indications, Priorities, and Damage Control

12

Selman Uranues and Abe Fingerhut

12.1 Introduction

Laparotomy for trauma has two essential roles, most often contemporaneous: diagnostic and therapeutic. In unstable patients, a trauma laparotomy is a life-saving measure and should not exceed 30–45 min. Only those measures that are essential to sustain life should be taken and protracted explorations that are not directly related to the life-threatening situation should be avoided. The surgeon should maintain constant communication with his/her most important partner, the anesthesiologist, to coordinate life-sustaining measures.

12.2 Indications and Priorities

In order to best perform exploratory laparotomy for trauma, the mechanisms of injury have to be analyzed. Energy transfer essentially determines the damage. Penetrating injuries are limited to the trajectory of low-velocity projectiles, whereas distant organs can be damaged by high-velocity projectiles. In blunt injury, the mechanisms are crushing, deceleration, and shearing (Fig. 12.1). Correct analysis of the mechanism of injury and/or the trajectory of penetrating projectiles can assist the trauma laparotomy surgeon in planning

the strategies of intra-abdominal exploration and prioritization of care.

Obvious indications for laparotomy include peritonism (progressive guarding; tenderness, including rebound tenderness; rigidity regardless of the bowel sounds), hypotension or signs of severe internal bleeding (increasing pulse rate, restlessness, pallor), or gunshot (projectile) and explosive (mines, grenades) wounds traversing the abdomen, visceral herniation through the diaphragm or abdominal wall, thoraco-abdominal wounds, hematemesis, blood in the gastric aspirate or rectal bleeding, penetrating anal or vaginal injuries, positive findings on paracentesis (positive diagnostic peritoneal lavage in the unstable patient) or gastric lavage, or increasing abdominal girth (Table 12.1).

Debatable indications, analyzed case by case on an individual basis, even include the stable patient with penetrating injury in some instances (stab wounds) [1]. One must remember that the confines of the abdomen are not limited to the belly and that the same penetrating wounds can involve the abdomen, the thorax, and the retroperitoneum.

Schematically, three different hemodynamic situations can be seen: (1) The moribund patient (absence of femoral pulse, no recordable blood pressure), in whom the goal is to perform laparotomy to clamp the aorta (at the diaphragm) and to stop the bleeding in order to obtain a blood pressure; (2) The unstable patient, for whom the basic "ABC" of ATLS must be quickly assured before undertaking exploratory laparotomy; and (3) The stable patient, for whom there is time for work-up, non-operative management, or sometimes laparoscopic exploration to rule out intra-abdominal lesions, especially in the setting of penetrating injury (Table 12.2).

Whenever laparotomy is indicated for abdominal trauma, three principles prevail, in order of importance: (1) stop the bleeding, (2) limit contamination, and (3)

S. Uranues (✉)
Department of Surgery, Medical University of Graz,
Graz, Austria
e-mail: selman.uranues@medunigraz.at

A. Fingerhut
Digestive and General Surgery Unit, Centre Hospitalier
Intercommunal, Poissy, France
e-mail: AbeFingerhut@aol.com

H.-J. Oestern et al. (eds.), *Head, Thoracic, Abdominal, and Vascular Injuries*,
DOI: 10.1007/978-3-540-88122-3_12, © Springer-Verlag Berlin Heidelberg 2011

Fig. 12.1 Blunt abdominal trauma with splenic injury caused by seat belt in a frontal car crash

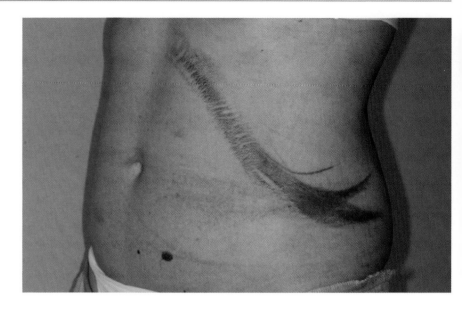

Table 12.1 Obvious indications for laparotomy in trauma

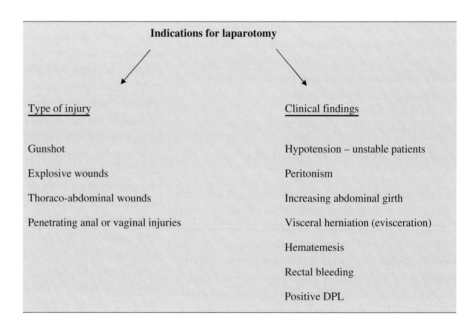

Indications for laparotomy

Type of injury	Clinical findings
Gunshot	Hypotension – unstable patients
Explosive wounds	Peritonism
Thoraco-abdominal wounds	Increasing abdominal girth
Penetrating anal or vaginal injuries	Visceral herniation (evisceration)
	Hematemesis
	Rectal bleeding
	Positive DPL

whenever possible and/or reasonable, reconstruct. Giving priority to hemostasis, however, is absolutely paramount to success: blood loss and need for transfusion are the important pejorative prognostic factors. Every effort must be made to stop or limit loss of blood, albeit by temporary means, while definitive hemostasis or reconstruction can take place later under better conditions: pressure, packing, sutures, and stents are preferred over blind attempts at instrumental arrest or ligation, but ligation may sometimes be the only life-saving alternative (Table 12.3). Temporary control of hemorrhage with pressure, packing, and then, patience, just taking the time to wait for natural hemostasis to take place, is golden and time-proven advice. This will give the anesthesiologist valuable time to stabilize the patient, particularly with respect to hemodynamic and metabolic indices. Once the crisis has passed, pressure or packs may be released slowly while the surgeon identifies the bleeding site.

Table 12.2 Therapeutic options according to the hemodynamic status in trauma patients

Hemodynamic status	Procedure
1 Stable	No time pressure, time for work-up
2 Unstable	"ABC" of ATLS, urgent exploratory laparotomy
3 Moribund	Life-saving measures, shock room laparotomy/thoracotomy

Table 12.3 Ligation site and incidence of necrosis

Ligation site	Incidence of necrosis (%)
Coeliac axis	< 5
Left gastric	0
Left hepatic	<10
Right hepatic	<10
Splenic	<10
Common hepatic	<10
Proper hepatic	<20
Gastroduodenal	0
Renal	>95
Superior mesenteric	>95
Inferior mesenteric	>95
Distal mesenteric	>50
Left colic	<25

Frantic efforts to clamp bleeding points may result in useless blood loss and possibly irreversible instrumental damage. If bleeding is so severe that in spite of the initial efforts, blood continues to fill up the abdomen, packing should be pursued, and pressure applied to the nearest major (feeding) vessel. This is when it is helpful to have an assistant. Stress reduction will make it easier to find the source of bleeding.

Contamination from the digestive tract can be limited by rapidly tying off or stapling the injured segment(s), leaving restoration of digestive continuity to later, as appropriate (Fig. 12.2).

One of the most important prognostic factors is the length of the interval between the decision to operate and the actual beginning of the intervention.

12.2.1 Adjunctive Measures

A nasogastric tube and gastric aspiration are always useful to deflate the stomach. A Foley catheter should be inserted in the bladder, in the absence of obvious or suspected lesions to the urethra; otherwise, a suprapubic catheter is advisable. Preoperative prophylaxis with a broad-spectrum antibiotic (first-generation cephalosporin usually suffices) during premedication or upon anesthesia induction but at the latest during the skin incision is the rule [2].

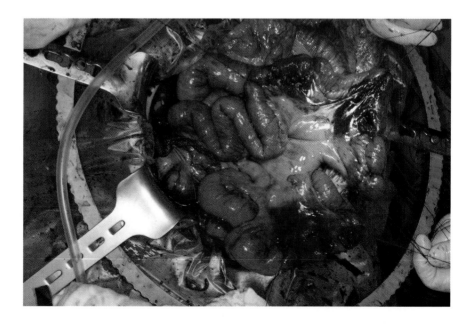

Fig. 12.2 Multiple small bowel injury caused by gunshot. The bowel is temporarily tied off

If there is no contamination upon laparotomy, antibiotics may be discontinued. If there is, or if the peritoneum is contaminated during surgery, but the contamination is present for less than 6–8 h and can be cleaned up with source control, such as closure or resection of a perforated segment of the intestinal tract, antibiotics may be discontinued after 24 h. The dose should be repeated after 10 units of transfusion and aminoglycosides should be avoided.

If there is established infection, or the perforation is of 8 h duration or more, antibiotics should be continued for at least 5 days.

The positive role of administration of Factor rVIIa has recently been underscored in both the blunt and penetrating trauma settings, but the exact timing and doses have not been established with a high level of evidence.

12.3 Associated Extra-Abdominal Lesions

The existence of head injury should not deter or delay a needed laparotomy. When multiple torso injuries are associated with cranial injury, priorities dictate this order of treatment:

1. Uncontained and uncontrolled hemorrhage, whether intraperitoneal or pleural
2. Neurosurgical emergencies (possibly, simultaneously)
3. Contained hemorrhage
4. Visceral injuries

High priority is given to establishing hemodynamic stability as soon as possible. Urgent cranial surgery can also only be undertaken after hemostasis and stabilization of the patient have been achieved, or synchronously with these measures. In this setting, there is little or no place for intra-abdominal preservation techniques.

Dyspnea due to hemo- and/or pneumohemothorax requires drainage, if need be under local anesthesia. If thoracic drainage does not improve the respiration status adequately, or if the bleeding rate is immediately alarming, or if a penetrating injury to the heart or greater vessels is suspected, a thoracotomy should be entertained before the laparotomy. In the case of associated thoraco-abdominal injuries, the intra-abdominal injuries take precedence, obviously excepting penetrating cardiothoracic or exsanguinating lesions.

Some penetrating back wounds might warrant exploration before the laparotomy, just to determine the degree of penetration. The prerequisite for dorsal exploration is the stability of the patient.

Pelvic fractures and major diaphysar fractures should be stabilized, especially when there is pelvic bleeding or nerve injury: this can be done quickly before the laparotomy or during the preparation for laparotomy depending on the patient's hemodynamics. Concomitant limb vessel injuries can be approached during the laparotomy: intralumenal stents may be preferred to definitive repair (vascular damage control).

The ideal order in which associated fractures and vascular lesions of limbs should be treated depends on the circumstances and the cooperation between orthopedic and general (vascular) surgeons: the expected duration of each procedure must be evaluated in order not to overrun the customary 1-h period of ischemia allowed in this setting. Several scenarios are possible: fractures that are more or less stable should be treated after vascular repair while those that are highly unstable and/or require important manipulations, can be treated either by a prompt external fixation followed by vascular repair or else insertion of a vascular shunt, with intraoperative monitoring during the treatment of the bone lesions. In case of severe pelvic injury with combined bone and vascular lesions, priority goes to arresting the bleeding (ideally, by embolization) before treating the bone injury.

12.4 Patient's Positioning and the Right Incision

Ideally, for trauma laparotomy the patient is supine with both arms extended to the sides.

The patient must be draped with the entire thorax, neck, and upper thighs in the operative field (Fig. 12.3). Large bore intravenous access to the upper (essential) and lower limbs is highly recommended. An arterial line is of secondary importance and should not be given high priority. The best incision to explore the abdomen in the case of trauma is midline, xyphoid to pubis. Two other incisions should be considered: extending the midline cephalad to a midline sternotomy, or performance of a right subcostal incision in the case of severe lesions to the right liver.

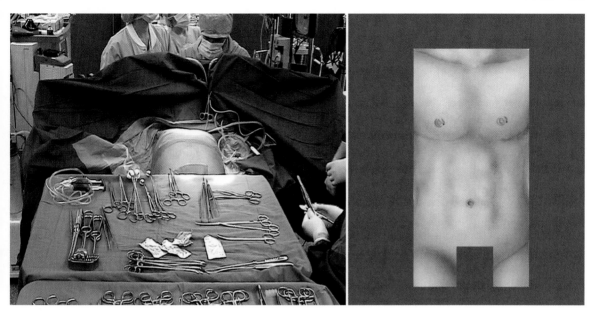

Fig. 12.3 Supine positioning and draping of the patient with both arms extended to the sides for a trauma laparotomy

A solid frame and/or set of fixed retractors are essential to obtain adequate exposure of the entire abdominal cavity.

12.4.1 Exploration

One essential point is to explore the abdomen with rigor and perform a systematic survey, in a specific and routine order, organ by organ, region by region, not forgetting to run the intestines, and view the three areas of the retroperitoneum (central, lateral, and the lesser pelvic cavity) (Fig. 12.4).

Therapeutic strategies in the multiple-injured depend on hemodynamic and cardiovascular status, metabolic status, and hemostatic capacity of the victim. Other priorities may be dictated by associated lesions and/or particular circumstances. The strategist should be the visceral surgeon.

Strategy and therapy, however, are often indistinguishable because finding the source of bleeding (diagnosis) and stopping it (therapy) must usually be accomplished simultaneously. All must be ready to deal with major vascular problems as soon as the peritoneum is entered, because once opened, the natural, temporary, counter-pressure buffer barrier will be released. The

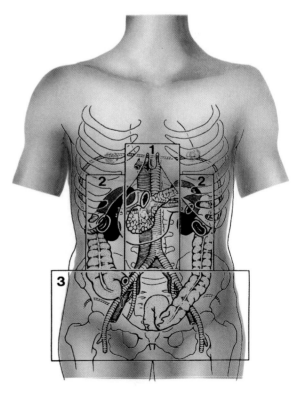

Fig. 12.4 Zones of the retroperitoneum: zone 1: central, zone 2: lateral, zone 3: pelvic

initial steps should be to pack as many abdominal pads as necessary in each of the four abdominal quadrants, the center of the abdomen, and the two paracolic gutters and pelvis, in order to stop or at least to limit, possibly with added manual compression, blood loss and gain control of major sources of bleeding.

Correct exploration of the liver as well as adequate packing of this organ may require mobilization (division of triangular or coronary ligaments, the falciform and round ligaments, as needed to ensure adequate placement of the pads to obtain hemostasis). As mentioned before, adequate exposure of the liver may require an additional incision, a combined midline-transverse surgical approach, especially in the case of severe right liver injuries. Complete exploration of the liver surface often requires taking down all the ligament attachments, but extreme caution should be exercised when these maneuvers, especially on the right, actually increase the bleeding, as this may indicate lesions of the hepatic veins or the retrohepatic vena cava. In this situation, the mobilized liver should be replaced immediately and pressure applied to try to stop the bleeding. Retrohepatic injuries to the inferior vena cava (IVC) are usually identified by the failure of manual compression and the Pringle maneuver to control bleeding from the liver. Of ill omen is dark blood that continues to well up from behind the liver despite these maneuvers.

Ideally, perihepatic packing should attempt to restore normal anatomy and replace the separated segments of the liver responsible for the hemorrhage. Unfolded abdominal pads can be placed between the bleeding lobe and the diaphragm, below the liver (never in the lesion), making use of the rigid rib cage whenever possible to provide counterpressure. A plastic sheet (e.g., "Steri-drape" occlusive dressing) between the parenchyma and the packs will prevent adherence of the pads to the hepatic capsule (Fig. 12.5) and further bleeding at the time of ablation of the packs, but this is not a priority.

No drains are necessary. Beware of creating an abdominal compartment syndrome (ACS) if the abdomen is closed with the packs inside.

Several intraoperative maneuvers will help access the retroperitoneum and most of the intra-abdominal organs including the Kocher and super Kocher (Fig. 12.6), Cattell-Braasch and Mattox maneuvers. Full mobilization of the left and right Toldt fascias is essential as well [3].

Kocher mobilization includes the mobilization of the right colonic flexure and duodenum. The Cattell-Braasch maneuver entails mobilization of the entire right hemicolon including the duodenum from caudal to cranial via incision of the peritoneum from parietal to visceral and slightly lateral to the reflection. The entire right hemicolon with the duodenum can then be

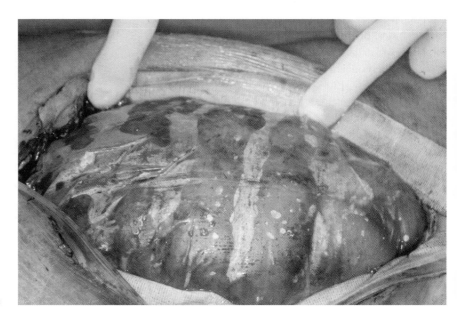

Fig. 12.5 Plastic dressing to cover the abdominal cavity and protect the bowel from additional damage from temporary abdominal closure

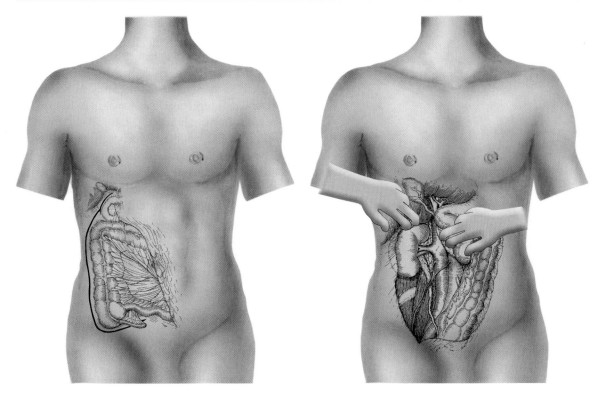

Fig. 12.6 Incision to open the right-sided retroperitoneum.

Fig. 12.7 Cattell-Braasch maneuver: mobilization of the entire right hemicolon including the duodenum from caudal to cranial giving access to the right-sided retroperitoneum

lifted medially, allowing access to the right half of the retroperitoneum and so to the IVC and the right kidney and ureter (Fig. 12.7).

The Mattox maneuver serves to mobilize the sigmoid and descending colon and the left colonic flexure, and so to shift the left hemicolon including the spleen and the left half of the pancreas medially. This provides a good access to the left retroperitoneum, abdominal aorta, and the left kidney and ureter (Fig. 12.8).

Other specific maneuvers to correctly visualize and treat lesions of the duodenum, pancreas, large vessels, celiac axis, portal and mesenteric vessels, liver and liver vessels must be known and used appropriately. Pelvic injuries are often combined (bony and intra-cavitary lesions). Initial (or contemporaneous) stabilization is usually required. Severe bleeding from the internal iliac vessels is best controlled by embolization but ligation may be necessary.

The abdominal pads are removed one by one, as the surgeon explores each quadrant of the abdomen in a routine and orderly fashion, space by space, organ by

organ, leaving nothing to chance. Systematic organ-by-organ exploration is the best way to treat all lesions properly and timely.

The upper left quadrant is explored first: in unstable patients with multiple injuries including the spleen, splenectomy usually cannot be avoided. If the patient becomes and remains stable after primary packing, however, spleen preservation can be an option even in patients who were initially unstable. In some cases, cupping the spleen laterally after incision of the lateral peritoneum to open the posterior mesogastrium will allow rapid clamping of the splenic pedicle, and the surgeon can continue the exploration. The decision for splenectomy, total or partial, or preservation, can be made later. Total splenectomy should always be entertained when the patient is in shock or has multiple severe intra-abdominal lesions (hepatic and other injuries); in this setting, there is no justification for preservation (see Chap. 8).

Most gastric lesions can be treated in a straightforward manner. Intestinal (small and large) injuries can be treated by suture or resection, followed or not by

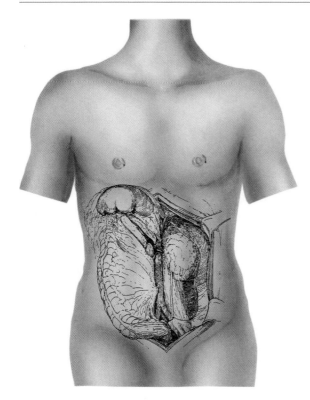

Fig. 12.8 Mattox maneuver: mobilization of the sigmoid and descending colon, the left colonic flexure, the spleen and the pancreatic tail, giving access to the left-sided retroperitoneum

anastomosis and/or derivation (see Chap. 9). Duodenal and pancreatic lesions constitute one of the most difficult challenges, but usually, as is the case with other intra-abdominal lesions, are not acutely life threatening except when associated with active bleeding. All severe edema, air bubbles or crepitation on palpation, or bile staining (or hematoma, see below) of the periduodenal tissues imply mandatory exploration to rule out duodenal or pancreatic injury; there is no place here for simple observation (see Chap. 9).

As simple and self-evident as any organ injury may seem, it is always necessary to thoroughly explore the adjacent structures in order not to miss any less obvious lesions.

12.4.2 Hematoma

Hematoma is defined as a swelling of collected blood contained within a closed cavity, organ, or compartment.

All pulsating hematomas, and, contrary to past dogmas, all juxta-intestinal or duodenopancreatic loge hematomas, even if nonexpanding in the stable patient, must be opened and explored in order to avoid missing a gastroduodenal or intestinal lesion hidden by the hematoma. All central retroperitoneal hematomas must be explored in the case of penetrating injury. Last, all upper midline retroperitoneal hematomas, both penetrating and blunt, must be explored. The presence of a central retroperitoneal hematoma suggests an injury to the midline vascular structures. A more right-sided, nonpulsatile lesion suggests an IVC injury rather than an aortic injury, but it can be difficult to determine this and of course, injuries may coexist. Conversely, it is not always necessary to routinely explore stable retroperitoneal hematomas in the case of blunt trauma.

12.4.3 Resuscitative Measures

During laparotomy for trauma, every possible means should be employed to prevent hypothermia and hemodilution, which aggravate coagulopathy and acidosis. Priority is then given to resuscitation maneuvers to complete hemodynamic stabilization. At this time, it becomes important to elaborate the therapeutic action to be undertaken and possibly to call for help from a colleague, order blood substitutes and/or is set up blood-saving devices.

12.5 The Indications for Abbreviated Laparotomy – Damage Control Surgery

The concept of "damage control" (also known as "staged laparotomy") has, as its objective, avoidance of additional surgical stress at a moment of physiological frailty. The concept is not new, but as the underlying rationale was not immediately well understood, the first results were not satisfying. Briefly stated, this is a technique in which the surgeon minimizes operative time and intervention in the grossly unstable patient. The primary reason is the physiologic instability that frequently results in a lethal triad of metabolic acidosis, hypothermia, and coagulopathy [4]. Damage control has proved to be life saving, with timely abortion of laparotomy after the intra-abdominal pack tamponade has been established and the bleeding stopped. The patient is returned to the operating room (OR) a few hours later, after stability has been achieved in an intensive care setting and coagulation has returned to an acceptable level. Although the principles are sound, extreme care has to be exercised to avoid secondary insults to viscera and so to minimize activation of the inflammatory cascade and the consequences of systemic inflammatory response syndrome (SIRS) and organ dysfunction. The concept of damage-control surgery applies to both routine and emergency procedures, and can apply equally well in the chest, pelvis, and neck as in the abdomen [5, 6].

The stages of damage-control surgery are:

1. Patient selection
2. Primary operation with hemorrhage and contamination control, packing, temporary abdominal closure
3. Secondary resuscitation and physiological restoration in the intensive care unit (ICU)
4. Reoperation and removal of packing, and definitive surgery
5. Permanent closure of the abdomen

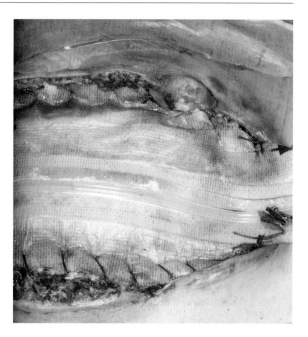

Fig. 12.9 Temporary abdominal zipper closure permitting multiple entries into the abdomen with the same dressing

12.5.1 Patient Selection and Primary Operation

Profound and seemingly irreversible hypothermia, coagulopathy, and acidosis may set in when operations last longer than 1.5 h and require more than 10 units of blood. Hemorrhage is controlled with vascular clamps and suture ligatures. Simple repairs and temporary intravascular shunts are other quick and easily implemented measures to arrest the bleeding. In solid organ injuries, time-consuming repairs should be avoided. In these situations, a rapid splenectomy may be the best solution in patients with splenic injuries. For pancreatic injuries, packing will generally suffice as temporary treatment. Complex hepatic injuries may require temporary vascular occlusion followed by pack compression and postoperative radiologic intervention. In this setting, the surgeon must rapidly and honestly assess whether the patient will tolerate further surgery or whether it is best to leave the packs in to maintain hemostasis. Pads are added until bleeding has stopped

or diminished as much as reasonable, interrupted intestinal segments are closed off (Fig. 12.2), and the abdomen is closed temporarily (Fig. 12.9). Abdominal closure can be achieved in several ways. The options range from towel clips over plastic bags to mesh closure. At this stage, closure of the fascia should not be taken into consideration to avoid unnecessary fascial loss. Temporary abdominal closure can be achieved very quickly and simply with an Opsite^R adhesive plastic membrane over laparotomy pads on the skin. For patients with incompletely controlled persistent bleeding from liver, pelvic or retroperitoneal injuries, angiographic embolization can be a worthwhile adjunct.

12.5.2 Physiological Restoration

When laparotomy has been aborted, vigorous secondary resuscitative measures are undertaken, including warming of the patient, correction of the coagulopathy, and maximal ventilatory support. These can be initiated in the OR and continued in the ICU. Special attention should be devoted to IAP, which can increase after circulatory restoration due to reperfusion damage and postresuscitation visceral edema and cause ACS. An

Table 12.4 Definition of Abdominal Compartment Syndrome (Zsolt B [2007] Crit Care Med 35(2):677–678)

Abdominal compartment syndrome (ACS)
Consensus Definitions (2004, Australia)
• Intra-Abdominal Pressure (IAP):   Normal range (<10 mmH-O)
• Intra-Abdominal Hypertension (IAH):   IAP>12 mmH-O, no organ dysfunction

• Abdominal Compartment Syndrome (ACS):
  IAH+organ dysfunction
  Cardiac, respiratory, renal

increased IAP causes splanchnic hypoperfusion and should be corrected immediately by enlarging the temporary abdominal closure or reopening the abdomen and decompressing it (Table 12.4).

Once the patient is stabilized, physiology is restored and the coagulopathy is corrected, the patient should be brought back to the OR, usually within the first 24 h after initial operation and not more than 48 h thereafter.

12.5.3 Reoperation

The reoperation should begin with careful removal of the packs and checking for further previously undiagnosed injuries. Solid organs require the most attention. The removal of packs should not cause new bleeding. Previously shunted vessels should be reconstructed. Repairs and anastomosis of the gastrointestinal organs can now be performed using traditional techniques. Drains should be placed if necessary.

12.5.4 Definitive Abdominal Wall Closure

When all lesions have been diagnosed and treated, the abdominal wall can be closed primarily. If possible, closure of the fascia is always the best option, keeping in mind that retraction may be a problem later on. It is, however, essential to monitor the IAP and to release the closure when the first signs of ACS appear or when pressure exceeds 20 mm H_2O. If primary closure of the fascia is not possible, a planned ventral hernia after skin closure is the best choice. Lateral separation of the fascia and other time-consuming techniques using skin graft or prosthetic materials may have the disadvantage of fostering wound infections and/or fistula. Once the patient has recovered, the ventral hernia can be repaired after 6 or more months.

References

1. Fabian TC (2007) Damage control in trauma: laparotomy wound management acute to chronic. Surg Clin North Am 87(1):73–93
2. Luchette FA, Borzotta AP, Croce MA et al (2000) Practice management guidelines for prophylactic antibiotic use in penetrating abdominal trauma: the EAST Practice Management Guidelines Work Group. J Trauma 48:508–518
3. Mattox KL, McCollum WB, Jordan et al (1974) Management of upper abdominal vascular trauma. Am J Surg 128(6):823–828
4. Mattox KL, Feliciano DV, Moore EE (2000) Trauma. McGraw-Hill, New York, pp 907–931
5. Moore EE, Burch JM, Franciose RJ (1998) Staged physiologic restoration and damage control surgery. World J Surgery 22:1184–1191
6. Rotondo MF, Schwab CW, McGonigal MD (1993) Damage control: an approach for improved survival in exsanguinating penetrating abdominal injury. J Trauma 35:375–383

Laparoscopic Procedures in Trauma Care

13

Selman Uranues, Abe Fingerhut, and Roberto Bergamaschi

13.1 Introduction

The first reports on the application of laparoscopy in trauma appeared in the 1970s, with a publication on laparoscopy for nonoperative management of penetrating trauma as early as 1970 by Heselson [5]. This was followed by the work of Gazzaniga et al. in 1976 [4] and Carnevale et al. in 1977 [2], who described their experience with diagnostic laparoscopy for penetrating abdominal injuries.

Minimally invasive techniques have assumed an important role in many areas of surgery, but it was only the developments of the last 15 years that have allowed laparoscopy and thoracoscopy to come into use as diagnostic and therapeutic tools in visceral trauma. Another important factor in this development is that the routine use of laparoscopy and thoracoscopy in elective surgery has furthered their application in other settings as well, even under the difficult circumstances posed by visceral trauma.

In most industrialized countries, trauma is the most common cause of death in the younger population under age 50. About one-half of the deaths take place within minutes at the site of the accident; these are usually severe head and cardiovascular injuries. Thirty percent of the deaths occur within a few hours of the injury and the remaining 20% after days to weeks due to infections and multiorgan failure. In the second group, in which victims die within a few hours, conservative estimates indicate that approximately 20–30% of them could be saved with timely diagnosis and proper treatment. Laparoscopy has come to play an increasing role in this concept. It is primarily a diagnostic measure, but when feasible, can also be applied therapeutically.

Although several diagnostic methods are available for evaluation of trauma patients, prompt recognition of intra-abdominal injury continues to pose a significant clinical challenge, particularly in patients who have no obvious indications for emergent surgery. The management of trauma patients should provide prompt diagnosis and appropriate timely treatment, and avoid complications.

13.2 Diagnosis with Blunt Abdominal Trauma

Obtaining information on the details of the accident is important for the understanding of the type of injuries. The clinical examination is an important part of the diagnostic work-up of trauma patients. Bruises and other marks on the body can point to organ injuries that may be present and should accordingly be carefully noted and examined (Fig. 13.1). Laboratory tests provide essential information on the extent of organ injuries and bleeding.

After the clinical examination, there are two radiological examinations that, owing to technological developments in the last two decades, provide high-quality information. These are ultrasound and CT, both

S. Uranues (✉)
Section for Surgical Research, Department of Surgery, Medical University of Graz, Graz, Austria
e-mail: selman.uranues@medunigraz.at

A. Fingerhut
Digestive and General Surgery Unit, Centre Hospitalier Intercommunal, Poissy, France
e-mail: abeFingerhut@aol.com

R. Bergamaschi
Division of Colon and Rectal Surgery, State University of New York, HSC T18-060, Stony Brook, NY, 11794-8191, USA
e-mail: lutz.sally@gmail.com

H.-J. Oestern et al. (eds.), *Head, Thoracic, Abdominal, and Vascular Injuries*,
DOI: 10.1007/978-3-540-88122-3_13, © Springer-Verlag Berlin Heidelberg 2011

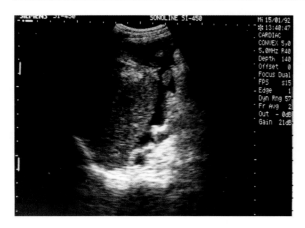

Fig. 13.1 Spleen injury with intra- and perisplenic fluid diagnosed by ultrasound

13.3 Why Laparoscopy?

Although these noninvasive methods provide high-quality information, there is still a degree of diagnostic uncertainty with blunt abdominal trauma, especially when the gastrointestinal tract and pancreas are involved. The considerable number of unnecessary exploratory laparotomies increases morbidity rates.

The literature shows that a variety of laparoscopic techniques can produce good results in patients with abdominal trauma. In a review by Villavicencio and Ancar [14], in two prospective studies, screening laparoscopy for blunt trauma showed a sensitivity of 90–100%, specificity of 86–100%, and accuracy of 88–100%. In nine prospective series, screening laparoscopy for penetrating trauma showed sensitivity of 85–100%, specificity of 73–100%, and accuracy of 80–100% with two procedure-related complications among 543 patients [11]. Diagnostic laparoscopy for blunt trauma had a sensitivity of 100%, specificity of 91%, and accuracy of 96%; for penetrating trauma, sensitivity was 80–100%, specificity 38–86%, and accuracy of 54–89% [14]. The rate of missed injuries at laparoscopy was 0.4% (6 of 1,708 patients). The rate of laparoscopy-related complications was 1.3% (22 of 1,672 patients) [14]. Laparoscopy may avoid laparotomy in 63% of patients presenting with a variety of injuries [14]. The laparoscopic approach avoids a negative laparotomy in 23–54% of stab wounds and blunt abdominal trauma patients [3]. Laparoscopy is cost effective when compared with negative laparotomy [12].

of which can be applied quickly and efficiently to trauma patients, although hemodynamic stability is a prerequisite for a CT.

Ultrasound can be performed in the emergency room with hand-held scanners, usually by general or trauma surgeons. The Focused Assessment for the Sonographic Examination of the Trauma Patient (FAST) protocol is intended to determine the presence of free fluid in the abdominal cavity and assess its quantity and location [1]. It is noninvasive and non-stressful and can be repeated as necessary. With portable equipment, ultrasound can be performed in emergency cases simultaneously with ongoing resuscitation without sedation, and can be done at the bedside without moving the patient. Rozycki et al. achieved a sensitivity of 83.3% and specificity of 99.7% in 1,540 patients with blunt and penetrating injuries [10].

CT is noninvasive and can provide valuable supplemental information on the size, number, and extent of pathological changes, and is operator independent. The findings can be determined precisely and reproducibly as opposed to ultrasound, which requires interpretation by an experienced operator at the time of scanning. CT has 97% sensitivity, 98% specificity, and 98% accuracy for peritoneal violation [11]. In detecting bowel injury, CT has an overall sensitivity of 94%, and 96% in detecting mesenteric injury [7].

Both ultrasound and CT are limited in diagnosing injuries to the diaphragm: Mihos et al. [9] achieved a correct preoperative diagnosis in only 26% of 65 patients with a diaphragmatic injury, and in 74% the diagnosis was made during the operation.

13.4 Selection of Patients

Patients should only undergo laparoscopy if trauma laparotomy is not indicated and when findings are unclear and require further investigation. Patients with blunt or penetrating trauma who are potential candidates for laparoscopy must have stable hemodynamic parameters. Those whose initial instability has been overcome relatively quickly in the process of resuscitation and who become and remain stable can also qualify for laparoscopy.

Laparoscopy candidates should have a CT study beforehand to increase the accuracy, reduce the rate of missed injuries, and prevent unnecessary surgeries.

13.5 Indications for Laparoscopy

The most common indications for laparoscopic diagnosis and treatment may be summarized as follows:

1. Blunt trauma – free fluid from unclear source
Patients who have free fluid in the peritoneal cavity after blunt abdominal trauma, but in whom the source of bleeding cannot be determined, can be treated conservatively. When the amount of free fluid increases or abdominal symptoms become more pronounced, an exploratory laparoscopy may be indicated. In these cases, a mesenteric laceration, often missed by CT scan, is usually found (Fig. 13.2).

2. Blunt trauma – suspected intestinal injury
When an intestinal laceration is suspected with blunt abdominal trauma, the extent of injury and/or of ongoing bleeding is usually unclear. Laparoscopy can provide a secure diagnosis with therapeutic potential (sewing over the laceration or resection) and so is a good and safe option.

3. Injury to the mesentery – vascular damage to the intestine
When CT has shown one or more mesenteric lacerations, but it is unclear whether the perfusion of the involved segment of the intestine is adequate or ischemic necrosis is a threat, laparoscopy can visualize the injury and help assess intestinal vitality, so that appropriate surgical measures can be taken (Fig. 13.3).

4. Unclear abdomen after blunt trauma
The term "unclear abdomen" indicates a discrepancy between the findings of imaging studies and clinical examination. In spite of conservative treatment, the patient's diffuse and unspecific symptoms do not improve. These symptoms may be due to pre-existing conditions such as volvulus or internal hernia that have nothing to do with the trauma. Laparoscopy can quickly clarify such situations and may also provide a therapeutic option.

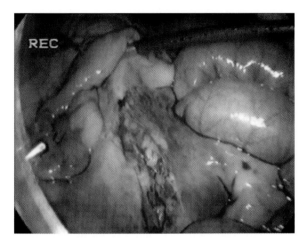

Fig. 13.2 Laparoscopic view of a mesenterial laceration in a case of blunt abdominal trauma

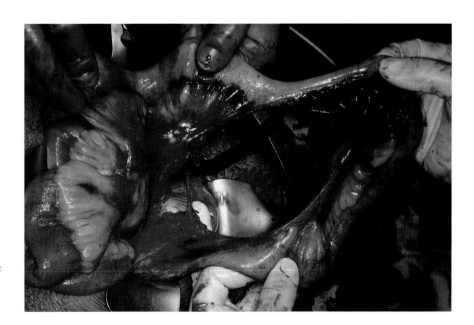

Fig. 13.3 Large mesenteric injury with devascularized small bowel primarily diagnosed by laparoscopy

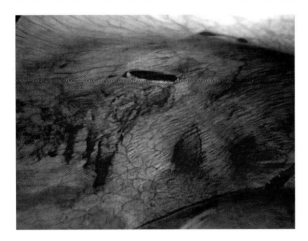

Fig. 13.4 Laparoscopic view of peritoneal damage by stab injury

5. Blunt trauma – solid organ injury – no time pressure
This is usually a matter of pancreas injury that does not require any immediate surgical or interventional radiologic treatment. If the clinical picture suggests it, these injuries can be debrided and drained laparoscopically.

6. Penetrating trauma – stable patient
With stab wounds, laparoscopy allows diagnosis of peritoneal penetration and subsequent exploration for other organ injuries (Fig. 13.4). Depending on severity, laparoscopic treatment of organ injuries such as those to the stomach wall or intestine may be possible. There is an increased advantage with diagonal thoraco-abdominal stab or gunshot wounds in the flank as a CT

diagnosis may miss an injury to the diaphragm. In these cases, the wound can be explored laparoscopically or thoracoscopically to determine whether laparotomy, thoracotomy, or a minimal access procedure is indicated.

13.6 How to Perform Laparoscopy in Trauma

The positioning and preparation of the patient for trauma laparoscopy are essentially the same as for a trauma laparotomy. Conversion to conventional open approach to the thorax and abdomen should be possible without delay or additional preparation. As for every trauma laparotomy, the inguinal region should be accessible (Fig. 13.5). The first access is achieved with open technique using a 10/11 mm trocar at the navel. Gas for the pneumoperitoneum should be insufflated slowly and carefully. If blood pressure drops or respiratory pressure suddenly rises, insufflation is to be stopped or the gas pressure reduced. In this case, laparoscopy can only be done with reduced gas pressure or gasless.

After a preliminary inspection of the entire abdominal cavity, two more 5–10 mm trocars are introduced on the right and left sides at the level of the umbilicus and lateral to the rectus muscle sheath (Fig. 13.6).

The abdomen is explored systematically, beginning with the right upper quadrant and proceeding clockwise.

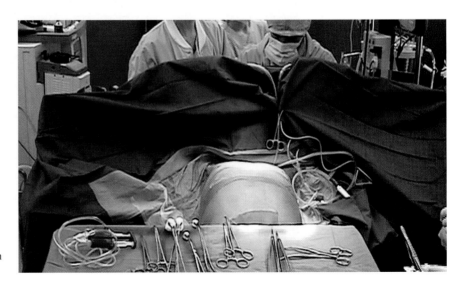

Fig. 13.5 Patient's position on operating table for laparotomy or laparoscopy in trauma case

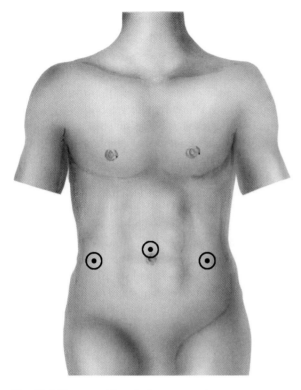

Fig. 13.6 Trocar positions for laparoscopy in trauma case

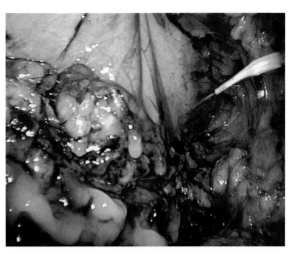

Fig. 13.7 Laparoscopic treatment of a pancreas lesion using fibrin glue

After a quick initial survey, the exploration continues in the same order for the second time. This time, blood is vacuumed off into a Cell Saver® device and the liver, including the subphrenic surface and the visceral fascia, is explored. It is advantageous during this phase of the operation to have the table in the anti-Trendelenburg position to shift the abdominal organs caudally because when the patient is in the supine position, the spleen is covered by the greater omentum and is not immediately visible. After the anterior wall of the stomach is inspected, the omentum is shifted caudally and the spleen is lifted from its bed with a blunt instrument. While the liver and spleen are being examined, the diaphragm can also be inspected. Even the most remote parts of the diaphragm can be seen much better laparoscopically than with open technique.

After the upper abdominal organs have been examined, the left flank with the left flexure, descending colon, and sigmoid are checked for injuries down to the left lower quadrant. The patient is placed in the Trendelenburg position for examination of the rectum, Douglas' space, urinary bladder, and, in women, the internal genital organs. The examination is continued in the right lower quadrant with the cecum and right hemicolon. The omentum is shifted cranially so that the small intestine can be examined. Using two atraumatic grasping forceps, the small intestine is followed from the ileocecal region in the oral direction to the duodenal-jejunal flexure (Fig. 13.3). Exploration of the duodenum, posterior gastric wall, and pancreas is only indicated when injury to these organs is suspected. It is justified when there are hematomas or thrombi adherent on these organs and/or on the basis of a CT image.

Treatment may depend on the equipment available and the surgeon's expertise. Simple lacerations of the intestine or mesentery can be sutured with monofilament 3/0 thread; however, extensive deceleration injuries to the intestines can only be treated quickly and safely with open technique. Small injuries to the diaphragm can be dealt with laparoscopically with sutures or suitable polytetrafluoroethylene (PTFE) prosthetic material. Active bleeding with blunt abdominal trauma requires open surgery. In stable patients, sources of bleeding, small vessels and those that have ceased bleeding, can be closed with 3/0 monofilament sutures or with modern coagulation devices (ultrasonic coagulator or Ligasure™). Large wound surfaces and lacerations of solid organs can be quickly and effectively sealed laparoscopically with autologous fibrin adhesive (Vivostat®, Vivolution, Allerød, Denmark) (Fig. 13.7) and tamponaded in combination with collagen fleece (Lyostypt®, B. Braun Melsungen AG, Melsungen, Germany) (Fig. 13.8). Laparoscopy is not

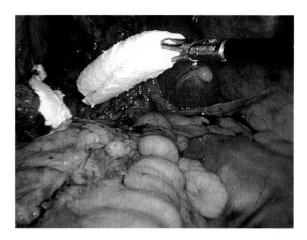

Fig. 13.8 Laparoscopic collagen fleece tamponade of the pancreas lesion shown in Fig. 13.7

indicated for surgery of actively bleeding spleen and liver injuries; this is still a domain of open surgery.

In the course of a laparoscopic exploration of the abdomen, nonbleeding or slightly oozing solid organ injuries can be treated laparoscopically with one of the above-mentioned techniques. The treatment of a solid organ injury should, however, never be the primary task of minimal access surgery. In stable patients, liver and spleen injuries that do not show active bleeding upon CT are handled conservatively without surgery [13]. If laparoscopy is required to rule out intestinal injury, the measures mentioned above can be applied to prevent renewed bleeding.

Trauma laparoscopy can be complicated in patients with extensive adhesions. In such cases, adhesiolysis should be limited, on the basis of CT findings, to the suspicious area. Extensive laparoscopic adhesiolysis can take more time than with the open technique and entail higher morbidity.

13.7 The Risks of Laparoscopy in Trauma

Laparoscopy in blunt abdominal trauma entails three risks, which, in order of their frequency and importance, are as follows:

1. Considerably increased morbidity when injuries, mainly involving the intestinal tract, are overlooked and their treatment so delayed

2. Laparoscopy-specific complications, such as vascular and intestinal injuries
3. Gas embolism

Missed injuries are the most common of these three problems and probably pose the most serious risk, though the data in the current literature are very unclear on this. Although some authors find that laparoscopy is inadequate for detecting intestinal injuries [6, 8], other centers, including ours, do not report any missed injuries [3]. Even a very experienced surgeon should not hesitate to convert to open technique if there is any uncertainty. Although it is theoretically possible, gas embolism has not yet been reported in trauma patients with intra-abdominal venous injuries.

The main benefits of laparoscopy are reduction in the rate of nontherapeutic and negative laparotomies, accurate identification of diaphragmatic injuries, and in some cases provision of a therapeutic option. It should be emphasized that the use of laparoscopy as a diagnostic or therapeutic method in trauma patients is strictly limited to hemodynamically stable patients. It should be noted that laparoscopy has limitations in the diagnosis of hollow viscus injury. Laparoscopy can detect and repair diaphragmatic injuries and exclude the risk of nontherapeutic laparotomy due to a nonbleeding injury of the spleen or liver. Further advantages are reduced morbidity, shortened hospital stay, and lower cost.

Minimal access surgery has become established as a useful tool in the management of trauma patients. Laparoscopy can be performed safely and effectively in stable patients with abdominal trauma. The future holds exciting prospects for this field of surgery through innovative developments in CT and robotic systems.

References

1. Ballard RB, Rozycki GS, Newman PG et al (1999) An algorithm to reduce the incidence of false-negative FAST examinations in patients at high risk for occult injury. J Am Coll Surg 189:145–151
2. Carnevale N, Baron N, Delany HM (1977) Peritoneoscopy as an aid in the diagnosis of abdominal trauma: a preliminary report. J Trauma 17:634–641
3. Chol YB, Lim KS (2003) Therapeutic laparoscopy for abdominal trauma. Surg Endosc 17:421–427
4. Gazzaniga AB, Stanton WW, Bartlett RH (1976) Laparoscopy in the diagnosis of blunt and penetrating injuries to the abdomen. Am J Surg 131:315–318

5. Heselson J (1970) Peritoneoscopy in abdominal trauma. S Afr J Surg 8:53–61

6. Ivatury RR, Simon RJ, Siahl WM (1993) A critical evaluation of laparoscopy in penetrating abdominal trauma. J Trauma 34:822–828

7. Killeen KL, Shanmunagathan K, Poletti PA et al (2001) Helical computed tomography of bowel and mesenteric injuries. J Trauma 51:26–36

8. Livingstone DH, Tortella BJ, Blackwood J et al (1992) The role of laparoscopy in abdominal trauma. J Trauma 33(3):471–475

9. Mihos P, Potaris K, Gakidis J et al (2003) Traumatic rupture of the diaphragm: Experience with 65 patients. Injury 34:169–172

10. Rozycki GS, Ballard RB, Feliciano DV et al (1998) Surgeon-performed ultrasound for the assessment of truncal injuries: lessons learned from 1540 patients. Ann Surg 228:557–567

11. Shanmunagathan K, Mirvis SE, Chiu WC et al (2004) Penetrating torso trauma: triple contrast helical CT in peritoneal violation and organ injury – a prospective study in 200 patients. Radiology 231:775–784

12. Smith RS, Fry WR, Morabito DJ et al (1995) Therapeutic laparoscopy in trauma. Am J Surg 170:632–636

13. Uranüs S, Pfeifer J (2001) Nonoperative treatment of blunt splenic injury. World J Surg 5:1405–1407

14. Villavicencio RT, Aucar JA (1999) Analysis of laparoscopy in trauma. J Am Coll Surg 189:11–20

Traumatic Injury of the Urogenital System

14

Corinne Wanner Schmid and Daniel Max Schmid

14.1 Introduction

Traumatic injuries to genitourinary organs are rare and mostly occur in patients with multiple injuries. Bony structures or truncal muscles protect the internal genitourinary organs, and the mobility of the penis and scrotum helps prevent injury to these organs. Traumatic lesions of the external organs are diagnosed clinically in most of the cases, whereas injury to the kidneys and bladder require radiologic and rarely operative evaluation. Therefore knowledge about the trauma mechanism leading to a specific kind of genitourinary organ lesion is important [1]. Involvement of an urologist in suspected injuries at an early stage of treatment should be advocated, as some trauma surgeons may not be familiar with specific requirements regarding diagnostic procedures and surgical techniques.

This chapter will give an insight into epidemiology, trauma mechanisms leading to specific genitourinary organ lesions, diagnostic procedures, and therapeutic strategies applied.

14.2 Epidemiology

There are few epidemiological data regarding trauma of the genitourinary tract. A prospective data collection in Scotland revealed that of 24,666 trauma patients, only 1.5% had injuries of the urogenital system [2]. Based on general population, this represents one case per 45,000 people per year. Of these, 14% had isolated genitourinary trauma; however, of all patients with abdominal trauma, 22% had associated genitourinary trauma. This survey included patients with blunt and penetrating trauma, with 79% of all genitourinary cases being due to blunt trauma mechanism.

A large survey from France including 43,056 victims of road traffic accidents showed that 0.46% of patients had suffered from genitourinary trauma, motorists being the largest group affected, followed by motorcyclists, cyclists, and pedestrians [3].

In the United States, approximately 10% of traumatic injuries involve the genitourinary organs [4]. Of all renal injuries, up to 4% and 16% are due to gunshots alone or gunshots and stabbing, respectively [5, 6].

The kidneys are, by far, the most commonly affected organ with up to 67% of all genitourinary trauma cases. In populations including penetrating trauma like gunshot wounds, bladder injuries are the second largest group, with up to 18 % of patients affected [2]. In populations with mainly road traffic accident victims, injuries to external genitourinary organs like testicles and penis are second and third most common, with up to 24% and 11% of patients concerned, respectively, followed by bladder injuries (9%) and scrotum injuries (8%) [3]. Injuries to the urethra (up to 4%) and ureters (approximately 1%) are rare in all populations [2, 3].

14.3 Trauma Mechanism and Related Urogenital Injuries

14.3.1 Kidneys and Ureter

The majority of kidney injuries are caused by blunt trauma from motor vehicle accident, assault or fall from

C.Wanner Schmid and D.M. Schmid (✉)
Department of Urology, University Hospital Zurich,
Frauenklinikstrasse 10, 8091, Zurich, Switzerland
e-mail: daniel.max.schmid@usz.ch

H.-J. Oestern et al. (eds.), *Head, Thoracic, Abdominal, and Vascular Injuries*,
DOI: 10.1007/978-3-540-88122-3_14, © Springer-Verlag Berlin Heidelberg 2011

heights. The amount of deceleration force can provide an indication of the extent of the lesion. With rapid and major deceleration from high speed or height, the kidney can be torn at the renal pedicle, one of the two of its fixing points, the other being the ureter. Injury to the renal vascular system has been seen in up to 4–10% of renal trauma cases [6, 7], leading to renal artery thrombosis due to intimal lesions, renal vein disruption or renal pedicle avulsion. Other possible injury mechanisms are lateral impact to the flank, flexion on the costal margin or crushing against the vertebral column, all of these leading to parenchymal laceration or disruption [3]. The extent of renal injuries by penetrating trauma depends on the velocity of the bullet entering the body. High velocity, small distance to target, bullet size and certain types of guns are risk factors for extended soft tissue damage [8]. In stab wounds, the length and width of the weapon provides information about the depth of the wound and the possible extent of the injury. Ninety percent of renal injuries are associated with abdominal trauma [9].

Ureteral injury is rare in nonmilitary settings and in most cases due to penetrating trauma. The majority of the patients have associated abdominal trauma, isolated injury is rare. Of all abdominal organs, the small and large bowels are the most frequently affected. Associated kidney injury can occur in up to approximately 20% of patients. Mortality is as high as 29% [10, 11]. Ureteral trauma from blunt force results from impact of great energy on the body and is associated with uncommon injury patterns of the vertebral column.

14.3.2 Bladder and Urethra

Blunt injuries to the bladder are caused by rapid deceleration in motor vehicle crashes, falls and assaults with impact on the lower abdomen. They are almost always associated with fracture of the pelvis, which normally is a natural protection to the bladder, and located extraperitoneally. Tear at its fascial fixing causes disruption, however direct injury by bone fragments can also be found [5, 12]. Intraperitoneal bladder rupture can occur after frontal impact with rapid deceleration of a full bladder. In one review of 111 patients with bladder trauma, 89% were due to blunt trauma, and 90% occurred after motor vehicle accident [13]. Penetrating bladder trauma from gunshot or stabbing is often associated with significant injury of other organs.

Injury of the posterior urethra can be found in patients with pelvic fracture involving the pubic part. The number of fractured pubic rami and involvement of the sacroiliac joint are risk factors for urethral involvement. Because of the anatomical fixation to the urogenital diaphragm and puboprostatic ligaments, the bulbomembranous part is the most vulnerable [14]. Multiple injuries of other organs are often associated.

Anterior urethral injuries are rare and often isolated, resulting from direct blunt impact of force, e.g. straddle injury, and involve mainly the bulbar urethra. The anterior urethra can also be injured with direct penetrating trauma to the penis or penile fracture.

14.3.3 Penis, Testicles, and Scrotum

Injuries to the penis and scrotum are commonly due to blunt trauma. In road traffic accidents, motor-cyclists typically suffer from crushing of the penis and testicles between the pelvis and the fuel tank, whereas in cyclists, penile and scrotal trauma from impact of the handlebars occurs [3].

Penis fracture can occur during sexual intercourse, when the erected penis slips out of the vagina and crushes against the bony pelvis (faux-pas du coït), causing a rupture of the corpus cavernosum. Other mechanisms leading to this pattern of trauma are seen after masturbation or crushing of the erected penis in various circumstances.

Gunshot wounds to the penis are associated with other injuries to the pelvis, abdomen, blood vessels or other genitourinary organs in the majority of cases. Other penetrating trauma mechanisms include animal and human bites, amputation due to self-mutilation and zipper injury, and strangulation.

Injuries to testes and scrotum can also arise from sports accidents, assaults, gunshots or impalement.

14.4 Diagnostic Procedures

14.4.1 Clinical Evaluation
            and Imaging Studies

Injury to the genitourinary system should be suspected in polytrauma patients, especially when great decelerating force has been present and the initial clinical evaluation shows fracture of lower ribs or vertebra in the thoracolumbar region; hematomas to the flank, abdomen or external genitalia; tenderness of the abdomen; fracture of the pelvis; stab or gunshot wounds to the lower thoracic region, flank, abdomen or pelvic region; and hematuria.

Hematuria is the main indicator of trauma to the genitourinary system [4]. However, the absence of hematuria does not exclude injuries to genitourinary organs.

If the patient is initially presenting with hemodynamic instability in spite of adequate resuscitation, hypotension with penetrating abdominal wounds, and overt bleeding from genitourinary tract with penetrating trauma, an emergency celiotomy is indicated.

14.4.2 Kidney

Fractures of lower ribs, thoracic or lumbar vertebras or hematomas to the lower thorax region or the flank are clinical signs suggestive of renal trauma. Urine should be collected promptly and the presence of gross or microscopic hematuria determined. The amount of hematuria, if present, does not correlate with the severity of genitourinary trauma [15]. With injuries of the renal vascular system, hematuria is absent in one-third of cases [16].

Computed tomography (CT) is the imaging method of choice (Fig. 14.6). Its high sensitivity and specificity, the ability of assessing concomitant injuries of other organs, and the possibility of precisely assessing the type and extent of injury make it far more valuable than the traditionally used intravenous urography. The presence and location of a renal hematoma with or without active arterial extravasation, the presence of urinary extravasation or of devascularized segments of renal parenchyma can be evaluated. Most important, CT can help determine whether the injury requires surgical intervention [17]. Early and delayed phase CT with contrast enhancement are needed to completely assess the renovascular system, and the excretory-phase CT imaging should be performed 3 or more min after contrast medium injection to assess an eventual collecting system injury [18].

Intravenous urography has mostly been replaced by CT but still can be helpful in intraoperative setting during abdominal exploration when unexpected findings have to be evaluated.

Ultrasonography is a valuable and readily available diagnostic tool in the emergency setting and has proven to be helpful in detecting free fluid in the intra- and retroperitoneum, but has proven to be unreliable in detecting renal parenchymal lesions of the kidney, as

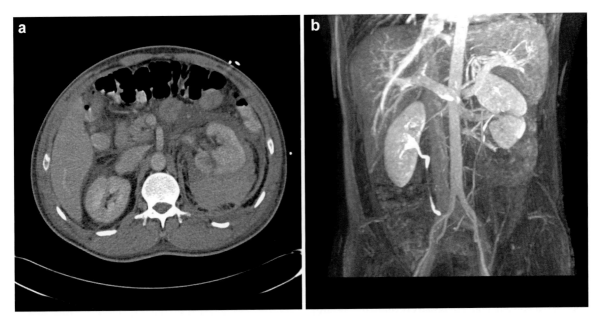

Fig. 14.1 (**a**) CT scan showing Grade III renal injury with deep parenchymal laceration through corticomedullary junction and perirenal hematoma on the left side (**b**) Angiography 5 months after conservative management, presenting complete renal healing

only four out of seven patients with such injury were initially diagnosed sonographically in a series of 121 trauma patients [19].

Arteriography can define renal lacerations (Fig. 14.8), extravasation, and pedicle injury as well as, renal venous injuries can best be evaluated thereby [17].

14.4.3 Ureter

Ureteral lesions are difficult to diagnose and a high index of suspicion is required in accidents involving gunshots, stab wounds or falls from great height resulting in injuries such as fractured lumbar process and thoracolumbar spinal dislocation. Hematuria is not a reliable finding; In one study including 20 patients, only 53% of initially detected ureteral lesions had gross or microscopic hematuria [10]. Therefore, recognition can be delayed and ureteral injury only detected after occurrence of secondary complications such as infection, sepsis or urinoma.

CT with late excretory- phase contrast-enhancement images is the diagnostic tool of choice. However, some patients will be diagnosed intraoperatively, as the associated injuries will require emergency celiotomy. Intraoperative intravenous urography can be helpful in this situation, as visual evaluation of the ureters can be difficult in patients with abdominal trauma.

14.4.4 Bladder

Clinical symptoms such as lower abdominal pain, suprapubic tenderness, and bruising are unspecific and can be masked by general abdominal tenderness in abdominal trauma. Differentiation from pelvic fracture sequelae can be difficult. Gross hematuria is present in nearly all (95–100%) patients with blunt bladder injury and is the most reliable clinical symptom [20, 21]. If diagnosis has been missed or delayed, fever, peritonitis, inability to void and elevated serum urea can occur. If the patient is hemodynamically stable, retrograde cystography with 350–400 ml of 30% iodine contrast medium, applied passively into the urethra catheter (40 cm H_2O water pressure), should be performed. Plain abdominal (a-p views), RX-ray films at

full bladder and after drainage should follow [22]: diagnostic accordance reaches up to 100% in detecting major bladder injuries. [20] (Fig.14.1 and Fig. 14.4).

Abdomen CT is generally inferior to retrograde cystography for detecting bladder leakage, unless injection of 2–4% contrast medium into the bladder is additionally given during CT scan [23]. In one study, conventional CT has an accuracy rate of only 60% for bladder injury [24]. However, whether or not a patient should undergo a retrograde cystogram examination depends mainly on his/her general condition rather than solely on the presence or absence of hematuria.

14.4.5 Urethra

The typical triad of urethral disruption is blood at the meatus, inability to urinate, and urinary retention with full bladder at palpation [25]. The pattern of distribution of hematoma can be useful in identifying the anatomical boundaries violated by the injury: Blood extravasation along the penile shaft indicates an injury confined by Buck's fascia, whereas disruption of the latter results in a pattern of extravasation limited by Colles' fascia, extending to the coracoclavicular fascia superiorly and the fascia lata inferiorly; this results in a characteristic butterfly pattern of bruising in the perineum. High-riding prostate is a relatively unreliable clinical finding in the acute phase, since pelvic hematoma often precludes adequate digital palpation of a small prostate in younger men.

An immediate retrograde urethrogram should be performed to rule out or demonstrate urethral injury, introducing a small (14–16 French) catheter into the fossa navicularis and blocked with 1–2 cl water; for fluoroscopy, the patient should be placed in an oblique/lateral declined position, then 25–30 ml contrast medium is gently injected [26]. In females, where a short urethra precludes adequate urethrography, urethroscopy is an important adjunct to physical examination [27].

14.4.6 Penis

Preoperative imaging for penile fracture should never delay surgical repair. If an associated urethral injury is

Fig. 14.2 (**a**) Selective catheterization and angiography of a bleeding renal cortical artery. (**b**) Bleeding stop after successful application of coils

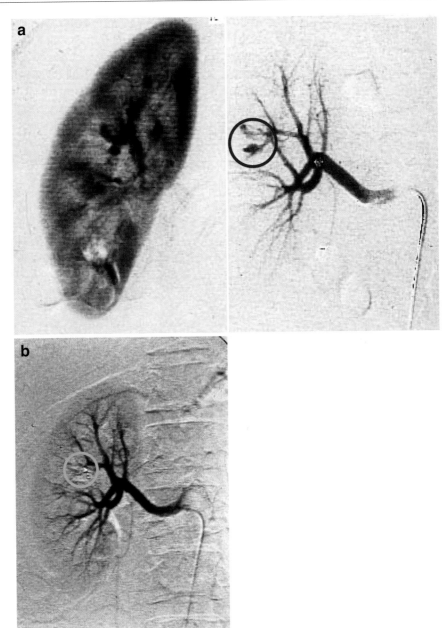

suspected, flexible cystoscopy is recommended in the OP room, as opposed to a retrograde urethrogram [28]. The typical clinical sign of a rupture of the tunica albuginea is local swelling of the penile shaft associated with progressive hematoma occurring along the fascia layers and giving the aspect of an eggplant. MRI and/or cavernosography can help identify or exclude a rupture of the tunica albuginea in unclear cases (Fig. 14.7).

14.4.7 Testes and Scrotum

Scrotal pain, nausea, tender swollen scrotum, and a palpatory indistinguishable testis are the clinical signs of blunt scrotal trauma. High-resolution ultrasonography (with 7.5–10 MHz probe) of the scrotum can help detecting injury of the testis (contusion or rupture of tunica albuginea) and hematoma after blunt scrotal trauma when it is not clinically visible, as this can be the

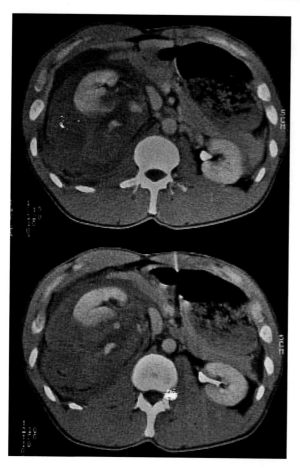

patients with isolated kidney injury showed increased mortality, need for operative repair, and length of stay for higher (grades IV&V) to lower grade injury [33], consistent with findings in previous studies [34, 35]. A retrospective survey including 8,465 patients found that increasing injury rate and age were predictive for nephrectomy, dialysis, and mortality rate in patients with blunt renal trauma, whereas for penetrating renal trauma only nephrectomy rates were higher in the multivariate analysis [36].

For ureter trauma, one survey including 57 patients found that higher injury grade was associated with more complex surgical repair procedure and mortality resulting from increased number of associated injuries. All except the five patients with grade I injury did require surgical repair [37].

Regarding trauma to male external genitalia, the data of 116 patients were collected and grading of injury retrospectively undertaken in one study [38]. The authors concluded that the grading scale helped to identify those with higher grade injury in need of surgical repair as well as selecting those in which nonoperative treatment can be attempted.

Fig. 14.3 Grade IV renal injury with gross perirenal hematoma and parenchymal laceration into collecting system of the right kidney

case in open scrotal lacerations (Fig. 14.10). Information regarding testicular perfusion may be increased by color Doppler-duplex ultrasonography [29].

14.4.8 AAST-Grading Scale of Renal Injury

The America Association for the Surgery of Trauma (AAST) has published an injury scaling and scoring system that provides a scaling system for injury to specific organs, including the kidneys (Table 14.1), ureter, bladder, urethra, penis, testes, and scrotum [30–32]. Studies regarding validation of these scales have been published for kidney, ureter, and male external genitalia. For kidney trauma, one large study including 9,433

14.4.9 EAU-Classification of Blunt Anterior and Posterior Urethra Trauma [Adapted according to EAU Guidelines 2007]

Type I comprises stretch injury that does not require treatment. Type II (Contusion with blood at meatus without extravasation) and Type III (partial disruption of anterior or posterior urethra with contrast extravasation at injury site with visualization of proximal urethra/bladder) can be managed conservatively with suprapubic cystostomy or urethral catheterisation. Type IV (complete disruption of anterior urethra with contrast extravasation at injury site without visualization of proximal urethra/bladder) and Type V (complete disruption of posterior urethra with contrast extravasation at injury site without visualization of bladder) will require open or endoscopic treatment, primary or delayed. Type VI (complete or partial disruption of posterior urethra with associated tear of the bladder neck or vagina) requires primary open repair.

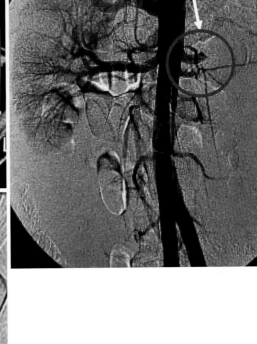

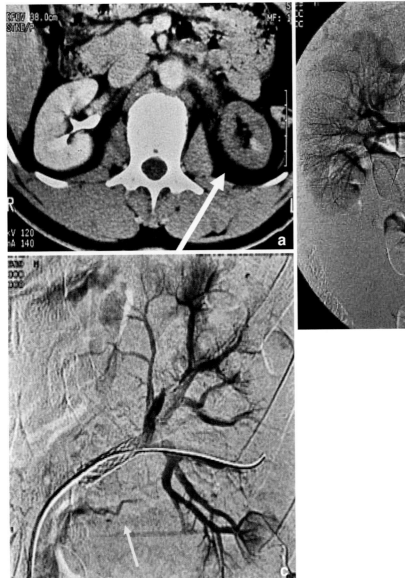

Fig. 14.4 Bike accident blunt trauma with Grade IV renal injury: (**a**) No perfusion of the left kidney on CT scan (*arrow*). (**b**) renovascular injury (thrombosis of **a** renalis) in angiography.

(**c**) The same patient after thrombolysis and stent application of **a** renalis and embolization of a bleeding pole artery (arrow)

14.5 Therapy

14.5.1 *Renal and Ureteral Trauma*

Due to improved radiographic techniques such as CT scans and validated injury-screening systems, nonoperative management of renal injuries increased in the past two decades [39]. Ninety-eight percent of blunt renal trauma can be managed nonoperatively, if the patient is hemodynamically stable with the injury well-staged in CT scan. Grades I-IV isolated blunt renal injuries, occurring commonly from blunt trauma, can be managed conservatively (nonoperatively) in most cases with bed rest, prophylactic antibiotics, and continuous monitoring of vital signs until hematuria resolves (Fig. 14.3). Stable patients with Grades I-III stab and low-velocity gunshot wounds should also be selected for expectant management after complete staging.

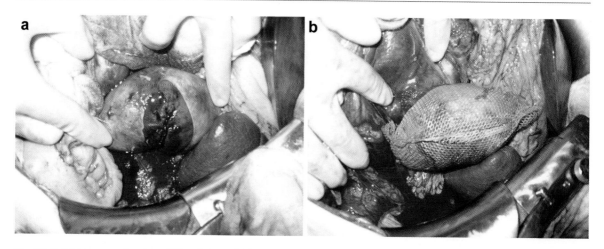

Fig. 14.5 (**a**) intraoperative situs of blunt left renal injury Grade III cortical laceration. (**b**) Operative repair with mesh wrapping of the renal wound

Table 14.1 Renal injury grading scale

Grade	Description of Injury
1	Contusion or non-expanding subcapsular hematoma. No laceration
2	Non-expanding perirenal hematoma; Cortical laceration >1 cm deep without extravasation
3	Cortical laceration >1 cm without urinary extravasation
4	Laceration: through corticomedullary junction into collecting system or: Vascular: segmental renal artery or vein injury with contained hematoma, or partial vessel laceration or vessel thrombosis
5	Laceration; shattered kidney or: Vascular: renal pedicle avulsion

However, there are some absolute indications for renal and renovascular explorations including: (1) hemodynamic instability (hypovolemic shock), (2) exploration for associated injuries, (3) expanding and/or pulsatile perirenal hematoma identified during laparotomy, whereas nonexpanding retroperitoneal hematoma can be managed successfully by nonoperative therapy [40, 41], (4) Grade V lesions with suspected renal pedicle avulsion, always presenting with hemodynamic instability, thus needing immediate operative exploration. Also, (5), incidental finding of pre-existing renal pathology requires surgical therapy (e.g., suspected renal tumors).

Renal exploration with reconstruction should be attempted in cases where the primary goal of controlling hemorrhage is achieved and a sufficient amount of renal parenchyma is viable [EAU Guidelines 2007]. In a study, 23.5% of patients with penetrating renal injuries of Grades III-V showed delayed bleeding and, therefore, had to undergo exploration and renal repair [42].

Absence of ureter visualization on delayed contrast medium CT scans or medial urine extravasation after major renal trauma is a sign of ureteropelvic junction avulsion/disruption or severe renal pelvis injury with consecutive massive urinoma that requires urgent operative repair. However, isolated urine extravasation can be occasionally observed, and spontaneous healing has been represented in up to 91% of these cases [43]. If extravasation persists in control CT scan 2 days after trauma, the indication is given for retrograde ureteral stent placement for the duration of about 6 weeks followed by placement of bladder-indwelling catheter for at least 1 week until hematuria resolves [40].

Persistent bleeding with hemodynamic instability, requiring >3 U RBC, urine extravasation, and devitalized renal parenchyma represent a relative indication to operative intervention [39]. In case of persistent hemorrhage, selective angio-embolization can be tried alternatively [44]. Low retroperitoneal urine extravasation can be managed by retrograde placement of a double-J ureteral stent.

Whereas exploratory laparotomy was commonly recommended for penetrating abdominal trauma with associated renal injuries, there is enough evidence today for a more selective management [42]. Absence of major blood loss as well as absence of intra-abdominal injury, major renal parenchyma and vessel trauma should allow conservative approach. On the other hand, penetrating renal vessel injuries lead to nephrectomy in 32% of

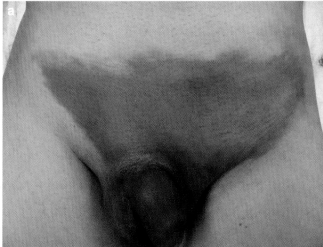
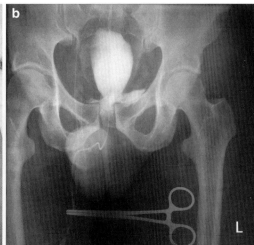
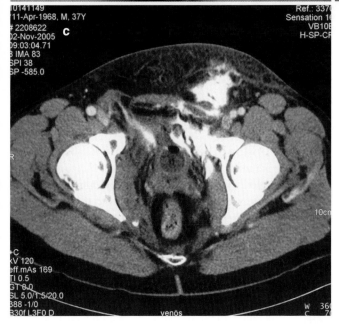

Fig. 14.6 (**a**) Clinical aspect of blunt posterior urethral trauma (pelvic injury with disruption of symphysis pubis) with subfascial hematoma/urinoma. (**b**) Retrograde contrast medium filling reveals extravasation at bladder neck. (**c**) CT scan showing contrast medium subfascial extravasation

patients studied, as vascular repair of grade V injuries is often rather challenging and has generally a negative outcome [45]. On the other hand, segmental arterial injuries show a better outcome, as need for blood transfusion is less common. Repair of isolated vein injuries is associated with good outcome and renal function.

The management of thrombosis of main renal artery is recommended, but repairs should only be attempted within an ischemia time of under 5 h in hemodynamically stable patients , the success rate being low; hence, nephrectomy should otherwise be performed [46]. Alternatively,

endovascular stents can be successfully placed during angiography in patients with renal artery thrombosis occurring from intimal flaps [47] (Fig. 14.11).

Still under controversial discussion is the standard management of grade IV renal injuries; In, but at least in cases of penetrating wounds with concomitant trauma operative exploration is undoubtedly the right approach. A renal salvage rate of 83% of grade IV trauma was achieved in a series of 153 patients managed operatively versus nonoperatively [41]. Grade IV parenchyma laceration with well-contained retroperitoneal hematoma

Fig. 14.7 Intraoperative aspect of bladder dome rupture

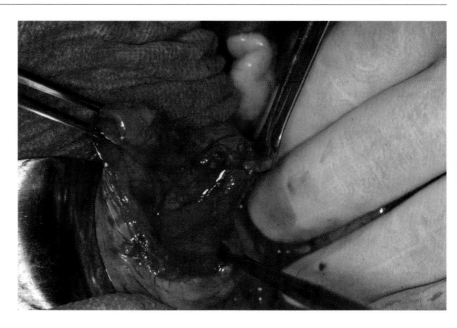

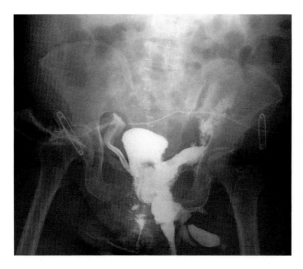

Fig. 14.8 Severe pelvic injury with disruption of symphysis pubis and bladder neck injury, proven by contrast medium extravasation in retrograde cystogram

can be treated non- operatively, though being closely monitored for delayed bleeding. Larger sections (>25%) of devascularized and devitalized renal parenchyma, associated with increased morbidity, should be removed operatively.

To avoid or lessen the possibility of perinephric abscess, use of antibiotics is strongly recommended [39]. Once gross hematuria clears, ambulation is allowed with close clinical follow-up.

14.5.1.1 OP-Technique

Kidney

A standard midline abdominal incision allows complete inspection of intra-abdominal organs and intentine and provides access to the retroperitoneum for renal exploration and repair. Renal exploration should be done in the following four general steps:

1. Isolation of the main renal vessels should be the first step to provide immediate capability to occlude them if massive bleeding ensues when Gerota's fascia is opened [48]. This procedure leads to lower nephrectomy rate by early controlling gross hemorrhage [49]. After lifting the transverse colon and small bowel onto the upper/right abdomen, an incision is made over the aorta from the inferior mesenteric artery to the ligamentum of Treitz, medial to the inferior mesenteric vein (Fig. 14.13). After identifying the renal vessels, vessel loops are used to mark them, allowing occlusion if needed (limited to <30 min. warm ischemia).

2. Complete exposure of the injured kidney by incising the peritoneum lateral to the colon, releasing of splenic splenic (Fig. 14.14) or hepatic (right) attachments, followed by mobilization and opening

of Gerota's fascia at this point. The kidney is completely dissected from the surrounding hematoma and fat tissue, followed by debridement of devitalized parenchyma. The isolated vessels can be temporally occluded, if gross hematuria occurs.

3. Watertight closure of the collecting system, if lesion is present, is provided by running 3–0 absorbable sutures. Diluted methylene blue solution can be retrogradely injected into the renal pelvis, the proximal ureter being temporally occluded, to check tightness and to rule out further collecting system injuries.

4. Hemostasis is obtained with absorbable 4–0 sutures on bleeding parenchymal vessels and with administering hemostatic agents. Closure of the parenchymal injuries and defects and approximation of the margins of the laceration is obtained by use of renal capsule, absorbable Gelatine bolsters, and absorbable 3–0 sutures allowing good hemostasis by renorrhaphy. A pedicle flap of omentum or absorbable mesh, placed around the kidney in a wrapping manner, can additionally be used to cover open parenchyma. (Fig. 14.12) If reconstruction of upper or lower polar injuries is impossible, partial nephrectomy and removal of nonviable tissue should be performed. Stab wounds can often be closed by simple approximation of entry wounds margins. If possible, Gerota's fascia should be readapted to provide hemostasis.

Renal vascular injuries are associated with gross blood loss. Therefore, main renal artery lacerations or avulsions commonly lead to nephrectomy; if the hemodynamic situation of the patient allows it, repair should at least be attempted. Main renal vein injuries can be closed by running 5–0 prolene sutures while temporarily occluding the main renal artery. Renal artery thrombosis due to disruption of intima can be successfully treated by the use of endovascular stents; however, the disadvantage of this procedure is the inability to begin anticoagulation.

In patients with extensive injuries, renal salvage can be improved by damage-control procedures. The injured kidney is packed with laparotomy pads and a second-look planned 24 h later to explore the extent of injury [50].

Immediate total nephrectomy is indicated in extensive renovascular injuries, especially when the patient's life would be threatened by attempted renal repair, in the presence of hemodynamic instability.

Follow-Up, Outcome, Complications

Guidelines on postoperative management and follow-up (adapted from EAU Guidelines 2007):

Strict bed rest is recommended, until gross hematuria resolves and serial hematocrit values keep stable. If gross hematuria in nonoperated patients persists more

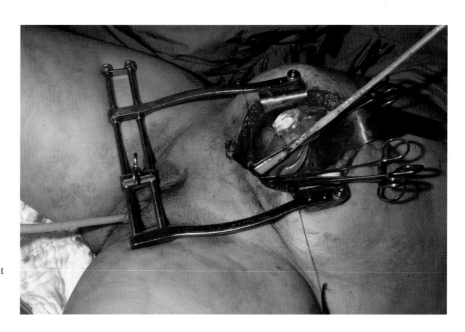

Fig. 14.9 Female patient with blunt pelvic injury and bladder neck disruption: intraoperative open alignment with catheter inserted transurethrally into the bladder

than 7–10 days, strict bed rest and selected angioembolization should be performed [51].

1. Repeated imaging (CT with 10 min. delayed films) is recommended within 2–4 days following significant renal trauma (grade IV/V injury), particularly in hospitalized patients with fever, flank pain or dropping hematocrit. Routine follow-up imaging is unnecessary for blunt renal injuries of grades I-III. Grade IV renovascular injury can be followed clinically without routine early follow-up imaging, but urine extravasation necessitates serial imaging to guide management decisions [52].
2. Nuclear scintigraphy before discharge is useful for documenting functional recovery.
3. Within 3 months of major renal injury, patients' follow-up should involve: physical examination, urinalysis, radiological investigation, serial blood pressure measurement, and serum determination of renal function.
4. Long-term follow-up at least involve monitoring for renovascular hypertension. Performance of other diagnostic procedures should be done according to the individual case.

Secondary hemorrhage (20% of nonoperatively managed stab wounds show delayed renal bleeding!), can occur several weeks (up to 21 days) after injury. Then, bed rest, hydratation, followed by angiography and, if needed, embolization, are indicated.

AV-fistulas and pseudoaneurysms are rare. In cases of perinephric abscess or infected urinoma, percutaneous drainage, antibiotics, and perhaps surgery and ureter stents are needed. Posttraumatic hypertension, mainly caused by renovascular injury, stenosis, and occlusion of the A. renalis are estimated to occur in less than 5% of cases [53]. Treatment is required if hypertension persists and may include drug treatment, vascular reconstruction or total nephrectomy.

Ureter

Minor ureteral injuries as external contusion often can be treated by retrograde placing of a stent for the duration of 6–8 weeks. Ureteral injuries often heal with stricture if microvascular injury results in necrosis of the mucosa. Therefore, severe or large contusion areas should be excised, followed by uretero-ureterostomy. Because of the tenuous blood supply of the ureter, mobilization should be done very carefully, widely sparing the adventitia, and debridement should be done until edges of the ureteral stumps bleed. Anastomosis then should be performed tension-free, stented, watertight and with ends of the ureter spatulated, using 5–0 resorbable sutures [54]. End-to-end uretero-ureterostomy repair is commonly used in the upper two-thirds of the ureter in up to 32% of cases with a high success rate of 90% [11, 55]. Delayed ureteral repairs, when a very large segment of ureter is destroyed, can be performed using bowel interpositions of tubularized ileum segments (Monti procedure) or appendix [56, 57]. Alternatively, the transuretero-ureterostomy technique (bringing the injured ureter across the midline and anastomosing it end-to-side into the contralateral ureter) is rarely used today but often successful (90–97%). This method can be problematic in patients with ureteral cancer or repeated stone formation though, possibly leading to surgery or the implantation of stents.

Distal ureteral injuries should be repaired by ureterocystoneostomy. If the distance between the bladder and the ureteral stump is too large, or if the injury being proximal of ureter vessels crossing, the psoas hitch and/or the Boari flap procedure can be used, with a high success rate of 95–100% for both techniques [58].

In cases of surgical injury, as ligation or transection, the former should be treated by removal of the ligature and placement of a stent, eventually by uretero-ureterostomy or reimplantation if viability is questionable; the latter should immediately be reanastomosed [59]. Nephrectomy is controversial and should only be performed in patients undergoing vascular prosthetic graft implantation because of potential urine leakage contaminating aortic or iliac vascular grafts.

In most cases of delayed recognition of an ureteral injury, an attempt to retrograde placement of ureteral stents is worth trying. Only if this is not possible, a neprostomy tube should be placed followed by an antegrade stenting attempt; if the latter is failing, an open reconstruction should not be done prior to 6 weeks later [60].

14.5.2 Bladder Trauma

Most of the uncomplicated *extraperitoneal* bladder ruptures are treated by non- operative management, using urethral catheter drainage (20–22 French) for 10–14 days (85% healing rate) and administration of antibiotics.

Then, cystography should be performed to help the healing process or to rule out persistent urinary leakage. Virtually, all leaks should be sealed within 3 weeks. Antibiotics should be given until 3 days after catheter removal. Blunt extraperitoneal bladder injuries with associated injuries of bladder neck or involvement of prostate or vagina that need immediate open exploration should be repaired during the same session [20]. (Fig. 14.5, Fig. 14.9). After midline transperitoneal incision, the access is through the anterior wall or bladder dome closing the tear intravesically with a single layer running absorbable suture (3–0) [61].

Debridement of bladder tissue is often not necessary due to rich blood supply, warranting excellent healing.

On the other hand, *intraperitoneal* bladder injuries or penetrating trauma should always result in immediate operative exploration and repair. (Fig. 14.2). Also, inadequate drainage or clots in urine, bladder neck injury, concomittant rectal or vaginal injury, open pelvic fracture or pelvic fracture requiring internal fixation, and bone fragments penetrating the bladder wall represent indications for immediate bladder repair. If there is concomitant injury of the intramural ureter or orifice, stents should be placed or the afflicted ureter should be reimplanted. Repair of the bladder laceration or rupture should be done in two layers (mucosa and muscularis) using 3–0 and 2–0 absorbable running sutures. If possible, the peritoneum should be closed in a separate layer with 3–0 absorbable running suture.

A large (24 French) suprapubic tube drainage is optional as it provides no clear benefit over urethral catheter drainage alone [62].

Antibiotics should be administered for 3 days and a voiding cystogram is obtained 7–10 days after surgery to ensure no further extravasation before catheter removal.

14.5.2.1 Follow-up

Patients sustaining extraperitoneal and complex (i.e. involving trigone or ureter) intraperitoneal bladder disruption require routine cystogram follow-up. In patients undergoing repair of simple intraperitoneal bladder disruption (bladder dome), routine follow-up cystogram did not affect clinical management in a study of 87 patients [63].

14.5.3 Posterior Urethral Trauma

Initial management and delayed reconstruction:

Initial suprapubic cystostomy is indicated in both posterior and anterior urethral disruption trauma [64].

The acute treatment of choice for patients presenting with both posterior and anterior urethral disruption trauma is placement of a suprapubic cystostomy tube

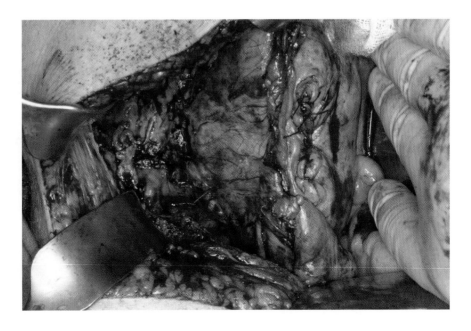

Fig. 14.10 Closure of intraperitoneal bladder rupture with interrupted sutures

Fig. 14.11 (**a**) Penile
fracture: clinical aspect of the
hematoma. (**b**) MRT of penis
presenting with rupture of
left corpus cavernosum and
subfascial hematoma

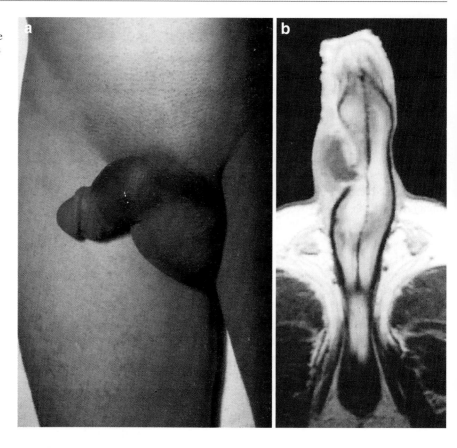

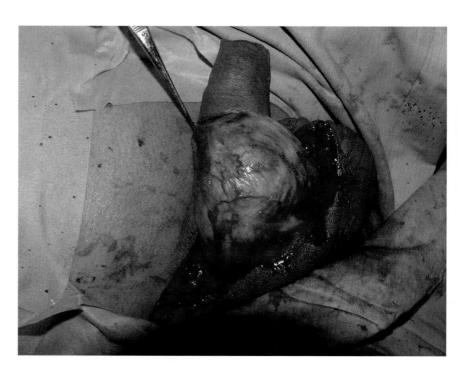

Fig. 14.12 Scrotal avulsion
trauma with right testicle
eventeration

with or without attempt to immediate realignment by urethral catheter placement under fluoroscopic or endoscopicy (by flexible cystoscope) control. Posterior urethral stenosis will occur in a high percentage of patients managed with suprapubic tube alone and also despite realignment and therefore will need posterior urethroplasty [65]. Posterior urethroplasty can be performed after a mean period of 1 month mostly 3 months after the trauma in the majority of cases, using 1-stage perineal anastomotic techniques, leading to excellent results in up to 95% of cases [66]. Immediate open urethroplasty of posterior injuries is not indicated because of poor visualization and the inability to assess accurately the degree of disruption, leading to higher rates of incontinence, impotence, and restricture.

Only in cases with associated bladder neck injury an open exploration with realignment is indicated. This immediate surgical reconstruction is often associated with poor outcome due to impotence, incontinence, restricture or intraoperative blood loss. [67].

Suprapubic tube placement is not contraindicated even in cases of pelvic fracture repair using anterior pubic hardware, as infection of the latter is a rare complication, when the catheter is placed high in the bladder dome and tunneled through the skin [68]. In cases of incomplete urethral tear, placement of a urethral catheter should be attempted. A complete transection of the urethra from this maneuver is not to be expected.

In females with urethral disruption, immediate repair is suggested because delayed anastomotic repair could be difficult in the short female urethra.

14.5.4 Anterior Urethral Trauma

Placement of an urethral catheter should be attempted only if contusion and/or incomplete disruption is shown by urethrography. In cases of major straddle injuries with complete disruption of the urethra, suprapubic cystostomy is the treatment of choice, followed by delayed secondary surgical repair (anastomotic urethroplasty). In cases of low-velocity urethral gunshot injuries, catheter alignment is useful, often resulting in urethral stricture.

Therefore, primary repair (end-to-end anastomosis) is recommended, leading to good results in >95% of cases [69, 70].

14.5.5 Penile Trauma

Rupture of the tunica albuginea should always immediately be explored and repaired by nonresorbable 2–0/3–0 interrupted sutures. Potential urethral injuries should be oversewn with 4–0 absorbable sutures over an indwelling catheter. In penetrating injuries, the urethra is often injured and prompt exploration and repair should follow. The urethra should be spatulated and an end-to-end anastomosis should be performed using 4–0 or 5–0 disrupted absorbable sutures. In case of complete penile amputation, microvascular replantation of dorsal veins, arteries and nerves (9–0 –11–0 nylon sutures), followed by reanastomosis of urethra and corpora cavernosa should be attempted. Even without microvascular reanastomosis, high success rates can be expected. [71, 72].

Technique: A subcoronal circumcision is recommended to deglove the entire penile shaft and have complete access to all the three corporal bodies as well as to nervous bundles. To evaluate surgical repair and detect any missed additional injuries, saline can be injected into the corporus cavernosum and spongiosum after a tourniquet has been placed at the penile basis.

14.5.6 Scrotal and Testicular Trauma

If a testis is injured, primary repair with readaptation of the tunica albuginea with running sutures should be attempted in order to preserve fertility and hormonal function [73]. Intratesticular hematoma that causes high pressure, entailing atrophy or necrosis, should be drained [74]. Scrotal injuries without testis involvement can be closed after debridement, inspection, irrigation, and drainage placement. In gunshot wounds of the scrotum, the vas deferens can be injured (9%) and must be ligated [75].

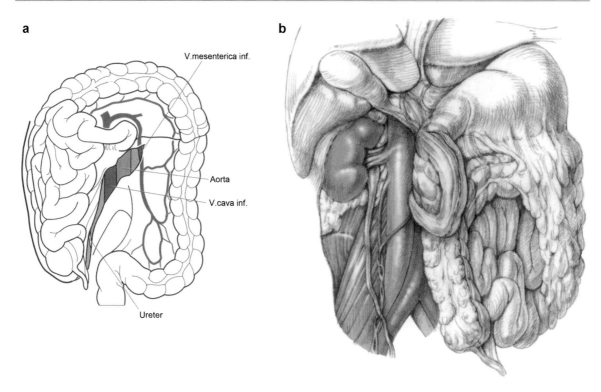

Fig. 14.13 (**a**) Incision line along the colon ascendens to get into the right retroperitoneal space. (**b**) After medialization of the right colon and small bowel there is access to the v. cava and right kidney and ureter.

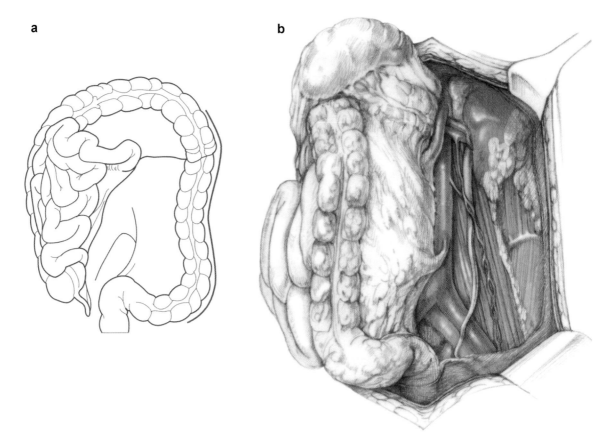

Fig. 14.14 (**a**) Incision line along the colon descendens to get into the left retroperitoneal space. (**b**) After mobilization of the left colon frame there is wide access to the aorta and left kidney and ureter.

References

1. Santucci RA, Fisher MB (2005) The literature increasingly supports expectant (conservative) management of renal trauma – a systematic review. J Trauma 59:493–503

2. Bariol SV, Stewart G, Smith RD et al (2005) An analysis of urinary tract trauma in Scotland: impact on management and resources needs. Surgeon 3:27–30

3. Paparel P, N'Diaye A, Laumon B et al (2005) The epidemiology of trauma in the genitourinary system after traffic accidents: analysis for a register of over 43 000 victims. BJU Int 97:338–341

4. McAninch JW, Santucci RA (2001) Genitorurinary injuries. In: Walsh, Retik, Vaugh, Wein (eds) Campbell's urology, 8th edn., vol IV. Chap. 105. Saunders: Elsevier Science, pp 3707–3744

5. McAninch JW, Carroll PR, Armenakas NA, Lee P (1993) Renal gunshot wounds: methods of salvage and reconstruction. J Trauma 35:279–283

6. Wessels H, Suh D, Porter JR et al (2003) Renal injury and operative management in the United States: results of a population- based study. J Trauma 54:423–430

7. Hammer CC, Santucci RA (2003) Effect of an institutional policy of nonoperative treatments of grades I to IV renal injuries. J Urol 169:1751–1753

8. Ordog GJ, Wasserberger J, Balasubramaniam S (1988) Shotgun wound ballistics. J Trauma 28:624–631

9. Rüter A, Trentz O, Wagner M (2004) Unfallchirurgie. 2. Urban and Fischer. Elsevier GmbH, München

10. Medina D, Lavery R, Ross SE (1998) Ureteral trauma: preoperative studies neither predict injury nor prevent missed injury. J Am Coll Surg 186:641–644

11. Elliott SP, McAninch JW (2003) Ureteral injuries from external violence: the 25 year experience at San Francisco General Hospital. J Urol 170:1213–1216

12. Corriere JN, Sandler CM (1999) Bladder rupture from external trauma: diagnosis and management. World J Urol 17:84–89

13. Corriere JN, Sandler CM (1986) Management of the ruptured bladder: 7 years of experience with 111 cases. J Trauma 26:830–833

14. Koraitim MM (1999) Pelvic fracture urethral injuries: the unresolved controversy. J Urol 161:1433–1441

15. Bright TC, White K, Peters PC (1978) Significance of hematuria after trauma. J Urol 120:455–456

16. Cass A (1989) Renovascular injuris from external trauma: Diagnosis, treatment, and outcome. Urol Clin North Am 16:213–220

17. Kawashima A, Sandler CM, Corl FM (2001) Imaging of renal trauma: a comprehensive review. Radiographics 21: 557–574

18. Kawashima A, Sandler CM, Corriere JN (1997) Ureteropelvic Junction injuries secondary to blunt abdominal trauma. Radiology 205:487–492

19. Mc Gahan JP, Rose J, Coates TL (1997) Use of ultrasonography in the patient with acute abdominal trauma. J Ultrasound Med 16:653–662

20. Carroll PR, McAninch JW (1984) Major bladder trauma: mechanisms of injury and a unified method of diagnosis and repair. J Urol 132:254–257

21. Cass AS (1984) The multiple injured patient with bladder trauma. J Trauma 24:731–734

22. Dubinsky TJ, Deck A, Maun FA (1999) Sonograpic diagnosis of a traumatic intraperitoneal bladder rupture. AJR Am J Roentgenol 172:770

23. Peng MY, Parisky YR, Cornwell EE et al (1999) CT cystography versus conventional cystography in evaluation of bladder injury. AJR Am J Roentgenol 173:1269–1272

24. Hsieh C-H, Chen R-J, Fang J-F et al (2002) Diagnosis and management of bladder injury by trauma surgeons. Am J Surg 184:143–147

25. Elliott DS, Barrett DM (1997) Long-term followup and evaluation of primary realignment of posterior urethra disruption. J Urol 157:814–816

26. Sandler CM, Jn CJN (1989) Urethrography in the diagnosis of acute urethra injuries. Urol Clin North Am 16:283–289

27. Chapple C, Barbagli G, Jordan G et al (2004) Consensus statement on urethral trauma. BJU Int 93:1195–1202

28. Kamdar C, Mooppan UMM, Kim H, Gulmi FA (2008) Penile fracture: preoperative evaluation and surgical technique for optimal patient outcome. BJU Int 102:1640–1644

29. Micallef M, Ahmad I, Ramesh N et al (2001) Ultrasound features of blunt testicular injury. Injury 32:23–26

30. Moore EE, Shackford SR, Pachter HL et al (1989) Organ injury scaling: spleen, liver and kidney. J Trauma 29: 1664–1666

31. Moore EE, Cogbill TH, Jurkovich GJ et al (1992) Organ injury scaling III: chest wall, abdominal vascular, ureter, bladder and urethra. J Trauma 33:337–339

32. Moore EE, Malangoni MA, Cogbill TH et al (1996) Organ injury scaling VII: cervical vascular, peripheral vascular, adrenal, penis, testis, and scrotum. J Trauma 41:523–524

33. Tinkoff T, Esposito TJ, Reed J et al (2008) American Association for the Surgery of Trauma Organ Injury Scale I: Spleen, liver and kidney, validation based on the national trauma databank. J Am Coll Surg 207:646–655

34. Santucci RA, McAninch JW, Safir M et al (2001) Validation of the American Association for the Surgery of Trauma organ injury severity scale for the kidney. J Trauma 50: 195–200

35. Shariat SF, Roehrborn CG, Karakiewicz PI et al (2007) Evidence based validation of the predictive value of the American Association for the Surgery of Trauma kidney injury scale. J Trauma 62:933–939

36. Kuan JK, Wright JL, Nathens AB et al (2006) American Association for the Surgery of Trauma Organ Injury Scale for kidney injuries predicts nephrectomy, dialysis, and death in patients with blunt injury and nephrectomy for penetrating injuries. J Trauma 60:351–356

37. Best CB, Petrone P, Buscarini M et al (2005) Traumatic ureteral injuries: a single institution experience validating the American Association for the Surgery of Trauma – organ injury grading scale. J Urol 173:1202–1205

38. Mohr AM, Pham AM, Lavery RF et al (2003) Management of trauma to the male external genitalia: the usefulness of American Association for the Surgery of Trauma organ injury scales. J Urology 170:2311–2315

39. Voelzke BB, McAninch JW (2008) The current management of renal injuries. Am Surg 74:667–678

40. Alsikafi NF, McAninch JW, Elliott SP, Garcia M (2006) Nonoperative management and outcomes of isolated urinary extravasation following renal lacerations due to external trauma. J Urol 176:2494–2497

41. Buckley JC, McAninch JW (2006) Selective management of isolated and nonisolated grade IV renal injuries. J Urol 176:2498–2502

42. Wessells H, McAninch JW, Meyer A, Bruce J (1997) Criteria for nonoperative treatment of significant penetrating renal lacerations. J Urol 157:24–27

43. Matthews LA, Smith EM, Spirnak JP (1997) Nonoperative treatment of major blunt renal lacerations with urinary extravasation. J Urol 157:2056–2058

44. Breyer BN, McAninch JW, Elliott SP, Master VA (2008) Minimally invasive ensovascular techniques to treat acute renal hemorrhage. J Urol 179:2248–2252

45. Elliott SP, Olweny EO, McAninch JW (2007) Renal arterial injuries: a single center analysis of management strategies and outcomes. J Urol 178:2451–2455

46. Haas CA, Dinchman KH, Nassrallah PF, Spirnak JP (1998) Traumatic renal artery occlusion: a 15-year review. J Trauma 45:557–561

47. Goodman DNF, Saibil EA, Kodama RT (1998) Traumatic intimal tear of the renal artery treated by insertion of a Palmaz stent. Cardiovasc Intervent Radiol 21:69–72

48. Scott RF Jr, Selzman HM (1966) Complications of nephrectomy: Review of 450 patients and a description of a modification of the transperitoneal approach. J Urol 95:307–312

49. Caroll PR, Klosterman P, McAninch JW (1989) Early vascular control for renal trauma: a critical review. J Urol 141:826–828

50. Coburn M (2002) Damage control surgery for urologic trauma: an evolving management strategy. J Urol 160:13

51. Pappas P, Leonardou P, Papadoukakis S et al (2006) Urgent superselected segmental renal artery embolization in the treatment of life-threatening renal hemorrhage. Urol Int 77:34–41

52. Malcolm JB, Derweesh IH, Mehrazin R et al (2008) Nonoperative management of blunt renal trauma: is routine early followup imaging necessary? BMC Urol 8:11–16

53. Monstrey SJ, Beerthuizen GI, vander Werken C et al (1989) Renal trauma and hypertension. J Trauma 29:65–70

54. Palmer LS, Rosenbaum RR, Gershbaum MD, Kentzer ER (1999) Penetrating ureteral trauma at an urban trauma center: 10-year experience. Urology 54:34–36

55. Presti JL Jr, Carroll PR, McAninch JW (1989) Ureteral and renal pelvic injuries from external trauma: diagnosis and management. J Trauma 29:370–374

56. Ali-el Dein B, Ghoneim MA (2003) Bridging long ureteral defects using the Yang-Monti principle. J Urol 169:1074–1077

57. Monti PR, Carvalho JR, Arap S (2000) The Monti procedure: applications and complications. Urology 55:616–621

58. Benson MC, Ring KS, Olsson CA (1990) Ureteral reconstruction and bypass: Experience with ileal interposition, the Boari flap-psoas hitch and renal autotransplantation. J Urol 143:20–23

59. Adamas JR, Mata JA, Culkin DJ, Venable DD (1992) Ureteral injury in abdominal vascular reconstructive surgery. Urology 39:77–81

60. Selzman AA, Spirnak JP (1996) Iatrogenic ureteral injuries: a 20-year experience in treating 165 injuries. J Urol 155:878–881

61. Morey AF, Iverson AJ, Swan A, Harmon WJ et al (2001) Bladder rupture after blunt trauma: guidelines for diagnostic imaging. J Trauma 51:683–686

62. Volpe MA, Pachter EM, Scalea TM et al (1999) Is there a difference in outcome when treating traumatic intraperitoneal bladder rupture with or without a suprapubic tube? J Urol 161:1103–1105

63. Inaba K, McKenney M, Munera F et al (2006) Cystogram follow-up in the management of traumatic bladder disruption. J Trauma 60:23–28

64. Park S, McAninch JW (2004) Straddle injuries to the bulbar urethra: management and outcomes in 78 patients. J Urol 171:722–725

65. Elliott DS, Barrett DM (1997) Long-term followup and evolution of primary realignment of posterior urethral disruptions. J Urol 157:814–816

66. Flynn BJ, Delvecchio FC, Webster GD (2003) Perineal repair of pelvic fracture urethral distraction: experience in 120 patients during the last 10 years. J Urol 170:1877–1880

67. Webster GD, Mathes GL, Selli C (1983) Prostatomembranous ureteral injuries: a review of the literature and rational approach to their management. J Urol 130:898–902

68. Brandes S, Borrelli J Jr (2001) Pelvic fracture and associated urologic injuries. World J Surg 25:1578–1587

69. Husman DA, Boone TB, Wilson WT (1993) Management of low velocity gunshot wounds to the anterior urethra: the role of primary repair versus diversion alone. J Urol 150:70–721

70. Santucci RA, Mario LA, McAninch JW (2002) Anastomotic urethroplasty for urethral stricture: Analysis of 168 patients. J Urol 167:1715–1719

71. Chapple C, Barbagli G, Jordan G et al (2004) Consensus statement on urethral trauma. BJU Int 93:1195–1202

72. Morey AF, Metro MJ, Carrey KJ et al (2004) Consensus on genitourinary trauma. BJU Int 94:507–515

73. Kukadia AN, Ercole CJ, Gleich P et al (1996) Testicular trauma: potential impact on reproductive function. J Urol 156:1643–1646

74. Cass AS, Luxenberg M (1988) Value of early operation in blunt testicular contusion with hematocele. J Urol 139:746–747

75. Brandes SB, Buckman RP, Cholsky MJ, Hanno PM (1995) External genital gunshot wounds: a ten-year experience with fifty-six cases. J Trauma 39:266–271

Abdominal Vascular Injuries

15

Juan A. Asensio, Tamer Karsidag, Aytekin Ünlü,
Juan M. Verde, and Patrizio Petrone

Every surgeon carries about him a little cemetery, in which from time to time he goes to pray, a cemetery of bitterness and regret, of which he seeks the reason for certain of his failures. (Rene Leriche [1879–1955])

15.1 Introduction

Abdominal vascular injuries are among the most lethal injuries sustained by trauma patients. Similarly, these injuries are also among the most difficult and challenging injuries encountered by modern-day trauma surgeons. For the most part, these patients arrive at trauma centers in profound shock secondary to massive blood loss, which is often unrelenting. Patients sustaining abdominal vascular injuries best exemplify the lethal vicious cycle of shock, acidosis, hypothermia, coagulopathy, and cardiac dysrythmias.

J.A. Asensio (✉)
Director, Trauma Clinical Research, Training and Community Affairs, Director, Trauma Surgery and Surgical Critical Care Fellowship; Director International Visiting Scholars/Research Fellowship; Division of Trauma Surgery and Surgical Critical Care; DeWitt Daughtry Family Department of Surgery, Medical Director for Education and Training, International Medical Institute, University of Miami Miller School of Medicine, Ryder Trauma Center, 1800 NW 10 Avenue, Suite T-247, Miami, Florida 33136, USA
e-mail: jasensio@med.miami.edu, asensio@att.blackberry.net

T. Karsidag, A. Unlu, J.M. Verde
International Visiting Scholars/Research Fellows;
Division of Trauma Surgery and Surgical Critical Care;
DeWitt Daughtry Family Department of Surgery;
University of Miami Miller School of Medicine; Ryder Trauma Center, Miami, Florida, USA

P. Petrone
Medical Advisor; Health Research Joint Commission;
Ministry of Health; 1120-51 Avenue, Suite 316, La Plata,
Province of Buenos Aires, Argentina

Many of these patients present in cardiopulmonary arrest and require drastic life-saving measures, such as emergency department thoracotomy, aortic cross-clamping, and open cardiopulmonary resuscitation to maximize any opportunity of reaching the operating room alive. To compound the problem, exposure of retroperitoneal hemorrhaging vessels is quite difficult and requires extensive dissection and mobilization of intraabdominal organs. These maneuvers are time-consuming and fraught with pitfalls, as rapid dissection through large retroperitoneal hematomas can lead to iatrogenic injuries in patients that can ill afford further uncontrolled hemorrhage.

Abdominal vascular injuries rarely occur as isolated entities; in fact, multiple associated injuries are the rule rather than the exception, thus increasing not only injury severity, but also the time needed to repair many critical associated injuries. Abdominal vascular injuries are also characterized by massive blood losses requiring large quantities of crystalloids, blood, and blood products for intravascular volume replacement. Coupled with the frequent need to crossclamp the aorta or other major intraabdominal vessels, this scenario predisposes these patients to the development of reperfusion injuries and if they survive, their sequelae.

The concept of "bail out" later renamed as "damage control" is usually applied in patients sustaining abdominal vascular injuries. Similarly, these patients often demand heroic abdominal-wall closures with prosthetic materials, which initiate a cycle of frequent surgical re-interventions adding multiple and additive physiologic and immunologic insults to an already compromised patient.

The classical dilemma encountered by trauma surgeons of how to repair vascular injuries in the midst of massive contamination while avoiding graft infections

H.-J. Oestern et al. (eds.), *Head, Thoracic, Abdominal, and Vascular Injuries*,
DOI: 10.1007/978-3-540-88122-3_15, © Springer-Verlag Berlin Heidelberg 2011

and vessel blow-outs remains one of the most difficult problems that face modern-day trauma surgeons. Septic processes and multiple systems organ failure (MSOF) are frequent complications encountered by these patients as profound shock, tissue hypoperfusion, massive blood volume replacement, generalized edema, and prolonged contamination places these patients at risk for these severe and often difficult to care for complications. All these factors clearly conspire to produce high morbidity rates for patients sustaining these injuries. Improved outcomes are generally the result of expedient and precise surgical interventions by trauma surgeons with extensive experience in the management of these injuries along with the vast surgical armamentarium needed to effectively deal with them.

arteriovenous fistulas exists either acutely or chronically; however, they are extremely rare.

The abdominal aorta may be injured at its suprarenal or infrarenal portions. The inferior vena cava (IVC) may be injured at its suprarenal or infrarenal portions or at its retrohepatic location, one of the most lethal injuries known to man. The superior mesenteric artery (SMA) may be injured in any of its four zones, just as the superior mesenteric vein (SMV) may be injured at its infra or retropancreatic location. The portal vein (PV) may be injured either at its origin at the confluence of the superior mesenteric and splenic veins (SV) or it may be injured alone within the confines of the portal triad. The renal artery (RA) may be injured in one of its three portions, whereas the renal veins (RV) may be injured either at their confluence with the inferior vena cava or at the renal hilum.

15.2 Anatomic Location of Injury

Abdominal vascular injuries associated with blunt trauma most commonly occur in upper abdominal vessels; however, penetrating injuries may occur in any of the retroperitoneal zones (Fig. 15.1), as missile trajectories are unpredictable, frequently injuring more than one vessel. The cumulative effect on mortality rises drastically as multiple vessels are usually injured. Because of proximity between abdominal arteries and veins, the potential for the development of

15.3 Operative Intervention

15.3.1 Pre-operative Preparations

In the operating room, the entire patient's torso, from the neck to mid-thighs, is prepared and draped. The area to the mid-thighs is quite important should the necessity arise to obtain an autogenous saphenous vein graft. The trauma surgeon must confirm that there are sufficient units of blood in the operating room for immediate

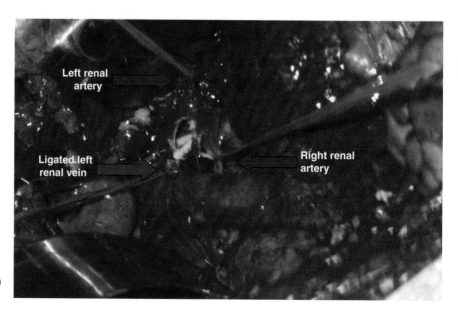

Fig. 15.1 Unreconstructable lethal aortic injury in the origin of SMA

transfusion via rapid infusion technology. They must also institute maneuvers to prevent hypothermia, which include placement of a warming blanket in the operating table, covering the patient's lower extremities with a circulating warm air mattress, covering the head to prevent heat loss, increasing the ventilator cascade temperature to 42°C, and providing an ample supply of microwave-heated irrigation fluids . In addition, the availability of autotransfusion apparatus and cell-saving technology is of great value. Appropiate instruments and shunts must always be available including the Argon beam coagulator and newer hemostatic agents.

15.3.2 Exposure and Incisions

Abdominal injuries should be explored through a midline incision extending from xiphoid to pubis. Immediate control of life-threatening hemorrhage, followed by immediate control of sources of gastrointestinal spillage, is the early goal to achieve. The next step in the management of abdominal injuries consists of a thorough exploration of the abdominal cavity. Since the abdominal vasculature resides in the retroperitoneum, a thorough exploration of these structures must be performed utilizing a systematic approach of the anatomic zones of the retroperitoneum. Exploration of the retroperitoneum is challenging and demands that the trauma surgeon be totally familiar with the complex anatomy of these zones.

15.3.3 Surgical Technique

The first and most important goal to achieve in the management of abdominal vascular injuries is hemorrhage control. As in all vascular injuries, proximal and distal control of the hemorrhaging blood vessel is required. However, in exsanguinating abdominal vascular injuries, achieving this rapidly may be difficult. Unfortunately, a significant number of patients succumb without vascular control.

Frequently, these patients experience severe and profound hypotension; therefore, crossclamping of the aorta is the first maneuver instituted to stop life-threatening hemorrhage. If the patient arrives profoundly hypotensive or experiences cardiopulmonary arrest in the OR, an immediate left anterolateral thoracotomy with aortic crossclamping and open cardiopulmonary resuscitation are performed prior to proceeding with the laparotomy.

For patients who arrive with hemodynamic stability, but decompensate during laparotomy, the abdominal aorta can be controlled at the aortic hiatus, either digitally or by the use of a Conn abdominal aortic root compressor or by crossclamping with a Crafoord–DeBakey or other aortic clamps. Placement of a crossclamp in this location is difficult, as the abdominal aorta is surrounded by the crura of the diaphragm, which often requires transection to reach of portion of the infradiaphragmatic aorta to place the aortic crossclamp.

Once the exsanguinating hemorrhage has been controlled, the trauma surgeon should classify the hemorrhage or hematoma into one of the three zones of the retroperitoneum. All trauma surgeons must be cognizant of the intricate anatomy and the anatomic boundaries of these zones. Zone I begins at the aortic hiatus and ends at the sacral promontory; it is located at the midline and courses on top of the spinal column. This zone is divided into supramesocolic and inframesocolic. There are two zone II, right and left, which are located at the pericolic gutters. Zone III begins at the sacral promontory and contains the major pelvic blood vessels.

Zone I supramesocolic contains the suprarenal abdominal aorta, the celiac axis (Tripod of Haller), and the first two parts of the superior mesenteric artery. The superior mesenteric artery (SMA) is divided into four parts. Part 1 has its origin at the aorta and ends at the point where the inferior pancreaticoduodenal artery emerges, Part 2 from the origin of the inferior pancreaticoduodenal to the origin of the middle colic artery, Part 3 is the trunk distal to the middle colic artery, and Part 4 encompasses the origins of the segmental jejunal, ileal, or colic branches. Zone I supramesocolic also contains the infrahepatic suprarenal inferior vena cava, the infrarenal inferior vena cava, as well as the proximal portion of the superior mesenteric vein (SMV).

Zone I inframesocolic contains the last two portions of the superior mesenteric artery (SMA), the inferior mesenteric artery (IMA), the infrarenal aorta and vena cava, as well as the distal superior mesenteric vein. Zone II is divided into right and left, each containing the renal vascular pedicle. Zone III contains the bifurcation of the aorta into the common iliac arteries and veins, which further bifurcate into the internal and external iliac vessels. It also contains the retroperitoneal venous plexus of the Batson. The portal–retrohepatic area is a special area, which contains the portal vein, hepatic artery, and retrohepatic vena cava.

As soon as the trauma surgeon has identified and classified the hemorrhage and/or hematoma into one of the zones of the retroperitoneum, they must approach this zone to obtain vascular control, expose the injured blood vessel, and attempt definitive repair and/or ligation. Each zone requires different and complex maneuvers for exposure of these vessels.

Zone I supramesocolic is generally approached utilizing a maneuver that rotates the left-sided viscera medially. This approach requires transection of the avascular line of Toldt of the left colon, along with incising the lienosplenic ligament and rotating the left colon, spleen, tail, and body of the pancreas, as well as the stomach medially. This exposes the aorta from its entrance into the abdominal cavity via the aortic hiatus and includes exposing of the origin of the celiac axis (Tripod of Haller), the first two zones of superior mesenteric artery, and the left renal vascular pedicle. This maneuver is difficult and time-consuming. The left kidney can be mobilized medially, although this is generally not done.

An alternative maneuver includes performing an extended Kocher maneuver along with transecting the avascular line of Toldt of the right colon, mobilizing medially the right colon, hepatic flexure, duodenum, and head of the pancreas to the level of the superior mesenteric vessels, elevating these structures in a cephalad direction and incising the loose retroperitoneal tissue to the left of the inferior vena cava. This maneuver exposes the suprarenal abdominal aorta between the celiac axis and the superior mesenteric artery. This maneuver has as a disadvantage that the exposure obtained is below the level of any injury to the supraceliac aorta and the aorta at the hiatus.

Maneuvers used to expose injuries in Zone I inframesocolic include displacing the transverse colon and mesocolon cephalad, eviscerating the small bowel to the right, locating the ligament of Treitz, transecting it along with the loose retroperitoneal tissue alongside the left of the abdominal aorta until left renal vein is located. This exposes the infrarenal aorta. Meticulous attention must be directed to avoid iatrogenic injuries to the IMV. To expose the infrarenal inferior vena cava, the avascular line of Toldt of the right colon is transected along while performing an extensive Kocher maneuver sweeping the pancreas and duodenum to the left and incising the retroperitoneal tissues covering the inferior vena cava.

Exposure to right and left zones II depends on whether the perirenal hematoma is actively bleeding and whether it is located laterally or medially. If active bleeding is found medially or if there is an expanding hematoma, vascular control of the renal artery and vein is required. Vessel loops should be used for control; alternatively, a Henley subclavian/renal clamp may also be used. On the right, this is achieved by mobilizing the right colon and hepatic flexure as well as performing a Kocher maneuver, exposing the inferior vena cava infrarenally and continuing the dissection cephalad by incising the tissues directly over the suprarenal infrahepatic inferior vena cava. This is continued until the right renal vein is encountered. Further dissection superiorly and posteriorly to the right renal vein will locate the right renal artery (Fig. 15.2).

On the left side, the left colon and splenic flexure are mobilized. The small bowel is than eviscerated to the right. The ligament of Treitz is located and the transverse colon and mesocolon are displaced cephalad. This should locate the intrarenal abdominal aorta. Cephalad dissection will locate the left renal vein as it crosses over the abdominal aorta. The left renal artery will also be found superiorly and posteriorly to the left renal vein. Once mobilized and controlled and if uninjured, the renal vessels may be retracted with a Cushing vein retractor. Alternatively, if a perirenal hematoma or active bleeding is found laterally with no extension into the hilum of the kidney, the lateral aspects of Gerota's fascia can be incised and the kidney elevated and displaced medially to locate the hemorrhage.

Exposure of the vessels in zone III can be achieved by transecting the avascular line of Toldt of both the right and left colons and displacing them medially. Utilizing a combination of blunt and sharp dissection, the common iliac vessels are located. Meticulous attention must be paid to locating and preserving the ureter as it crosses the common iliac artery. Avoidance of devascularization of the ureter's blood supply is a must. A vessel loop should be passed around the ureter to retract it. Dissection is then extended in a caudad direction opening the retroperitoneum over the vessels.

Structures in the portal-retrohepatic area are very difficult to expose and require extensive dissections. The portal vein is formed by the confluence of the superior mesenteric vein (SMV) and the slightly smaller splenic vein (SV) posterior to the neck of the pancreas. This confluence is located just to the right of the body of the second lumbar vertebra (L2) and immediately anterior to the left border of the inferior vena cava. The inferior mesenteric vein (IMV) is the third major tributary to the inferior vena cava indirectly

Fig. 15.2 Dissection of both renal veins and supra and infrarenal inferior vena cava (IVC)

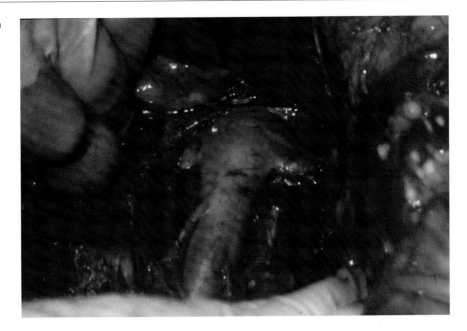

contributing its flow to the portal vein, by entering either the splenic vein generally, or SMV in the immediate vicinity of the major confluence rarely. In as many as 30% of cases, the IMV enters at the angle of the major confluence. In contrast to the suprapancreatic portal vein, the retropancreatic confluence zone is not intimately related to the bile duct or hepatic artery.

Sound knowledge of the anatomy of the portal confluence is of utmost importance to trauma surgeons. From its origin, the valveless portal vein passes cephalad, inclining slightly rightward over its course of 7.5–10 cm to reach the hilum of the liver, where it divides extrahepatically into right and left branches. During its course, it passes in succession behind the upper pancreatic neck and the first portion of the duodenum. Then, upon entering the hepatoduodenal ligament, it forms a relationship with the hepatic artery and bile duct, lying behind these structures and forming the anterior border of the foramen of Winslow. Throughout its length, the portal vein lies immediately anterior to the suprarenal segment of the inferior vena cava (IVC). The portal vein receives, in addition to its main tributaries, the pyloric vein from the pancreas and duodenum, left gastric (coronary) vein, and the superior pancreaticoduodenal vein. A cystic vein, if present, also drains into the portal vein.

Wounds of the suprapancreatic portal vein can be exposed by an extensive Kocher maneuver, with mobilization and rotation of the hepatic flexure of the colon. Preliminary hepatic inflow occlusion and the division of the cystic duct facilitate the exposure. Retropancreatic wounds involving the portal confluence or its major tributaries and suprapancreatic wounds with suspected additional injury of the IVC or other vessels are exposed by a combination of an extensive Kocher maneuver and mobilization of the entire right colon and mesenteric base, from the cecum to the duodenojejunal flexure. This maneuver, when combined with leftward mobilization of hepatic flexure, provides access to the entire portal vein and the proximal portions of its major tributaries. It also exposes the entire infrahepatic vena cava and the aorta up to the origin of the SMA.

Surgical transection of the neck of the pancreas can also be utilized to expose the retropancreatic portal vein. An avascular plane exists between the neck of the pancreas and the anterior surface of the portal vein, as there are no venous tributaries draining into the anterior surface of the portal vein. Transection of the neck of the pancreas can be achieved either with a GIA or TIA stapler. This maneuver is recommended when there is an associated pancreatic injury, which will mandate distal pancreatectomy or as completion pancreatectomy for an almost totally transected pancreas at its neck. It may be utilized as the last ditch effort, if hemorrhage containment cannot be accomplished in any another way. All these maneuvers as well as direct dissection of the portal triad will also expose the hepatic artery and its branches.

One of the most difficult vascular structures to expose is the retrohepatic vena cava. This segment of the inferior vena cava has unique anatomic features such as multiple tributaries draining anteriorly at the level of the caudate lobe. This portion of the vena cava measures approximately 7–12 cm in length and lies in a groove on the posterior aspect of the liver. The retrohepatic cava is joined by the major hepatic veins: the right, middle, and left hepatic veins. Frequently, the left and the middle hepatic veins join in a short 1–2 cm common trunk prior to entering the retrohepatic IVC. Similarly, other major accessory hepatic veins of different sizes may also drain into the retrohepatic IVC.

Exposure of the retrohepatic IVC and the major hepatic veins is both difficult and fraught with pitfalls. Prior to any direct attempts at exposure, a wide right-sided visceral rotation is undertaken by transecting the avascular line of Toldt of the right colon and performing an extensive Kocher maneuver, thus exposing both infrarenal as well as the suprarenal infrahepatic IVC. Similarly, the falciform ligament is sharply transected toward its origin at the bare area of the liver where meticulous transection of the coronary ligaments will expose 1–2 cm of the retrohepatic IVC.

One of the ways to expose the retrohepatic IVC is by directly approaching it via an extensive hepatotomy through the interlobar plane at Cantlie's line; frequently, this is done as completion of a massive fracture. Alternatively, sharp transection of the right triangular ligament with extensive right to left mobilization of the right lobe of the liver will expose the right hepatic vein as well as the retrohepatic IVC. The left hepatic vein can be exposed by transecting the left triangular ligament and rotating laterally the lateral segment of the left lobe of the liver. At times, a median sternotomy is necessary to control the intrapericardial portion of the IVC at the space of Gibbons. Alternatively, the utilization of atriocaval shunts may be used as adjuncts to expose the retrohepatic IVC. This is a very difficult procedure, usually unsuccessful and not recommended.

Once exposure and proximal and distal control have been obtained, all abdominal vascular injuries should be graded utilizing the American Association for the Surgery of Trauma – Organ Injury Scale for vascular injuries (AAST – OIS) (Table 15.1). Routine principles of vascular surgery apply to the management of all abdominal vascular injuries. Adequate exposure, proximal and distal control, debridement of injured vessel wall, prevention of embolization of clot, debri, or plaque, irrigation with heparinized saline, judicious use of Fogarty catheters,

meticulous arteriorraphy or venorraphy with monofilament vascular sutures, avoiding narrowing of the vessel during repair, insertion of an autogenous or prosthetic graft when applicable, and rarely intraoperative angiography when feasible are the mainstays of successful repair. Occasionally, the use of temporary vascular shunts as part of damage control may be required.

The management of vascular injuries in zone I, supramesocolic will consist of primary arteriorraphy of the suprarenal abdominal aorta when feasible (Fig. 15.3), and in rare occasions the insertion of a Dacron or PTFE graft (Fig. 15.4). Injuries to the celiac axis are usually dealt with primary repair if simple, or ligation if destructive. Management of injuries to the first two parts of the superior mesenteric artery should be dealt with by primary repair whenever possible. Intense vasoconstriction makes this quite difficult. These injuries can also be ligated, as theoretically there are sufficient collaterals to preserve the viability of the small and large bowel; however, profound vasospasm may lead to intense ischemia and bowel necrosis. The first two zones of the superior mesenteric artery can also be repaired either with an autogenous or prosthetic graft (Fig. 15.5). Insertion of a shunt may be utilized as a temporary measure.

The management of injuries in zone I inframesocolic employs the same techniques as in zone I supramesocolic. Parts 3 and 4 of the superior mesenteric artery should also be repaired, although the main jejunal ileal, and colic branches of Part 4 may be ligated. The management of inferior mesenteric artery injuries is usually by ligation, as they rarely require reconstruction. The management of injuries to be infrahepatic suprarenal inferior vena cava, as well as the infrarenal inferior vena cava will consist of lateral venorraphy whenever feasible. If through and through injuries are found in these vessels, both anterior and posterior aspects of the vessel must be repaired. This can prove quite challenging. Complex infrarenal IVC injuries not amenable to repair will require ligation.

Although the infrahepatic suprarenal inferior vena cava has no venous tributaries, it is very difficult to mobilize. In general, these repairs are accomplished by extending the injury in the anterior wall and repairing the posterior wall from within. This vessel can be mobilized by rotating the right kidney from medial to lateral outside of the renal fossa; however, this maneuver is quite treacherous and not recommended.

When there has been massive destruction of the infrahepatic suprarenal inferior vena cava, ligation can be considered; however, survival rates are quite low.

Table 15.1 American Association for the Surgery of Trauma (AAST) abdominal vascular organ injury scale

	OIS grade	ICD-9	AIS-85	AIS-90
Grade I[a]				
Nonnamed superior mesenteric artery or superior mesenteric vein branches	I	902.20/902.39	NS	NS
Nonnamed inferior mesenteric artery or inferior mesenteric vein branches	I	902.27/902.32	NS	NS
Phrenic artery/vein	I	902.89	NS	NS
Lumbar	I	902.89	NS	NS
Gonadal	I	902.89	NS	NS
Ovarian	I	902.81/902.82	NS	NS
Other nonnamed small arterial or venous structures requiring ligation	I	902.90	NS	NS
Grade II[a]				
Right, left, or common hepatic artery	II	902.22	3	3
Splenic artery/vein	II	902.23/902.34	3	3
Right or left gastric arteries	II	902.21	3	3
Gastroduodenal artery	II	902.24	3	3
Inferior mesenteric artery, trunk or inferior mesenteric vein, trunk	II	902.27/902.32	3	3
Primary named branches of mesenteric artery (e.g., ileocolicartery) or mesenteric vein	II	902.26/902.31	3	3
Other named abdominal vessel requiring ligation/repair	II	902.89	3	3
Grade III[a]				
Superior mesenteric vein, trunk	III	902.31	3	3
Renal artery/vein	III	902.41/902.42	3	3
Iliac artery/vein	III	902.53/902.54	3	3
Hypogastric artery/vein	III	902.51/902.52	3	3
Vena cava, infrarenal	III	902.10		3
Grade IV[a]				
Superior mesenteric artery, trunk	IV	902.25	3	3
Celiac axis proper	IV	902.24	3	3
Vena cava, suprarenal and infrahepatic	IV	902.10	3	3
Aorta, infrarenal	IV	902.00	4	4
Grade V[a]				
Portal vein	V	902.33	3	3
Extraparenchymal hepatic vein	V	902.11	3 (hepatic vein)	3 (hepatic vein)
			5 (liver vein)	5 (liver vein)
Vena cava, retrohepatic or suprahepatic	V	902.19	5	5
Aorta, suprarenal, subdiaphragmatic	V	902.00	4	4

[a]Increase one grade for multiple grade III or IV injuries involving >50% vessel circumference. Downgrade one grade if <25% vessel circumference laceration for grades IV and V

This classification system is applicable for extraparenchymal vascular injuries. If the vessel injury is within the 2 cm of the organ parenchyma, refer to specific organ injury scale

Fig. 15.3 Suprarenal aorta stab wound (SW). Primarily repair of SMA origin

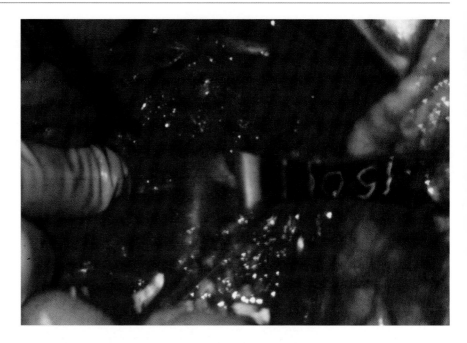

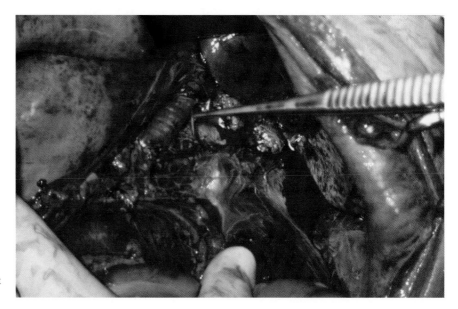

Fig. 15.4 Suprarenal aortic injury secondary to GSW. Suprarenal aortic replacement with Dacron graft

Rarely prosthetic grafts have been utilized in this position. The management of injuries to the infrarenal inferior vena cava generally consists of lateral venorraphy after placement of a partially occluding Satinsky or Derra vascular clamp. In the presence of through and through injuries, primary repair can be accomplished either by extending the laceration or rotating the vessel. However, this involves ligating many of its lumbar veins, which are quite fragile. We recommend performing the repair from within the vessel. The infrarenal inferior vena cava can be ligated in cases of massive destruction. Ligation is generally well tolerated. Injuries to the superior mesenteric vein should be primarily repaired although they can also be ligated; serious sequelae to the circulation of the small and large bowel may result.

Injuries to either right or left Zone II can be quite challenging. Injuries to the renal artery can be either

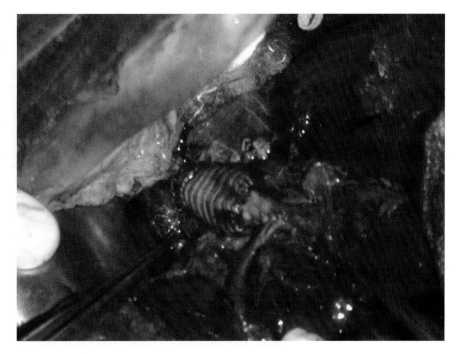

Fig. 15.5 Abdominal GSW. Celiac axis ligature + superior mesenteric artery (SMA) replacement

primarily repaired or resected and grafted utilizing either an autogenous or prosthetic graft. This is technically challenging. Rarely an aortorenal bypass can be performed utilizing a distal site in the anterior wall of the abdominal aorta. Primary repair of the renal arteries is difficult. Generally, ligation of the renal artery is performed with subsequent nephrectomy. Injuries to the renal veins can also be repaired with primary venorraphy or ligation. An injury to the right renal vein that cannot be successfully repaired requires ligation and will demand that a nephrectomy be performed secondary to the lack of venous collaterals. Ligation of the left renal vein is generally well tolerated provided that it is performed proximally and close to the inferior vena cava as the venous collaterals such as the gonadal, adrenal, and renolumbar veins handle the venous outflow.

Injuries to Zone III can also be quite challenging to manage, as they are often associated colonic and genitourinary injuries resulting in significant contamination. Injuries to the common iliac arteries can be primarily repaired via arteriorrhaphy. Occasionally, resection and primary anastomosis can be performed. Prosthetic (Fig. 15.6) and very rarely autogenous grafts can also be utilized to repair common iliac arteries. Internal iliac artery injuries are generally dealt with by ligation. Injuries to the external iliac artery can be primarily repaired via arteriorraphy and occasionally by resection and primary anastomosis. Iliofemoral bypasses can be performed usually with prosthetic and extremely rarely with autogenous grafts (Fig. 15.7), as it is uncommon to find a saphenous vein of adequate size to perform an iliofemoral repair. In the presence of massive contamination, it is strongly recommended that all grafts, be it autogenous or prosthetic, be covered by reperitonealization with autogenous tissues to avoid graft blow-outs. Insertion of shunts may be utilized as a temporary measure in either the iliac artery or vein.

When there has been massive destruction of either the common or internal iliac artery, ligation may be needed. Arterial flow can be restored utilizing a crossover femoro-femoral or axillo-femoral bypass. These bypasses have the disadvantages of having to involve uninjured vessels and have a high incidence of thrombosis. Injuries to the iliac veins, either common, external, or internal, can be dealt with by ligation, as this is frequently well tolerated, although they can also be dealt with by lateral venorraphy.

Fig. 15.6 Abdominal GSW with secondary laceration of right common, external, and internal veins + right iliac artery injury. Ligated vein + iliac artery repair with 8 mm PTFE graft

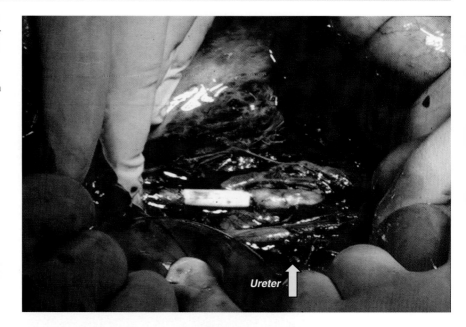

Fig. 15.7 Left external iliac artery injury + colon and bladder injuries secondary to abdominal GSW. Primary iliofemoral bypass with autogenous reverse saphenous vein graft (Extremely rare as generally saphenous vein cannot be used for bypasses in this location)

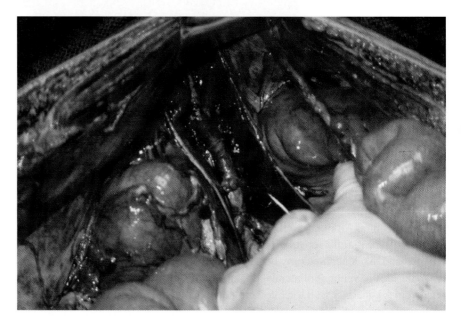

Injuries to the portal vein should be primarily repaired whenever possible. Lateral venorraphy, although technically difficult, should be attempted even if the repair narrows the portal vein. Alternatively, if the patient is acidotic, hypothermic, and coagulopathic, the portal vein can be ligated. This very frequently results in the splanchnic hypervolemia and systemic hypovolemia syndrome. Other techniques that have been employed with little success are resection of the damaged segment and primary end to end of

anastomosis, autogenous and prosthetic grafts, end-to-side portacaval shunts, and transposition of the splenic vein to the SMV. Injuries to the hepatic artery can be primarily repaired or ligated.

The management of injuries to the retrohepatic IVC consists of primary venorraphy, as this represents the only chance for survival in these patients. Ligation is not an option as patients will not survive. In a few reported cases in the literature, the entire liver has been extirpated and a number 36 or 40 Fr chest tube

Fig. 15.8 Hartman procedure with left colon colostomy + rectal injury primarily repaired

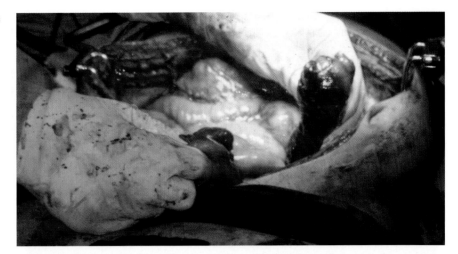

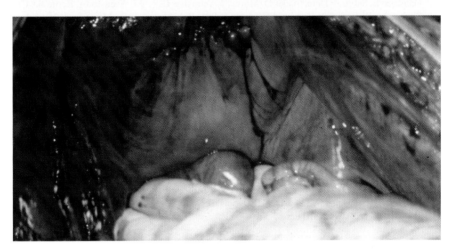

Fig. 15.9 (Bladder injury Primarily required)

has been placed in the retrohepatic IVC as a shunt in anticipation of a hepatic transplant. Injuries to the hepatic veins should be primarily repaired; ligation will most often result in hepatic necrosis as there are literally no collateral venous channels between the hepatic lobes.

Whenever a trauma surgeon performs an abdominal vascular repair, serious considerations must be given to "second look" operation to assess for bowel viability. This is particularly of importance after repair of any of the parts of the superior mesenteric artery and should be considered after repair or ligation of the portal vein or superior mesenteric vein. Contamination from gastrointestinal or genitourinary injuries (Figs. 15.8 and 15.9) pose great risks for the development of infections in prosthetic grafts inserted to bypass injured vessels. Whenever possible, all grafts, either autogenous or prosthetic, should be reperitonealized. Similarly,

for all vascular repairs adjacent to gastrointestinal suture lines, an effort should be made to interpose viable tissue, generally omentum between the suture lines to prevent vascular-enteric fistulas, anastomotic dehisances, and blow-outs.

References

1. Asensio JA, Petrone P, Garcia-Nuñez L, Healy M, Martin M, Kuncir E (2007) Superior mesenteric venous injuries: to ligate or to repair remains the question. J Trauma 62(3): 668–675, discussion 675
2. Asensio JA, Kuncir EJ, García-Núñez LM, Petrone P (2006) Femoral vessel injuries: analysis of factors predictive of outcomes. J Am Coll Surg 203(4):512–520, Epub 2006 Aug 23
3. Asensio JA, Petrone P, Kimbrell B, Kuncir E (2005) Lessons learned in the management of thirteen celiac axis injuries. South Med J 98(4):462–466, Review

4. Kumar SR, Rowe VL, Petrone P, Kuncir EJ, Asensio JA (2003) The vasculopathic patient: uncommon surgical emergencies. Emerg Med Clin North Am 21(4):803–815, Review

5. Asensio JA, Petrone P, Roldán G, Kuncir E, Rowe VL, Chan L, Shoemaker W, Berne TV (2003) Analysis of 185 iliac vessel injuries: risk factors and prediction of outcome. Arch Surg 138(11):1187–1193, discussion 1193–1194

6. Asensio JA, Petrone P, Karsidag T, Ramos-Kelly JR, Demiral S, Roldan G, Pak-Art R, Kuncir E (2002) Abdomianal vascular injuries: a continuing challenge. Ulus Travma Derg 8(4):189–197, Review

7. Rowe VL, Salim A, Lipham J, Asensio JA (2002) Shank vessel injuries. Surg Clin North Am 82(1):91–104, xx. Review

8. Asensio JA, Forno W, Roldán G, Petrone P, Rojo E, Ceballos J, Wang C, Costaglioli B, Romero J, Tillou A, Carmody I, Shoemaker WC, Berne TV (2002) Visceral vascular injuries. Surg Clin North Am 82(1):1–20, xix. Review

9. Asensio JA, McDuffie L, Petrone P, Roldań G, Forno W, Gambaro E, Salim A, Demetriades D, Murray J, Velmahos G, Shoemaker W, Berne TV, Ramicone E, Chan L (2001) Reliable variables in the exsanguinated patient which indicate damage control and predict outcome. Am J Surg 182(6):743–751

10. Tillou A, Romero J, Asensio JA, Best CD, Petrone P, Roldan G, Rojo E (2001) Renal vascular injuries. Surg Clin North Am 81(6):1417–1430, Review

11. Asensio JA, Forno W, Roldan G, Petrone P, Rojo E, Tillou A, Murray JA, Feliciano DV (2001) Abdominal vascular injuries: injuries to the aorta. Surg Clin North Am 81(6):1395–1416

12. Asensio JA, Soto SN, Forno W, Roldan G, Petrone P, Gambaro E, Salim A, Rowe V, Demetriades D (2001) Abdominal vascular injuries: the trauma surgeon's challenge. Surg Today 31(11):949–957, Review

13. Asensio JA, Britt LD, Borzotta A, Peitzman A, Miller FB, Mackersie RC, Pasquale MD, Pachter HL, Hoyt DB, Rodriguez JL, Falcone R, Davis K, Anderson JT, Ali J, Chan L (2001) Multiinstitutional experience with the management of superior mesentery artery injuries. J Am Coll Surg 193(4):354–365, discussion 365–366. Erratum in: J Am Coll Surg 2001 Dec;193(6):718

14. Asensio JA, Chahwan S, Hanpeter D, Demetriades D, Forno W, Gambaro E, Murray J, Velmahos G, Marengo J, Shoemaker WC, Berne TV (2000) Operative management and outcome of 302 abdominal vascular injuries. Am J Surg 180(6):528–533, discussion 533–534

15. Asensio JA, Forno W, Gambaro E, Steinberg D, Tsai KJ, Rowe V, Navarro Nuño I, Leppäniemi A, Demetriades D (2000) Abdominal vascular injuries: the trauma surgeon's challenge. Ann Chir Gynaecol 89(1):71–78, No abstract available

16. Velmahos GC, Demetriades D, Chahwan S, Gomez H, Hanks SE, Murray JA, Asensio JA, Berne TV (1999) Angiographic embolization for arrest of bleeding after penetrating trauma to the abdomen. Am J Surg 178(5):367–373

17. Asensio JA, Berne JD, Chahwan S, Hanpeter D, Demetriades D, Marengo J, Velmahos GC, Murray J, Shoemaker WC, Berne TV (1999) Traumatic injury of the superior mesenteric artery. Am J Surg 178(3):235–239

18. Cornwell EE 3rd, Velmahos GC, Berne TV, Tatevossian R, Belzberg H, Eckstein M, Murray JA, Asensio JA, Demetriades D (1998) Lethal abdominal gunshot wounds at a level I trauma center: analysis of TRISS (Revised Trauma Score and Injury Severity Score) fallouts. J Am Coll Surg 187(2):123–129

19. Fabian TC, Richardson JD, Croce MA, Smith JS Jr, Rodman G Jr, Kearney PA, Flynn W, Ney AL, Cone JB, Luchette FA, Wisner DH, Scholten DJ, Beaver BL, Conn AK, Coscia R, Hoyt DB, Morris JA Jr, Harviel JD, Peitzman AB, Bynoe RP, Diamond DL, Wall M, Gates JD, Asensio JA, Enderson BL et al (1997) Prospective study of blunt aortic injury: multicenter trial of the American Association for the Surgery of Trauma. J Trauma 42(3):374–380, discussion 380–383

Vascular Injuries of the Neck

16

Juan A. Asensio, Juan M. Verde, Aytekin Ünlü, Daniel Pust, Mamoun Nabri, Tamer Karsidag, and Patrizio Petrone

16.1 Introduction

Penetrating neck trauma accounts for approximately 5–10% of all penetrating trauma patients. Approximately 30% of those admitted to a Trauma Center with penetrating neck injuries incur vascular injuries. Majority of the population affected are young males who have sustained injuries due to interpersonal violence. Vascular injuries are most frequently caused by penetrating trauma. Most affect zone II of the neck, with the jugular vein and carotid artery and its branches as the most frequently injured vessels. Vascular injuries of the neck from blunt trauma are quite uncommon. Their overall mortality of 20–40% and morbidity rates are significantly higher than for those patients who sustain penetrating trauma.

J.A. Asensio (✉)
Director, Trauma Clinical Research, Training and Community Affairs; Director, Trauma Surgery and Surgical Critical Care Fellowship; Director International Visiting Scholars/Research Fellowship; Division of Trauma Surgery and Surgical Critical Care; DeWitt Daughtry Family Department of Surgery, Medical Director for Education and Training, International Medical Institute; University of Miami Miller School of Medicine; Ryder Trauma Center, 1800 NW 10 Avenue, Suite T-247, Miami, Florida 33136, USA
e-mail: jasensio@med.miami.edu, asensio@att.blackberry.net

J.M. Verde, A. Ünlü, D. Pust, M. Nabri,
T. Karsidag
International Visiting Scholars/Research Fellows; Division of Trauma Surgery and Surgical Critical Care; DeWitt Daughtry Family Department of Surgery; University of Miami Miller School of Medicine; Ryder Trauma Center, Miami, Florida, USA

P. Petrone
Medical Advisor; Health Research Joint Commission; Ministry of Health; 1120-51 Avenue, Suite 316, La Plata (C.P. 1900), Province of Buenos Aires, Argentina

In 1552, Paré reported the first carotid artery injury, ligated due to a tangential laceration of the common carotid artery. The patient survived with extensive neurologic deficit. Fleming performed the same procedure in a suicidal sailor 250 years after with a successful outcome.

The controversy of mandatory surgical intervention versus selective management has been put to rest; as of now, most patients are managed selectively.

The greatest advances in injury management are always made during wars. During the Civil War, the mainstay of treatment was observation with a mortality rate of 15% for penetrating neck injuries. During World War I, observation remained the mainstay of therapy, with sporadic exploration and ligation becoming more common. Overall mortality rates ranged from 11% to 18%. However, during World War II, the dictum changed to mandatory exploration and attempted repair of vascular injuries with a subsequent decrease in mortality rates to 7%. During both the Korean and Vietnam conflicts, mandatory exploration with routine use of vascular repair became commonplace; however, mortality rates increased to 15% most likely due to greater injury severity caused by automatic weapons. In the civilian arena, mandatory exploration has been replaced by selective management or observation alone with mortality rates that range from 0% to 11%.

The most common clinical presentation for patients who reach trauma centers alive are shock, active bleeding, hematoma, neurologic deficit, and bruit. Once diagnosed, the patient's clinical condition guides treatment.

16.2 Operative Interventions

16.2.1 Pre-Operative Preparations

All patients requiring neck exploration, including those sustaining vascular injuries of the neck, are placed in a

H.-J. Oestern et al. (eds.), *Head, Thoracic, Abdominal, and Vascular Injuries*,
DOI: 10.1007/978-3-540-88122-3_16, © Springer-Verlag Berlin Heidelberg 2011

supine position with the head extended and rotated to the opposite side of the area to be explored. Both the face and neck as well as the supraclavicular and chest areas are included in the operating fields, should an extension of the incision high above the angle of the mandible or thoracotomy be necessary for exposure and management of vascular injuries in zones I and III, respectively. If at all possible, it is recommended that a towel roll be placed on the patients back at the interscapular area to facilitate neck extension and exposure.

The neck is explored through the standard incision starting on the anterior border of sternocleidomastoid muscle (SCM) extending from the angle of the mandible to the sternoclavicular junction. An extension of the incision toward the origin of the SCM may be made if the injury is located in zone III. Additional exposure may be obtained by dislocation of the mandible anteriorly. The neck incision may be extended as a median sternotomy for the management of most zone I injuries; similarly, the neck incision may also be extended as a supraclavicular incision for the management of associated subclavian vessel injuries, which occur with an incidence of 1–2% and are located within zone I (Figure 16.1).

Rarely, bilateral neck explorations may be required. In these cases, the standard incisions on the anterior borders of both SCM may be connected by a transverse incision, which will allow the trauma surgeon to elevate a flap, thus exposing structures in the midline of the neck. In these cases, serious consideration must be given to performing a protective tracheostomy.

16.2.2 Anatomy of the Neck

The anatomy of the neck is unique. No other part of the body contains so many vital structures in such proximity. The neck comprises the narrow portion of the body between the head and the trunk and is limited superiorly by mandible, mastoid process, and superior nuchal line, and inferiorly by the sternum, clavicles, and the seventh cervical vertebra (C7) spinous process. Deep into the skin lies the subcutaneous tissue and the superficial layer of the cervical fascia, which splits to surround both the SCM and the trapezius muscles. The cervical fascia consists of two more layers, the pretracheal layer that invests the strap muscles and the prevertebral layer that invests the prevertebral muscles. The aero-digestive tract components are located in the midline, whereas the neck vessels including the carotid artery and its branches and the internal jugular vein along with the vagus nerves are found on both sides of zone II. These structures are found in proximity and lie immediately under the skin. Musculoskeletal structures such as the cervical muscles and components of the vertebral column provide support. Such tight fascial compartmentalization of the neck structures limits external bleeding from vascular injuries, thus minimizing the possibility of exsanguination. This apparent beneficial effect is countered by the effects of bleeding within these closed spaces, which frequently compromises the airway and in essence creates a compartment syndrome of the neck.

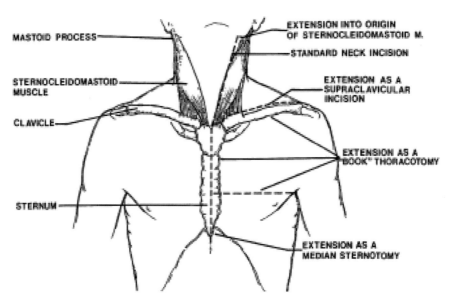

Fig.16.1 Incisions from Asensio JA, Valenziano CP, Falcone KE, Grosh JD (1991). Management of penetrating neck injuries: the controversy surrounding zone II injuries. In: Asensio JA, Weigelt J (eds). Surg Clin North Am 71, 267–296.

For the purposes of surgical management of penetrating neck injuries, the neck is classified into three anatomic zones, which are anterior to the sterno-cleidomastoid muscles (Figure 16.2). *Zone I* begins at the level of the clavicles and sternal notch and extends to the cricoid cartilage. The proximal carotid arteries (CA), subclavian vessels, great vessels of the chest, esophagus, and trachea are found in this zone. *Zone II* extends from the level of cricoid cartilage to the angle of the mandible; included here are the carotid arteries and their branches, jugular veins (JV), larynx, and hypopharynx. Zone III begins at the angle of mandible and extends to the base of the skull and contains the distal internal carotid artery (ICA), distal JV, and hypopharynx. Zone II is the easiest to clinically evaluate, and is also the easiest to approach surgically; it is also the most frequently injured zone. Zones I and III frequently mandate radiologic investigation prior to surgical intervention to determine the optimal surgical approach and fortunately are less frequently injured (Figures 16.3 and 16.4).

Knowledge of neck anatomy, coupled with an effort to conceptualize which structures lie within each zone, allows the surgeon to institute a systematic diagnostic search for injuries to the three key anatomic components of the neck: the cardiovascular, respiratory, and digestive systems.

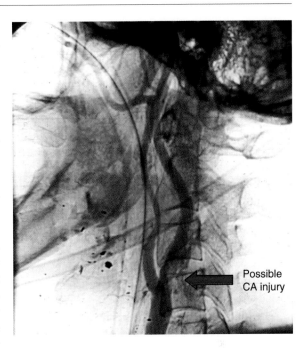

Fig. 16.3 GSW junction Zone II-III. Angiogram reveals mandibular fracture and possibly carotid artery injury

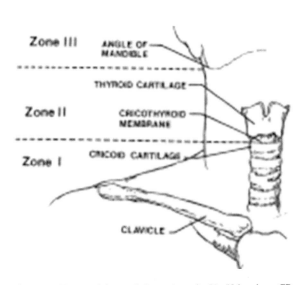

Fig. 16.2 Zones of the neck from Asensio JA, Valenziano CP, Falcone KE, Grosh JD (1991). Management of penetrating neck injuries: the controversy surrounding zone II injuries. In: Asensio JA, Weigelt J (eds). Surg Clin North Am 71, 267–296

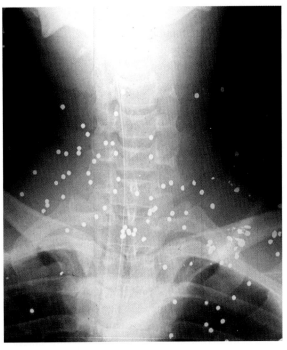

Fig. 16.4 Cervical X-ray shows multiple injuries secondary to shotgun

16.2.3 Vascular Anatomy of the Neck

16.2.3.1 Carotid Artery

The carotid vessels include both the common carotid artery (CCA) and its terminal branches, the internal (ICA) and external carotid arteries (ECA). In immediate relation with the arterial axis lie the internal jugular vein (IJV) and its tributaries; therefore, the most frequently associated injuries are those to the IJV. Each common carotid artery ascends within the carotid sheath along the IJV and vagus nerve to the level of the superior border of the thyroid cartilage. In this location, each common carotid artery bifurcates into the internal carotid artery (ICA) and external carotid (ECA). Branches of the ECA supply structures within the neck; however, the ICA gives rise to no branches in the neck and all of its branches are intracranial.

The right common carotid artery (CCA) begins at the bifurcation of the brachiocephalic trunk (the right subclavian artery is the other branch of this trunk). The left CCA originates on the arch of the aorta prior to ascending in the neck. Consequently, the left common carotid follows a course of approximately 2 cm in the superior mediastinum before entering the neck.

Both ICA are direct continuations of the CCA once the CCA bifurcates into an ICA and ECA at the level of the superior border of the thyroid cartilage. The ICA enter the cranium through carotid canal in the temporal bones and become the main arteries supplying blood flow to brain, while branches of ECAs supply most structures external to the cranium (ascending pharyngeal, occipital, posterior auricular, superior thyroid, lingual and facial arteries).

16.2.3.2 Jugular Vein

The internal jugular vein (IJV) serves as the main venous drainage conduit for the brain, face, cervical structures, and deep muscles of the neck. It originates at the jugular foramen as direct continuation of the sigmoid sinus, from a dilatation at its origin (superior bulb). The IJV descends in the carotid sheath with ICA superior to the carotid bifurcation and the CCA and vagus nerve inferiorly. The vein lies laterally within the sheath and the nerve is located posteriorly. The IJV leaves the anterior cervical region by coursing deep to the sternocleidomastoid muscle (SCM) ending between the sternal and clavicular heads of this muscle. At this point, the IJV merges with the subclavian vein to form the brachiocephalic or innominate vein. The inferior end of the IJV dilates to form the inferior bulb of the IJV.

16.2.3.3 Vertebral Artery

The vertebral artery (VA) arises from the superior aspect of the first part of subclavian artery. It ascends in the intervertebral foramina starting at the level of the sixth cervical vertebra (C6). It exits at the second cervical vertebra (C2) and curves medially behind its lateral mass entering the cranium via the foramen magnum to merge with the contralateral VA to give rise to the basilar artery. Classically, the VA is divided into four parts, the first originates in the subclavian artery and courses upward between the longus colli and scalenus anterior muscles, behind the CCA. It is crossed by thoracic duct on the left and right lymphatic duct on the right side. The second part begins once the VA enters the transverse foramina of the sixth cervical vertebrae and it is accompanied by paired vertebral veins. Third part begins when it exits the transverse foramina at the level of the second cervical vertebrae (C2) medial to the rectus capitis lateralis and curves backwards and medially behind the lateral mass of the atlas, with the first ventral spinal ramus lying on its medial side. In this position, it enters the vertebral canal through atlanto-occipital membrane in the suboccipital triangle. The fourth and last part ascends to the medulla oblongata and unites with contralateral VA to form the midline basilar artery at the lower border of the pons.

16.2.4 Exposure and Incisions

16.2.4.1 Surgical Exposure Carotid Artery and Internal Jugular Vein

The carotid sheath is directly approached via the standard incision anterior to the SCM. For the management of proximal injuries, a median sternotomy incision is required. Exposure of high ICA lesions at the base of the skull is one of the most difficult operations in trauma surgery. Anterior subluxation of the mandible improves exposure by 1–2 cm. For very high injuries, an osteotomy of the mandibular ramus may be required and is the preferred approach as it is simpler and safer.

Fortunately, these approaches are rarely needed. For severe intraoperative bleeding near the base of the skull, insertion of Fogarty balloon catheter in the distal carotid may be effective in controlling and/or tamponading the bleeding.

In the absence of neurologic deficits, carotid arterial repair should be performed whenever possible. If an interposition graft is required, the saphenous is the preferred conduit, although prosthetic grafts can also be used. It is important to remember that autogenous saphenous veins should not be reversed when used for carotid interposition bypasses as the flow in the saphenous vein follows the same direction of the flow in the carotid artery. The segment selected for bypass should not have any valves.

Ligation in neurologically intact patients is reserved for those sustaining very high ICA and for the patients in which the trauma surgeon experiences significant difficulties in controlling bleeding. The presence of coma and/or profound neurological deficits has a grave prognosis, irrespective of the type of operative management. On the basis of available data, the best chance for improvement even in patients with coma or profound neurological deficit seems to be immediate revascularization. The same approach should be undertaken for patients admitted in shock, which renders the preoperative neurologic assessment inaccurate. Currently, the consensus strongly supports primary repair while ligation is reserved for those in whom repair is technically impossible, for those with complete cessation of blood flow at the time of surgery, and for those with intraluminal thrombus in the distant segment of vessel as restoration of blood flow may cause cerebral embolization.

Carotid injuries that are amenable to repair with simple arteriorraphy may not require shunts. However, for more complex injuries requiring either bypass or circumferential end-to-end anastomosis, shunts are extremely useful to prevent ischemia. We recommend shunting for any complex injuries and for all complex repairs. When shunting, systemic heparinization is required. Debridement of the carotid injury to remove damaged portions of the vessel is a must. Reconstruction is either with primary end-to-end anastomosis or graft interposition (autogenous or prosthetic).

Injuries of IJV remain the most common vascular injuries in penetrating neck trauma and are frequently associated to CA injuries. The exposure and approach is the same as for carotid arteries. The clinical presentation is similar to other vascular injuries, with expanding hematomas and significant bleeding. There seems to be complacency with regard to the management of IJV injuries. The management of these injuries consists of venorrhaphy or ligation if repair is not feasible. We strongly recommend careful venorraphy with meticulous attention to surgical technique to prevent luminal narrowing. Ligation may be performed ipsilaterally. However, bilateral ligature is contraindicated as cerebral edema may rapidly develop and is invariably lethal.

16.2.4.2 Surgical Exposure Vertebral Artery

Vertebral artery (VA) injuries are being recognized with increasing frequency secondary of the liberal use of diagnostic angiography. The clinical presentation depends on the nature of the injury and, most importantly, on the presence of other associated injuries. Generally, isolated VA injuries are asymptomatic in about 30% of the patients. Rarely occlusions of VA result in neurologic deficit.

Hemodynamically stable patients with a thrombosed VA will not require surgical intervention, they may only need a late follow-up to exclude delayed complications such as an arteriovenous fistula. Angiographic embolization remains the treatment of choice in the majority of patients with VA injuries while operative management should be reserved for patients presenting with active bleeding or in cases where embolization has failed.

Positioning for VA exposure requires turning the head away from the injured side extending the neck. A long incision is made along the anterior border of the SCM, from the mastoid process to the sternoclavicular junction. This incision provides adequate exposure to the first and second parts of the VA. The SCM is retracted laterally and if necessary may be retracted cephalad after division at its insertion on the clavicle. The omohyoid should always be divided and the carotid sheath is thus exposed and retracted exposing the space between the anterior tubercle of the transverse processes and the vertebral bodies. Once removed, the longus cervicis colli muscle, the anterior rim of the vertebral foramen, the VA, is exposed. The rim will require removal with bone rongeurs to expose the vertebral vessels.

Fastidious hemorrhage from the venous plexus surrounding the VA not amenable to surgical ligation or application of fine silver clips should be controlled by packing and damage control approach to the injured VA followed by angiographic embolization. The utilization of bone wax to pack the vertebral canal is very useful in this situations. In cases of high VA injuries, a suboccipital craniectomy may be necessary to gain distal control.

16.2.5 Surgical Techniques

There are a number of critical surgical maneuvers that are standard in the management of all vascular injuries. They include:

1. Application of direct pressure for control of active bleeding.
2. Prepping the person holding pressure into the operative field.
3. Choosing the appropriate surgical exposure and plan to expose the injured vessel widely.
4. Obtain proximal and distal control of both arteries and veins, as combined injuries are common.
5. Isolate the injured vessels with meticulous dissection (Figure 16.5).
6. Retraction of injured or uninjured vessels can be carried out by looping them with vessel loops (Figure 16.6) or Cushing vein retractors.

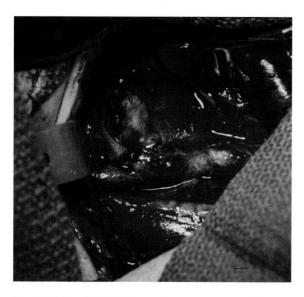

Fig. 16.5 Cervical GSW impacting common carotid artery (CCA)

7. To retract nerves, utilize gentle dissection while placing two vessel loops at distal points for retraction to distribute the pressure required to retract the nerve evenly and avoid neuropraxia.
8. Identify the injury and approach directly after proximal and distal control have been obtained (Figures 16.7 and 16.8).
9. Expose the injured vessel widely with meticulous surgical dissection. This may require taking down some of their branches and/or collaterals; however, care must be exercised to preserve as many collateral branches as possible.
10. Except for some stab wounds and/or lacerations in which the vessel can be directly repaired and/or anastomosed, resect appropriate length of the injured vessel, until normal proximal and distal cleared margins with uninjured intima are obtained. In the case of arteries, resection should avoid raising intimal flaps.
11. Inspect the transected edges of the artery. If there are intimal flaps re-resect. In cases in which there is an extensive flap and further resection is not possible, tack the intimal flap with internal horizontal mattress sutures of Halsted, placing the sutures from the inside of the vessel lumen tying the knots outside of the vessel. This should be done utilizing the finest monofilament polypropylene sutures.
12. Flush the proximal and distal ends of the transected vessel with heparinized saline. Check for distal back bleeding. Flush frequently and gently.
13. If there is no distal back bleeding, pass Fogarty catheters of the appropriate size and length, gently, and if possible, under direct vision of the vessels being thrombectomized. Do not hyperinflate the balloon and do not pass the catheter more than necessary to achieve good back bleeding as this will increase the risk of intimal damage.
14. Arterial injuries may be repaired by primary arteriography or by end-to-end anastomosis (Figure 16.9). They may also require a bypass or interposition graft either with an autogenous reverse saphenous vein graft (Figure 16.10) or with a prosthetic graft (Figure 16.11). Repairs and/or bypasses should never be under tension. They also should not be excessively long in order to prevent kinking. Most bypasses placed across a joint have their length properly selected with consideration of the range of motion (flexion) of the

Fig. 16.6 Cervical exploration reveals on CA injury (CA endarterectomy was performed)

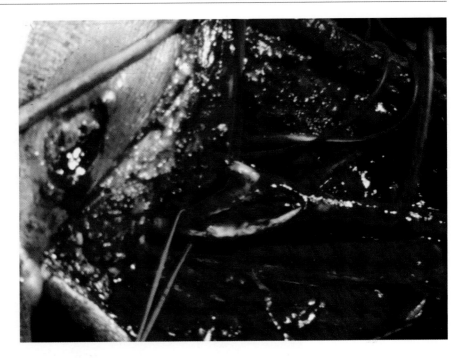

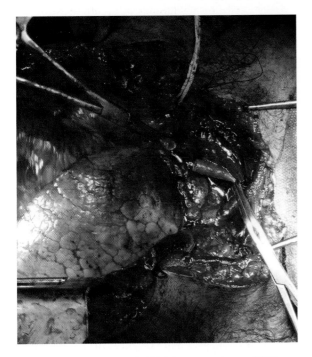

Fig. 16.7 Left intrathoracic CA injury secondary to GSW

joint to prevent kinking or graft occlusion. All anastomosis should be performed end to end with fine double-armed 5–0 or 6–0 polypropylene sutures preferably in a running fashion. Although it has been commonly thought that straight anastomosis might eventually develop stenosis, this is not the case.

15. Vessel discrepancies may be addressed by spatulating and/or fish-mouthing the graft. For small end-to-end vessel anastomosis, simple interrupted sutures of polypropylene may be used circumferentially and for difficult anastomosis the tri-partite suture technique of Carrel may be used.

16. Bypasses performed to smaller vessels such as distal, radial, and ulnar arteries may require their distal anastomosis to be end to side, which increases both the size of the anastomosis as well as its flow characteristics. This concept also applies to shank vessel such as the anterior and posterior tibial vessels. Obviously, this does not apply to carotid arteries.

Fig. 16.8 Intrathoracic left CA injury

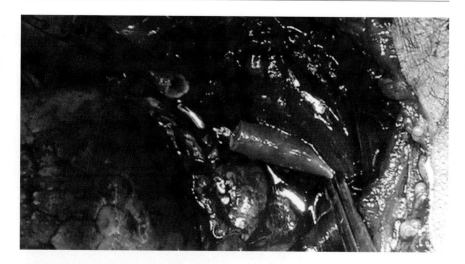

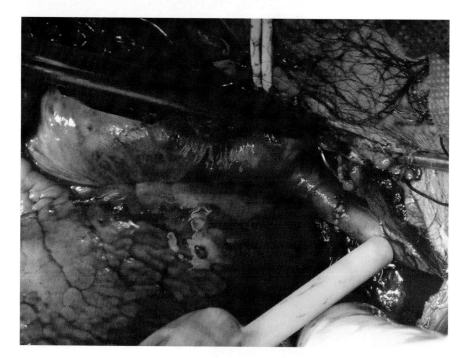

Fig. 16.9 Primary repair performing end-to-end anastomosis

17. Venous injuries may be ligated or primarily repaired. Double ligation with silk sutures is preferred for all veins. Primary venorraphy should be carried out with fine monofilament polypropylene sutures preventing narrowing the repaired vein. Very rarely, veno-venous bypass may be required.

18. Fasciotomies should be performed early, expediently, and when indicated. The more soft tissue injury there is, the shorter amount of ischemic time is tolerated. We recommend utilizing either cadaveric and/or porcine skin as biological dressings.

19. At the completion of the arterial repair and/or bypass, pulses should be checked by digital palpation and interrogated by a hand-held Doppler probe including the proximal and distal anastomosis of the bypass, the bypass itself, as well as all distal vessels.

20. The use of completion angiography should be individualized; however, it is highly recommended to detect correctable defects intraoperatively, which will prevent a vessel and/or bypass failure.

Fig. 16.10 Arterial bypass with 6-mm PTFE graft

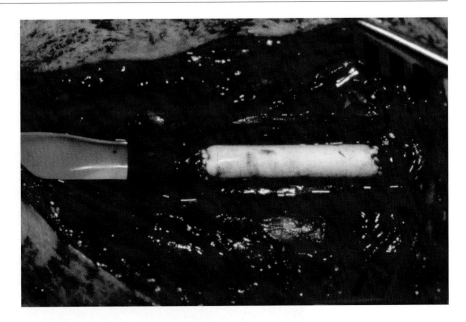

Fig. 16.11 Carotid repair with autogenous saphenous vein)

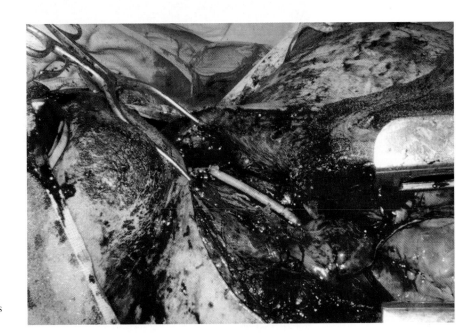

Although the majority of these critical maneuvers can be applied to most vascular injuries, the carotid artery requires special maneuvers to prevent cerebral ischemia. Shunting (Figure 16.12) is highly recommended for complex repairs and those requiring bypass grafting either with autogenous saphenous veins and/or PTFE. We recommend using straight shunts (Argyle), which are easier to place. Other shunts include the Pruitt–Inahara shunt (Figure 16.13), which are held in place by inflating balloons proximally and distally within the vessel lumen. Both the Sundt and Javid shunts require special clamps to secure them in place. When shunting, we strongly recommend systemic heparinization with either 5,000 or 7,500 units of heparin (the number of units of heparin follow surgeon's preferences) as a preventive measure to avoid cerebral

Fig. 16.12 Cervical exploration and arterial shunt

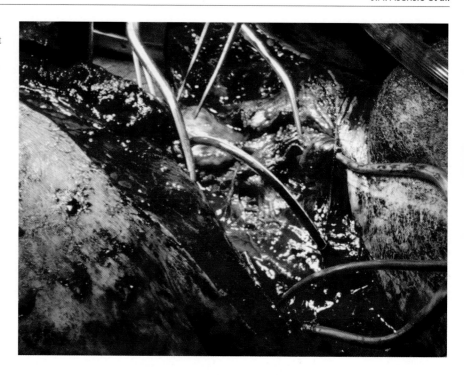

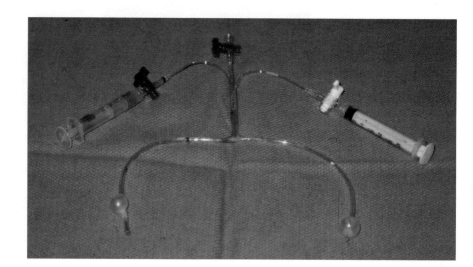

Fig. 16.13 Pruitt-Inahara shunt

thrombosis and are willing to accept the sequelae of soft tissue bleeding. Similarly, we recommend using either the Kitzmiller right or left carotid clamps (Figure 16.14) for very distal control, Castaneda (Figure 16.15), or 45° angled De Bakey clamps for vascular control.

After the completion of the carotid arterial repair, the ECA clamp is first removed while maintaining the ICA clamp in place, then the CCA clamp is removed to vent clots or arterial plaque into the ECA and not the ICA. Having performed this procedure, the ICA clamp can be removed. Mannitol may be administered as a preventive measure to decrease cerebral edema.

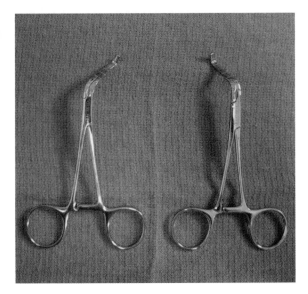

Fig. 16.14 Kitzmiller carotid clamps

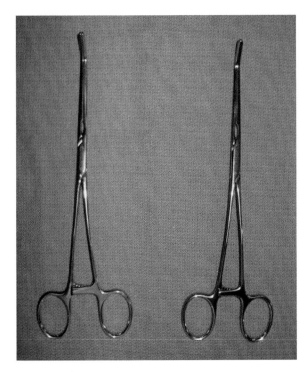

Fig. 16.15 Castaneda clamp

References

1. Asensio JA, Valenziano CP, Falcone RE et al (1991) Management of penetrating neck injuries. Surg Clin North Am 71(2):267–282
2. Elerding SC, Manart FD, Moore EE (1980) A reappraisal of penetrating neck injury management. J Trauma 20(8):695–697
3. Demetriades D, Asensio JA, Velmahos G (1996) Complex problems in penetrating neck trauma. Surg Clin North Am 76(4):661–684
4. Pate JW, Herwell W (1964) Arterial Injuries of the Base of the Neck. Arch Surg 89:1106–1110
5. Mutze S, Rademacher G, Matthes G et al (2005) Blunt cerebrovascular injury in patients with multiple blunt trauma. Radiology 237:884–892
6. Dragon R, Saranchak H, Lakin P et al (1981) Blunt injuries to the carotid and vertebral arteries. Am J Surg 141:497–500
7. Brown MF, Graham JM, Feliciano DV et al (1982) Carotid artery injuries. Am J Surg 144:748–753
8. Perry MO, Snyder WH, Thal ER (1980) Carotid artery injuries caused by blunt trauma. Ann Surg 192(1):74–77
9. Hayes P, Gerlock AJ, Cobb CA (1980) Cervical spine trauma, a cause of vertebral artery injury. J Trauma 20(10):904–905
10. Steenburg RW, Ravitch MM (1963) Cervico-thoracic approach for subclavian vessel injury from compound fracture of clavicle. Ann Surg 157(6):839–846
11. Munera F, Soto JA, Palacio D et al (2000) Diagnosis of arterial injuries caused by penetrating trauma to the neck. Radiology 216:356–362
12. Kuzniec P, Kauffman LJ, Molnar R et al (1998) Diagnosis of limbs and neck arterial trauma using duplex US. Cardiovasc Surg 61(4):358–366
13. Meissner M, Paun M, Johansen K (1991) Duplex scanning for arterial trauma. Am J Surg 161:552–555
14. Fry WR, Dort JA, Smith S (1994) Duplex scanning replaces arteriography and operative exploration in the diagnosis of potential cervical vascular injuries. Am J Surg 168:693–696
15. Rathlev NK, Medzon R, Bracken ME (2007) Evaluation and management neck trauma. Emerg Med Clin North Am 25:679–694
16. Roon AJ, Christensen N (1979) Evaluation and treatment of penetrating cervical injuries. J Trauma 19(6):391–397
17. Demetriades D, Theodorou D, Cornwell E, Berne TV, Asensio JA, Belzberg H, Velmahos G, Weaver F, Yellin A (1997) Evaluation of penetrating injuries of the neck, prospective study of 223 patients. World J Surg 21:41–48

18. Matthew JM, Mullneix PS, Steele SR et al (2005) Functional outcome after blunt and penetrating carotid artery injuries. J Trauma 59:860–864

19. Eddy JA (2000) Is routine arteriography mandatory for penetrating injuries to zone 1 of the neck. J Trauma 48(2): 208–214

20. Watson WL, Silverstone SM (1939) Ligature of the common carotid artery in cancer of the head and neck. Ann Surg 109(1):1–27

21. Wright GA (1888) Ligature of the subclavian artery for axillary aneurism. Ann Surg 8(5):362–367

22. Demetriades D, Theodorou J, Asensio JA et al (1996) Management options in vertebral artery injuries. Br J Surg 83:83–86

23. Thavendran A, Wijemanne NY, Soysa A et al (1975) Penetrating injuries of the neck. Injury 7(1):58–60

24. Thompson EC, Porter JM, Fernandez LG (2002) Penetrating neck trauma, an overview management. J Oral Maxillofac Surg 60:918–923

25. Jurkovich GJ, Zingarelli W, Wallace J et al (1986) Penetrating neck trauma, diagnostic studies in the asymptomatic patient. J Trauma 25(9):819–822

26. Saletta JD, Lowe RJ, Lim LT et al (1976) Penetrating tauma of the neck. J Trauma 16(7):579–587

27. Kuehne JP, Weaver FA, Papanicolau G (1996) Penetrating trauma of the internal carotid artery. Arch Surg 131:942–948

28. Fogelman MJ, Stewart RD (1956) Penetrating wounds of the neck. Am J Surg 91:581–586

29. Stein A, Seaward PD (1967) Penetrating wounds of the neck. J Trauma 7(2):238–247

30. Stain SC, Yellin AE, Weaver FA et al (1989) Selective management of nonocclusive arterial injuries. Arch Surg 24:1136–1141

31. Rich NM, Baugh JH, Hughes CW (1970) Significance of complications associated with vascular repairs performed in Vietnam. Arch Surg 100:646–651

32. Demetriades D, Asensio JA (2001) Subclavian and axillary vascular injuries. Surg Clin North Am 81(6):1357–1373

33. Murphy JB (1897) Surgical case-histories from the past. Harold Ellis. Royal Soc of Medicine, Chap. 28; Successful repair of GSW of the femoral artery, pp. 163–169.

34. Biffl WL, Moore EE, Elliot JP et al (2000) The devastating potential of blunt vertebral arterial injuries. Ann Surg 231(5):672–681

35. Weaver FA, Yellin AE, Wagner WH et al (1988) The role of arterial reconstruction in penetrating carotid artery injuries. Arch Surg 123:1106–1111

36. Cogbill TH, Moore EE, Meissner M et al (1994) The spectrum of blunt injury to the carotid artery. J Trauma 37(3): 473–479

37. Cogbill TH, Moore EE, Meissner M (1994) The spectrum of blunt injury to the carotid artery. J Trauma 37(3): 473–479

38. Ginzburg E, Montalvo B, LeBlang S et al (1996) The use of duplex ultrasonography in penetrating neck trauma. Arch Surg 131:691–693

Vascular Injuries of the Lower Extremities

17

Juan A. Asensio, Tamer Karsidag, Aytekin Ünlü,
Juan M. Verde, and Patrizio Petrone

17.1 Introduction

Vascular injuries to the extremities are relatively uncommon. They are generally seen in most major trauma centers (Figure 17.1). The majority of these injuries are the result of penetrating trauma such as gunshots (GSW), stab wounds (SW), and shotgun wounds (SGW). Similar mechanisms prevail in military arenas of warfare. In addition, in combat conditions, vascular injuries are also caused by antipersonnel devices including landmines and improvised explosive devices as well as by shrapnel or missile fragments. In contrast to civilian extremity vascular injuries, military injuries are usually accompanied by extensive soft tissue destruction.

The clinical presentation of extremity vascular injuries may range from cardiopulmonary arrest secondary to exsanguination, severe active arterial and/or venous bleeding to difficult-to-diagnose occult vascular injuries. Rarely, undetected and untreated vascular injuries may present on a delayed fashion even years after trauma in the form of pseudoaneurysms or arterial insufficiency.

Vascular injury of lower extremity incurs low mortality, and patients rarely exsanguinate, but these injuries are generally associated with significant morbidity and long-term disability. Femoral vessel injuries are among the most common vascular injuries treated in urban trauma centers, and may account for up to 70% of all peripheral vascular injuries in some series.

17.2 Operative Interventions

17.2.1 Pre-Operative Preparations

In the case of vascular injuries of lower extremities, the affected extremity is prepped widely including the feet, which should be covered with stockinettes. In cases of lower extremity injuries, the contralateral lower extremity is also prepped widely. The area to the mid-thighs is quite important should the necessity arise to obtain an autogenous saphenous vein graft. Before the operation, the surgeon has to be sure that there is enough blood supply, patient is kept warm, and specific instruments for vascular surgery are ready.

17.2.2 Vascular Anatomy of Lower Extremities

17.2.2.1 Common Femoral Artery

The common femoral artery is the direct continuation of the external iliac artery. It enters the femoral triangle

J.A. Asensio (✉)
Director, Trauma Clinical Research, Training and Community Affairs, Director, Trauma Surgery and Surgical Critical Care Fellowship, Director International Visiting Scholars/Research Fellowship, Division of Trauma Surgery and Surgical Critical Care, DeWitt Daughtry Family Department of Surgery, Medical Director for Education and Training, International Medical Institute, University of Miami Miller School of Medicine, Ryder Trauma Center, 1800 NW 10 Avenue, Suite T-247, Miami, FL 33136, USA
e-mail: jasensio@med.miami.edu, asensio@att.blackberry.net

T. Karsidag, A. Ünlü, J.M. Verde
International Visiting Scholars/Research Fellows, Division of Trauma Surgery and Surgical Critical Care, DeWitt Daughtry Family Department of Surgery, University of Miami Miller School of Medicine, Ryder Trauma Center, Miami, FL 33136, USA

P. Petrone
Medical Advisor; Health Research Joint Commission; Ministry of Health; 1120-51 Avenue, Suite 316, La Plata (C.P. 1900), Province of Buenos Aires, Argentina

H.-J. Oestern et al. (eds.), *Head, Thoracic, Abdominal, and Vascular Injuries*,
DOI: 10.1007/978-3-540-88122-3_17, © Springer-Verlag Berlin Heidelberg 2011

of Scarpa behind the inguinal ligament, midway between the anterior superior iliac spine and the symphysis pubis. The femoral triangle of Scarpa is bounded by the inguinal ligament superiorly, medial border of the sartorius muscle laterally, medial border adductor longus, and pectineus muscle medially. The floor of the triangle is formed by the iliacus, psoas major, pectineus, and adductor longus muscles. Within the triangle, the femoral artery is related laterally to the femoral nerve, medially to the femoral vein and femoral canal, and posteriorly to the psoas and pectineus muscles. Early in its course, the femoral artery gives rise to several branches: the superficial epigastric, superficial circumflex iliac, superior geniculate, and superficial, and deep external pudendal arteries. After traveling about 4 cm, the artery bifurcates within the femoral triangle into superficial femoral artery and profunda femoris artery.

17.2.2.2 Superficial Femoral Artery

This is usually the larger of the two terminating branches. It exits the femoral triangle at the apex and descends into the adductor canal. This canal is bordered by the sartorius muscle medially, vastus medialis anterolaterally, and the adductor longus and magnus muscle posteriorly. Within the canal, the artery is bound closely to the femoral vein by connective tissue. The saphenous nerve lies anterior to the vessel. The artery then pierces the adductor magnus at the adductor hiatus at the adductor canal of Hunter to become the popliteal artery.

17.2.2.3 Profunda Femoris Artery

The profunda femoris artery provides the main blood supply to the thigh. It usually arises from the posterolateral aspect of the femoral artery and descends first laterally, and then posterior to the superficial femoral artery. Subsequently, the artery runs down the thigh deep to the adductor longus muscle, in close relation to the linea aspera of the femur, and pierces the adductor magnus muscle to become the fourth perforating artery. The medial and lateral circumflex femoral arteries arise soon after the origin of the profunda femoris artery, although they branch out from the common femoral artery at the level of bifurcation in 20% of patients. These important vessels can flow in either direction. They serve as collaterals via cruciate anastomosis around the hip when either the internal or external iliac

artery is occluded. Three perforating arteries are also given out along the course of the profunda femoris artery to supply the muscle of the thigh. They are also connected by a rich anastomotic network.

17.2.2.4 Common Femoral Vein

The common femoral vein is a direct continuation of the external iliac vein; it accompanies the common femoral artery as it enters the femoral triangle of Scarpa. It is related medially to the common femoral vein. It is generally a short trunk measuring approximately 4 cm.

17.2.2.5 Superficial Femoral Vein

This is the larger of the two terminating branches of the common femoral vein as it bifurcates into the superficial femoral vein and the profunda femoris vein. It courses along the superficial femoral artery.

17.2.2.6 Popliteal Artery

The popliteal artery begins at the adductor hiatus at Hunter's canal as the direct continuation of the superficial femoral artery. It travels downward and slightly laterally to go behind the distal femur to enter the popliteal fossa. The popliteal fossa is an important anatomical area because all neurovascular structures passing from the thigh to the leg traverse this space. It is filled with tissues that offer protection to the neurovascular structure and yet allow the movement at the knee joint. It is a diamond-shaped fossa located behind the knee. The floor consists of popliteal surface of the femur above, and the posterior surface of the joint capsule with overlying popliteus muscle below. The superior border is made up of the bicep femoris muscle and tendon laterally, and four muscles, the semimembranosus, semitendinosus, gracilis, and sartorius muscles medially. The inferior boundaries are formed by the lateral and medial head of the gastrocnemius muscle, respectively. The roof consists of a strong sheet of deep investing fascia, which is pierced in the center by the short saphenous vein, subcutaneous tissue, and skin. This unites with the muscles and tendons forming the boundaries to form a well-enclosed space.

The popliteal artery runs on the floor of the popliteal fossa between the condyles of the femur until it reaches the distal border of fossa and tibioperoneal trunk.

Throughout the course, it is in direct contact with the posterior ligament of the knee joint. Two pairs of branches are given out to supply the knee and these form important collaterals. These are the paired superior and inferior (lateral and medial) geniculate arteries.

17.2.2.7 Popliteal Vein

The popliteal vein begins at the adductor hiatus at Hunter's canal as the direct continuation of the superficial femoral vein. It travels downward in slightly lateral to go behind the distal femur to enter popliteal fossa. The popliteal vein is a delicate structure and although it is usually described as a single vessel of large caliber more often it consists of two large venous trunks. It receives multiple venous tributaries including the soleal plexus, which is generally a large vein and not a plexus itself.

17.2.2.8 Tibioperoneal Trunk

The tibioperoneal trunk is the larger terminating branch of the popliteal artery. It originates and descends from just behind the soleal plexus. The trunk lies on the tibialis posterior muscle and is covered by the gastrocnemius and soleus muscles. A network of complex and thin-walled venous vessels surrounds the artery. The tibial nerve accompanies the artery below the arch of the soleus muscle. It runs a variable length, ranging from 0 to 5 cm before bifurcating into posterior tibial and peroneal artery.

17.2.2.9 Anterior Tibial Artery

The anterior tibial artery is the smaller terminating branch of the popliteal artery that arises from the lower border of the popliteus muscle. It passes forward through the interosseous membrane into the anterior compartment of the leg. At first, it lies close to the medial aspect of the neck of the fibula, but inclines medially and forward on the membrane as it descends and rests against the anterior surface of the shaft of tibia in the lower third of the leg. It lies deep between anterior tibialis and extensor digitorum longus muscle proximally and extensor hallucis longus muscle distally. In the final part of its course, it is covered only by skin, fascia, and the extensor retinaculum. At the level of the ankle, the tendon of the extensor hallucis longus muscle crosses in front of the artery to become medially related. The artery then continues on as the dorsalis pedis.

Throughout the course, the anterior tibial artery is surrounded by two interlacing venae comitantes and the deep peroneal nerve. The deep peroneal nerve, after winding around the neck of the fibula, joins the anterior tibial artery soon after the artery enters the anterior compartment. Initially, the nerves lie laterally to the artery, but from about the middle of the leg, the nerve takes up an anterolateral relationship to the artery for the rest of its course.

17.2.2.10 Posterior Tibial Artery

The posterior tibial artery is the direct continuation of the tibioperoneal trunk. It descends in the posterior compartment, lying on the posterior tibialis for most of its course and covered by the gastrocnemius and soleus muscles. In the upper two thirds, the posterior tibial artery lies deep in the covering muscles. For the rest of the course, the artery takes a superficial course. At its termination, the artery lies midway between the medial malleolus and the medial tubercle of the calcaneus, among the tendons of the deep leg muscles and under the cover of the flexor retinaculum. A pair of deep veins accompanies the artery as venae comitantes. Throughout the course, the posterior tibial nerve runs alongside the artery. The nerve takes a medial relationship initially and becomes posterior in the lower part of the leg. The posterior tibial artery terminates by dividing into medial and lateral plantar arteries.

17.2.2.11 Peroneal Artery

The peroneal artery descends laterally toward the fibula after branching off from the tibioperoneal trunk. It then follows the medial edge of the fibula, between flexor hallucis longus and tibialis posterior muscles, in close relation to the posterior aspect of the fibula and the interosseous membrane throughout the course. At the ankle, the artery gives off a branch that perforates the interosseous membrane.

This anterior malleolar branch of the peroneal artery descends in front of the lateral malleolus, and forms an anastomotic network around the malleolus with the lateral and posterior malleolar branches of the peroneal artery. A pair of deep veins accompanies the artery, but there is major nerve that travels with the artery.

17.2.3 Adjuncts

Essential to good vascular surgical technique is adequate illumination generally with a fiber-optic head lamp, as well as visualization with optical loupes with a 2.5× or 3.5× magnification. Other important adjuncts include vessel loops, shunts, heparin for systemic administration, heparinized saline for irrigation, papaverine and embolectomy catheters (Fogarty catheters), as well as biological dressings such as cadaver and/or porcine skin to cover fasciotomies and act as biological dressings. Other important adjuncts include prosthetic grafts generally made from polytetrafluroethylene (PTFE). Availability of hand-held Doppler probes and intraoperative angiography are a must. It is always important to set up two sets of electrocautery and two suction devices.

17.2.4 Lower Extremities Vessels' Surgical Exposure

17.2.4.1 Common Femoral Artery and Vein

Exposure can be achieved via a longitudinal incision over the femoral pulse over the femoral triangle of Scarpa. In the absence of a pulse, the incision can be placed inferior to the midpoint between anterior superior iliac spine and pubic tubercle. Proximal control of the external iliac artery and vein can be achieved through either a separate incision that runs parallel to the inguinal ligament or by retracting or extending the longitudinal incision superiorly and laterally through the inguinal ligament.

The incision is deepened to expose the deep fascia covering the femoral triangle. Incision of the fascia will allow the retraction of sartorius and adductor magnus to expose the femoral sheath. The sheath is then sharply incised to expose the common femoral artery within. Exposure of the femoral vein is carried out in similar fashion as it lies medial to the artery.

17.2.4.2 Superficial Femoral Artery and Vein

Exposure can be achieved by longitudinal incision over the femoral pulse at the femoral triangle Scarpa. In the absence of a pulse, the incision can be placed inferior to the midpoint between anterior superior iliac spine and pubic tubercle.

The incision is deepened to expose the deep fascia covering the femoral triangle. Incision of the fascia will allow the retraction of sartorius and adductor magnus to expose the femoral sheath. The sheath is then sharply incised to expose the superficial femoral artery within. Exposure of the superficial femoral vein is carried out in a similar fashion as it lies medially.

The superficial femoral artery and vein can be approached through an incision along the line joining the anterior superior iliac spine and medial femoral condyle. The incision is deepened through the superficial fascia, carefully retracting the greater saphenous vein. The fascia covering of the sartorius is divided and the muscle can be retracted medially to expose the superficial femoral vessels with the saphenous nerve on the anterior surface. The incision and dissection are carried out distally to achieve full exposure of the vessel.

17.2.4.3 Popliteal Artery and Vein

The approach to the popliteal artery can be carried out in a posterior or a medial incision. A posterior S-shaped incision requires the patient to be placed in a prone position and have limited access to the anterior compartment of the leg; thus, it is seldom used for vascular injury unless there is a certainty that the popliteal injury is an isolated injury. Therefore, it is usually not recommended. The medial approach tends to be more versatile (Figure 17.2), and lacks the disadvantages of the posterior approach. The leg is adducted and flexed at the knee while it is being propped with several surgical towels. The incision is placed from the medial femoral condyle across the knee down to the leg. The incision of the superficial fascia will expose the underlying muscles. Anterior retraction of vastus medialis muscle and posterior retraction of sartorius muscle will expose the popliteal vessels and the saphenous nerve. This incision can also be extended distally behind the bony prominence of the tibia, to approach the origin of the anterior tibial artery and the tibioperoneal trunk. The exposure can be further enhanced by dividing the medial head of the gastrocnemius muscle, the tendon of the adductor magnus, sartorius and the tendinous insertions of the semimembranosus, and semitendinosus (the pes anserinus).

17.2.4.4 Tibioperoneal Trunk

This vessel is exposed by dividing the medial head of the gastrocnemius and continuing the dissection in a downward fashion.

17.2.4.5 Anterior Tibial Artery

The anterior tibial artery in the anterior compartment lies in front of the interosseous membrane. Exposure can be gained by a longitudinal lateral incision between the tibia and fibula. The incision is carried through the intermuscular septum between the tibialis anterior and extensor hallucis muscles, without disrupting the belly of the muscles. The extensor hallucis longus can be retracted laterally to facilitate exposure. Care must be taken to preserve the venae comitantes and the deep peroneal nerve. This approach, coupled with resection of fibula, will also facilitate exposure of the peroneal vessels that lie just behind the fibula in the posterior compartment. The anterior tibial artery in the lower part of the leg lies superficial. The incision placed over the pulse, dissection of the subcutaneous tissue, and investing fascia will allow for exposure of the vessel.

17.2.4.6 Posterior Tibial Artery

The posterior tibial artery is accessed through a medial approach. An incision is placed behind the posterior border of the tibia. The deep investing fascia is incised for the length of the wound and the intermuscular plane between the flexor digitorum longus anteriorly, and the medial head of gastrocnemius and soleus muscles posteriorly. This will also allow exposure of the peroneal vessels, which lie in a more lateral position. Care must be taken to avoid injuring the tibial nerve, which lies adjacent to the posterior tibial artery. In the lower third of the calf, the posterior tibial artery takes a superficial course after emerging from under the soleus and gastrocnemius muscles. It is only covered by skin, subscutaneous tissue, and the deep investing fascia. The incision can be made directly over the pulse or about an inch anterior to the Achilles tendon and deepened to expose the vessel.

17.2.4.7 Peroneal Artery

This vessel can be exposed utilizing the approaches for both the anterior and posterior tibial arteries.

17.2.5 Surgical Techniques

Rapid surgical intervention with immediate exposure to obtain proximal and distal control and stop the rapid blood loss experienced by these patients is key to their survival.

Fluid resuscitation and application of direct pressure or tourniquet occlusion technique for control of active bleeding benefit life and limb salvage as prehospital treatment. Do not blindly attempt to clamp a vessel.

Critical surgical maneuvers:

1. Application of direct pressure for control of active bleeding.
2. Prepping the person holding pressure into the operative field.
3. Choosing the appropriate surgical exposure and plan to expose the injured vessel widely.
4. Obtain proximal and distal control of both arteries and veins, as combined injuries are common.
5. Isolate the injured vessels with meticulous dissection.
6. Retraction of injured or uninjured vessels can be carried out by looping them with vessel loops or Cushing vein retractors.
7. To retract nerves, utilize gentle dissection and place two vessel loops at distal points for retraction to distribute the pressure required to retract the nerve evenly.
8. Identify the injury and approach directly after proximal and distal controls have been obtained.
9. Expose the injured vessel widely with meticulous surgical dissection. This may require taking down some of their branches and/or collaterals; however, care must be exercised to preserve as many as possible.
10. Except for some stab wounds and/or lacerations in which the vessel can be directly repaired and/or anastomosed, resect appropriate length of the injured vessel, until normal proximal and distal vessel is obtained. In the case of arteries, resection should avoid raising intimal flaps.
11. Inspect the transected edges of the artery. If there are intimal flaps re-resect. In cases in which there is an extensive flap and further resection is not possible, tack the intimal flap with internal horizontal mattress sutures of Halsted, placing the sutures from the inside of the vessel lumen tying the knots outside of the vessel. This should be done utilizing the finest monofilament polypropylene sutures.

12. Flush the proximal and distal ends of the transected vessel with heparinized saline. Check for distal back bleeding. Flush frequently and gently.

13. If there is no distal back bleeding, pass Fogarty catheters of the appropriate size and length, gently and, if possible, under direct vision of the vessels being thrombectomized. Do not hyperinflate the balloon and do not pass the catheter more than necessary to achieve good back bleeding as this will increase the risk of intimal damage. If there is no arterial flow return, papaverine may be instilled to break vasospasm.

14. Arterial injuries may be repaired by primary arteriography or by end-to-end anastomosis. They may also require a bypass or interposition graft either with an autogenous reverse saphenous vein graft or with a prosthetic graft (Figures 17.3–17.6). Repairs and/or bypasses should never be under tension. They also should not be too long in order to prevent kinking. Bypasses placed across a joint most have their length properly selected with consideration of the range of motion (flexion) of the joint to prevent kinking or graft occlusion. All anastomosis should be performed end to end with double-armed polypropylene sutures preferably in a running fashion. Although it has been commonly thought that straight anastomosis might eventually develop stenosis, this is not the case.

15. Vessel discrepancies may be addressed by spatulating and/or fish-mouthing the graft. For small end-to-end vessel anastomosis, simple interrupted sutures of polypropylene may be used circumferentially and for difficult anastomosis the tripartite suture technique of Carrel may be used.

16. Bypasses performed to smaller vessels such as the posterior tibial, anterior tibial, or rarely the peroneal arteries may require their distal anastomosis to be end to side, which increases both the size of the anastomosis as well as its flow characteristics.

17. Venous injuries may be ligated or primarily repaired. Double ligation with silk sutures is preferred for all veins. Larger veins in the lower extremity should be repaired, if possible. Primary venorrhaphy should be carried out with fine monofilament polypropylene sutures preventing narrowing of the repaired vein. Very rarely will a veno-venous bypass be required (Fig. 17.3).

18. Fasciotomies should be performed early, expediently, and when indicated. The more soft tissue injury there is, the shorter is the amount of ischemic time that is tolerated.

19. At the completion of the arterial repair and/or bypass, pulses should be checked by digital palpation and interrogated by a hand-held Doppler probe including the proximal and distal anastomosis of the bypass, the bypass itself, as well as all distal vessels.

20. The use of completion angiography should be individualized; however, it is highly recommended to detect correctable defects intraoperatively, which will prevent a vessel and/or bypass failure.

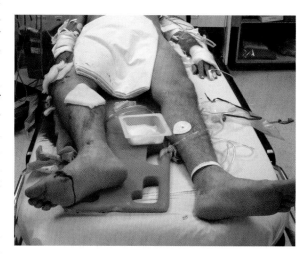

Fig. 17.1 Motor vehicle collision (MVC) with secondary femur/tibial fracture associated to ischemic signs

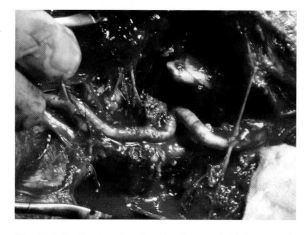

Fig. 17.2 Popliteal exploration showing arterial injury associated to femur fracture

Fig. 17.3 Femoropopliteal
bypass with autogenous
inverse saphenous vein graft
(Proximal anastomosis)

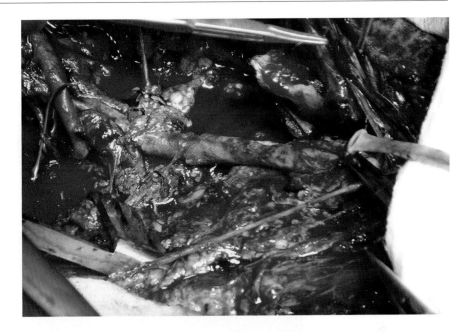

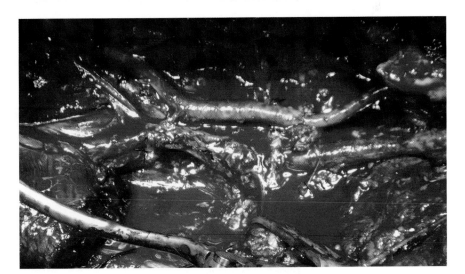

Fig. 17.4 Femoropopliteal
bypass with autogenous
inverse saphenous vein graft

Fig. 17.5 MVC with secondary femur fracture and superficial femoral artery injury. Femorofemoral bypass with autogenous inverse saphenous vein graft

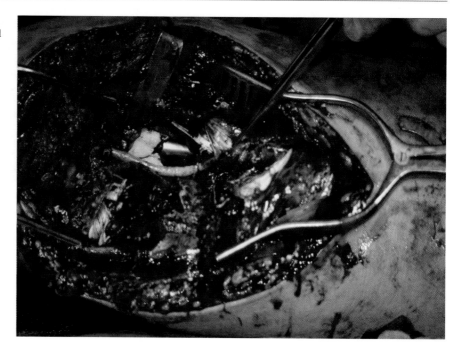

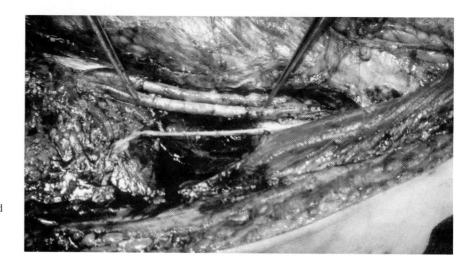

Fig. 17.6 Femoral vein and artery injuries due to GSW. Arterial and vein primary repair (bypass)

References

1. Asensio JA, Kuncir EJ, García-Núñez LM, Petrone P (2006) Femoral vessel injuries: analysis of factors predictive of outcomes. J Am Coll Surg 203(4):512–520, Epub 2006 Aug 23
2. Kumar SR, Rowe VL, Petrone P, Kuncir EJ, Asensio JA (2003) The vasculopathic patient: uncommon surgical emergencies. Emerg Med Clin North Am 21(4):803–815, Review
3. Asensio JA, Petrone P, Roldán G, Kuncir E, Rowe VL, Chan L, Shoemaker W, Berne TV (2003) Analysis of 185 iliac vessel injuries: risk factors and prediction of outcome. Arch Surg 138(11):118–193, discussion 1193-1194
4. Asensio JA, Petrone P, Karsidag T, Ramos-Kelly JR, Demiral S, Roldan G, Pak-Art R, Kuncir E (2002) Abdominal vascular injuries: a continuing challenge. Ulus Travma Derg 8(4):189–197, Review
5. Rowe VL, Salim A, Lipham J, Asensio JA (2002) Shank vessel injurie. Surg Clin North Am 82(1):91–104, xx. Review
6. Asensio JA, McDuffie L, Petrone P, Roldán G, Forno W, Gambaro E, Salim A, Demetriades D, Murray J, Velmahos G, Shoemaker W, Berne TV, Ramicone E, Chan L (2001) Reliable variables in the exsanguinated patient wich indicate damage control and predict outcome. Am J Surg 182(6):743–751

7. Asensio JA, Soto SN, Forno W, Roldan G, Petrone P, Gambaro E, Salim A, Rowe V, Demetriades D (2001) Abdominal vascular injuries: the trauma surgeon's challenge. Surg Today 31(11):949–957, Review

8. Asensio JA, Britt LD, Borzotta A, Peitzman A, Miller FB, Mackersie RC, Pasquale MD, Pachter HL, Hoyt DB, Rodriguez JL, Falcone R, Davis K, Anderson JT, Ali J, Chan L (2001) Multiinstitutional experience with the management of superior mesentery artery injuries. J Am Coll Surg 193(4):354–365, discussion 365-366. Erratum in: J Am Coll Surg 2001 Dec;193(6):718

9. Asensio JA, Chahwan S, Hanpeter D, Demetriades D, Forno W, Gambaro E, Murray J, Velmahos G, Marengo J, Shoemaker WC, Berne TV (2000) Operative management and outcome of 302 abdominal vascular injuries. Am J Surg 180(6):528–533, discussion 533-4

10. Asensio JA, Forno W, Gambaro E, Steinberg D, Tsai KJ, Rowe V, Navarro Nuño I, Leppäniemi A, Demetriades D (2000) Abdominal vascular injuries: the trauma surgeon's challenge. Ann Chir Gynaecol 89(1):71–78, No abstract available

11. Velmahos GC, Demetriades D, Chahwan S, Gomez H, Hanks SE, Murray JA, Asensio JA, Berne TV (1999) Angiographic embolization for arrest of bleeding after penetrating trauma to the abdomen. Am J Surg 178(5):367–373

12. Asensio JA, Berne JD, Chahwan S, Hanpeter D, Demetriades D, Marengo J, Velmahos GC, Murray J, Shoemaker WC, Berne TV (1999) Traumatic injury of the superior mesenteric artery. Am J Surg 178(3):235–239

13. Cornwell EE 3rd, Velmahos GC, Berne TV, Tatevossian R, Belzberg H, Eckstein M, Murray JA, Asensio JA, Demetriades D (1998) Lethal abdominal gunshot wounds at a level I trauma center: analysis of TRISS (Revised Trauma Score and Injury Severity Score) fallouts. J Am Coll Surg 187(2):123–129

14. Fabian TC, Richardson JD, Croce MA, Smith JS Jr, Rodman G Jr, Kearney PA, Flynn W, Ney AL, Cone JB, Luchette FA, Wisner DH, Scholten DJ, Beaver BL, Conn AK, Coscia R, Hoyt DB, Morris JA Jr, Harviel JD, Peitzman AB, Bynoe RP, Diamond DL, Wall M, Gates JD, Asensio JA, Enderson BL et al (1997) Prospective study of blunt aortic injury: multicenter trial of the American Association for the Surgery of Trauma. J Trauma 42(3):374–380, discussion 380-383

Vascular Injuries of the Upper Extremities

18

Juan A. Asensio, Tamer Karsidag, Aytekin Ünlü,
Juan M. Verde, and Patrizio Petrone

I think the ligature of main arteries for arrest of bleeding in distant parts is often somewhat blindly advised and possibly too frequently carried out. (Sir Frederick Treves [1853–1923])

18.1 Introduction

Upper extremity injuries are increasingly common among peripheral vascular injuries, as a result of penetrating trauma (Figure 18.1). Blunt trauma may also result in significant vascular injury primarily due to associated injuries such as fractures and dislocations. Injuries to the brachial artery are most commonly reported.

Vascular injuries of the upper extremity cause significant morbidity with severe consequences on motor function of the extremities. Death is generally due to exsanguination from uncontrolled hemorrhage. However, these injuries may be associated with significant morbidity secondary to failed vascular repairs and/or associated soft tissue, nerve or bone injuries, which may result in limb loss or permanent disability. Management with good outcomes depends on early diagnosis and prompt surgical approach.

18.2 Operative Interventions

18.2.1 Pre-Operative Preparations

In the operating room, the patient's entire torso, from the neck to mid-thighs, is prepared and draped. In the case of upper extremity vascular injuries, the affected extremity is prepped widely including the hands. In cases of upper extremity injuries, it is important to prep the contralateral (lower extremity, as one can harvest a saphenous vein from the opposite side of the table if there are two teams working simultaneously). The trauma surgeon must confirm that there are sufficient units of blood in the operating room for immediate transfusion via rapid infusion technology. They must also institute maneuvers to prevent hypothermia which include: placing a warming blanket in the operating table, covering the patient's unaffected extremities with a circulating warm air mattress, covering the head to prevent heat loss, increasing the ventilator cascade temperature to 42°C, and insuring that an ample supply of warmed irrigation and intravenous fluids are available. In addition, the availability of auto-transfusion apparatus and cell-saving technology is of great value. Appropriate vascular instruments and shunts must always be available. The authors also favor having the newer hemostatic agents available.

J.A. Asensio (✉)
Director, Trauma Clinical Research, Training and Community Affairs, Director, Trauma Surgery and Surgical Critical Care Fellowship, Director International Visiting Scholars/Research Fellowship, Division of Trauma Surgery and Surgical Critical Care, DeWitt Daughtry Family Department of Surgery, Medical Director for Education and Training, International Medical Institute, University of Miami Miller School of Medicine, Ryder Trauma Center, 1800 NW 10 Avenue, Suite T-247, Miami, FL 33136, USA
e-mail: jasensio@med.miami.edu, asensio@att.blackberry.net

T. Karsidag, A. Ünlü, J.M. Verde
International Visiting Scholars/Research Fellows, Division of Trauma Surgery and Surgical Critical Care, DeWitt Daughtry Family Department of Surgery, University of Miami Miller School of Medicine, Ryder Trauma Center, Miami, FL 33136, USA

P. Petrone
Medical Advisor; Health Research Joint Commission; Ministry of Health; 1120-51 Avenue, Suite 316, La Plata (C.P. 1900), Province of Buenos Aires, Argentina

H.-J. Oestern et al. (eds.), *Head, Thoracic, Abdominal, and Vascular Injuries*,
DOI: 10.1007/978-3-540-88122-3_18, © Springer-Verlag Berlin Heidelberg 2011

18.2.2 Vascular Anatomy Upper Extremity

18.2.2.1 Axillary Artery

The axillary artery starts from the lateral border of the first rib, as a direct continuation of the subclavian artery. In enters the axilla at its apex and crosses the first intercostal space to run along the lateral wall of the axilla. As the artery emerges from beneath the costoclavicular passage, it becomes closely related to the brachial plexus, divisions, and cords. These nerves surround the artery and exchange fibers to eventually become the median, ulnar, and radial nerves at the distal portion of the axillary artery. This neurovascular bundle is enclosed in the axillary sheath, which separates it from the axillary vein. Distally, the axillary artery continues on as brachial artery at the lateral edge of the teres major muscle tendon.

Anteriorly, the axillary artery follows a course under the pectoralis minor muscle as it inserts into the coracoid process. The muscle divides the artery into three anatomical portions: the first portion runs from lateral edge of the first rib to the upper border of the tendon of the pectoralis minor muscle, behind the clavipectoral fascia and the clavicular head of the pectoralis major muscle. It gives rise to a single branch in this portion, the supreme thoracic artery. The second portion lies behind the pectoralis minor muscle. This is the shortest portion and it has two branches of clinical significance, the thoracoacromial artery and the lateral thoracic artery. The cords of the brachial plexus surround the axillary artery at this section. The third portion starts from the lateral border of the pectoralis muscle to the lateral border of the teres major muscle. The axillary artery gives rise to three branches at this portion, the subscapular, the lateral humeral circumflex, and the medial circumflex artery. At this level, the brachial plexus becomes the median nerve, which is anterior, the radial nerve, which is posterior, and the ulnar nerve, which is inferior to the axillary in the axillary sheath.

18.2.2.2 Axillary Vein

The basilic vein continues on at the lower edge of the teres major muscle as the axillary vein. Its main tributaries are brachial veins, which accompany the named

arteries while they ascend in the axilla, and the cephalic vein, which courses through the deltopectoral groove, just below the clavicle. The axillary vein then becomes the subclavian vein as it courses above the lateral border of the fist rib by the ligament of Halsted. The axillary vein lies medial to the axillary artery. It is separated from the artery by the medial pectoral nerve, medial cord of the brachial plexus, and the ulnar nerve. It is separated from the axillary sheath by a pad of fat pad.

18.2.2.3 Brachial Artery

The brachial artery originates at the lower border of the teres major muscle as a direct continuation of the axillary artery. It follows a course toward the antecubital fossa, together with the median nerve, and bifurcates into the radial and ulnar arteries opposite the neck of the radius. The medial bicipital sulcus, which separates the coracobrachialis and biceps muscle anteriorly from the triceps muscle posteriorly, marks the course of the basilic vein toward the axillary vein and provides the surface marking of the brachial vessels.

The proximal part of the brachial artery lies on the medial aspect of the arm, anterior to the long and median head of the triceps and bordered laterally by the coracobrachialis muscle. The median nerve lies between the coracobrachialis muscle and the brachial artery, whereas the ulnar nerve separates the artery from the basilic vein. The brachial artery gives rise to the profunda brachii artery posteriorly, which passes backward and accompanies the radial nerve in the radial groove to the lateral condyle of the humerus. This artery collateralizes about the shoulder with the circumflex humeral arteries arising from the axillary artery.

The brachial artery gradually inclines forward and outward and eventually comes to lie below the medial border of the biceps muscle. The median nerve crosses the artery obliquely at this part of the arm. The basilic vein and the medial cutaneous nerve are separated from the artery by the deep fascia sheath. The branches arising from this portion of the brachial artery include the nutrient artery to the humerus, muscular branches, and superior ulnar collateral artery, which accompanies the ulnar nerve to the groove on the posterior surface of the medial epicondyle. This artery subsequently takes part in the rich anastomosis around the elbow joint.

The distal part of the brachial artery is overlapped by the medial border of the biceps muscle and biceps tendon and eventually comes to lie medial to the biceps tendon before the bifurcation of the artery. The median nerve lies medial to the brachial artery. This inferior ulnar collateral artery arises near the elbow and forms a rich network of collaterals around the elbow joint. The brachial artery bifurcates opposite the next of the radius bone to give rise to ulnar artery medially and the radial artery laterally. The artery is closely accompanied by a pair of venae comitantes that drain into the axillary vein.

18.2.2.4 Radial Artery

The radial artery is usually the smaller branch that follows the general direction of the brachial artery. It is a fairly superficial vessel, covered mainly by skin, subcutaneous tissue, and fascia, save for the muscle. The artery takes a course that travels laterally gradually, and after emerging from under the brachioradialis muscle, it comes to lie between the brachioradialis and the flexor carpi radialis muscles. The distal part, which is the most superficial part of the radial artery, travels between the tendon of flexor pollicis longus and the lateral border of the radius, until it passes behind the flexor retinaculum to enter the hand. The radial artery gives rise to two major branches, the radial recurrent branch near the origin and the superficial palmar branch, which takes part in the formation of the superficial palmar arch.

18.2.2.5 Ulnar Artery

The ulnar artery is the larger of the two terminal trunks of the brachial artery. It runs downward and medially to reach the medial aspect of the forearm from the bifurcation. During its course, the artery lies on the brachialis muscle in the upper part and then on the flexor digitorum profundus as it progresses distally. It is covered by the pronator teres muscle, flexor carpi radialis, and flexor digitorum superficialis. The median nerve lies medial to the ulnar artery for the first 2.5 cm before it crosses in front of the artery to take up a lateral relationship. After the crossing over, the nerve is separated from the artery by the ulnar head of the pronator teres. At the distal part, the ulnar artery emerges between the tendon of the flexor digitorum superficialis medially and flexor carpi ulnaris laterally to be covered by skin and fascia only. It subsequently passes behind the palmaris brevis to determine in the superficial palmar arch. The branches that give out near the origin of the ulnar artery include the anterior and posterior ulnar recurrent arteries and the common intersseous artery.

18.2.2.6 Basilic Vein

The basilic vein receives tributaries from the ulnar component of the dorsal venous network. It runs up the posterior surface of the forearm and curves around the ulnar border below the elbow to the anterior surface of the forearm. In the elbow, it is joined by the vena mediana cubiti, a branch from the cephalic vein. The vein takes a medial and superficial relation to the brachial artery and the medial cutaneous nerve in this part of the course. It then runs upward along the medial border of the biceps brachii muscle, and perforates the deep fascia to run along the medial side of the brachial artery. At the lower border of the teres major muscles, the vein continues on as the axillary vein.

18.2.2.7 Cephalic Vein

The cephalic vein begins as the coalescence of the radial part of the dorsal venous network and winds upwards around the radial border. In the antecubital fossa just below the elbow, the cephalic vein gives off the vena mediana cubiti, which receives a perforating branch from the deep veins of the forearm and passes across to join the basilic vein. In the elbow, it crosses superficial to the musculocutaneous nerve and ascends along the lateral border of the biceps brachii muscle. In the upper part of the arm, the cephalic vein runs in the deltopectoral groove, where it is accompanied by the deltoid branch of the thoracoacromial artery. It then pierces the clavipectoral fascia to drain into the axillary vein just below the clavicle.

18.2.3 Adjuncts

Essential to good vascular surgical technique is adequate illumination generally with a fiber-optic head lamp, as well as visualization with optical loupes with a 2.5× or 3.5× magnification. Other important adjuncts include vessel loops, shunts, heparin for systemic administration, heparinized saline for irrigation, papaverine and embolectomy catheters (Fogarty catheters), as well as biological dressings such as cadaver and/or porcine skin to cover fasciotomies as biological dressings. Other important adjuncts include prosthetic grafts generally made from polytetrafluoroethylene (PTFE). Availability of hand-held Doppler probes and intraoperative angiography are a must. It is always important to set up two sets of electrocautery and two suction devices.

18.2.4 Upper Extremities Vessels' Surgical Exposure

18.2.4.1 Surgical Exposure Axillary Artery and Vein

The axillary artery lies anterior to the capsule of the shoulder joint and might be injured when the shoulder is dislocated anteriorly. Fractures of the surgical neck of the humerus will also risk lacerating the vessel as it runs over the fusion of the subscapularis tendon and the joint capsule. The axillary artery can be exposed through an infraclavicular incision placed 2 cm below and parallel to the mid-point of the clavicle, following a gentle curve along the anterior axillary line and then along the anterior border of the deltoid muscle. The first portion of the artery is the simplest to expose because it is medial to the pectoralis muscle and contains only one branch. Exposure of the second portion will require the detachment of the pectoralis minor tendon from the coracoid process. The cords of the brachial plexus surround this portion of the axillary artery, arranged medially, laterally, and posteriorly. From the posterior cord arises the axillary nerve, which follows a posterolateral course on the neck of the humerus. This nerve can be easily injured by dislocation causing atrophy of the deltoid muscle and numbness of an area over the deltoid region. The third portion becomes superficial after emerging from under the pectoralis minor muscle prior to becoming the brachial artery. Great care must be taken while exposing this portion as the nerves to the upper extremities run alongside it. The median nerve runs anterior to the artery and is frequently involved in axillary injuries resulting from its superficial position.

18.2.4.2 Surgical Exposure Brachial Artery

In the arm, exposure in any part of the artery can be achieved by a longitudinal incision along the bicipital sulcus. This sulcus can be easily identified by grasping the head of the biceps and lifting it up to reveal the groove. The artery, along with the accompanying vein and nerves, is immediately visible after dividing the skin, subcutaneous tissue and, investing fascia, followed by splitting the biceps and triceps muscle. The basilic vein runs a superficial course along the bicipital sulcus. It can be identified and retracted laterally to prevent injury to the vein.

Just above the elbow, the brachial artery passes behind the bicipital aponeurosis, which may be divided to facilitate exposure of the vessel. The brachial artery is juxtaposed to the median nerve. Extension of the incision across the antecubital fossa should be made with an S-shaped incision to reduce the risk of joint contracture. Care has to be exercised to prevent injury to the accompanying nerves and veins.

18.2.4.3 Surgical Exposure of the Ulnar and Radial Arteries

Exposure of the ulnar artery is made through an incision over the medial volar aspect of the forearm, over the course of the vessel. The incision can be extended proximally to reach the antecubital fossa to gain control of the brachial artery. The skin incision is deepened to the subcutaneous tissue, and the tissue between flexor carpi radialis and flexor digitorum superficialis can be split to facilitate exposure.

The radial artery can be exposed throughout its length via a longitudinal incision made on the medial aspect of the brachioradialis muscle. This will allow lateral retraction of the muscle to facilitate exposure. The artery runs superficially at the wrist, and exposure over the pulsation. However, this artery is very susceptible to the development of spasm. Papaverine can be used to infiltrate the radial sheath, before sharp dissection and mobilization.

18.2.5 Surgical Techniques

There are a number of critical surgical maneuvers that are standard in the management of all vascular injuries. They include:

1. Application of direct pressure for control of active bleeding.
2. Prepping the person holding pressure into the operative field.
3. Choosing the appropriate surgical exposure and plan to expose the injured vessel widely.
4. Obtain proximal and distal control of both arteries and veins (Figure 18.2), as combined injuries are common.

5. Isolate the injured vessels with meticulous dissection.

6. Retraction of injured or uninjured vessels can be carried out by looping them with vessel loops or Cushing vein retractors.

7. To retract nerves, utilize gentle dissection and place two vessel loops at distal points for retraction to distribute the pressure required to retract the nerve evenly.

8. Identify the injury and approach directly after proximal and distal control has been obtained.

9. Expose the injured vessel widely with meticulous surgical dissection. This may require taking down some of their branches and/or collaterals; however, care must be exercised to preserve as many as possible.

10. Except for some stab wounds and/or lacerations in which the vessel can be directly repaired and/or anastomosed, resect appropriate length of the injured vessel, until normal proximal and distal vessel is obtained. In the case of arteries, resection should avoid raising intimal flaps.

11. Inspect the transected edges of the artery. If there are intimal flaps re-resect. In cases in which there is an extensive flap and further resection is not possible, tack the intimal flap with internal horizontal mattress sutures of Halsted, placing the sutures from the inside of the vessel lumen tying the knots outside of the vessel. This should be done utilizing the finest monofilament polypropylene sutures.

12. Flush the proximal and distal ends of the transected vessel with heparinized saline. Check for distal back bleeding. Flush frequently and gently.

13. If there is no distal back bleeding, pass Fogarty catheters of the appropriate size and length, gently and, if possible, under direct vision of the vessels being thrombectomized. Do not hyperinflate the balloon and do not pass the catheter more than necessary to achieve good back bleeding as this will increase the risk of intimal damage. If there is no arterial flow return, papaverine may be instilled to break vasospasm.

14. Arterial injuries may be repaired by primary arteriography (Figure 18.3) or by end-to-end anastomosis. They may also require a bypass or interposition graft either with an autogenous reverse saphenous vein graft (Figure 18.4) or with a prosthetic graft. Repairs and/or bypasses should never be under tension. They also should not be excessively long in order to prevent kinking. Bypasses placed across a joint most have their length properly selected with consideration of the range of motion (flexion) of the joint to prevent kinking or graft occlusion. All anastomosis should be performed end to end with double-armed polypropylene sutures preferably in a running fashion. Although it has been commonly thought that straight anastomosis might eventually develop stenosis, this is not the case.

15. Vessel discrepancies may be addressed by spatulating and/or fish-mouthing the graft. For small end-to-end vessel anastomosis, simple interrupted sutures of polypropylene may be used circumferentially and for difficult anastomosis the tri-partite suture technique of Carrel may be used.

16. Bypasses performed to smaller vessels such as distal, radial, and ulnar arteries may require their distal anastomosis to be end to side, which increases both the size of the anastomosis as well as its flow characteristics.

17. Venous injuries may be ligated or primarily repaired. Double ligation with silk sutures is preferred for all veins. Primary venorraphy should be carried out with fine monofilament polypropylene sutures preventing narrowing the repaired vein. Very rarely, veno-venous bypass may be required.

18. Fasciotomies should be performed early, expediently, and when indicated. The more soft tissue injury there is, the shorter is the amount of ischemic time that is tolerated. We recommend utilizing either cadaveric and/or skin as biological dressings.

19. At the completion of the arterial repair and/or bypass, pulses should be checked by digital palpation and interrogated by a hand-held Doppler probe (Figure 18.5) including the proximal and distal anastomosis of the bypass, the bypass itself, as well as all distal vessels.

20. The use of completion angiography (Figures 18.6 and 18.7) should be individualized; however, it is highly recommended to detect correctable defects intraoperatively, which will prevent a vessel and/or bypass failure.

Fig. 18.1 Multiple injuries secondary shotgun

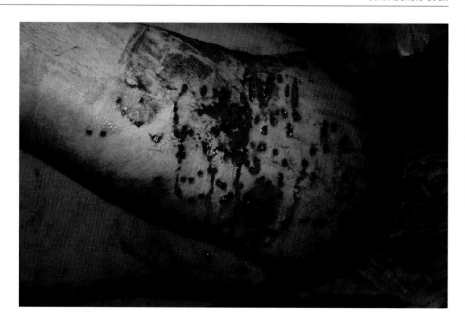

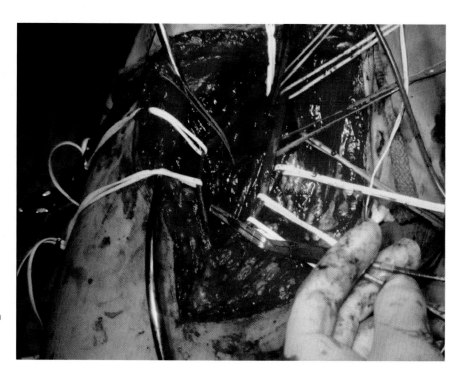

Fig. 18.2 GSW brachial with associated vascular injury. Brachial exploration reveals brachial artery injury

Fig. 18.3 Axillar exploration and primarily arterial repair

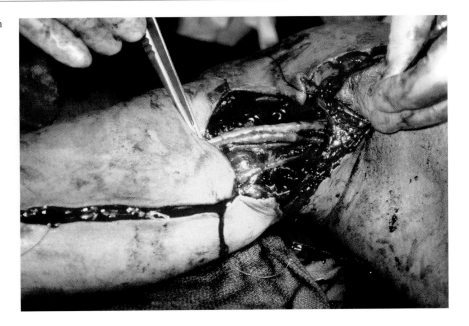

Fig. 18.4 Brachial artery primary repair with autogenous saphenous vein graft

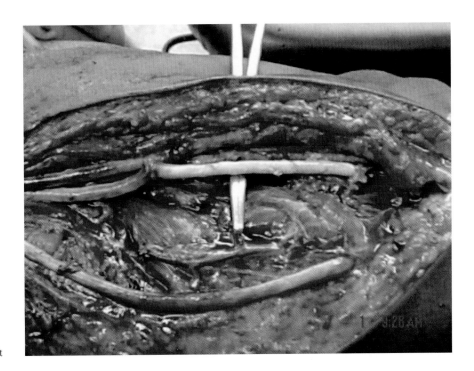

Fig. 18.5 Doppler signal
control

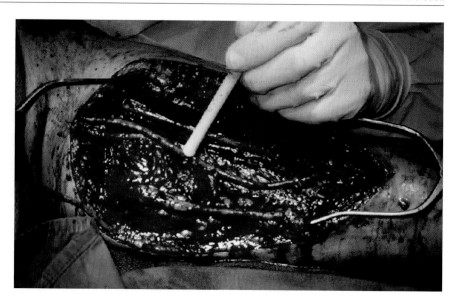

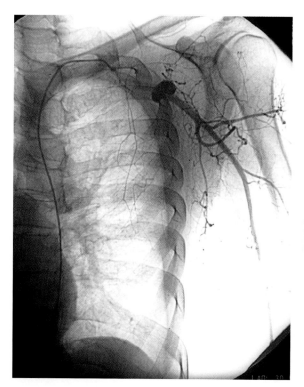

Fig. 18.6 Angiogram reveals aneurysm secondary to GSW

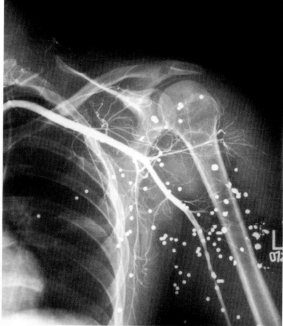

Fig. 18.7 Angiogram reveals vascular injury secondary to shotgun wound

References

1. Asensio JA, McDuffie L, Petrone P, Roldań G, Forno W, Gambaro E, Salim A, Demetriades D, Murray J, Velmahos G, Shoemaker W, Berne TV, Ramicone E, Chan L (2001) Reliable variables in the exsanguinated patient which indicate damage control and predict outcome. Am J Surg 182(6):743–751

2. Demetriades D, Asensio JA (2001) Subclavian and axillary vascular injuries. Surg Clin North Am 81(6):1357–1373

3. Kumar SR, Rowe VL, Petrone P, Kuncir EJ, Asensio JA (2003) The vasculopathic patient: uncommon surgical emergencies. Emerg Med Clin North Am 21(4):803–815, Review

4. Asensio JA, Petrone P, Roldán G, Kuncir E, Rowe VL, Chan L, Shoemaker W, Berne TV (2003) Analysis of 185 iliac vessel injuries: risk factors and prediction of outcome. Arch Surg 138(11):1187–1193, discussion 1193–1194

5. Rowe VL, Salim A, Lipham J, Asensio JA (2002) Shank vessel injuries. Surg Clin North Am 82(1):91–104, xx. Review

6. Asensio JA, Forno W, Roldán G, Petrone P, Rojo E, Ceballos J, Wang C, Costaglioli B, Romero J, Tillou A, Carmody I, Shoemaker WC, Berne TV (2002) Visceral vascular injuries. Surg Clin North Am 82(1):1–20, xix. Review

7. Asensio JA, Forno W, Roldan G, Petrone P, Rojo E, Tillou A, Murray JA, Feliciano DV (2001) Abdominal vascular injuries: injuries to the aorta. Surg Clin North Am 81(6): 1395–1416

8. Asensio JA, Soto SN, Forno W, Roldan G, Petrone P, Gambaro E, Salim A, Rowe V, Demetriades D (2001) Abdominal vascular injuries: the trauma surgeon's challenge. Surg Today 31(11):949–957, Review

9. Asensio JA, Britt LD, Borzotta A, Peitzman A, Miller FB, Mackersie RC, Pasquale MD, Pachter HL, Hoyt DB, Rodriguez JL, Falcone R, Davis K, Anderson JT, Ali J, Chan L (2001) Multiinstitutional experience with the management of superior mesentery artery injuries. J Am Coll Surg 193(4):354–365, discussion 365–366. Erratum in: J Am Coll Surg 2001 Dec;193(6):718

10. Asensio JA, Chahwan S, Hanpeter D, Demetriades D, Forno W, Gambaro E, Murray J, Velmahos G, Marengo J, Shoemaker WC, Berne TV (2000) Operative management and outcome of 302 abdominal vascular injuries. Am J Surg 180(6):528–533, discussion 533–534

11. Asensio JA, Forno W, Gambaro E, Steinberg D, Tsai KJ, Rowe V, Navarro Nuño I, Leppäniemi A, Demetriades D (2000) Abdominal vascular injuries: the trauma surgeon's challenge. Ann Chir Gynaecol 89(1):71–78, No abstract available

12. Velmahos GC, Demetriades D, Chahwan S, Gomez H, Hanks SE, Murray JA, Asensio JA, Berne TV (1999) Angiographic embolization for arrest of bleeding after penetrating trauma to the abdomen. Am J Surg 178(5): 367–373

13. Asensio JA, Berne JD, Chahwan S, Hanpeter D, Demetriades D, Marengo J, Velmahos GC, Murray J, Shoemaker WC, Berne TV (1999) Traumatic injury of the superior mesenteric artery. Am J Surg 178(3):235–239

Index

H.-J. Oestern et al. (eds.), *Head, Thoracic, Abdominal, and Vascular Injuries*,
DOI: 10.1007/978-3-540-88122-3, © Springer-Verlag Berlin Heidelberg 2011

Printing and Binding: Stürtz GmbH, Würzburg